D1608711

CEREBROSPINAL FLUID IN DISEASES OF THE NERVOUS SYSTEM

ROBERT A. FISHMAN, M.D.

Professor of Neurology
Chairman of the Department of Neurology
School of Medicine
University of California, San Francisco

1980

W. B. SAUNDERS COMPANY
Philadelphia   London   Toronto

W. B. Saunders Company: West Washington Square
Philadelphia, PA   19105

1 St. Anne's Road
Eastbourne, East Sussex BN21, 3UN, England

1 Goldthorne Avenue
Toronto, Ontario M8Z 5T9, Canada

Library of Congress Cataloging in Publication Data

Fishman, Robert A

Cerebrospinal fluid in diseases of the nervous system.

1. Cerebrospinal fluid — Examination.   2. Cerebrospinal
   fluid.   3. Central nervous system — Diseases — Diagnosis.
   I. Title.

RB55.F53   616.8'04'756   79–67304

ISBN 0–7216–3686–1

Cerebrospinal Fluid in Diseases of the Nervous System   ISBN   0-7216-3686-1

Last digit is the print number: 9   8   7   6   5   4   3   2   1

To Peggy
and
Mary, Alice, and Elizabeth

PREFACE

Clinicians interested in diseases of the central nervous system have long envied their colleagues in other fields of medicine. Not only do they have ready access to blood, urine, and the other body effluents, they can even examine biopsy specimens of liver, kidney, or muscle in the pursuit of knowledge about systemic diseases. In contrast, the student of diseases of the brain and spinal cord generally has to make do with indirect methods and postmortem material. The introduction of lumbar puncture into clinical medicine almost 90 years ago at last provided access to a fluid in close proximity to the central nervous system. Ever since then, the cerebrospinal fluid (CSF) has been analyzed extensively to elucidate the physiological and biochemical bases of neurological disease. The data derived from such investigations comprise a major part of this book.

For many years, the CSF was studied chiefly by clinicians, neurologists, and neurosurgeons, who asked mainly clinical questions. Recently, there has been a gratifying increase in attention to the CSF by physiologists, neurochemists, and neurobiologists, because of its unique composition and its special relevance to neurological function. In the last 15 years, the plethora of publications dealing with basic and clinical aspects of the fluid has made it difficult to keep abreast of important advances in our knowledge. There have been extensive modifications and additions to our understanding of the physiology and chemistry of the CSF. Major technical advances in the analysis of biological fluids have been applied to the study of the CSF. The goal of this book is to summarize and interpret our expanding knowledge of the CSF, emphasizing data which are derived from patient studies and are of special relevance to the understanding of neurological disease. It is intended for neurologists and neurosurgeons, as well as for internists, pediatricians, neuroradiologists, and other physicians interested in diseases of the nervous system.

Following a brief historical introduction, the early chapters review the anatomy, physiology, and chemistry of the CSF and its special relationship to the brain, including the blood-brain barrier. The normal and disordered physiology of the intracranial pressure is discussed, with application to the clinical problems of intracranial hypertension, pseudotumor, hydrocephalus, and brain edema. The technical aspects of spinal puncture and its indications, contraindications, and complications are reviewed. The composition of the CSF is described in detail, including its physical features, cytology, and chemical constituents, using data from patient studies. The last part of the book deals with alterations of the composition of the CSF in specific diseases of the nervous system, emphasizing the data that are clinically useful.

A rather lengthy bibliography has been included, the selection of which posed special problems. About 1500 relevant papers have been published yearly for the last

20 years, in addition to the extensive earlier literature, and it was impossible to include all of these references. In compiling the bibliography, therefore, I tried to choose papers which contained primary data or had good bibliographies, but papers of historic importance were also included. In the text, I made extensive use of tables to condense and summarize data on various topics.

In writing this book, I often returned affectionately to the classic monograph by Merritt and Fremont-Smith (1938), "The Cerebrospinal Fluid", for many years the authoritative clinical sourcebook, published more than 40 years ago by Saunders. It contained the copious data collected by the CSF laboratory of the Boston City Hospital between 1926 and 1938, based on the study of 21,000 samples of fluid. Some of these data are unique (e.g., the findings in purulent meningitis, poliomyelitis, and pernicious anemia) and are still quite relevant to clinical practice. I tried to salvage them (and to pay homage to my teacher, the late H. Houston Merritt) by including some of the well-validated information in the present book.

Much of this book was written in London during a sabbatical leave in 1978 spent at the National Hospital, Queen Square, and the Institute of Neurology. I am most grateful to Professor Roger W. Gilliat, Dean Peter Gautier-Smith, and their associates for their very kind hospitality. The preparation of the book was helped greatly by a grant from the Commonwealth Fund of New York, for which I express my appreciation to Dr. Reginald H. Fitz, Vice President. Joan M. Mello of San Francisco and Norma Walker of London provided very expert assistance in the production of the manuscript. The staff of the W. B. Saunders Company has been very helpful, and I wish to thank Mrs. Anna Congdon for editorial assistance and Mr. Albert E. Meier, editor-in-chief for health sciences, for his guidance. I am in debt to the many authors who kindly gave me permission to use their published figures. I also wish to thank my colleagues and students who stimulated me to write this book.

Finally, I wish to express my special gratitude to my wife, Peggy, who encouraged the effort, cheerfully tolerated the preoccupied weekend and evening hours, and assisted greatly in preparation of the text.

ROBERT A. FISHMAN

San Francisco

CONTENTS

Chapter 7
CEREBROSPINAL FLUID FINDINGS IN DISEASES OF THE NERVOUS SYSTEM

CHAPTER 1

HISTORICAL INTRODUCTION

In order to summarize and discuss contemporary knowledge of the cerebrospinal fluid (CSF) in normal and disease states, it is useful to examine the roots of our current information. This short historical summary is intended to point out some of the major early advances and the investigators involved; these contributions have served as the prologue to contemporary knowledge. Woollam (1957), Clarke and O'Malley (1968), and McHenry (1969) summarized the early history of the cerebrospinal fluid, providing excellent guides to the historical literature.

The presence of a fluid within the cavities of the brain was known to the ancients. Its existence was first recorded in the Edwin Smith Surgical Papyrus, which was probably written in the 17th century B.C. Hippocrates, in the 4th century B.C., recorded the presence of fluid within the cavities of the brain and is credited with tapping the ventricles in hydrocephalus, probably after death. The nature of the fluid was not understood, and its occurrence was considered pathological in origin.

Galen, in the 2nd century A.D., provided the first description of ventricular cavities. For more than a millenium, galenic theory persisted, and the ventricles were thought to be filled with a vital spirit. Much later, Vesalius, Valsalva, and Haller contributed more detailed observations of the anatomical features of the ventricular system. Vesalius, in 1543, drew attention to the presence within the ventricles of a watery humor as opposed to a gaseous one. Valsalva, in 1672, according to Billanchoni (Woollam,1957), found "an ounce of a certain liquid in cutting the cord membrane of a dog, a fluid resembling that seen in articulations." Willis, in 1664, believed that the fluids of the brain passed through the pituitary body, mamillary bodies, and cribriform plate to enter the circulation, whereas Lower, in 1669 (Brisman, 1970), suggested brain fluid could enter the venous system directly. Pacchioni, in 1705, considered the dura to be contractible and the intracranial fluid to be secreted by the arachnoid granulations that bear his name. Haller, in 1757, described the cerebrospinal fluid as a "viscous fluid, coagulable by a heat of about 150 degrees, by alcohol, and by strong acid."

The first satisfactory account of the cerebrospinal fluid was given in 1764, by Contugno, who described its appearance within the cerebral ventricles and subarachnoid space, studying the bodies of 20 adults with dissections and lumbar taps. Viets (1935) provided a translation of this innovative work. Contugno pointed out that earlier anatomists had failed to find the fluid because decapitation was performed before dissection, causing the fluid to escape from both the cranial and spinal cavities. His observations, embedded in a treatise on sciatica, were not appreciated, and for many years most authors considered that the arachnoid membrane formed a closed sac analogous to the pleural or peritoneal cavities.

Systematic studies of the CSF began with the early papers of Magendie (1825), who first tapped the cisterna magna in animals. It owes its names, *liquide céphalo-rachidien* or *cérébro-spinal*, to Magendie, who initiated chemical and physiological studies of the fluid. He established the existence of a communicating foramen between the fourth ventricle and the subarachnoid space as well as the continuity of the subarachnoid space around both the brain and spinal cord. Magendie considered the fluid to be a secretion of the pia-arachnoid with the direction of the fluid flow from the subarachnoid space to the ventricles; the basis for this curious conclusion is not clear. He noted the movement of the fluid which occurred with respiration, and he concluded that the fluid was under a positive pressure.

Alexander Monro, in 1783, had deduced that the cranium was a rigid box filled with a "nearly incompressible" brain and that therefore the quantity of blood within the head must be the same or nearly the same at all times, whether in health or disease. Monro's concepts were confirmed by the experimental work of George Kellie (1824), who noted that the brains of animals killed by exsanguination still contained blood except when he had broken the integrity of the skull by trephination before death. Kellie also noted that cerebral congestion was not observed in those who died by hanging. These observations were the basis of the "Monro-Kellie hypothesis," which postulated that the volume of blood within the brain did not change. Burrows (1846) later modified this concept by adding that the blood volume of the brain could change, but only change reciprocally with the volumes of brain and CSF within the cranial cavity. Subsequent workers have provided substantial support for this view, and contemporary studies of intracranial pressure-volume relationships and cerebrovascular autoregulation still allude to the Monro-Kellie hypothesis.

The first definitive work on the CSF was carried out by the Swedish anatomists Axel Key and Magnus Retzius (1875). They made a detailed investigation of the membranes and cavities of the brain and spinal cord. With the injection of gelatin and dyes, they confirmed the existence of the lateral foramina of Luschka and the medial foramen of Magendie. They showed that the CSF passes from the subarachnoid space through the pacchionian bodies into the cerebral venous sinuses. Their magnificent atlas and monograph formed the basis on which much modern work on this subject is built. Dixon and Halliburton (1913) investigated the effects of drugs and anesthetics on spinal fluid outflow through a cisternal catheter, and in the following decades there was an expanding literature about the physiology of the CSF and of the blood brain barrier. These experiments provided a basis for much of the subsequent experimental work regarding the pathophysiology of hydrocephalus.

Lewis Weed (1935), in a long series of innovative papers beginning in 1914, elaborated the earlier concepts of Retzius and Key which demonstrated that the fluid originated in the choroid plexus, then passed through the ventricles into the subarachnoid space to be absorbed by the arachnoid villi. He first emphasized the dual origin of the CSF, from both the choroid plexus and the perivascular spaces (interstitial fluid) of the brain. Dandy and Blackfan's work (1914) supported the view that the fluid originated from the choroid plexus, and first showed the development of hydrocephalus by blocking the aqueduct of Sylvius. Weed's early work (Weed and McKibben, 1919) also dealt with the effects of solutions with various osmolarities upon the intracranial pressure and was the basis for the subsequent introduction of hyperosmolar intravenous solutions in the treatment of intracranial hypertension.

Spinal Puncture in Patients

Corning (1885), after experiments in animals, first injected a solution of hydrochlorate of cocaine between the spinous processes of the 11th and 12th thoracic vertebrae in a man with "spinal weakness." He observed transient sensory impairment in the patient's legs, and he thus demonstrated the possibility of spinal anesthesia prior to any interest in the diagnostic value of the study of the fluid. Corning did not describe his technique, nor was he concerned about the hazards of so high an injection. Wynter (1891) reported the use of spinal fluid drainage in a patient with tuberculous meningitis, making a skin incision to enable passage of a trocar (Levinson, 1918; Gray, 1921).

Quincke (1891) first developed the technique of spinal puncture as a diagnostic method. He introduced the use of a percutaneous needle with stylet, a procedure which has changed little since. He was the first to examine the constituents of the fluid and to record the pressure with a manometer. His studies included cell counts and the measurement of protein and sugar content. Quincke focused on the role of spinal fluid drainage in the treatment of tuberculous meningitis and hydrocephalus. His reports prompted much clinical interest, and by the turn of the centry spinal puncture was generally adopted in American and European hospitals as a routine diagnostic procedure. There was rapid development of cytological techniques by Widal (1901) and others. Froin described the syndrome of spinal block in 1903, and thereafter a flurry of papers dealt with various aspects of the fluid during the early years of the century. Mestrezat's monograph (1912) first summarized the analyses of the chemical constituents of the fluid in various diseases, and this volume was the standard clinical reference for many years. In 1913, Lange described the colloidal gold curve, an empirical technique for measuring qualitative changes in the composition of the cerebrospinal fluid proteins. Dandy introduced ventriculography and pneumoencephalography in 1918, and myelography with iodized oil (lipidol) was introduced by Sicard and Forester in 1921.

There was an extraordinary interest in the clinical aspects of the fluid in the early decades of this century. Much of the literature dealt with changes in the fluid in bacterial meningitis and neurosyphilis. Levinson (1929) provided a list of 30 monographs, written chiefly in French and German, reflecting this clinical interest. The monographs of Levinson, published between 1919 and 1929, served as a major American reference for many years. Merritt and Fremont-Smith (1938) summarized the 20 year experience of the spinal fluid laboratory of the Boston City Hospital, as well as the earlier literature, providing a definitive reference regarding the clinical aspects of the fluid. Their work still stands as a valuable resource, and some of their data are included in the present volume. An analogous book by Lups and Haan (1954) was the most recent volume in English devoted to the CSF that was written for clinicians. Schmidt (1968) edited a comprehensive book on clinical aspects of the CSF that was published in Germany.

Intrathecal Therapy

There was an early interest in the potential value of the intrathecal injection of various medications. Kocher, in 1899, first used this route, injecting anti-tetanic serum into the ventricles in a case of tetanus. Levinson (1929) summarized the early history of intrathecal therapy in some detail. In the pre-antibiotic era there were many efforts to treat meningitis with the intrathecal injection of immune serum. Levinson (1929) tabulated the results in several clinical reports, totaling 4500 patients with meningococcal meningitis, which indicated that such therapy appeared to reduce the mortality to one third or one half that observed in untreated cases. The complications of the treatment included shock, aggravation of symptoms due to "serum meningitis," and the development of serum sickness. There were reports of the futile treatment of tuberculous meningitis with intrathecal injections of carbolic acid, creosol, tuberculin, and air!

Poliomyelitis was treated with intraspinal adrenalin, and both tetanus and chorea with intraspinal injections of magnesium sulfate. There was extensive use of the intrathecal route in the treatment of neurosyphilis. Both arsenicals and mercurial compounds were used, at times causing cord necrosis. The Swift-Ellis method made use of the blood serum of luetic patients treated with heavy metals, which was injected intrathecally as a 40 per cent solution in normal saline at weekly intervals for four to five weeks. One cringes at the thought of the chemical meningitis that attended such therapies!

Intrathecal therapy, using a wide variety of agents, has periodically been advocated. In the 1930's and 1940's there was an interest in spinal barbotage, introduced by Speranski in Russia (Savage, 1948). This technique involved repeated withdrawal and re-injection of lumbar CSF in the treatment of rheumatoid arthritis. In contemporary practice few pharmacological agents have an established role when administered by the intrathecal route.

Recent History

Since 1950, extraordinary advances in the study of the physiology and chemistry of the CSF have paralleled progress in the biomedical sciences in the study of body fluids. These have included (a) application of radioisotopes to the study of the formation and absorption of the fluid; (b) development of isovolumetric pressure transducers to study pulsations of the CSF; (c) better understanding of the principles of membrane transport of ions, sugars, amino acids, and proteins; *(d)* improved analytical methods for the separation and measurement of proteins, enzymes, and metabolites in dilute solutions; *(e)* ultra-structural studies of the relationships of CSF to blood and to the extracellular fluid of brain; and *(f)* the method of ventriculo-cisternal perfusion, which has provided a means for measuring the rates of CSF formation and absorption and has established that the choroid plexus has bidirectional transport systems analogous in function to the proximal renal tubule. Various aspects of the extensive experimental literature regarding the physiology of the CSF have been well summarized in the several monographs by Davson (1967), Katzman and Pappius (1973), and Rapoport (1976), and in the symposia edited by Cserr, Fenster-macher, and Fencl (1975), and Bito, Davson, and Fenstermacher (1977). Many of the arguments of earlier years have been resolved, although there are still many unanswered questions.

In the ensuing chapters, emphasis will be placed on contemporary knowl-edge of the anatomy, physiology, chemistry, and pharmacology of the CSF. The pathophysiology of the fluid in various disorders will be described, including intracranial hypertension, brain edema, and hydrocephalus. The composition of the CSF will be described, including its cellular components and chemical con-stituents. Finally, the characteristic changes in the CSF associated with various diseases of the nervous system will be summarized, and the interpretation of such changes in differential diagnosis will be discussed.

CHAPTER 2

ANATOMICAL ASPECTS OF THE CEREBROSPINAL FLUID

Recent advances in the study of the anatomy of cerebrospinal fluid pathways have made important contributions to our knowledge of the physiology and pathophysiology of the fluid. The anatomical features of the ventricular system, choroid plexus, and subarachnoid spaces have been described in detail by Millen and Woollam (1962), and most of this information will not be duplicated here. Figure 2–1 illustrates the CSF pathways schematically. The sites for CSF absorption at the arachnoid villi of the cranial and spinal subarachnoid spaces are indicated. Recent work, particularly the application of ultrastructural techniques to the study of CSF pathways, has greatly expanded our understanding of the morphological basis for CSF production and absorption, as well as the relationships of the CSF to the extracellular fluid of the brain and to the blood-brain barrier. Therefore, pertinent aspects of the morphology of the choroid plexus, capillary endothelial cells, the ependyma, the pial and arachnoid membranes, the arachnoid villi, the dura, and the interstitial space will be briefly summarized in this chapter as a prelude to more detailed discussion of the physiology of the fluid.

Anatomy of the Choroid Plexus

The choroid plexus includes the choroidal epithelium, blood vessels, and interstitial connective tissue (Voetmann, 1949). There has been a great interest in recent years in its development, structure, and function, well summarized in a monograph by Netsky and Shuangshoti (1975), which includes reviews of its ultrastructure by Tennyson (1975) and by Brightman (1975).

The plexus is formed as a result of the invagination of the ependyma into the ventricular cavities by the blood vessels of the pia mater. Thus, the choroidal epithelium is continuous at its margins with the ependymal lining of the ventricles. The choroid plexus of each lateral ventricle is continuous with the choroid plexus of the third ventricle. The choroid plexus of the fourth ventricle is T-shaped, with two vertical segments projecting into the cavity from the roof,

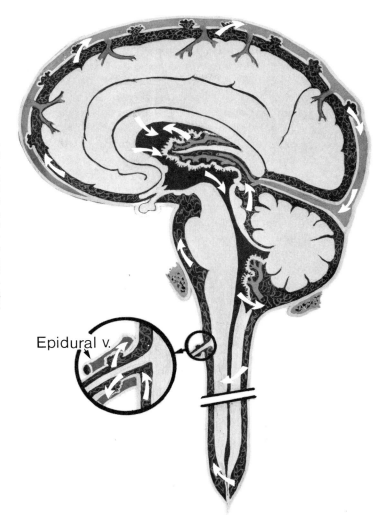

Figure 2-1 The CSF pathways. This diagram illustrates the sites of formation, circulation, and absorption of the CSF. Both choroidal and extrachoroidal sources of the fluid within the ventricular system are indicated. The circulation of the CSF to the subarachnoid space and its absorption into the venous system via the arachnoid villi are shown. The presence of arachnoid villi adjacent to the spinal roots supplements the absorption that takes place into the intracranial venous sinuses.

Epidural v.

one on either side of the midline, and two horizontal segments, at right angles to the vertical segments, extending to the lateral recesses of the ventricle and protruding through the lateral foramina of Luschka into the subarachnoid space (Millen and Woollam, 1962). Although functional differences between the choroid plexus of the lateral and third ventricles and that of the fourth ventricle were suggested by Pappenheimer *et al*. (1961), no morphological differences have been found. There is an ovoid swelling of the plexus as it crosses over the thalamus, called the glomus choroideum, whose specific function is not known. Histological study of the plexus has revealed the presence of psammoma bodies and the frequent appearance of cysts with aging.

The arterial supply to the choroid plexus of the lateral ventricle originates from the anterior and posterior choroidal arteries. The anterior choroidal artery, a small branch of the internal carotid artery, supplies the posterior part of the plexus in the temporal horn; the posterior choroidal artery, a small branch of the posterior cerebral artery, supplies the anterior portion of the plexus. Within the plexus there are multiple branches and anastomoses of both arteries. The plexus within the third ventricle is supplied by choroidal branches of the posterior cerebral artery. The plexus within the fourth ventricle is supplied chiefly by the posterior inferior cerebellar artery, with an occasional supply from the anterior inferior cerebellar artery and internal auditory artery. The venous drainage from the choroid plexus of the lateral and third ventricles enters the thalamostriate veins and the internal cerebral veins. The venous drainage from the fourth ventricular plexus enters the basal veins. Thus, the choroid plexus has an extensive blood supply which reflects its high metabolic activity (to be discussed in Chapter 3).

Woollam and Millen (1962) referred to the early recognition that the choroid plexus had a nerve supply, which Benedikt in 1874 had termed the "13th cranial nerve." Subsequent work has revealed an extensive perivascular innervation derived in part from the cervical sympathetic chain, from the neural plexus of the internal carotid and posterior cerebral arteries, and from the vagal nuclei (Cooper, 1958). The precise role of these nerves is not known; it has been presumed that the innervation is chiefly vasomotor in function. However, recent studies indicate that the sympathetic innervation inhibits secretion by the choroidal epithelium independent of its vasomotor effects (Lindvall *et al.*, 1978). The mechanism of neurogenic modulation of CSF secretion and its physiological role require elucidation.

Ultrastructural Studies

The choroidal epithelium is composed of a single row of epithelial cells, folded into villi around a core of blood vessels and connective tissue. The ventricular surface of the epithelial cells has a brush border composed of a series of microvilli. There are numerous basal and lateral infoldings which, with the microvilli, indicate that structurally the choroid resembles other epithelia noted for fluid transport. There are also occasional cilia on the apical surface. Curiously, in developing brain, the cilia are far more numerous than in maturity. Pinocytic vesicles are present at both the apical and basal surfaces of the cell and even along the lateral borders. Other inclusions are present, including dense bodies (probably lysosomes), the Golgi complex, ribosomes, tubular endoplasmic reticulum, and mitochondria, as well as fat droplets and pigment granules (Tennyson, 1975; Becker and Sutton, 1975; Dohrmann, 1970).

Vesicular Transport

Brightman (1975) has studied the permeability characteristics of the choroid plexus, using the electron microscopically dense marker horseradish peroxidase (HRP). This is a metalloenzyme with a molecular weight of about 40,000 (compared with albumin, MW 69,000). Both pinocytosis and vesicular transport have been observed in choroidal cells. Brightman (1975) has pointed out the distinction between pinocytosis and vesicular transport. Pinocytosis or "drinking by cells" occurs when the cell membrane invaginates to form a small flask-like pit which fuses to form a round or oval vesicle. The vesicle engulfs a small volume of fluid and solute, and it then moves within the cell to fuse with a larger membrane-bound vacuole or multivesicular body. The whole process of pinocytosis ends inside the cell.

Vesicular transport resembles pinocytosis but differs in that the vacuole moves across the cell to fuse with the opposite cell membrane. Vesicular transport is an active process by which fluid and solutes move across the cell from one fluid compartment to another. The structural basis for the barriers to HRP movement in the choroid plexus are analogous to those seen in the eye, the testis, and other special vascular beds. A special form of vesicular transport has been described also in the arachnoid villi (to be discussed later in this chapter). Van Deurs (1978) has studied the removal of microperoxidase from the ventricular fluid by the choroidal epithelium. These data support the view that the plexus plays a role in the removal of molecules from the CSF by micropinocytosis and lysosomal sequestration. The functional importance of bidirectional choroidal transport is discussed in Chapter 3.

Tight Junctions

The perivascular and epithelial basement membranes of the choroid plexus are permeable to HRP. However, there is a barrier at the choroid plexus to the movement of HRP and other macromolecules (ferritin, lanthanum) from blood to the ventricular cavity, and from the ventricular cavity to blood. The membrane barrier to the movement of macromolecules is the *tight junction*, which joins adjacent choroidal epthelial cells (Brightman, 1975). Tight junctions also characterize brain endothelial cells and the cells of the arachnoid membrane. The area of fusion has a pentalaminar structure forming a continuous "zonula" around each cell (Brightman and Reese, 1969). The electrical resistance found on the apical surface of the choroidal epithelium has been attributed to such tight junctions (Bennett, 1969).

Although vesicular transport of large molecules appears to be quite active in choroidal epithelial cells, it is not clear whether this normally serves to bypass the zonular junctions and thus allow the small leakage of serum proteins into the ventricular fluid. There is evidence of bidirectional vesicular transport in the plexus, but the functional importance of vesicular transport and the factors that determine its directional preponderance are not known. So far, the ultrastructural studies have not defined the morphological basis (whether transjunctional, transendothelial, or vesicular) for the transport of smaller conpounds, ions, and organic acids, which are known to be transported bidirectionally across the choroidal epithelium (see Chapter 3).

Histochemistry

The choroid plexus has also been studied extensively with histochemical and cytochemical techniques (Becker and Sutton, 1975). These observations indicate that most of the non-mitochondrial granules in the choroidal epithelium are lysosomal in nature and probably related to the process of pinocytosis. There are high activities within the choroidal cells of several plasma membrane nucleoside phosphatases and of many oxidative enzymes, which reflect the role of the choroid plexus in the active transport of electrolytes and other solutes (Cserr, 1971).

Capillary Endothelial Cells

Brain capillaries have a number of morphological differences from capillaries in other organs. Unlike systemic capillaries, endothelial cells in brain capillaries are joined by tight junctions, which are present around the lateral circumference of the capillary tube. This results in a continuous layer of endothelial cells, which effectively separate the plasma from the extracellular fluid of the brain (Brightman, 1977). The tight junctions serve as a barrier to the movement of water soluble ions and molecules, so that they move across the endothelial cells by vesicular transport or transendothelial diffusion, rather than between them. In systemic capillaries many pinocytotic vesicles are seen, but normally in brain endothelial cells few are seen. This probably accounts for the relative exclusion of plasma proteins from the CSF. Brain endothelial cells also have three to five times more mitochondria than systemic endothelial cells, reflecting the high energy demands of brain endothelial cells for active transport (Oldendorf, 1977)

Another feature of brain capillaries is that they are surrounded by a well-defined basement membrane, which is approximately 25 per cent the width of the endothelial cell. The basement membrane contains collagen residues and glycoproteins arranged in an amorphous pattern that appears to serve as a skeleton for the capillary wall. Goldstein (1979) considers the basement membrane sufficiently rigid to help maintain the integrity of the capillary tube under adverse conditions, such as severe osmotic stress or exposure to increased hydrostatic pressure from abrupt elevations in cerebral blood flow. The capillary is also largely surrounded by the astrocytic feet, which have a functional role, with the capillary endothelial cells and the choroid plexus, in maintaining the ionic composition of CSF (Katzman, 1976).

Ependyma

The cerebral ventricles are lined with a continuous single layer of ependymal cells, beneath which is usually a subependymal layer of glial fibers and often a deeper layer of glial cells (Tennyson and Pappas, 1968). The morphology of the ependymal cells varies in different locations (Knigge *et al.*, 1975). Over most of the ventricular system the cuboidal endothelial cells are ciliated, unlike the choroidal cells which have many microvillus-like protrusions. The cilia are easily destroyed with routine fixation but are readily seen with the scanning electron microscope. However, the ependymal cells have a different structure in several specialized regions (Weindl and Joynt, 1972). Thus, ependymal cells in the following areas are lacking in cilia: over the circumventricular organs, including the median eminence; the neurohypophysis; the pineal body; the subcommissural organ; the organum vasculosum of the lamina terminalis; the subfornical organ; the paraventricular organ; and the area postrema. The median eminence, neurohypophysis, and pineal body are thought to play a role in neuroendocrine regulation, but the functions of the other structures are still not well defined. Ultrastructural studies of ependymal cells have shown many features, including pinocytotic vesicles, similar to those seen in the choroidal epithelium. The structure of the cilia is similar to that of other ciliated cells. However, the conspicuous tight junctions of the choroidal epithelium are not seen in most areas of the ependyma, where discontinuous gap junctions are characteristic (Brightman *et al.*, 1975).

The lining of the ventricle is not uniform in its regional permeability to dye. When trypan blue was injected into the cisterna magna, the periventricular neuropile was stained except for the infundibular recess, median eminence, area postrema, and choroid plexus (Feldberg and Fleischhauer, 1960). Recent studies by Brightman *et al.* (1975) have shown that the ependymal epithelium overlying these special regions is impermeable to macromolecules. This reflects the presence between these cells of tight junctions, unlike most of the ependyma where the cells are connected by discontinuous gap junctions. Similarly, horseradish peroxidase injected intravenously crosses the fenestrated capillaries of the median eminence, but its flow is halted at the tight junctions of the adjacent ependymal surface. These structural findings are in accord with the observation that most of the ependyma is readily permeable to the bidirectional transfer of molecules as large as inulin, MW 5000 (Katzman and Pappius, 1973). Both thorium and ferritin particles are incorporated into pinocytotic vesicles in the ependymal cells after intraventricular injection (Brightman, 1977). However, the relative importance of pinocytosis compared with that of intercellular and intracellular diffusion in the transport of various solutes is not known.

Tanycytes

The functional importance of the specialized ependymal regions just described is of special interest. The ependymal wall at the level of the median eminence of the hypothalamus consists of two cell types. Dorsally, there are

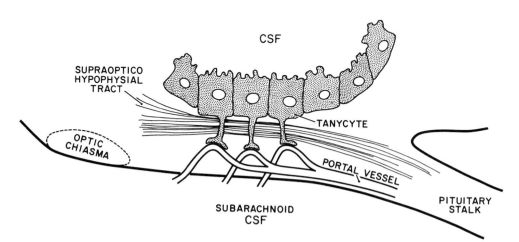

Figure 2–2   Tanycytes. These specialized ependymal cells, which lack cilia, are located in the floor of the third ventricle. The soma is directed toward the ventricle, and the neck and tail extend to make contact with a capillary wall. They are considered to transport hypophysiotropic hormones, such as luteinizing hormone and other releasing factors formed in the hypothalamus, to the portal circulation of the hypophysis (from Porter *et al.*, 1975).

frequently ciliated cuboidal cells with central nuclei similar to ependymal cells elsewhere. Ventrally, there are cells of the second type, called *tanycytes* (Knigge *et al.*, 1975; Millhouse, 1975). These cells lack cilia and have dense, elongate nuclei. With Golgi staining, these cells are seen to have a soma directed toward the ventricle, and a neck and tail that extend to make contact with a capillary wall. There is evidence to support the hypothesis that the tanycytes serve to transport hypophysiotropic hormones, such as luteinizing hormone–releasing factor, and probably other releasing factors formed in the hypothalamus. The releasing factors then diffuse into the third ventricle and are transported by tanycytes to the portal circulation of the hypophysis. This anatomical arrangement has been illustrated by Porter et al., (1975); see Figure 2–2. Thus, the ependymal epithelium, although readily permeable in most regions, appears to have specialized functions overlying the hypothalamus and other specialized areas that require further definition.

Pia-Arachnoid Membranes

The leptomeninges form a complete investment for the brain and spinal cord. They are divided into an outer layer, the arachnoid mater, and an inner layer, the pia mater. The two membranes encompass the subarachnoid space, which contains the extraventricular cerebrospinal fluid. The membranes are structurally similar and probably develop from the same embryonic layer; they are connected by the dentate ligaments in the spinal canal and by numerous trabeculae. In the past, they have often been regarded as forming a single structure, the leptomeninges or pia-arachnoid (Millen and Woollam, 1962).

The leptomeninges are relatively avascular, i.e., they contain few capillaries and probably depend upon the adjacent CSF and the extracellular fluid of the underlying cortex for nutrition. Many cortical blood vessels run along the surface of the pia mater and protrude into the subarachnoid space. Where blood vessels enter or leave the central nervous system, the pia is invaginated into the nervous system to form the outer surface of the perivascular space, and tissue derived from the arachnoid forms the inner wall of the perivascular space. The filaments of the spinal motor and sensory roots, as well as those of the cranial nerves, are similarly invested with a reticular sheath derived from the pia which forms the endoneurial sheath as they traverse the subarachnoid space. The pia mater also forms the roof (tela choroidea) of the third ventricle and the lower part of the roof of the fourth ventricle, as well as the medial wall of the lateral ventricle, the choroidal fissure. In these regions, the pia adheres closely to a single layer of ependymal cells. There appear to be no nerves within the pia-arachnoid, apart from the numerous small nerves seen within blood vessel walls.

In the older literature, several spaces within the brain were described (Millen and Woollam, 1962). These included the perineuronal, pericapillary, and subpial spaces, with a variety of eponyms. They are now considered artifacts, except for the perivascular space of Virchow-Robin, which has recently been restudied by Cserr (1971). This space extends from the subarachnoid space to a variable depth. The problem of the changes in tissue volume that accompany fixation for pathologic study makes it difficult to ascertain the precise size of the Virchow-Robin space. The prominence of perivascular cuffing in inflammatory lesions illustrates the potential for enlargement of the perivascular space. Cserr (1971) has provided evidence that this perivascular space allows the free diffusion of solutes below 100 to 200 angstroms in diameter between the interstitial and cerebrospinal fluid. This facilitates the movement of metabolites from deep within the hemisphere to the cortical subarachnoid spaces as well as to the ventricular system.

Ultrastructural Studies

The fact that the subarachnoid space is filled with an almost protein-free CSF has long been attributed to the presence of a blood-CSF barrier (Rapoport, 1976). As will be discussed later, this in part reflects the special permeability characteristic of brain endothelial cells and of the choroid plexus. There has been speculation in the past as to how materials in the dura were prevented from reaching the fluid and the brain. Weed (1938) and later Broman (1949) suggested that the arachnoid membrane might serve as such a barrier.

Recently, Nabeshima *et al.* (1975) restudied the ultrastructure of the meninges, using electron microscopy and freeze fracture techniques with various species of laboratory animals. Their studies showed that the dural border cells (the innermost surface of the dura) had no tight junctions of any type that might be expected to form an effective barrier to the diffusion of substances from the dura into the CSF; instead, rather large clefts were found between these cells. However, the adjacent arachnoidal cells were shown to have a dense intercellular matrix and conspicuous tight junctions. The freeze fracture studies showed that these junctions form an extensive branching network clearly compatible with the role of serving as an effective membranous barrier to the entry of large molecules.

The structure of the inner layer (pia) of the pia-arachnoid differed in that tight junctions appeared to be absent, although *gap junctions*, which are structurally distinct from tight junctions, were seen. Gap junctions have frequently been described as sites of electrical coupling, although how this actually occurs is not known. Although there is no direct evidence for electrical coupling between pial cells, it has been presumed that many of these cells are coupled in order to explain the high electrical capacitance of the pial membrane when current is applied to its surface (Bennett, 1969). The extensive system of gap junctions between pial cells allows intercellular transport of small molecules. It will be seen that the special ultrastructural features of the pia-arachnoid are functionally important in its role as an integral component of the blood-brain barrier.

Anatomy of the Arachnoid Villi

The arachnoid villi and granulations (pacchionian bodies) are herniations of the arachnoid membrane which penetrate gaps in the dura and protrude into the lumen of the superior saggital sinus and other venous structures. The villi may be seen only microscopically, but the granulations are large, macroscopic structures composed of multiple villi, which actually indent the inner surface of the calvarium. The granulations become visible at age 6 months, and by age 4 there are usually more than 50 large granulations (Millen and Wollam, 1962). There is considerable interest in the structure and function of the villi, because since the work of Weed (1923) they have been considered a major route for spinal fluid reabsorption.

The morphology and function of the villus have been the subject of much controversy. It was long assumed that the boundary between the CSF and the venous blood at the villus was membrane bound. This was the conclusion of the early work of Weed (1923), which was later supported by ultrastructural studies indicating that the endothelium of the venous sinus and the endothelial surface of the villi were continuous (Shabo and Maxwell, 1968; Alksne and Lovings, 1972). These morphological data were consistent with Weed's view that CSF absorption took place by filtration across an intact membrane. On the other hand, Welch and Friedman (1960) and Welch and Pollay (1963) regarded the villi as a "labyrinth of coupled tubes" allowing a direct flow of fluid from subarachnoid space to venous sinus, a view compatible with the valve-like function of the villi. The work of Potts and associates (1972) suggested that the granulations have both a tubular system and an endothelial cap.

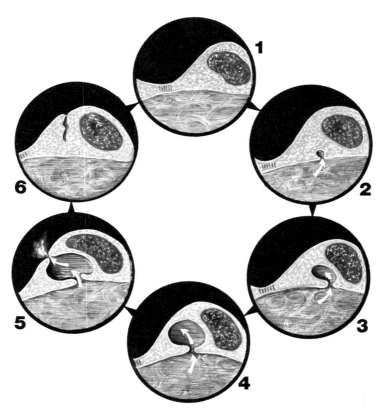

Figure 2–3 The arachnoid villus. Schematic representation of giant vacuolar transport, by which bulk flow reabsorption of CSF occurs from the subarachnoid space to the venous system. The arachnoidal cells have tight intercellular junctions. The vesicles are large enough to encompass red blood cells. This figure is a modification of Tripathi and Tripathi's published schema (1974, 1977).

Another mechanism has been proposed more recently by Tripathi and Tripathi (1974; 1977), namely, the presence in the arachnoid villous membrane of multiple vacuoles, which allow vesicular transport analogous to the absorptive system of the aqueous humor. These studies appear to have resolved the two apparently opposing views of a "closed" and an "open" system. This work has revealed an intact mesothelial lining of the arachnoid membrane, joined by tight junctions. However, the villous cells have giant vacuoles, some of which have both basal and apical openings, thus constituting a system of transcellular channels or pores. It is presumed that these giant vacuoles provide the mechanism for bulk reabsorption of fluid into the venous system. Intact red blood cells have been seen within some vacuoles, which would account for the reported transfer of isotopically labelled red cells from the CSF to the blood (Bradford and Johnson, 1962). Figure 2–3 illustrates *giant vacuolar transport*. This mechanism is presumed to be directly influenced by hydrostatic pressures, which increase bulk absorption of CSF. The precise cellular mechanisms that allow such a remarkable membrane dislocation require further study.

It is noteworthy that the arachnoid villi are not located only in the intracranial venous sinuses. Clusters of arachnoidal cells adjacent to the emerging spinal nerve roots are attached to and also penetrate the dura of the root sleeves extending into small spinal veins (Elman, 1923; Welch and Pollay, 1963; Welch, 1975). Figure 2–4 illustrates these anatomical relationships. The quantitative importance of the spinal villi in CSF absorption is not known. The occurrence of

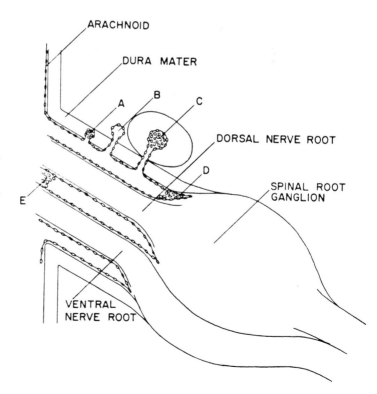

Figure 2-4 Arachnoid villi adjacent to spinal roots: schematic representation. At *A*, growth of arachnoidal cells within the dura mater is represented. *B* represents complete penetration of the dura by arachnoidal cells. *C* represents protrusion of an arachnoid villus into a radicular vein. *D* and *E* are arachnoidal cellular proliferations (from Welch and Pollay, 1963).

hydrocephalus in association with the absence of intracranial arachnoid villi has been reported (Gutierrez *et al.*, 1975), and the spinal absorptive system may be important in various pathological states associated with intracranial hypertension. The physiology of CSF absorption will be discussed in Chapter 3.

Anatomy of the Extracellular Fluid Space

The extracellular interstitial fluid of the brain has been a subject of much controversy in efforts to define its precise size, composition, and relationship to blood and cerebrospinal fluid. The intimate contact of the extracellular fluid with neurons has made its composition of special concern to neurophysiologists; deviations in its volume have been of special interest to clinicians concerned with the pathogenesis of brain edema and hydrocephalus. Before the development of physiological markers, there was great uncertainty about the magnitude of the extracellular fluid because of the limitations of conventional microscopic techniques, as well as the artifactual distortions of tissue fixation (Van Harreveld, 1972). The term "ground substance" was the usual appellation for the diffusely stained matrix of the brain that appeared distinct from clearly defined nuclear structures or cellular membranes that were recognized with light microscopy. More recently, there have been three approaches to the problem which have clarified the extent and functional importance of the extracellular (interstitial) fluid space. These are: (1) the use of extracellular markers *in vivo* and *in vitro*, (2) the use of the electrical impedance of the cerebrum to measure its extracellular fluid volume, and (3) the use of electron microscopy.

Extracellular Markers

The use of extracellular markers to determine the volumes of both the intracellular and extracellular spaces has depended upon using a marker that cannot enter cells and whose concentration can be measured precisely both in plasma and in the tissue, i.e., concentration in brain/concentration in plasma $\times 100$ = extracellular space (per cent). This technique has been used with muscle, liver, and other tissues, but there are special problems when it is applied to brain. Initially, calculations were made using either brain sodium or chloride as the marker, showing an extracellular fluid space of 35 per cent and 25 per cent, respectively. Both ions are known to be present within cells, and therefore both figures must be considered erroneously high.

Other markers were used, including sulfate, bromide, and non-metabolized sugars like inulin and sucrose. Various figures were obtained, as low as 4 per cent with sulfate and even lower with inulin and sucrose. A limiting factor in such calculations was the failure to consider the role of the very low concentrations of these markers obtained in the cerebrospinal fluid. This served as a constant sink for the diffusion of the marker from the brain. When similar concentrations of the marker were maintained in both blood and CSF for sufficient time to approach a "steady" state, the concentrations of the marker in the brain were much higher. With the latter technique, an extracellular fluid space in the brain of about 15 to 20 per cent has been calculated.

The technical difficulties have been critically analyzed by Katzman and Pappius (1973) and by Van Harreveld (1972). Their reviews are excellent summaries of the extensive literature. It is clear that even the most reliable figures are at best approximations which have proved useful experimentally. Data obtained with markers have shown that there is a functionally important extracellular fluid space in brain that is modified in disease states, best exemplified in the various forms of brain edema.

Electrical Impedance

Measurement of the electrical impedance of the brain was developed as an index of its extracellular fluid volume by Van Harreveld (1972). The technique is based on the principle that the resistance of brain tissue to the passage of a low frequency alternating current is dependent upon: (1) the relative volume enclosed by cellular membranes with high electrical resistance, and (2) the extracellular fluid volume with low electrical resistance. Thus, when cells swell the impedance is increased; conversely, cellular shrinkage is associated with a decreased impedance. The advantage of the technique is that it allows the recording of very rapid changes in cellular volume; its major disadvantage is that the changes recorded are technically difficult to express in quantitative terms because of the complex structure of the tissue and uncertainty about the specific resistance of its various cellular elements. Van Harreveld (1972) considered that the available data using impedance measurements were compatible with an extracellular fluid space in cortex of about 15 per cent.

Electron Microscopy

Early electron microscopic reports in the 1950's indicated little or no extracellular fluid space in brain. This view was paralleled by the then current view that the inulin space was only about 3 to 5 per cent. The technical problems involved in the fixation of brain tissue for electron microscopy have been critically reviewed by Van Harreveld (1972). His studies indicated that cellular swelling at the expense of the extracellular fluid occurred rapidly because of the dehydration of tissue samples and the direct effects of many fixatives upon the permeability of cell membranes to sodium. The artifactual loss of the extracellular fluid space was minimized by using the method of freeze substitution, in which fixation with acetone was done at −85°C. It is clear that in the past electron microscopy underestimated the size of the extracellular fluid space. The use of electron microscopic markers, metallo-enzymes like horseradish peroxidase (MW 40,000) and microperoxidase (MW 2000), has allowed visualization of the normal extracellular space and qualitative assessment of changes in its volume in pathological conditions.

In summary, the appropriate use of markers, impedance studies, and electron microscopy with the method of freeze substitution lead to the conclusion that the extracellular fluid space in normal brain has a volume in the range of 15 to 20 per cent. The space is greater in gray matter than in white matter, the former having a much higher water content than the latter.

Dura Mater

The dura mater is a rough, thick, inelastic membrane that serves as a sheath completely encompassing the brain, spinal cord, and lumbar sac. It consists of two layers formed of collagenous bundles, joined together to form thin longitudinal lamellae interlaced with an elastic network. The cerebral dura has two layers, an outer periosteal layer that forms the inner periosteum of the skull, and an inner meningeal layer that corresponds to the spinal dura mater. The meningeal layer is the protective envelope of the brain; it surrounds the cranial nerves as they pierce the dura. The two dural layers split to form the intracranial venous sinuses. The falx, the tentorium, and the diaphragm of the sella are formed by reduplication of the inner meningeal layer of the dura. The dura is well drained by lymphatics, and it has an extensive nerve supply derived from the parasympathetic and sympathetic nervous systems. An excellent description of the classical anatomy of the dura is given by Millen and Woollam (1962). Anatomical variations of the dura mater and the dural sinuses have been studied by Hempel and Elmohamed (1977) in 200 autopsies. There was considerable variation in the sinuses; five main patterns were described, including asymmetry in the size of the transverse sinuses, the right being much larger than the left in 66 per cent of cases. The great vein of Galen was subject to much variation in size and could not be identified in 30 of 70 cases. These major differences in venous structure contribute to the variable clinical manifestations of dural sinus and venous occlusions.

The ultrastructure of the dura of various mammals was examined by Nabeshema *et al.* (1975) electron microscopically, using thin sections and freeze techniques. The dural endothelial cells were fenestrated and had the features of general somatic vessels rather than tight junctions like cerebral capillaries and arachnoidal membranes. These observations were supported by Broman's (1949) earlier work, which showed that intravascular dyes, such as trypan blue, stained the dura but did not stain the arachnoid. Thus, the dura is clearly outside the blood-brain barrier, the features of which will be discussed in Chapter 3.

PHYSIOLOGY OF THE CEREBROSPINAL FLUID

This chapter deals with the physiology of cerebrospinal fluid formation and absorption. The relationship of the CSF to the extracellular fluid of the brain and the functional importance of the CSF will be discussed. The morphology and physiology of the blood-brain barrier will be reviewed, and changes in the barrier in pathological conditions will be summarized. In recent years these topics have been the subject of widespread interest, resulting in several monographs and reviews dealing with various facets of the subject. These include the publications of Davson (1967, 1972); Cserr (1971); Leusen (1972); Milhorat (1972); Katzman and Pappius (1973); Welch (1975); and Rapoport (1976). The publication of several symposia has also provided additional source material, including those edited by Siesjo and Sorenson (1971); Cserr, Fenstermacher, and Fencl (1975); and Bito, Davson, and Fenstermacher (1977). Valuable reviews of an earlier time include those of Flexner (1934); Weed (1935); Davson (1956); Bakay (1956); Bering (1958); and Tschirgi (1960). The physiology of the intracranial pressure in normal and pathological conditions will be considered in Chapter IV.

Prior to discussion of the physiology of CSF formation, it will be useful to define several terms regarding the movement of solutes across membranes. *Passive diffusion* across a membrane or in solution is movement of a solute down a chemical or electrical potential gradient or both, from a higher to a lower level in accord with Fick's law, without the expenditure of energy. *Active transport,* which is an energy-dependent process, is movement of a solute "uphill" against a concentration gradient. Perhaps the best example of active transport is the action of the sodium-potassium ion exchange pump, namely, the enzyme sodium-potassium activated ATPase, which is widespread in cell membranes. It is responsible for the normal distribution of sodium as a chiefly extracellular ion and of potassium as a chiefly intracellular ion; the energy for this ionic distribution is derived from adenosine triphosphate (ATP).

Facilitated diffusion is movement of a solute that depends on its combination with a specific membrane carrier on one side of the membrane which then "shuttles" across the membrane to release the solute on the other side. Facilitated (carrier) diffusion is characteristically stereo-specific, i.e., the carrier binds only those solutes which have a highly specific configuration. Similarly, competitive inhibition between analogous molecules for binding to the membrane carrier can be demonstrated. In addition, the rate of facilitated diffusion can be saturated, i.e., it reaches a maximum with increasing concentrations of the solute. This differs from simple passive diffusion, in which the rate increases linearly with increasing concentration. There are clear-cut similarities between carrier transport and the kinetics of enzyme-substrate interactions (Michaelis-Menton kinetics). Facilitated diffusion is not energy dependent; it usually occurs "downhill," that is, down a concentration gradient. Carrier transport is bidirectional and demonstrates the phenomenon of counter-flow, indicating that the carrier is mobile within the membrane. The movement of specific hexoses and amino acids (both water soluble compounds) across the lipid structure of cellular membranes of brain cells and the blood-brain barrier demonstrates these features of carrier-facilitated diffusion.

Vesicular transport was described in Chapter 2; it has been defined electron microscopically as a specialized means of transcellular transport of macromolecules and other solutes that depends upon vesicle formation reminiscent of pinocytosis. Rapoport (1976) has provided a very concise and lucid summary of the several mechanisms of membrane transport.

FORMATION OF THE CEREBROSPINAL FLUID

Methods of Study

Spinal Drainage

Early investigators estimated the rate of spinal fluid formation in patients by measuring the time needed for the spinal fluid pressure to return to its initial level following removal of a known volume of CSF by drainage. Masserman (1935) calculated that after removal of 20 to 35 ml of fluid in patients, the fluid was replaced at a rate of about 0.32 ml/min, and with a similar technique Sjoqvist (1937) reported a formation rate of 0.36 ml/min. This technique is open to criticism because it assumes that neither fluid formation nor fluid absorption is altered by drainage. It is of special interest that the rates determined are strikingly similar to the average formation rates of 0.35 ml/min obtained in patients by Cutler *et al.*(1968), and 0.37 ml/min obtained by Rubin *et al.* (1966) using the better validated but technically more difficult technique of ventriculo-cisternal perfusion developed thirty years later. Results of the different techniques agree that the normal rate of CSF formation is about 500 ml per day. However, the older drainage method is subject to error, and therefore the data so obtained would be difficult to interpret in pathological or experimental conditions with major changes in pressure-volume relationships in the craniospinal axis.

Isotopic Exchange

With the availability of radioisotopes, there were attempts to determine the rate of spinal fluid formation by studying the rate of exchange of its individual constituents. Greenberg *et al.* (1943), in pioneer studies of the entry of radioisotopes into cerebrospinal fluid, demonstrated that each isotope, whether that of an endogenous ion such as sodium, potassium, or iodine or of an exogenous ion such as rubidium or bromide, entered the fluid at a different rate. Investigators, optimistic that the use of deuterated or tritiated water would clarify the pathophysiology of hydrocephalus and related disorders, were soon disappointed when the very rapid flux of labelled water was shown to depend upon exchange diffusion of the marker rather than upon bulk flow formation or absorption of the CSF (Sweet *et al.*, 1950). Although Davson (1967) indicated that rate of sodium turnover might be used as a measure of CSF turnover, the method has been little used in humans, in part because of the limitations inherent in the use of high-energy isotopes in patients.

The early clinical investigations of Sweet and colleagues (1953) provided information regarding the comparative exchanges of isotopes of sodium, potassium, chloride, and water from blood to various levels along the spinal fluid pathways, as did the studies of protein exchange of Fishman *et al.* (1958). These studies threw some light on the permeability of the blood-CSF barrier at various levels with regard to the flux of several solutes (see regional differences in isotopic exchange, later in this chapter). However, there were no quantitative data available regarding the rates of CSF formation or absorption until the advent of the method of ventriculo-cisternal perfusion.

The Method of Ventriculo-Cisternal Perfusion

Pappenheimer and colleagues (1961) established the method of ventriculo-cisternal perfusion as a quantitative technique for measuring CSF turnover (*bulk formation* and *bulk absorption*) in animals and humans. While Leusen (1949) had already used ventriculo-cisternal perfusion to study the effects of various ions on the brain, Pappenheimer first adapted the method to the study of the cerebrospinal fluid in accordance with concepts underlying renal clearance techniques. Thus, by knowing (1) the concentration of the solute and (2) the volume of fluid both entering and leaving the compartment, a clearance of that substance could be calculated. The technique of ventriculo-cisternal perfusion requires perfusion of the ventricular system, using an artificial CSF with its special ionic composition, and precise measurement of the volume of fluid entering the lateral ventricle and leaving the cisterna magna.

The perfusate contains a known concentration of a non-metabolized marker that does not escape across the ventricular walls, and its concentration is also measured in the cisternal fluid outflow. Inulin, a non-metabolized polymer of fructose (MW about 5000), was used initially, but because it diffuses across the ependyma, the larger molecule of radioiodinated serum albumin (MW 70,000) is preferred.

The calculations for determining CSF formation, reabsorption, and volume are as follows (Heisey *et al.*, 1962; Lorenzo *et al.*, 1970; Welch, 1975):

$$\text{Formation rate (Vf)} = \text{Vi} \frac{(\text{Ci-Co})}{\text{Co}}$$

where Vi is the rate of perfusion and Ci and Co are concentrations of the test substance, inulin or albumin, in the inflow and outflow fluid, respectively.

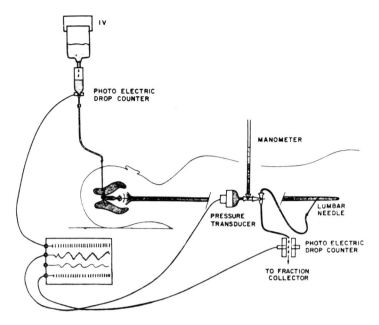

Figure 3–1   The method of ventriculo-lumbar perfusion applied to the study of patients. The placement of drop counters (used to determine influx and efflux rates), pressure transducer, and manometer to measure mean CSF pressure is illustrated. See text (from Lorenzo *et al.*, 1970).

$$\text{Absorption rate (Va)} = \text{Vi} + \text{Vf} - \text{Vo}$$

where Vo is the outflow rate.

This method also allows calculation of the CSF volume, as follows:

$$\text{CSF volume} = \sum_{0}^{n} \left[\frac{\text{Vi Ci} - (\text{Vo} + \text{Va})\,\text{Co}}{\text{C steady state}} \right] dt$$

which represents the area under the curve describing replacement of existing CSF by artificial CSF.

The rate of formation varies with the species, from 0.002 ml/min in rats to 0.35 ml/min in humans, with a good correlation in the various species of formation rate per unit weight of choroid plexus, 0.2 to 0.5 ml/min/gm (Welch, 1975).

The Pappenheimer (1961) method is described in the original papers and has been dealt with further by Davson (1967), Cserr (1971), Katzman and Pappius (1973), and Welch, (1975). It has also been adapted for ventriculo-lumbar as well as ventriculo-ventricular studies. Figure 3–1 illustrates the ventriculo-lumbar technique as applied to the study of patients by Lorenzo *et al.* (1970). The studies must be done with great precision, because there are many pitfalls which have been the subject of published errors, as discussed by Welch (1975).

Radiographic Contrast Studies

Potts and colleagues (1977) have developed radiographic techniques for estimating the rates of CSF formation in animals and humans. After either air or iodinated contrast media were positioned into the lateral ventricle posterior to the foramen of Monro, the ascent of the air fluid level or contrast fluid level was radiographically measured and its estimated volume used as an estimate of CSF formation. Similarly, Rottenberg *et al.* (1977) have used computed tomography to study the disappearance of metrizamide after its intraventricular injection as a measure of CSF bulk flow. These radiographic techniques might be suitable for serial studies in the same patient, but they appear to have inherent limitations as quantitative methods.

Animal Studies In Vivo

Rougemont *et al.* (1960) and Ames and colleagues (1964, 1965) clarified the function of the choroid plexus by developing a technically difficult method for sampling ventricular fluid as it is newly formed at the surface of the choroid plexus. Welch *et al.* (1966) developed an even more demanding technique, which used micropuncture of the principal vein of the choroid plexus in rabbits to measure choroidal blood flow. Rates of choroidal fluid formation were calculated based on the change in hematocrit as the blood passed through the plexus. The method characterized the choroid plexus in terms of its diffusional permeability coefficient and the coefficient of osmotic flow. For an appraisal of these techniques and the experimental data so derived, see the reviews of Cserr (1971) and Welch (1975).

In Vitro Studies

Major advances in our understanding of transport functions of the choroid plexus have been made possible by use of a flux chamber for *in vitro* studies. A variety of such techniques has been used by Czaky (1969), Wright (1972), Pollay *et al.* (1972), Miner and Reed (1972), Wright *et al.* (1977), and others. The contribution of these studies to current understanding of the cellular events underlying CSF formation will be discussed further.

Formation by the Choroid Plexus

The likelihood that the choroid plexus was the site of CSF formation, suggested in the 19th century, was supported by the early studies of Dandy and Blackfan (1914). Dandy (1919) later showed that the removal of choroid plexus from one lateral ventricle prevented the hydrocephalus obtained by occlusion of the ipsilateral foramen of Monro. This early experiment has been the subject of much controversy. Hassin and colleagues (1937) could not reproduce the experiment, and Bering (1958, 1962, 1963) reported that hydrocephalus was prevented because choroid plexectomy obliterated the pulsatile pressures originating from the plexus rather than because of removal of the secretory epithelium. To further complicate the interpretation of these experiments, Milhorat (1972) found that hydrocephalic dilatation of the ventricle occurred despite plexectomy with obstruction of the foramen of Monro. This favored extrachoroidal fluid formation as the cause of the hydrocephalus. Thus, the precise role of choroid plexus in the genesis of the hydrocephalus associated with foraminal obstruction is not clear. (The mechanism of ventricular dilation in hydrocephalus is discussed in Chapter 4.)

TABLE 3–1   Compounds Actively Transported by the Choroid Plexus Demonstrated with *in Vivo* or *in Vitro* Methods

Cations
>   Sodium, potassium, calcium, magnesium

Anions
>   Iodide, thiocyanate, sulfate

Organic Acids
>   5-Hydroxyindoleacetic acid, para-aminohippurate, penicillin, methotrexate,
>   phenolsulfonthalein, salicylic acid, prostaglandin PGE

Organic Bases
>   Primary amines (serotonin and norepinephrine)
>   Tertiary amines (morphine, nalorphine, codeine, levorphan)
>   Quaternary amines (hexamethonium, choline)

Monosaccharides
>   Glucose, galactose

Purines
>   Xanthine

Amino Acids
>   Basic, acidic and neutral amino acids

Vitamins
>   Vitamin A, thiamine, nicotinamide, riboflavin, pyridoxine, folic acid

However, there is substantial and convincing evidence that the choroid plexus serves as a major site for the secretion of ventricular fluid. While Cushing's (1914) observation that fluid drops leak from the surface of the exposed choroid plexus at operation is subject to other interpretations, the studies of Ames and colleagues (1964, 1965) provided direct and conclusive evidence for the secretion of ventricular fluid by the choroid plexus. Their technique (Rougemont *et al.*, 1960 for direct sampling of newly formed choroidal fluid in cats made possible the study of its chemical composition and of the factors affecting the rate of fluid production.

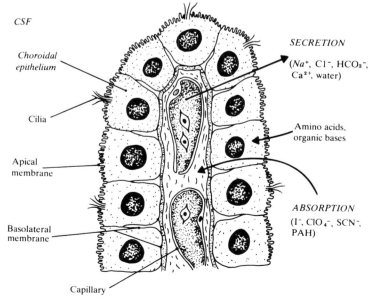

CSF

Choroidal epithelium

Cilia

Apical membrane

Basolateral membrane

Capillary

SECRETION

(*Na*$^+$, Cl$^-$, HCO$_3$$^-$, Ca^{2+}, water)

Amino acids, organic bases

ABSORPTION

(I$^-$, ClO$_4$$^-$, SCN$^-$, PAH)

Figure 3–2 The functional organization of the choroid plexus. The choroidal cells have tight apical junctions. The major solutes that are secreted and absorbed are indicated. Capillary filtration is the first step in CSF formation (Wright, 1978).

As noted earlier, the rate of CSF formation in various species, measured with ventriculo-cisternal perfusion, varies between 0.002 ml/min in the rat to 0.35 ml/min in humans. There is a close correlation between the formation rate and the weight of the choroid plexus; the formation rate in various species varies between 0.2 and 0.5 ml/min per/gram of choroid plexus (Welch, 1975). There have been extensive studies of the isolated choroid plexus both *in vivo* and *in vitro*. Specific transport systems for a variety of compounds, including ions, organic acids and bases, sugars, purines, amino acids, and vitamins have been identified, the data are summarized in Table 3–1. Figure 3–2 illustrates the functional organization of the choroid plexus as a secretory and absorptive epithelium. The importance of the choroid plexus in CSF formation and absorption, and its contribution to blood-brain barrier effects, will be discussed later.

Choroidal Secretion

The enzyme sodium-potassium activated ATPase plays a key role in the formation of ventricular fluid. The existence of this mechanism has been supported by observations that perfusion of the cerebral ventricles with a solution containing ouabain, a specific inhibitor of the enzyme, greatly inhibited the formation of choroidal fluid *in vivo*, and perfusion of the plexus *in vitro* had similar effects (Vates *et al.*, 1964, Cserr, 1971). The cellular mechanisms for secretion of the fluid have been illuminated by the studies of Wright (1972) using frog choroid plexus. Wright's view of choroidal secretion is based upon the "standing gradient" hypothesis of Diamond and Bossert (1967), which considers local osmotic forces within secretory epithelia to be responsible for the movement of water.

The mechanism of choroidal fluid secretion may be summarized as follows. Secretion is dependent upon the active transport of sodium via the sodium pump. This pump is probably present at the apical surface as well as at the intercellular clefts. The transport of both bicarbonate and chloride is in some way coupled to the transport of sodium and thereby to the formation of the fluid. The precise mode of action of the sodium pump, as well as the factors controlling secretory rate and epithelial permeability, require further elucidation. Figure 3–3, from Segal and Pollay (1977) (a modification of an earlier figure of Wright, 1972), summarizes these events. The figure indicates that hydrostatic pressure derived from the choroidal capillaries initiates the transfer of water and ions to the choroidal epithelium. The further transfer of ions and water from the intercellular cleft proceeds in two ways: (1) into the ventricular cavity across the tight apical junction and (2) intracellularly and then across the plasma membrane of the apical villus into the ventricular cavity. Both of these transmembranal transfers are probably dependent upon the sodium pump. It is noteworthy that the small electrical potential between blood and CSF does not appear to have a significant role in choroidal secretion (Welch, 1975).

Another enzyme, carbonic anhydrase, present in the choroid plexus, plays an important role in the secretion of choroidal fluid. The enzyme, distributed widely in many tissues, catalyzes the formation of carbonic acid from water and carbon dioxide (Maren, 1967). Carbonic acid dissociates to form bicarbonate and hydrogen ions. Studies have been made of the effects of acetazolamide (Dia-

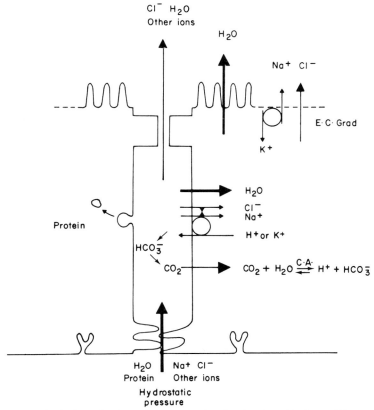

Figure 3–3 Hypothetical mechanism of CSF secretion by the choroid plexus. The entry of water and solutes at the base must be balanced by an equal movement at the apical microvilli and via the tight junctions. Water and salts enter the intercellular clefts by capillary hydrostatic pressure. Specific transport systems responsible for the transfer of sodium and potassium are shown. The role of carbonic anhydrase and the movement of protein by pinocytosis are indicated. See text (after Segal and Pollay, 1977).

mox), an inhibitor of the enzyme, on spinal fluid formation and the intracranial pressure. It was first shown by Tschirgi *et al.* (1954) that the drug substantially reduced CSF flow or formation, or both, in several species. Several investigators showed the reduction of CSF sodium exchange by acetazolamide to 50 to 100 per cent of control values (Davson and Luck, 1957, Fishman, 1959). Davson (1967) has summarized the literature leading to the conclusion that the rate of sodium exchange directly parallels the rate of spinal fluid formation. A good correlation between these rates has been demonstrated, but the quantitative relationship between the two is not certain. (An unresolved problem is the differentiation between bulk transfer of the sodium ion from blood to CSF, and simple exchange of labelled sodium ions with the sodium pool of the brain, plasma, and cerebrospinal fluid.) Despite extensive study, the mechanism has been elusive whereby inhibition of the enzyme carbonic anhydrase slows sodium flux, as well as bicarbonate and chloride uptake, to result in inhibition of bulk formation of CSF (Ames *et al.*, 1965; Davson and Segal, 1970; Maren and Broder

1970; Maren, 1971; Wright, 1972, 1978). The drug furosemide also slows the rate of CSF formation. It is considered to have a primary influence on chloride flux which is independent from the effect of acetazolamide on carbonic anhydrase.

Both drugs have been shown to have other effects besides their reduction of CSF formation (Reed, 1969; Sahar and Tsipstein, 1978). In addition to its ability to reduce CSF secretion, acetazolamide has secondary effects on the intracranial pressure, which will be discussed in Chapter 4 (Knopp et al., 1957; Birzis et al., 1958; Atkinson and Ward, 1958; Fishman, 1959; and Rubin et al., 1966).

CSF Filtration and Secretion

Early arguments about whether CSF was formed as a simple filtrate of plasma or as a result of active transport by the choroidal epithelium (Merritt and Fremont-Smith, 1938) were resolved by analysis of the ionic composition of the fluid. Davson's (1967) studies of the cisternal fluid of rabbits and Rougemont and colleagues' (1960) studies of newly formed choroidal fluid in cats supported older studies of the ionic composition of the CSF by Flexner (1934) and others which indicated that its ionic composition was different from that of a plasma filtrate.

While the sodium content of both fluids is about the same, CSF has an excess of chloride and magnesium and a deficit of potassium and bicarbonate compared with the concentration of these ions in a plasma filtrate. When the two fluids are compared, their ionic concentrations should be corrected for differences in the water content; plasma is 93 per cent water, and CSF is 99 per cent water. The effect of binding of some cations, notably calcium and magnesium, to serum albumin also influences their distribution ratio, CSF/plasma. The concentration ratios of the major ions in CSF are different from those in a protein-free filtrate; this indicates that the composition of the fluid is dependent upon a secretory process (Davson, 1967). It is noteworthy that the osmolalities of plasma, CSF, and plasma ultrafiltrate are very similar; that is, in the steady state they are isosmotic (Katzman and Pappius, 1973). This indicates the ready equilibration of water between the two fluids.

Welch (1975) has critically reviewed the literature and concluded that choroidal fluid formation involves two distinct processes that occur in series: first, filtration across the choroidal capillary wall, and second, secretion by the choroidal epithelium. The regulation of these two processes in maintaining the normal rate of CSF formation needs further elucidation. The special chemical composition of CSF will be discussed in Chapter 6. The data document that the chemical composition of CSF can be explained only as a consequence of active transport processes adjacent to the CSF, in the choroidal epithelium and in other cellular elements of the nervous system.

Extrachoroidal Formation

Although there is substantial evidence for the secretion of CSF by the choroid plexus, there is considerable support for its extrachoroidal formation as well. Weed (1935) wrote of the dual origin of the cerebrospinal fluid, and Wallace and Brodie (1940) actually considered all of the CSF to arise from the brain. Bering and Sato (1963) later reported that ventricular fluid was formed within the plexectomized ventricle at about half the rate seen in a normal ventricle. Curl and Pollay (1968), using the method of ventriculo-cisternal perfusion in rabbits, estimated that transependymal formation was responsible for about one third of the intraventricular fluid formation. Milhorat (1972) reported that choroid plexectomy did not affect the rate of formation or the composition of the fluid 2 to 6 months later.

While the evidence for a dual source is convincing, there are no data available which establish the relative contributions of the choroidal and the transependymal routes of formation in humans. The view that lateral choroid plexectomy does not alter ventricular fluid formation and composition requires further substantiation with particular reference to the function of the remaining choroid plexus of the fourth ventricle in such experiments. The source of the CSF found in the subarachnoid space in cases of obstruction of the ventricular outflow is not clear. Fluid within the cortical sulci has been seen by neurosurgeons in such cases, and it seems likely that such fluid originates in the adjacent cerebrum. Pollay and Curl (1967) have demonstrated the formation of CSF in the isolated sylvian aqueduct; it originated transependymally in the absence of the choroid plexus. Lorenzo *et al.* (1970) and Hochwald *et al.* (1967) were unable to detect CSF formation by perfusion of the isolated spinal subarachnoid space of cats. However, patients with complete high thoracic or cervical cord block clearly have CSF below the level of the block, at times with only mild or moderate elevations of protein content. This clinical observation supports the presence of extrachoroidal formation of CSF within the adjacent spinal cord in this pathological situation, although there are no experimental data to support this view.

Factors Influencing the Rate of CSF Formation

The various techniques just described are used to determine the normal rate of CSF formation. They have also been used to examine several factors that might modify this rate. Although both increased and decreased formation rates have been induced, there is a great tendency for formation to be maintained at a rather constant rate. The effects of some drugs, hydrostatic pressures, and changes in osmolality upon the rate of CSF formation will now be summarized.

Cardiac Glycosides

The inhibitory effects of ouabain, a potent inhibitor of sodium-potassium activated ATPase, on choroidal secretion of CSF have been described earlier. The drug has proved effective in reducing CSF formation only when used to perfuse the plexus directly, either by the intraventricular route *in vivo* or by addition to the perfusate *in vitro* (Welch, 1975). The cardiac effects of the digitalis glycosides limit the dosage that can be given systemically; with the usual systemic dosages only trace amounts have been detectable in CSF. While there is a single report that parenteral digoxin slowed the flow of ventricular fluid in 3 hydrocephalic children (Neblett *et al.*, 1972), this has not been confirmed subsequently (Schott and Holt, 1974).

Carbonic Anhydrase Inhibitors

The inhibitory effects of acetezolamide, an inhibitor of carbonic anhydrase, on choroidal secretion have been described earlier. The systemic administration of the drug reduces the rate of CSF formation by about 50 per cent in several species, measured by several methods including ventriculo-cisternal perfusion, direct sampling of choroidal fluid, and using the sodium exchange rate as a measure of CSF formation (Davson and Luck, 1957; Fishman, 1959; Ames *et al.*, 1965; and Rubin *et al.*, 1966). It is important to note that intravenous acetazolamide may cause an acute transient increase in intracranial pressure even while inducing a decrease in the rate of CSF formation (Knapp *et al.*, 1957; Birzis *et al.*, 1958; Fishman, 1959; Rubin *et al.*, 1966). This pressure increase is probably secondary to the effects of carbon dioxide accumulation in the cerebral tissue resulting in vasodilatation and a secondary increase in intracranial pressure. *It also illustrates the general rule that the intracranial pressure is far more dependent upon cerebral hemodynamics than upon the rate of CSF formation.*

Furosemide

Furosemide, a potent inhibitor of the renal tubular reabsorption of salt and water, also slows CSF formation. Its mode of action in the ascending loop of Henle is considered to be independent of the role of carbonic anhydrase and the mineralocorticoids. Reed (1969) and Buhrley and Reed (1972) showed that both furosemide and acetazolamide independently reduced CSF formation in rabbits by about 50 per cent; when both drugs were given together, CSF formation fell about 75 per cent. They concluded that furosemide inhibited the formation of CSF by a different mechanism than did acetazolamide. Furosemide has direct effects on chloride transport in the renal tubular epithelium, and this may be the basis for its effects on the choroid plexus. Domer (1969) found that furosemide had no immediate effect on CSF formation in cats. However, Sahar and Tsipstein (1978) reported that the drug caused reduction in CSF function in cats measured by ventriculo-cisternal perfusion, 2 hours after intravenous injection and immediately after intraventricular administration. However, large doses were used, from 0.9 to 2.0 mg/kg, and there are insufficient data available in patients to validate the clinical effectiveness of the drug. The drug has been used in clinical trials with recent reports that it proved effective in reducing intracranial pressure (see Chapter 4).

Steroids

The literature regarding the effects of glucocorticoids on CSF formation is inconsistent. Fishman (1959) found that neither glucocorticoids nor mineralocorticoids in dogs had an effect on sodium exchange time (which serves as an index of bulk formation of CSF). On the other hand, Garcia-Bengochea (1965) found that cortisone inhibited CSF flow in cats, and Weiss and Nulsen (1970) found that dexamethasone acutely reduced CSF flow in dogs, measured by spinal drainage. More recently, Vela *et al.* (1979) have systematically studied the effects of various glucocorticoids in CSF formation and absorption in dogs, using the method of ventriculo-cisternal perfusion. No significant effects on CSF formation or absorption were demonstrated. It seems likely that the benefits of glucocorticoids in brain edema reflect chiefly their beneficial effects on endothelial cell permeability rather than any direct effects on CSF formation. The possibility that glucocorticoids modify CSF absorption in inflammatory diseases of the meninges is discussed in Chapter 4.

Drugs and Procedures without Effect on CSF Formation

A diverse group of drugs and procedures has been shown to have an insignificant effect on CSF formation, measured with various techniques that include simple outflow, sodium exchange time, and ventriculo-cisternal perfusion. The drugs studied include norepinephrine, insulin, chlorothiazide, meralluride, neostigmine, diphenylhydantoin (Fishman, 1959), and the inhibitors of protein synthesis, actinomycin D, puromycin, and cycloheximide (Davson and Segal, 1970). These drugs were studied in acute experiments; long-term studies might elicit changes. Oppelt *et al.* (1964) showed that neither metabolic nor respiratory acidosis affected CSF formation, although respiratory and metabolic alkalosis had inhibitory effects the mechanism of which is obscure.

Effects of Hydrostatic Pressure

The rate of formation of CSF is probably independent of moderate, brief variation in the level of the intraventricular pressure. Heisey *et al.* (1962), using ventriculo-cisternal perfusion in goats, showed that varying the intraventricular pressure acutely from -100 to $+300$ mm H_2O did not change the rate of fluid formation. Cutler *et al.* (1968) confirmed this observation in clinical studies. In studies of chronically hydrocephalic animals, Sahar (1972) and Hochwald *et al.* (1972) reported a definite reduction in CSF formation with increasing intraventricular pressure. Welch (1975) has critically reviewed the literature and has concluded that the rate of CSF formation declines as intraventricular pressure is elevated to sufficient duration and degree. As discussed earlier, it seems likely that choroidal fluid formation involves two processes that occur in series: first, filtration across the capillary endothelial cell wall, and second, secretion by the choroidal epithelium. Increases in hydrostatic pressures would be expected to affect chiefly the first process but might also adversely affect the secretory epithelium. Atrophy of the choroid plexus has been seen in chronic hydrocephalus (Russell, 1949). The quantitative relationship between choroidal filtration and secretion requires further study in hydrocephalus.

Effects of Changes in Osmolality

Heisey *et al.* (1962) and Welch *et al.* (1966) have studied the effects of altered osmolality of the ventricular fluid on the rate of CSF production. The theoretical implications of these studies have been reviewed by Welch (1975). In experiments of more direct clinical relevance, DiMattio *et al.* (1975) and Hochwald *et al.* (1976) studied the effects in cats of acute serum hyperosmolality, obtained with hypertonic sucrose or glucose, and acute serum hypo-osmolality obtained with water loads. CSF formation was clearly reduced when the serum osmolality was increased, and CSF formation was increased when the serum was made hypotonic. The relationship was approximately linear, with a 1 per cent change in serum osmolality causing a 6.7 per cent change in CSF formation. Whether such striking effects occur in clinical situations has not been determined. The serum osmolality may be depressed 10 per cent (30mOsm) or more in patients with symptomatic hyponatremia, and the osmolality may be elevated 10 to 20 per cent or more in hypernatremic states. The therapeutic use of hypertonic solutions commonly elevates the serum osmolality 5 to 10 per cent (15 to 30 mOsm). However, there are no data available in patients regarding the effect on CSF formation of such acute or chronic changes in osmolality. In light of the adaptation of the brain to chronic alterations in osmolality (Fishman, 1974), it is possible that the choroid plexus also would adapt to chronic osmotic derangement with a return to a normal rate of CSF secretion.

Homeostasis in Cerebrospinal Fluid Composition

The relative constancy of the rate of CSF formation just described is paralleled by the relative constancy of its ionic composition despite major changes in the serum ion concentration. This occurs in both clinical studies and animal experiments. The homeostatic processes differ with each of the major ions, and the precise mechanisms involved are not well understood. They include active transport by the choroidal epithelium as well as within the brain parenchyma, probably by the endothelial cells and glia. The Donnan effect, also, influences the distribution in CSF of the major anions chloride and bicarbonate. It is attributable to the high concentration of anionic proteins in plasma compared to CSF. Its role has been discussed in detail by Davson (1967) and by Katzman and Pappius (1973). The factors maintaining homeostasis of the major ions of CSF will be discussed separately.

Sodium

The concentration of sodium in plasma and in CSF is very similar, with little species variation. When the concentrations are expressed in terms of the differences in water content of the two fluids, the concentration of sodium is a few per cent higher, except in rabbits, in which, curiously, it is slightly lower (Davson, 1967). As noted earlier, the concentration of sodium is slightly higher in CSF than in a plasma ultrafiltrate. Although the level of CSF sodium is dependent upon active transport processes (Davson and Segal, 1970), it is also dependent upon osmotic forces between plasma and CSF. Thus, in experimental hyponatremia and hypernatremia, the CSF sodium level varies directly with the plasma level, although there is a delay in equilibration between the two compartments. In dogs, the half-time for radiosodium exchange varied between 90 and 260 minutes (Fishman, 1959). In cats with acute hypernatremia, the CSF sodium lagged behind the plasma sodium level by about 60 minutes, and the change in CSF sodium was modulated, i.e., it approached but did not reach the plasma level (Pape and Katzman, 1970; Katzman and Pappius, 1973). However, in chronic states of hypernatremia, the CSF level more closely approximates the plasma level. This has been well supported by clinical observations (see Chapter 6). Sodium differs from potassium, calcium, and magnesium because the concentrations of the latter ions are more narrowly maintained, whereas the level of sodium, the major osmotically active cation in CSF, readily parallels the sodium level in serum.

Potassium

The potassium level in CSF is maintained within narrow limits. Bradbury and Kleeman (1967) and others have shown a remarkable constancy of the CSF potassium level despite marked hypokalemia or hyperkalemia. Thus, during changes in plasma potassium that varied from 1.58 to 7.09 meq/l, the CSF level remained unchanged at about 2.9 meq/l. There is an extensive literature dealing with the effects of various drugs and manipulations, e.g., shock, hyperthermia, glucose, insulin, and death, which confirms the remarkable constancy of the concentration of potassium in CSF in life (Katzman and Pappius, 1973). It appears biologically necessary to maintain within very narrow limits the concentration of potassium in CSF and in the contiguous extracellular fluid of the central nervous system. The two control mechanisms involved are (1) active transport of potassium from the blood to the CSF by the choroid plexus, and (2) active transport processes in brain that remove potassium from the CSF. Ames *et al.* (1964, 1965) have studied the potassium concentration in newly formed choroidal fluid and found that it was about 3.15 meq/l, a concentration about one third less than that of the plasma level. However, they noted that fluid from the cisterna magna sampled simultaneously had an even lower concentration, 2.66 meq/l. Bito (1969) also confirmed the fall in potassium content as the fluid moved away from the choroid plexus, for the potassium level in fluid from the cortical sulci was even lower, 2.51 meq/l.

These observations lead to the conclusion that there is an active process for the removal of potassium ions in cerebral tissue distal to the choroid plexus. There is considerable electrophysiological data indicating that glial cells function as a sink for potassium ions in the extracellular fluid space (Tower, 1972; Katzman, 1976). Intracellular potassium levels are in the range of 100 meq per kg wet weight. If potassium ions are continuously removed from CSF and brain extracellular fluid, the glial cells are inadequate alone to serve this function, and it is an attractive hypothesis that the capillary endothelial cells of the brain may serve as an important site for the active transport of potassium from the extracellular fluid to the blood. The recent work of Goldstein (1979) and Betz and Goldstein (1978), using brain capillaries *in vitro*, supports such a function for amino acids, organic acids, and potassium ions. Further study is required of the joint roles of the glial and capillary endothelial cells in maintaining the CSF and extracellular fluid potassium levels between very narrow limits.

Calcium

The normal level of the CSF calcium in various species is reported to range between 2.3 and 3.2 meq/l with serum levels ranging between 4.3 and 5.4 meq/l (Katzman and Pappius, 1973). There is probably little difference in the calcium levels of fluid obtained from different levels, e.g., ventricular, cisternal, lumbar. Since about one third to one half of the serum calcium is bound to plasma proteins, chiefly albumin, it was suggested early that the CSF level might represent the ionized, diffusible calcium fraction present in the serum. However, Merritt and Bauer (1931) showed that the concentration ratio of CSF to plasma calcium, about 0.50, was independent of the plasma protein level. It was subsequently shown that the CSF calcium was little or not at all affected by parathyroidectomy, intravenous infusions of calcium or parathormone, or administration of EDTA to deplete the plasma calcium (Katzman and Pappius, 1973). Thus, the available data indicate that in the choroid plexus and other cellular elements comprising the blood-brain barrier there is a homeostatic mechanism that maintains the CSF calcium level within very narrow limits. The studies by Graziani *et al.* (1967) of radioactive calcium flux indicate that the entry of calcium into the ventricular fluid depends on a carrier-mediated transport system that is inhibited by ouabain but not affected by acetazolamide. Parathormone may play a role in maintaining CSF calcium level in the presence of marked hypocalcemia. The cellular mechanisms that stabilize the concentration of calcium in CSF and brain clearly require further study.

Magnesium

There has long been an interest in the CSF magnesium level because it is normally maintained at higher levels than in plasma. Cohen (1927) showed that the CSF concentration fell toward the serum level in meningitis. While there is some variation in the literature, the reliable method of atomic absorption gives the normal serum level as 1.67 ± 0.14 (S.D.) meq/l and the normal CSF level as 2.24 ± 0.10 (S.D.) meq/l (Woodbury *et al.*, 1968; Katzman and Pappius, 1973). Moreover, magnesium is about 35 per cent bound to serum protein, increasing the concentration ratio of the *diffusible* magnesium in the CSF relative to serum to about 2.0. A higher magnesium level in ventricular fluid than in cisternal or lumbar fluid has been reported in monkeys (Bito and Myers, 1970), suggesting that, like potassium, magnesium is transported into cellular elements as the fluid moves distally from the choroid plexus.

The CSF level varies little despite marked elevations in the serum level. Thus, Oppelt *et al.* (1963) elevated the serum levels threefold with magnesium salt infusions, but the CSF level was increased only about 20 per cent. Similarly, chronic hypomagnesemia induced with a low magnesium diet resulted in only a minor fall in CSF magnesium (Chutkow and Meyers, 1968; Bradbury and Kleeman, 1969). The CSF magnesium rises rapidly after death. Thus, it is clear that complex active transport systems in the choroid plexus, as well as other cellular elements (glial or endothelial cells, or both) in the nervous system, modulate the CSF magnesium and maintain it within narrow limits at a level exceeding that of blood.

Chloride

The chloride concentration of CSF is higher than in the plasma of all vertebrates studied (Katzman and Pappius, 1973). The chloride concentration in human CSF is about 115 meq/l, approximately 15 meq/l higher than in the plasma. Ames *et al.* (1965) found a slightly higher chloride concentration in the cisternal fluid than in the newly formed choroidal fluid. This indicates that the CSF chloride, the major anion in extracellular fluid, has both a choroidal and an extrachoroidal origin. The higher concentration of chloride ions in CSF reflects the Donnan equilibrium and is determined by the relative absence of proteins (anionic in charge) from the CSF. The Donnan effect is reflected in the slight reduction in CSF chloride observed when the CSF protein is very high (Merritt and Fremont-Smith, 1938). The CSF chloride is in osmotic equilibrium with the plasma chloride, and parallel changes occur in CSF chloride with both hypochloremia and hyperchloremia, although the 15 meq/l higher concentration in the CSF persists.

The transfer of chloride from plasma to CSF has been considered a passive process which maintains electrochemical neutrality. However, data reviewed by Maren (1971, 1972) and by Bourke and Nelson (1972) indicate that bicarbonate and chloride transport are directly linked to the active transport of sodium and that carbonic anhydrase influences the transfer of each ion into the CSF. This indicates that the transfer of chloride, like that of other ions, depends upon a specific membrane transport system, although its higher concentration in CSF than in plasma is in part passive because of its dependence on the electrochemical gradient between the two compartments.

Glucose

The transfer of glucose between blood and CSF (Fishman, 1964) as well as between blood and brain (Crone, 1965) is dependent upon carrier transport (facilitated diffusion), the features of which were described earlier. Carrier transport enables lipid insoluble compounds like glucose and specific amino acids to cross cell membranes by combining with a mobile carrier in the membrane, a specific protein or proteolipid, which moves the compound across the membrane and releases it on the other side. Figure 3–4 demonstrates the effect of 2-deoxy-D-glucose, an analog of glucose, in inhibiting the entry of glucose into the cisternal fluid of dogs when both sugars were given intravenously at the same time. Such competitive inhibition between two analogous molecules is a characteristic feature of carrier-mediated transport.

Carrier transport of glucose has also been demonstrated in choroid plexus, brain capillaries, cortical brain slices, synaptosomes, and glial cells in culture (Pardridge and Oldendorf, 1977; Lorenzo, 1977; Lund-Andersen, 1979). The kinetics vary in these systems, probably reflecting, in part, differences in the

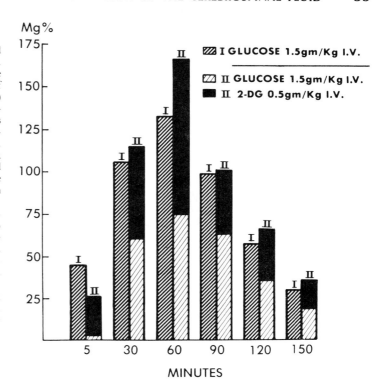

Figure 3-4 Carrier-mediated transport of glucose into CSF. Experiment I shows that the intravenous administration of glucose in a dog (1.5 gm/kg) resulted in an increase in cisternal fluid glucose that was maximal at 60 minutes and largely dissipated at 150 minutes. In experiment II, one week later, the same dog received the same intravenous dosage of glucose concomitant with 2-deoxy-D-glucose (0.5 gm/kg). The presence of the 2-DG inhibited the entry of glucose into the cisternal fluid. Note that the total increase in hexose was about the same in the two experiments. This study illustrates some of the features characteristic of carrier-mediated transport of sugars across the blood-brain barrier, including competitive inhibition of analogous compounds. See text (from Fishman, 1964).

functional characteristics of the various membrane carriers, in terms of their stereospecificity and affinity.

Glucose does not enter the CSF solely in the ventricles; it was shown to be elevated above and below a spinal ligature following intravenous injection (Riser, 1929). The CSF concentration of glucose is about 60 per cent of the blood glucose in humans in the steady state. This is caused not only by its utilization in the nervous system, Sadler and Welch (1967) found that newly formed choroidal fluid also had reduced concentrations. However, brain tissue contains only about 20 mg per cent glucose in the steady state. This fact supports the view that the low level of glucose in CSF is, in part, due to its movement "downhill" into the tissue. Although such CSF to brain transfer of glucose accounts in part for the normal CSF/blood glucose ratio of 0.6, it is probably of minor importance in providing for the brain's need for glucose, which is largely supplied by the circulation.

Other Solutes

The chemical composition of the CSF, including its acid-base characteristics, will be considered at length in Chapter 6.

Regional Differences in Isotopic Exchange

The evidence favoring the cerebral ventricles as the site for the formation of both choroidal and extrachoroidal fluid has been summarized earlier. However, soon after the introduction of isotopes for the study of the CSF, investigations, largely performed in patients, established that there was a ready exchange of various tracers between blood and CSF all along the neuraxis. Following intravenous injection in animals, labelled water reached equilibrium with all the brain water and CSF water very rapidly, essentially as a function of blood flow (Oldendorf, 1977).

In studies using isotopically labelled water, sodium, potassium, and albumin administered intravenously, three different patterns of isotopic exchange were observed when the ventricular, cisternal, and lumbar fluids were sampled simultaneously. (1) The ions entered the ventricular fluid more rapidly than the cisternal or the lumbar fluid (Sweet *et al.*, 1950). (2) Labelled water entered the cisternal fluid most rapidly (Sweet *et al.*, 1953). (3) Albumin entered the lumbar fluid more rapidly than either the cisternal or the ventricular fluid (Fishman *et al.*, 1957). The rapid entry of ions into the ventricular fluid reflects their derivation from the choroid plexus as well as their entry from the extracellular fluid space of the cerebrum. The exchange of water occurs most rapidly in the cisternal fluid, because this small volume of fluid is in contiguity with the extensive membrane surfaces of the cerebellar folia and cortical gyri, facilitating the entry of a compound (such as nitrous oxide) whose transfer is dependent chiefly upon the cerebral blood flow. The most rapid entry of iodinated albumin into the lumbar fluid suggests that the endothelial cell barrier to large molecules, which normally limits the entry of proteins, is less effective in the blood vessels of the lumbar subarachnoid region than in the brain. The effect of such regional permeability differences on the normal gradient in CSF protein concentration is discussed Chapter 6. Although minor differences in vascular permeability to large molecules may occur along the neuraxis, there is no evidence for bulk formation of CSF in the lumbar region of cats (Lorenzo *et al.*, 1970a).

ABSORPTION OF THE CEREBROSPINAL FLUID

In the steady or equilibrium state, by definition, the rate of absorption of CSF equals its rate of formation. The data summarized earlier indicate that the dual rates are about 0.35 ml per minute or 500 ml per day. These rates represent the bulk flow or turnover of the fluid. The bulk turnover of the fluid must be distinguished from the turnover or exchange of individual constituents of the fluid, e.g., ions, sugar, proteins, or drugs, each of which exchanges at a different rate. (The turnover of radiosodium has been used as an index of the rate of bulk flow formation of the fluid, as discussed earlier, but it does not provide quantitative data regarding bulk flow.) The rate of absorption of each individual solute depends upon three factors: (1) the rate of bulk flow absorption of the fluid, (2) the active transport of many solutes from the CSF by the choroid plexus and by other cellular elements, including capillary endothelial cells, and (3) the disappearance by diffusion into brain and brain capillaries of each solute. These mechanisms will now be considered.

Bulk Flow Absorption

The early studies by Key and Retzius (1875) and by Weed (1914) of the fate of intrathecal dyes implicated the pacchionian granulations as a site for CSF absorption. There has been a lingering controversy over how the arachnoid villus system functions to allow for the bulk absorption of fluid, already summarized in the discussion of the anatomy of the arachnoid villi (see Chapter 2). Several investigations in the early 1960's greatly clarified the physiology of absorption. Prockop *et al.* (1962) studied the disappearance from the ventricular fluid of four non-metabolized sugars: mannitol, sucrose, inulin, and dextran. Despite marked differences in molecular weight, these compounds left the subarachnoid space at about the same rate. Furthermore, the rate of inulin clearance was directly proportional to the pressure difference between the CSF and the dural venous sinus. These data documented that the existence of a mechanism for the bulk flow reabsorption of the CSF depended upon the hydrostatic pressure within the subarachnoid space.

The studies of Welch and Friedman (1960) further clarified the process. They placed the dural sinus of monkeys in an *in vitro* flux chamber, which allowed the study of the flow of fluids across the arachnoid villi. They found that the flow was unidirectional, from the arachnoidal side to the venous side, and that flow in the reverse direction did not occur. Thus, it was quite appropriate to conclude that the arachnoid villi functioned like a system of one-way valves. These investigations also showed that there was a critical opening pressure of 20 to 50 mm H_2O at which flow could be initiated from the arachnoidal side. In addition, as the pressure gradient increased, there was a steep increase in flow rate. Welch and Pollay (1961) also studied the size of particles that could cross the villi in the *in vitro* preparation. A variety of particles ranging in diameter from that of colloidal gold (0.2 μm) to those of polystyrene (1.8 μm), yeast (3.6 μm), and erythrocytes (7.5 μm) could pass through the valves, but larger polystyrene spheres (6.4 to 12.8 μm) were excluded. The early ultrastructural data of Shabo and Maxwell (1968) and others, indicating that the villi were membrane bound, have been clarified by Tripathi (1977). He has demonstrated a specialized system of giant vesicular transport, which appears to be the basis for the valve-like function of the arachnoid villi in the bulk reabsorption of CSF (see Chapter 2, Anatomical Aspects).

The method of ventriculo-cisternal perfusion *in vivo* provided quantitative information about the rate of CSF absorption in ml per minute and about its dependency upon the CSF pressure. Heisey *et al.* (1962) first reported that in the goat, bulk absorption (defined as the inulin clearance rate) was directly related to the CSF pressure over a range of -100 to $+300$ mm H_2O. Bering and Sato (1963) found a similar relationship in dogs, at CSF pressures ranging from -100 to $+400$ mm H_2O. Prockop and Fishman (1968) studied the effect of increased protein concentration in canine CSF upon the bulk absorption of the fluid. A CSF protein of about 300 mg per cent only slightly slowed the rate of inulin clearance. In a model of human disease, however, inflammatory changes due to

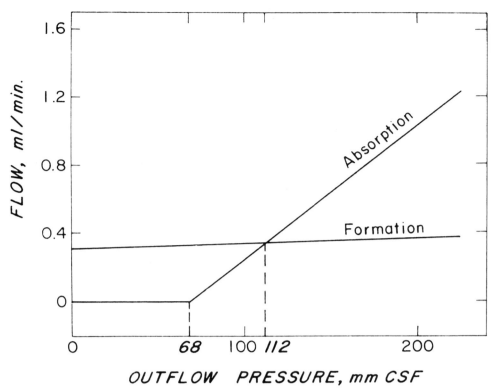

Figure 3-5   Schema illustrating the relationships between CSF formation and absorption in humans with regard to the intracranial (outflow) pressure. The data were obtained with the method of ventriculo-lumbar perfusion. Note the relative constancy of CSF formation, about 0.35 ml/min. over the pressure range, 0 to 220 mm. In contrast, CSF absorption is directly dependent upon intracranial pressure. CSF absorption begins at a pressure of about 68 mm. At a pressure of about 112 mm, the rates of CSF formation and absorption are equal. See text (from Cutler *et al.*, 1968).

experimental pneumococcal meningitis markedly slowed inulin clearance and, to an even greater degree, the clearance of albumin, indicating impairment of bulk flow reabsorption by the arachnoid villi.

Rubin *et al.* (1966) first applied to patients the method of ventriculo-lumbar perfusion, that is, the method of ventriculo-cisternal perfusion using lumbar CSF instead of cisternal CSF. The patients had cerebral glioma or meningeal leukemia. Data obtained from 25 perfusions in 8 patients led the observers to conclude that bulk flow increased linearly only at pressures from 0 to 100 mm and that it was constant from 100 to 160 mm. It seems likely that meningeal leukemia interferes with CSF absorption, and these data probably reflect the pathology present.

Cutler *et al.* (1968) studied CSF turnover, using ventriculo-lumbar perfusion, in 12 children aged 5 to 14 years with subacute sclerosing panencephalitis or pontine glioma. Such patients do not have inflammatory changes in the leptomeninges and thus were suitable for study of CSF turnover. They found that CSF absorption began at an average CSF pressure of +68 mm H_2O and that the absorption increased linearly with pressure up to 250 mm H_2O, at which point the absorption rate was 1.5 ml/min. Formation and absorption were equal at a pressure of about 112 mm. Figure 3–5 summarizes these data regarding the relationship between CSF formation and absorption in humans. These relationships are quite analogous to Pappenheimer and colleagues' (1961) observations in goats. However, there are data which indicate that the constant rate of CSF formation may be reduced in chronic states of intracranial hypertension such as hydrocephalus, which will be discussed later.

The low resistance to CSF absorption in humans indicates that a very large increase in its rate of formation would be required to result in an elevated CSF pressure. This has not been shown to occur in any condition apart from choroid plexus papilloma (Eisenberg et al., 1974). The reduction in CSF absorption that results from intracranial hypotension is a homeostatic response to help preserve intracranial pressure and CSF volume. Similarly, the increase in CSF absorption that occurs with intracranial hypertension is also a homeostatic response to obtain a normal intracranial pressure.

Katzman and Hussey (1970) developed the manometric infusion technique to estimate the rate of CSF absorption in patients (the "flush test" to be described in Chapter 5). The response of the CSF pressure to the infusion of normal saline at a constant rate into the lumbar space was determined. The test serves as a measure of CSF absorptive capacity. During lumbar infusion of saline at 0.76 ml/min (twice the normal rate of CSF formation), a steady level of intracranial pressure was reached within about 20 to 30 minutes. The upper limit of pressure obtained in normal subjects was 295 mm. There was considerable variation in the absorptive capacity of the patients studied. Katzman and Hussey (1970) found that in some patients, the absorptive capacity became overloaded when infusion rates corresponded to 5 to 6 times the normal rate of CSF absorption (0.35 ml/min); i.e., with infusion rates of 1.75 ml/min to 2.1 ml/min, the intracranial pressure increased to pathological levels. With infusions of 3.5 ml/min, the absorptive capacity was overloaded in all patients, causing an excessive rise in intracranial pressure. Changes in CSF absorption in hydrocephalus and other pathological conditions will be discussed later.

Absorptive Function of the Choroid Plexus and Other Cellular Elements

While Hassin et al. (1937) and other early workers suggested that the choroid plexus had an absorptive function, the first convincing support for such a role was obtained using the method of ventriculo-cisternal perfusion by Pappenheimer and colleagues (1961). They showed that the organic acids Diodrast and phenolsulfonphthalein were cleared from the ventricular system by an active transport system, which was analogous to their transport by the proximal renal tubular epithelium. (The data suggested that this might occur chiefly in the fourth ventricle. The possibility that the choroid plexus of the fourth ventricle and that of the lateral ventricle might have functional differences regarding the absorption of various substances requires further study.) Penicillin was shown to be actively transported from the CSF following cisternal injection (Fishman, 1966). Subsequent reports, using the method of ventriculo-cisternal perfusion, have confirmed the active transport of a variety of compounds from the CSF, including para-aminohippurate, 5-hydroxyindoleacetic and homovanillic acids, sulfate, iodide, thiocyanate, cycloleucine, and some quanternary ammonium compounds (Lorenzo, 1977).

In addition to these *in vivo* studies, the transport systems of the choroid plexus have been further established and delineated by *in vitro* studies of its absorptive functions. Cserr (1971) has summarized this literature well. *In vitro*, against a concentration gradient, choroid plexus accumulates and concentrates a variety of substrates for which highly specific membrane carriers have been identified. Table 3–1 (p. 24) summarizes the classes of compounds that are actively transported from the ventricular system by the choroid plexus as demonstrated by *in vivo* and *in vitro* techniques. These observations do not necessarily exclude the role of transependymal movement of some of these compounds into glial or endothelial cells as additional active transport systems for clearing such compounds from the CSF and extracellular fluid with which it is contiguous. The possible role of astrocytes and endothelial cells as sites for the active transport of potassium and other solutes has been discussed earlier. The absorptive functions of endothelial cells in normal and pathological conditions require further elucidation.

Diffusion into Brain and Brain Capillaries

As noted, bulk flow absorption via the arachnoid villi allows for the removal of about 500 ml per day of CSF with its dissolved solutes. The choroid plexus has highly specific transport systems for polar (water soluble) solutes, and endothelial cells probably have an analogous function (Goldstein *et al.*, 1979). In addition, some solutes disappear by diffusion from the CSF into the adjacent brain and capillaries to be removed by the circulation. This is the normal route of disappearance of carbon dioxide, which is highly lipid soluble. Other physiological metabolites, such as lactate, hydrogen ions, and ammonia, probably leave the brain and CSF at least in part by simple diffusion. (At body pH, ammonia is present as ammonium, much of which is fixed as glutamine in brain.) The CSF glucose level follows changes in the blood glucose level, whether increased of decreased; its equilibration depends upon carrier-mediated diffusion. These parallel changes reflect the bidirectionality of the carrier-mediated transport system in the capillary endothelial cells, which makes possible such rapid exchanges. Lipid soluble drugs leave the subarachnoid space more rapidly than can be accounted for by bulk flow (Rall and Zubrod, 1962). Thus, the disappearance of anesthetics such as procaine or of the active form of glucocorticoids is an examples of the rapid diffusion of the lipid soluble forms of drugs from the CSF into the blood. In summary, the reabsorption of CSF and its solutes depends upon (1) simple and carrier-mediated diffusion of small molecules, (2) active transport of specific solutes, and (3) bulk flow reabsorption.

FUNCTIONS OF THE CEREBROSPINAL FLUID

Four major functions of the CSF have been defined: (1) physical support, (2) excretory function and sink action, (3) intracerebral transport, and (4) control of the chemical environment of the central nervous system.

Physical Support

The most obvious function of the CSF is its provision of physical support or buoyancy for the brain. When suspended in CSF, a 1500 gm brain which has a water content of 80 per cent weighs only 50 gm, reflecting the specific gravity of the brain and CSF, i.e., 1.040 and 1.007 respectively (Cserr, 1971). The value of keeping the brain afloat is illustrated by the painful disability associated with pneumoencephalography, which results in stretching of the meninges and blood vessels, the pain-sensitive structures within the cranium. The water jacket is protective also because the CSF volume fluctuates reciprocally with changes in intracranial blood volume when the skull is intact (the Monro-Kellie hypothesis). The CSF is important in protecting the brain from the acute changes in central venous pressure that are associated with postural and respiratory changes, and from changes in arterial and pulse pressure. These physiological events will be discussed again later; they are mentioned now as illustrations of the protective functions of the CSF.

Excretory Function and Sink Action

The CSF was considered to serve an excretory function for the brain by early investigators (Hassin *et al.*, 1937); more recently, there is increasing experimental support for this function. The absence of a lymphatic system in the brain indicates that the products of brain metabolism may be removed only by two routes, by either capillary blood flow or transfer into the CSF, then allowing their removal by bulk flow reabsorption or by the choroid plexus. It is difficult to quantify the respective contributions of these routes in the normal state.

The cerebral circulation is responsible for removing the chief products of cerebral metabolism, which include carbon dioxide, lactate, and hydrogen ions. The magnitude of the cerebral circulation, almost 800 ml/min, supports the quantitative importance of the transcapillary route. Studies of cerebral metabolism utilize the jugular venous blood to measure the metabolites cleared from the brain (Siesjo,1978). However, the jugular venous outflow includes metabolites derived from the CSF, as well as those from the cerebral circulation. The CSF route, which includes choroidal transport and bulk flow, may be more important in pathological states when increased amounts of lactic acid are produced in the brain. For example, with convulsive seizures, ischemia, and purulent meningitis, increased lactate concentrations are present in lumbar CSF; it is not clear whether these levels would be higher or lower in the ventricular fluid in these disorders.

The quantitative role of the choroid plexus and the arachnoid villi in the removal of various brain metabolites under normal or pathological conditions is not known. The accumulation of organic acids in uremia (Fishman, 1970) and of ammonia and other amines in both hepatic failure (Plum, 1971) and hyperosmolality (Chan and Fishman, 1979) might have inhibitory effects on the transport systems of the choroid plexus, the arachnoid villi, and the capillary endothelial cells. Thus, changes in the excretory function and sink action of the CSF could be important in the pathogenesis of these metabolic encephalopathies. This is an important area for further study.

The concept of the *sink action* of the CSF, a term introduced by Davson *et al.*

(1962) was based on the observation that the concentration of polar (water soluble) markers such as iodide, thiocyanate, and sucrose was lower in CSF than in the brain. These solutes entered brain slowly, and reached only low equilibrium state distribution ratios (brain/plasma ratios) as the solutes moved freely from the brain into the ventricles. This led to the generalization that normally there is diffusion of endogeneous water soluble metabolites (which have restricted entry across the barrier) from brain to CSF, from which they are removed by bulk flow and, in some cases, by choroid plexus transport. The CSF pulsations (and to a minimal extent the activity of the ependymal cilia) would account for mixing within the ventricles.

Cserr *et al.* (1977) have studied the disappearance of substances injected into the cerebrum and their entry into the ventricles to determine whether the transfer of solutes is due only to simple downhill diffusion or whether there is also a bulk flow of interstitial fluid into the ventricular system accounting for extrachoroidal fluid formation. These studies of the disappearance of various macromolecules following injection into the caudate nucleus provide evidence for the bulk drainage of interstitial fluid. This interstitial fluid is presumably produced at the "capillary-glial complex"; it then flows via the perivascular and the subependymal regions into the ventricular system and subarachnoid space. The quantitative role of such extrachoroidal CSF formation in removing metabolites from the brain is unknown.

Intracerebral Transport

There is substantial evidence that the CSF serves to distribute biologically active substances within the central nervous systems. The possible role of the CSF as a route of intracerebral transport was suggested by Cushing and Goetsch (1910) with regard to the discharge of pituitary hormones into the third ventricle. In recent years, a fundamental issue in neuroendocrinology has been the question of how thyrotropin releasing factor (TRF), luteinizing hormone releasing factor (LRF), and other releasing factors which originate in the hypothalamus are delivered to the pituitary gland. Knigge *et al.* (1975) have provided evidence that the CSF of the third ventricle serves as a path for the diffusion of the releasing factors from their cells of origin in the hypothalamus to their effective sites in the cells of the median eminence. Evidence for this mechanism was provided by finding, in the ventricular fluid, significant levels of TRF and LRF which fluctuated with changes in the physiological state of the animal. Reference was made in Chapter 2 to the role of tanycytes, specialized ependymal cells overlying the median eminence, which appear to transport the hypophysiotropic hormones from the third ventricle to the portal circulation.

Whether the CSF normally serves to distribute other neuroactive substances requires further study. Pappenheimer and associates (1974) have been studying a sleep promoting factor which appears in CSF during sleep deprivation, The factor is composed of several peptides that have been only partially characterized. It is uncertain whether the sleep promoting factors in the CSF represent only by-products of brain metabolism which have diffused from brain to CSF for ultimate excretion or metabolic degradation by the kidney and liver. Are they functionally active in the brain, and does their appearance in CSF reflect higher tissue levels? Or, are they secreted into CSF to act as chemical messengers lower down in the brain stem? Further investigations are needed to answer these questions regarding the transport functions of the CSF.

Control of the Chemical Environment of the Central Nervous System

The important role of the CSF in maintaining a stable chemical environment for the central nervous system has been reviewed earlier in the discussion of homeostasis of the ionic composition of the fluid. The CSF contributes to the role of the blood-brain barrier in regulating the composition of the extracellular fluid of the brain in normal and pathological conditions.

BLOOD-BRAIN BARRIER

It is necessary to consider the role of the blood-brain barrier in order to understand the functional basis of the CSF abnormalities associated with various neurological diseases. The literature regarding this subject is very extensive; various aspects have been reviewed recently by Lee (1971), Katzman and Pappius (1973), Rapoport (1976), Ford (1976), Davson (1976), Oldendorf (1977) and Bradbury (1979). Earlier publications by Friedemann (1942), Bakay (1956), Barlow (1964), Davson (1967), and Lajtha and Ford (1968) provide useful source material as well. The concept of a barrier that limited exchange between blood and brain was initiated by Ehrlich's (1885) observation that certain aniline dyes, given intravenously, failed to stain the brain, although other tissues were rapidly stained. Goldman (1913) later showed that trypan blue, injected intracisternally, would stain the brain. Subsequently the exclusion of trypan blue following systemic administration was often used to indicate the presence of an intact blood-brain barrier. The term, *blood-brain barrier,* introduced by Stern and Gautier (1921), was formerly differentiated from *blood-CSF barrier* and *brain-CSF barrier.* In contemporary thought, the concept of the blood-brain barrier encompasses consideration of the bidirectional exchanges occurring at the interfaces between blood, brain, and CSF; the term blood-brain barrier is used all-inclusively. Fundamental to the concept of the barrier is the relative stability, i.e., lack of net change, in the chemical composition of brain and CSF compared with that of other organs in response to changes in the blood. It is essential to distinguish net change or accumulation from entry rate. Thus, many compounds, like glucose and amino acids, may enter brain (exchange) rapidly, but there is no net change in the brain concentration.

It is important to avoid using the term *barrier* without specifying the molecule in question. Thus, the barrier to protein differs from the barrier to organic acids. Barrier effects depend upon: (1) morphological constraints to the transfer of solutes, (2) the biochemical characteristics of the solute, and (3) specific transport systems in the choroidal epithelium and cerebral capillary endothelium. These aspects of the blood-brain barrier will be discussed first. Then some pharmacological aspects of the barrier will be summarized, and, finally, changes in the barrier in pathological conditions will be described.

Morphological Aspects

The anatomical features of the choroidal epithelium, arachnoid membranes, and capillary endothelial cells have been described in Chapter 2. Each of these structures is characterized by endothelial tight junctions, which serve as the morphological basis for the barrier to macromolecules. However, there are portions of the hypothalamus, the area postrema, and the sub-fornical and sub-commisural organs where the endothelial barrier is not found. These areas serve as "windows" in the brain and allow greater proximity of the plasma to the hypothalamic osmoreceptors and the chemoreceptors of the area postrema and the sub-fornical and sub-commissural organs. Except for the specialized ependymal cells over the median eminence, the tanycytes (see Chapter 2), the ependymal cells are largely free of tight junctions, allowing for the ready diffusion of molecules as large as inulin (MW 5000) between the ventricular fluid and the adjacent brain (Katzman and Pappius, 1973). Thus, the CSF and brain interstitial (extracellular) fluid are contiguous and have a similar chemical composition.

The use of trypan blue dye as a test substance for the integrity of the barrier depends upon its binding to albumin (MW 69,000), which is largely excluded by tight intercellular junctions. However, other morphological features characterize the blood-brain barrier apart from these features.

Intracellular clefts, pinocytotic vesicles, and fenestrae, which allow ready transcapillary exchange in most systemic capillaries, are virtually not seen in normal brain endothelial cells. Their absence helps explain the relative exclusion of macromolecules from the CSF and the extracellular fluid of the brain. Olden-

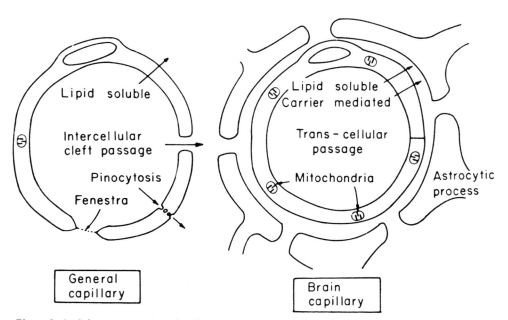

Figure 3–6 Schema comparing the ultrastructural features of general (systemic) capillaries and the capillary endothelial cells of the brain. Note the relative absence of pinocytotic vesicles, the greatly increased number of mitochondria, and the presence of tight junctions in brain capillaries, unlike general capillaries which have clefts, fenestrae, and prominent pinocytotic vesicles (from Oldendorf *et al.*, 1977).

TABLE 3–2   The Blood-Brain Barrier

MORPHOLOGICAL FEATURES

1. Tight junctions between capillary endothelial cells.
2. Tight junctions between the cells of the choroid plexus epithelium and of the arachnoid membrane.
3. Glial foot processes surrounding capillaries.
4. Few pinocytotic vesicles in the endothelial cells.
5. Increased number of mitochondria in endothelial cells.

PHYSIOLOGICAL AND BIOCHEMICAL FEATURES

1. Permeability characteristics of endothelial cells *restricts* the entry of macromolecules and polar (lipid insoluble) compounds; the entry of lipid soluble compounds is relatively *unrestricted.*
2. Osmotic differences are sustained for brief periods only, i.e., brain and CSF osmolality vary directly with changes in plasma osmolality.
3. *Bidirectional* active transport by choroid plexus and endothelial cells of ions, organic acids, and bases which serves to stabilize the composition of CSF and the brain's extracellular fluid.

---

dorf (1977) has shown that brain endothelial cells have additional major structural differences from the cells in most systemic capillaries, such as those in muscles. Many mitochondria are observed in brain endothelial cells; in systemic endothelial cells they are rare. Their presence reflects the high metabolic activity of the former cells (Oldendorf *et al.*, 1977). In addition, brain capillaries are largely surrounded by the processes of astrocytes, the astrocytic feet. The function of astrocytic foot processes is obscure, it has been suggested that they also have a transport function, carrying materials bidirectionally between endothelial cells and neurons. In view of the evidence that astrocytes take up potassium from the extracellular fluid (discussed earlier), it is of special interest to consider that the foot process might serve as a means of transferring this cation and other metabolic products to the capillary. Unfortunately, there is no evidence now available to establish such a role for the astrocytic foot. Figure 3–6 shows Oldendorf's (1977) schema of the comparative differences between general and cerebral capillaries. Table 3–2 summarizes the morphological features that characterize the blood-brain barrier.

Physiological and Biochemical Aspects

The blood-brain barrier has special permeability characteristics with regard to various solutes. The molecular weight greatly influences their entry into or exclusion from CSF. Thus, as noted earlier, the entry of sucrose (MW 360), inulin (MW 5000), and albumin (MW 69,000) is inversely proportional to their molecular weight. The relative exclusion of large molecules from the CSF is illustrated by the 1:200 ratio of the concentration of albumin in CSF to that in blood. The exclusion of large molecules is even more closely correlated with their molecular hydrodynamic volume (Stokes-Einstein radius) than with their molecular weight (see Table 6–8b, page 193) (Felgenhauer, 1974).

There is relatively more albumin (MW 69,000) than gamma globulin (MW 150,000) in normal CSF than would be expected from their concentration ratios in plasma. This suggests that proteins normally cross the endothelial cells to enter CSF, in part by filtration and not solely by vesicular transport, because the latter would not be expected to discriminate between these two macromolecules on the basis of their size. It is possible that both filtration and vesicular transport are responsible for protein entry from the serum. Additional data are needed to clarify this issue.

Other physical properties of solutes are also of major importance. In general, their rapid entry and equilibration between blood and brain or CSF depends upon a high degree of lipid solubility, low ionization at physiological pH, and the absence of binding to plasma albumin and other plasma proteins (Rapoport, 1976). Calcium and magnesium ions and other metabolites such as bilirubin, which are bound to albumin or other serum proteins, are restricted in their entry into CSF and brain. Carbon dioxide, oxygen, and many neuroactive drugs are highly lipid soluble; this enables them to cross the barrier with great rapidity. Their rates of entry are dependent chiefly upon blood flow.

Low equilibrium levels and slower entry into brain and CSF are obtained with water soluble, polar compounds because of their difficulty in crossing lipid membranes in the absence of a specific membrane transport system such as that demonstrated for glucose and some amino acids. This principle holds true for endogenous metabolites, such as the bicarbonate ion, which only slowly exchange from the blood, unlike carbon dioxide, whose transfer is very rapid (Leusen 1972). Similarly, the corticosteroids that are able to rapidly enter the CSF are the active, lipid soluble forms of the hormone, whereas the biologically inactive steroids that are conjugated with glucuronic acid are largely excluded (Christy and Fishman, 1961).

The following observations are also of fundamental importance in explaining water and electrolyte exchange as well as osmotic equilibration across the barrier. First, the blood-brain barrier is very permeable, although not freely permeable to water molecules. Labelled water rapidly reaches equilibrium in the brain following intravenous administration, almost as a function of blood flow. Raichle *et al.* (1976) reported that 93 per cent of an injected bolus of labelled water freely exchanges with brain compared to 97 per cent of ethanol. Second, the movement of ions and other polar metabolites is restricted; it takes many hours for the major cations sodium and potassium to reach equilibrium in brain (Katzman and Pappius, 1973). It took 6 hours for radiosodium and 48 hours for radiopotassium to reach equilibrium in rat brain (Fishman and Raskin, 1967). Third, the osmolality of CSF, brain tissue, and blood are approximately equal under normal conditions; when osmolality is deranged in either compartment, an osmotic equilibrium with the other compartment is re-established within hours. Thus, brain and CSF osmolality vary directly with changes in plasma osmolality. The responses in brain are examples of "isosmotic intracellular regulation"; the mechanisms involved and their relevance to the regulation of the intracranial pressure are discussed in Chapter 4.

Capillary Endothelial Transport Systems

In addition to the physical properties of solutes that affect their movement across the endothelial and choroidal cell barriers, there are also highly specific transport systems in the brain endothelial cells which selectively facilitate the entry

of certain solutes. Oldendorf (1977) has developed a technique that eluci-
dates the mechanism of capillary transport. This method, a modification of
Crone's (1965) indicator diffusion technique, uses tritiated water as a measure of
both blood flow and free diffusion (exchange diffusion) into rat brain. Tritiated
water (^{3}H) and a radiocarbon-labelled test substance (^{14}C) are simultaneously
injected into the carotid artery, and the rats are decapitated 15 seconds later, after
approximately two circulation times. The extraction ratio of ^{14}C/^{3}H gives an
estimate of the extraction of the test compound, the entry of the tritiated water
being assigned a value of 100 per cent. (Levin [1977] has pointed out the
differences between studies of the initial versus steady-state uptake of substances
by the brain and some limitations of the Oldendorf method.) Recently, Oldendorf
(1977) has further improved the sensitivity of the method based on the same
principle, using different indicators and decapitating at five seconds. The
technique has enabled Oldendorf and others to identify a number of independent, highly specific transport systems in brain capillaries for sugars, several
organic acids, choline, nucleic acid precursors, and neutral, basic, and acidic
amino acids.

Conceptually, study of the blood-brain barrier has focused on the restrictions
imposed on the entry of many compounds. However, the présence within
capillary endothelial cells of these highly selective carrier systems, which acceler-
ate the entry across the endothelium of specific metabolites essential to the brain,
supports a broader function for the endothelial cell barriers. These carrier
transport systems are probably all bidirectional; this has been clearly demonstrated for sugars, and it can be inferred that other metabolites also leave the brain by

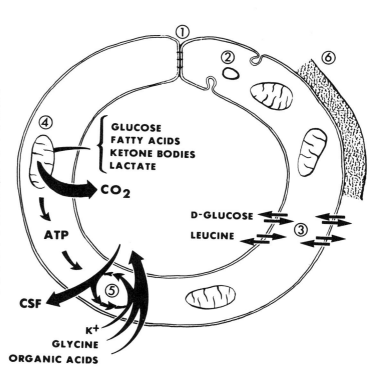

Figure 3-7 Brain capillary
endothelial cell structure and
function. (1) Endothelial cell
tight junction. (2) Pinocytotic
vesicles, which are greatly increased in number in disease.
(3) Specific bidirectional transport systems for glucose and
amino acids. (4) Importance of
mitochondrial metabolism and
utilization of fatty acids and
ketone bodies. (5) Bidirectional
transport systems responsible
for CSF secretion and the absorption of potassium and
organic acids. (6) Basement
membrane surrounding the
capillary. See text (from Goldstein, 1979).

GLUCOSE
FATTY ACIDS
KETONE BODIES
LACTATE

CO_2

ATP

D-GLUCOSE

LEUCINE

CSF

K$^+$
GLYCINE
ORGANIC ACIDS

an endothelial transport system (Goldstein, 1979). It also seems likely that endothelial cells transfer potassium from brain to blood, as discussed earlier. There are also several enzymes in cerebral capillary endothelial cells. These include several nucleoside phosphatases, presumably related to ion transport, as well as gamma glutamyl transpeptidase, probably related to amino acid or peptide transport (Orlowski *et al.*, 1974). The presence of specific carrier systems has been shown to determine the transcapillary passage of some amino acids (Betz and Goldstein, 1978). This is evident in the observation that dihydroxyphenylalanine (dopa) will enter brain, whereas dopamine is excluded. New techniques for the study of brain capillary metabolism have become available, and they should elucidate further the functions of these cells as key components of the blood-brain barrier (Goldstein et al., 1975). Figure 3–7 summarizes current concepts of capillary endothelial cell structure and function (Goldstein, 1979).

Choroidal Transport Systems and Other Factors

The bidirectional transport systems of the choroid plexus have been discussed earlier with regard to their participation in CSF formation and absorption. The choroid plexus plays an integral role in determining the special chemical composition of the CSF as well as its stability. The choroid plexus contributes to the excretory function and sink action of the CSF, which was discussed earlier. In addition, the choroid plexus has specific transport systems for transferring the essential vitamins, thiamine, ascorbic acid, pyridoxine, and folate into the ventricular fluid (Spector, 1978). Lorenzo (1977) has summarized the evidence that choroid plexus has a regulatory role in maintaining adequate concentrations in the CSF of ascorbic acid, thiamine, and folic acid (5-methyltetrahydrofolic acid). Thus, choroidal transport systems contribute to the various effects which together constitute the blood-brain barrier as outlined in Table 3–2. *The blood-brain barrier and the CSF serve as a system for preserving homeostasis for the central nervous system, facilitating both the entry of needed metabolites and the removal or exclusion of toxic or unnecessary metabolites.*

Differences in Electrical Potential

There is a complex literature regarding the small difference in electrical potential present between CSF and blood (Loeschcke, 1971; Welch, 1975). The potential has been measured usually by placing a salt bridge between the CSF and the jugular venous system. The size of the electrical potential has been variously reported in different laboratories, ranging between 0 to +15 mV, although some investigators have found it to be slightly negative. The small gradient in potential between the two compartments has been considered to be due to diffusion potentials arising from differences in the selective permeabilities of ions across the separating membranes. The potential varies with pH changes of the blood, and it has been considered to be a blood-brain barrier potential (across capillary endothelial cells) rather than a reflection of a potential gradient across the choroid plexus, which is close to zero. Welch (1975) has concisely reviewed the subject and concluded that neither the genesis nor the functional importance of the electrical potential has been established. The reader is referred to his review for detailed analysis of the subject.

Pharmacological Aspects of the Blood-Brain Barrier

The permeability characteristics of the blood-brain barrier, as well as the physical properties of various drugs, greatly influence their entry into or exclusion from brain and CSF. Three physical properties affect drug entry; molecular size, protein-binding, and lipid solubility. The pH of the body fluids also influences the entry of ionized drugs (Rall and Zubrod, 1962; Rapoport, 1976).

Molecular Size and Protein Binding

The relative exclusion of macromolecules determines also the relative exclusion of drugs that are bound to serum protein (Desgnez and Traverse, 1966). Of these, albumin is the most important in binding a large number of drugs and normal metabolites, including bilirubin, adrenal steroids, calcium, and magnesium. Drugs that bind to albumin are variously dissociated and are present in plasma in a protein-bound and a free form. Only the free, or dissociated, form of a drug in plasma is available for entry into brain or CSF. Thus, many drugs like penicillin, methyltrexate, long-acting barbiturates, and diphenylhydantoin are in part excluded from brain and CSF because of their binding to albumin.

Lipid Solubility

Highly lipid soluble drugs rapidly cross membranes and therefore rapidly enter brain and CSF. Thus, for example, the rate of equilibration of nitrous oxide in brain is a direct function of the blood flow to the organ, as is the case with other volatile anesthetics like ether, chloroform, and alcohol. Another example is the behavior of diphenylhydantoin. This highly lipid soluble drug enters brain rapidly, and its concentration in the brain exceeds that in the plasma 60 minutes after intravenous injection (Firemark *et al.*, 1963). Although the concentration of diphenylhydantoin in human CSF is equal to the non–protein bound, diffusible fraction in plasma (Triedman *et al.*, 1960), a much higher concentration in brain of this lipophilic drug would be expected. Thus, the concentration of a lipid soluble drug in CSF is not an accurate guide to its concentration in the brain. Ionized, polar drugs are relatively excluded because of the poor lipid solubility of dissociated compounds. The degree of dissociation of such compounds is dependent upon the pH of the plasma, CSF, and intracellular compartments of the brain.

The Role of pH

The effect of pH on the distribution of organic acids and bases across cellular membranes has been termed the pH partition hypothesis (Rall *et al.*, 1959; Rall and Zubrod, 1962). Drugs that are organic acids or bases occur in solution in an ionized (charged) and an nonionized (uncharged) form. The relative amounts of each form depend upon the pH of the solution and the dissociation constant of the drug. The nonionized drug is far more soluble in lipids and readily crosses membranes, whereas the polar, ionized form is largely excluded because of its lipid insolubility. The ionic dissociation constant of a compound, the pK, refers to the pH at which 50 per cent of the compound is ionized. The degree of ionization of a compound in biological fluids may be calculated from the Henderson-Hasselbalch equation:

$$\text{For weak acids: pH} = \text{pKa} + \log \frac{\text{(salt)}}{\text{(acid)}}$$

$$\text{For weak bases: pH} = 14\text{-pKb} - \log \frac{\text{(salt)}}{\text{(base)}}$$

For drugs whose pK is the same as the normal pH of the plasma (7.4), 50 per cent will be nonionized and available for entry into brain and CSF, while 50 per cent will be ionized and restricted in its entry. For a weak acid, like phenobarbital, an increase in plasma acidity results in an increased concentration of the nonionized form, and therefore greater entry of the drug into brain and CSF occurs. Conversely, a weak base is distributed in the opposite direction (Rall *et al.*, 1959). A drug like diphenylhydantoin, with a pKa of 8.3, is almost entirely nonionized at a pH of 7.4 and is very lipid soluble. Hence, it rapidly enters brain and CSF, and in the steady state the concentration of diphenylhydantoin in CSF is equal to the free (non–protein bound) fraction in serum (Triedman *et al.*, 1960).

In normal subjects the arterial pH is about 7.40 and the CSF pH about 7.32. This small pH difference across the barrier of about 0.08 influences the distribution of weak acids and weak bases. Weak acids are relatively excluded from compartments with a low pH and are concentrated in compartments of high pH, whereas weak bases are distributed in opposite fashion. The level of the plasma pH greatly influences the entry of an acidic drug into the CSF. Figure 3–8

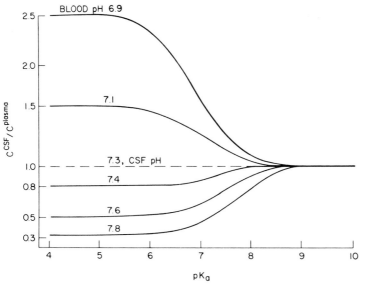

Figure 3–8 Effect of pH upon the distribution of drugs between plasma and CSF. The calculated CSF/plasma ratios of an acidic drug at different blood pH values are shown as a function of its ionization constant (pKa) (from Rapoport, 1976).

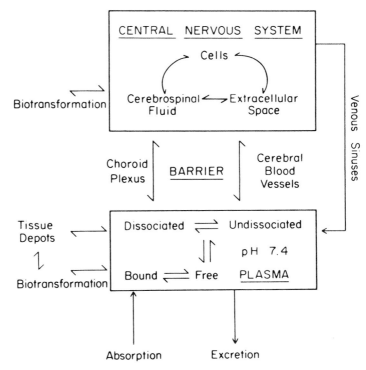

Figure 3-9 Schema illustrating the factors which regulate the distribution of drugs in the central nervous system. Drugs may undergo biotransformation, ionization, excretion, and binding in any of the compartments of the body. Drugs leave the CNS by the sink action of the CSF, passing into the blood at the arachnoid villi and with transport by the choroid plexus and endothelial cells. (from Rapoport, 1976).

illustrates the CSF/plasma concentration ratio for such a drug with a CSF pH of 7.3 and the plasma pH varying between a pH of 6.9 and 7.8 (Rall *et al.*, 1959; Rapoport, 1976). Thus, the CSF/plasma ratio would vary between 0.3 and 2.5. This explains the aggravation of barbiturate poisoning by systemic acidosis, because it results in a substantial increase in the barbiturate levels in CSF and brain. Figure 3-9 illustrates the factors regulating drug distribution in the central nervous system (Rapoport, 1976). These principles enable one to predict whether a given drug is likely to enter the brain or CSF as well as what concentration might be obtained.

Paradoxical pH Responses

The rather unexpected, parodoxical responses of the CSF pH, following acute changes in the blood pH in metabolic alkalosis and acidosis, illustrate the consequences of the different permeabilities of lipid soluble and polar compounds (Leusen, 1972). When sodium bicarbonate was infused intravenously, the plasma pH rose acutely but the CSF pH fell. However, if dilute hydrochloric acid was injected intravenously, the CSF pH rose acutely despite the fall in plasma pH. These paradoxical responses were transient because sustained systemic acidosis and alkalosis subsequently resulted in parallel changes in the CSF. The duration of the paradoxical responses varied from minutes to hours in various species. The occurrence of the paradoxical responses reflects the rapid exchange of carbon dioxide and the very much slower exchange of bicarbonate, the pH being dependent upon the bicarbonate/carbonic acid ratio in accord with the Henderson-Hasselbalch equation. Such a paradoxical response has been reported by Posner and Plum (1967) in patients with compensated metabolic acidosis following the intravenous infusion of sodium bicarbonate, which may rapidly induce coma. Analogous paradoxical responses in CSF pH have occurred with the rapid intravenous infusion of ammonium chloride (Katzman and Pappius, 1973).

Pharmacokinetics

Other sources should be consulted for a detailed discussion of the pharmacokinetics of the many neuroactive drugs in general use. To illustrate the complex effects of the blood-brain barrier on drug distribution, the pharmacokinetics of penicillin will be summarized. Penicillin was early recognized to be largely excluded from normal CSF, even though therapeutic levels could be reached in the presence of purulent meningitis. The drug, like other related organic acids, was convulsant when injected into the CSF (10,000 units in patients) or placed on the cortex in experimental animals. What is the mechanism for the limited entry of penicillin across the blood-brain barrier? Penicillin is excluded for three reasons; (1) it is an organic acid with poor lipid solubility; (2) it is bound in part to albumin, and only the unbound drug is available to cross cellular membranes; and (3) the drug that does enter CSF is actively transported by the choroid plexus to the blood (Fishman, 1966).

An even more complex drug interaction is evident when the effects of benemid on the kinetics of penicillin exchange are examined. Benemid, a sulfonamide derivative, is a competitive inhibitor of penicillin transport by the renal tubular epithelium and, therefore raises blood penicillin levels. Benemid and penicillin also compete for a common binding site on albumin, and therefore benemid administration increases the concentration of free penicillin in plasma available for transfer into CSF and brain. Benemid also competitively inhibits the active removal of penicillin from CSF by the choroid plexus; this contributes to higher CSF levels of the antibiotic. At first glance, it would appear that benemid administration is a logical way to obtain higher penicillin levels in the CSF. However, both drugs compete also for entry into the brain. This competition is analogous to that between the drugs for transport by the choroid plexus and the renal tubular epithelium, and for binding with plasma albumin. The simultaneous administration of both drugs results in a reduction in the penicillin concentration in the brain relative to the concentration in the blood (Fishman, 1966). Therefore, to obtain high brain levels, it is better to increase the penicillin dosage to obtain a higher blood level than to give both drugs together, which reduces penicillin concentration in the brain despite a higher blood level.

While the physical characteristics of a drug help predict its distribution, it is necessary to know the kinetics of the drug in detail as well as its interactions with other drugs and metabolites. *It is difficult to predict with any degree of accuracy the concentration of a drug in the brain from its concentration in the CSF!*

Intrathecal Therapy

The rather dreary early history of intrathecal therapy was briefly summarized in the historical introduction (Chapter 1). The major complications of intrathecal therapy have included chemical meningitis, transverse myelitis, arachnoiditis, convulsive seizures, and hydrocephalus (Wishler, 1978). With the advent of effective systemic chemotherapy for bacterial meningitis, intrathecal therapy has been relatively little used. However, there are several chemotherapeutic agents whose physical characteristics greatly limit their entry into CSF, and, when necessary, the intrathecal route appears appropriate.

The rate of disappearance of various agents following their intrathecal injection also depends upon their physical characteristics. Thus, lipid soluble agents, such as procaine, diffuse from the CSF rapidly at a level close to their site of injection. Koster *et al.* (1938) studied the disappearance of 3.5 ml of procaine injected into the lumbar sac in adult patients. They found the drug was absent, or present in trace concentrations only, in the cisternal fluid despite the use of the Trendelenburg position, after injection of a solution with a density greater than that of CSF. Rieselbach *et al.* (1962) studied the subarachnoid distribution of substances injected into the lumbar sac of humans and monkeys by three-dimensional external scanning and with autoradiographic techniques. The volume of the injected solution was very important in attaining widespread subarachnoid distribution. When compounds were injected in a volume approximately 10 per cent of the estimated CSF volume (130 ± 30 ml in humans), substantial concentrations were obtained in the basal cisterns. When about 25 per cent of the estimated CSF volume was injected in monkeys, distribution was obtained throughout the cerebral subarachnoid space and ventricular cavities.

The method of isotopic cisternography, developed for the study of patients with suspected hydrocephalus, follows the disappearance of radioiodinated albumin after intrathecal injection (Harbert, 1972). Cisternography has revealed that normally little of the injected tracer enters the ventricular system despite accumulation in the basal cisterns prior to flow over the hemisphere toward the sagittal sinus. Thus, it is difficult to get thorough mixing of drugs with the CSF and to uniformly expose the brain to drugs following intraspinal injection. The technique of ventricular perfusion using the Ommaya reservoir was developed to circumvent this problem. It has been used widely for intrathecal therapy with amphotericin in the treatment of fungal meningitis (Ratcheson and Ommaya, 1968).

Increasing interest in finding suitable chemotherapeutic agents for central nervous system malignancies prompted the study of the kinetics of several such drugs following intrathecal injection in monkeys (Blasberg *et al.* (1975). The drugs studied included methotrexate, cytosine arabinoside, thiotepa, and a nitrosourea derivative (BCNU). Several factors that determine the "concentration profile" in the brain following ventriculocisternal perfusion of the drugs were examined, including diffusion through the extracellular fluid of the brain, loss across the capillaries into the blood, and uptake, binding, and/or metabolism by brain cells. The results confirmed that lipid solubility, charge, binding affinities, and metabolic transformation determined the concentration profile in brain tissue. These factors must be evaluated to determine whether the intrathecal route is likely to achieve satisfactory therapeutic concentrations.

Two drugs appropriate for intrathecal therapy are methotrexate, in meningeal leukemia, and amphotericin B, in the fungal meningitides (Utz, 1974; Shapiro *et al.*, 1975; Yen *et al.*, 1978). Both of these polar drugs are excluded by the barrier, and significant levels are not obtained despite the increased barrier permeability induced by the disease processes. The complications of intrathecal therapy include acute and chronic meningitis (arachnoiditis), hydrocephalus, and convulsive seizures. Their occurrence emphasizes the need to avoid intrathecal therapy unless it is essential.

There is a controversial, older literature regarding the use of intrathecal steroids in the treatment of multiple sclerosis (Goldstein *et al.*, 1962). A study of the kinetics of steroid transfer revealed that the free glucocorticoids are highly soluble compounds that enter and leave the nervous system rapidly (Christy and Fishman, 1961). By the injection of free steroid in the subarachnoid space, a high concentration can be maintained in the CSF or adjacent tissue for brief periods only. Sixty minutes after intracisternal injection of cortisol in dogs, the same plasma level was obtained as that observed 60 minutes after an intravenous injection of the same dosage (Fishman and Christy, 1965). Thus, the intrathecal injection of cortisol was like a slow intravenous injection. Depot preparations of the glucocorticoids are suspensions in a micellar form, which retards their solubility in body fluids. The ability of such preparations to induce arachnoiditis is considered a contraindication to their intrathecal injection (Fishman and Christy, 1965; Cohen, 1979). Intrathecal administration of steroids lacks a pharmacological rationale in disorders like multiple sclerosis. Higher drug levels in the brain are expected after systemic administration. The high levels reached acutely in the spinal cord and roots after lumbar injection are transient because of the rapid diffusibility of free steroids.

Blood-Brain Barrier in Pathological Conditions

There is an extensive experimental and clinical literature regarding pathological alterations in the blood-brain barrier (Katzman and Pappius, 1973; Rapoport, 1976). The early experimental studies focused chiefly on the exclusion of trypan blue as a measure of normal permeability of the barrier. The entry of the dye into pathological lesions in the brain was shown to represent increased permeability to albumin, to which trypan blue is bound. Since then, various radioisotopic markers (including iodinated albumin, fluorescein-labelled protein, inulin, sulfate, and sucrose) have been used in experimental studies of vascular permeability. The distribution of inulin, sulfate, and sucrose in brain has been used as a measure of the extracellular fluid volume. These studies coupled with changes in brain composition, most notably water and electrolyte content, have allowed estimation of the electrolyte concentration of the extracellular fluid in various experimental conditions.

Vascular Permeability

Increased permeability of the endothelial cell barriers to various markers characterizes many pathological conditions. However, there has been uncertainty whether these markers enter brain in pathological conditions by (1) interendothelial passage across tight junctions, (2) transendothelial flow, or (3) vesicular transport across endothelial cells, or whether the three routes may be variably important. A fourth possible mechanism should be considered to explain the delay in time often observed after trauma prior to the appearance of increased endothelial cell permeability. In such cases, the appearance of newly formed endothelial cells (neovascularization) may be responsible for the leakage of proteins. In clinical practice these four possible mechanisms are relevant to explanations of the increased passage of isotopes and radiographic contrast media into regions of stroke, tumor, and abscess. In cases of brain tumor, the appearance of positive scans is often associated with evidence of neovascularization. The delay in appearance of a positive scan frequently observed following ischemic infarction may also be secondary to this mechanism (Verhas *et al.*, 1975).

The use of horseradish peroxidase, an electron microscopically dense metalloprotein, has facilitated study of vesicular transport. Vesicular transport may be more important in the pathological leak of proteins than are defective tight junctions, although this point remains controversial (Beggs and Waggener, 1976; Brightman, 1977; Westergaard *et al.*, 1978; Petito, 1979). Vesicular transport has

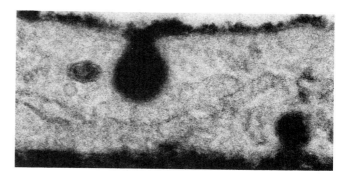

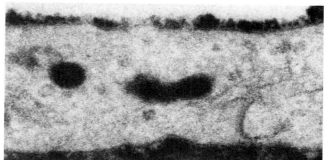

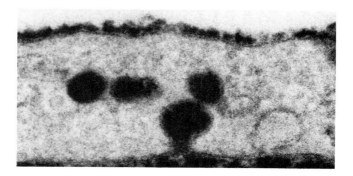

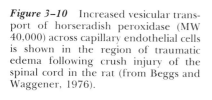

Figure 3-10 Increased vesicular transport of horseradish peroxidase (MW 40,000) across capillary endothelial cells is shown in the region of traumatic edema following crush injury of the spinal cord in the rat (from Beggs and Waggener, 1976).

been reported to be increased by ischemia, arterial hypertension, and convulsive seizures (Westergaard *et al.*, 1976, 1977, 1978). Figure 3–10 illustrates vesicular transport of horseradish peroxidase (MW 40,000) in the region of traumatic edema following crush injury of the spinal cord in the rat (Beggs and Waggener, 1976). This is presumed to take place in the vasogenic edemas and in the diverse pathological conditions associated with an increase in CSF protein. This mechanism occurred also in the opposite direction, from brain extracellular fluid to capillary lumen, when horseradish peroxidase was injected into the cerebral ventricle (van Deurs, 1977). Luminal vesicular transport might be important in the resolution of pathological conditions like cerebral hematoma, by removing macromolecules from the tissue. However, a quantitative assessment of the relative importance of bidirectional vesicular transport, transendothelial cell flow, interendothelial cell leakage, and neovascularization in various pathological conditions is not yet available.

Many substances and metabolic and toxic disorders have been shown to alter the barrier. They include the following: osmotic changes, hypertension, carbon dioxide, acidosis, seizures, chemical toxins, uremia, brain tumor, purulent meningitis, radiation injury, hormones, immaturity, and kernicterus (Rapoport, 1976). Selected aspects of the relevant literature will be summarized briefly. The effects of various physical injuries on the barrier will be discussed also, in the section devoted to vasogenic brain edema.

Osmotic Changes

Both acute and chronic hyperosmolality have been shown to alter the blood-brain barrier. The therapeutic role of hypertonic solutions in the management of brain edema and intracranial hypertension will be discussed in Chapter 4. Experimentally, the administration of hypertonic salt solutions or hypertonic solutions of various iodine-containing radiologic contrast media has been shown to increase the entry of dyes and other markers (Almen, 1971). Hyperosmolality also induces encephalopathy with seizures, coma, and pathological evidence of intracerebral bleeding and subdural hematoma (Swanson, 1976). This has been observed in patients, particularly in infancy, and in experimental animals

The effects of brief periods of acute hyperosmolality on the permeability of capillary endothelial cells have been studied extensively by Rapoport (1976), who has termed the resultant changes "osmotic opening" of the blood-brain barrier. This was obtained by injecting small volumes of hypertonic urea, sodium chloride, sucrose, and other solutes directly into the carotid artery. Osmotic opening produced transfer of intravascular protein (horseradish peroxidase) between the cells but not through them. The endothelial cells were reduced in volume, and the tight junctions appeared widened. This change appears not to occur in other forms of injury, such as crush injury and ischemia, which activate vesicular transport (Beggs and Waggener, 1976; Petito, 1979). Osmotic opening was shown to be reversible. Rapoport (1976) has suggested that the technique may prove therapeutically useful in facilitating the entry of drugs and antibodies otherwise excluded from the brain, but this has not yet been demonstrated.

Hypo-osmolality has profound effects on brain and on electrolyte and amino acid metabolism; it also induces intracranial hypertension and cellular (cytotoxic)

brain edema, which will be discussed in Chapter 4. However, it has not been shown to have specific effects on the permeability of the barrier.

Anoxia and Ischemia

Alterations in the permeability of the barrier have been studied, using various animal models of anoxia and ischemia. (The changes in the autoregulation of the microcirculation associated with infarction will be omitted from this discussion.) There is substantial evidence that endothelial cells are more resistant to anoxia and ischemia than are neurons and glia. Hossman and Olsson (1971) confirmed observations by Broman *et al.* (1949) that exudation of protein tracers did not occur after transient cerebral ischemia, even when the duration of ischemia was much longer than necessary to irreversibly damage the brain. In acute experiments, with electron microscopic evidence of severe damage to endothelial cells, the tight junctions continued to exclude the passage of horseradish peroxidase. There was little evidence of vesicular transport; this may be related to the observation that pinocytosis is dependent upon an adequate oxygen supply.

With prolonged periods of ischemia, increased vesicular transport and protein leakage have been demonstrated (Hossman and Olsson, 1971; Petito, 1979). Cerebral ischemia in patients is commonly associated with an increase in CSF protein. This increase is a reflection of increased barrier permeability. It is noteworthy that clinical studies have shown that isotopic brain scans are often normal for a week or more after cerebral infarction, then show increased permeability (Verhas *et al.*, 1975). In light of the observation that newly formed endothelial cells are more permeable to proteins, the delay in the onset of increased permeability seen following stroke may depend partly upon the time needed for the endothelial cell proliferation and neovascularization that occur in the margins of an area of infarction.

Hypertension

Defects in barrier permeability induced by hypertension have been studied with several animal models, under conditions which include renal ischemia, aortic ligation, and the infusion of angiotensin, metaraminol, and noradrenaline. Byrom (1954) developed a rat model of hypertensive encephalopathy, obtained with renal ischemia, which allowed observation of the cortical circulation through a window in the calvarium. Hypertension induced segmental arterial constrictions and a leakage of trypan blue into the cortex. This process was reversible when the renal artery clamp was removed. In rabbit brain, protein extravasation occurred chiefly in the arterial boundary zones between the major cerebral arteries. Rodda and Denny-Brown (1966) suggested that the changes were due to excessive arteriolar constriction causing focal areas of hypoxia.

The relative importance of such changes and those due to increased intravascular pressure *per se* have been the subject of controversy regarding their possible roles in the pathogenesis of hypertensive encephalopathy and the increased permeability of brain endothelial cells to proteins. The argument has hinged on whether increased intraluminal pressure brings about these effects by excessive autoregulation (vasospasm) and distal ischemia or by excessive vasodilatation and overstretching of the capillary wall. The time course of the permeability change was studied by Johansson (1976), who noted that it could be observed 30 seconds after the rise in blood pressure induced by metaraminol. This rapid response supports the conclusion that the early increase in permeability observed with acute hypertension is related to dilatation and overstretching of the capillary wall. This increase would be a manifestation of defective cerebral autoregulation observed with acute hypertension, rather than of excessive autoregulation (vasospasm). While the role of excessive vasoconstriction with distal ischemia cannot be excluded, there are few data available to support this possibility, other than Byrom's original observations of the pial circulation. It is noteworthy that animals with chronic and sustained hypertension appear more resistant to developing increased vascular permeability than animals with acute hypertension of similar magnitude. The mechanism of such adaptation is not known.

The mechanism of the increased permeability of endothelial cells to protein observed in hypertension and seizures has also been a subject of controversy. The main route for protein was considered to be interendothelial cell passage by Hedley-Whyte *et al.* (1976), whereas Petito *et al.* (1977) and Westergaard *et al.* (1977) have favored increased vesicular transport. Ultrastructural studies in hypertensive animals have shown (1) a prominent increase in vesicular transport and (2) separated or incomplete junctional complexes between endothelial cells. While the former changes were more striking, the quantitative importance of each is not known. The experimental models used appear to be reasonable analogies of the acute hypertensive encephalopathy seen with eclampsia, pheochromocytoma, and malignant hypertension. However, in patients with chronic essential hypertension, the blood-brain barrier is usually normal when examined with computed tomography or isotope encephalography, and the CSF protein is also normal.

Carbon Dioxide

Carbon dioxide is a potent cerebral vasodilator that causes an acute increase in cerebral blood flow, intracranial hypertension, and respiratory acidosis. Moreover, hypercarbia has been demonstrated *per se* to produce, in guinea pigs, a reversible increase in barrier permeability to sulfate and albumin. Preferential involvement of some cerebral regions such as the brain stem, and relative sparing of the cortex were demonstrated (Cutler and Barlow, 1966). The changes in blood flow (vasodilation) and the acidosis were not considered responsible for the permeability changes, although the regional vulnerability was not explained. In contrast to the view of Cutler and Barlow (1966), Rapoport (1976) suggested that CO_2 might open the tight junctions of endothelial cells, perhaps as a consequence of capillary stretching. The differential effects of intracranial hypertension and tissue acidosis on endothelial cell function are not clear. The influence of hypercarbia on vesicular transport, interendothelial cell leakage, and endothelial cell metabolism requires elucidation.

Convulsive Seizures

Convulsive seizures, whether produced by electrical stimulation, convulsive drugs, or hypoglycemia, have been responsible for a reversible increase in barrier permeability (Westergaard et al., 1978). With electrically induced seizures and drug-induced seizures caused by metrazol, strychnine, or methionine sulfoximine, and using albumin or sulfate to measure permeability, the changes have been focally more marked in the thalamus than in other areas of the brain (Petito *et al.*, 1977). During convulsive seizures, brain metabolism is greatly stimulated, with marked increases in brain lactate production and a fall in brain pH. The focal increases in permeability indicate that such changes are greatest in the thalamus and diencephalon, in areas considered to be sites of increased neuronal activity underlying convulsions. Although Westergaard *et al.* (1978) have emphasized the importance of vesicular transport, there is uncertainty regarding the roles of interendothelial cell transport (leaky tight junctions) in the pathogenesis of the increased endothelial permeability induced by seizures. Following a bout of status epilepticus, patients may show a transient elevation in CSF protein. It is necessary to differentiate between the cerebral effects of seizures and the systemic effects (hypertension, acidosis, and hypoxia) that occur with generalized convulsions; both may alter the barrier.

Chemical Toxins

There is an extensive literature regarding the effects of toxins on the barrier (Katzman and Pappius, 1973; Rapoport, 1976). Diverse chemical toxins injected into the carotid artery have been responsible for increased barrier permeability, determined with trypan blue, fluorescent dyes, and radioactive markers (Steinwall and Klatzo, 1966; Rapoport, 1976). The agents used have included mercuric chloride, penicillin, and sulfhydryl blocking agents. Graded increases in permeability have been described with increasing dosages. There is also evidence of molecular sifting, with greater entry of small molecules like sucrose than of larger molecules like albumin. The vulnerability of the barrier, presumably a capillary endothelial cell change, to a variety of toxins has been demonstrated, but the cellular and molecular mechanisms involved are not clear. Experimentally, lead encephalopathy has been attributed to endothelial cell damage (Goldstein *et al.*, 1977). Radiologic agents used in cerebral arteriography and computed tomography are usually given as hyperosmolal solutions. These include derivatives of triiodobenzoic acid such as iodopyracet (Diodrast) and sodium diatrizoate (Hypaque). These agents have been shown to increase barrier permeability because of their direct toxic effects, which are further increased when hyperosmolal solutions are used. The cellular and biochemical basis for the toxicity is not known, nor have their relative effects on vesicular transport, interendothelial leakage, and endothelial cell metabolism been delineated.

Uremia

The metabolic encephalopathy that accompanies renal insufficiency has been shown to be associated with increased permeability of the blood-brain barrier. In a rat model of uremia, increased permeability to sucrose and inulin was demonstrated (Fishman and Raskin, 1967). However, the changes in permeability are complex. Thus, the normally limited entry of penicillin into brain was *inhibited* further in experimental uremia, suggesting that the organic acids that accumulate in uremia may compete with penicillin for transport across the barrier (Fishman, 1970). There are complex changes in brain energy metabolism, calcium metabolism, ion exchange, and amino acid concentration in uremia, and the role of changes in barrier function in the pathogenesis of the encephalopathy in not known (Arieff and Massry, 1974; Raskin and Fishman, 1976).

Tumors

Many primary and metastatic human brain tumors, as well as experimental tumors in animals, are associated with increased endothelial cell permeability to proteins and other markers. Tumors are responsible for endothelial cell proliferation (neovascularization); the new vessels have open clefts between adjacent endothelial cells, and fewer tight junctions are seen. Long (1970) has reported the occurrence of fenestrae, small round windows, in the newly formed endothelial cells of tumors. Hirano *et al.* (1974) have shown that the capillaries of malignant cerebral lymphoma have the same ultrastructural features of systemic capillaries rather than those of cerebral endothelial cells. Such features in the newly formed endothelial cells within tumors would account for their increased permeability to macromoleceles. It is not clear whether the protein leak characteristic of tumors occurs via open junctions or via the fenestrae, or whether vesicular transport is also responsible for the defective barrier to macromolecules. It is possible that with malignant tumors, the several mechanisms operate in concert.

Purulent Meningitis

Changes in the composition of the CSF that characterize purulent meningitis have long been attributed to increased permeability of the blood-brain barrier (Levinson, 1929). The composition of the CSF in meningitis more closely resembles the composition of the plasma. The nature of the permeability changes associated with inflammation has been studied in experimental models (Shabo and Maxwell, 1971). Leukocytes cross capillary endothelial cells to enter the interstitial fluid and CSF by the process of *emperipolesis*. The term describes a form of cellular transmigration by which the white cell moves to the abluminal side of the capillary by being engulfed by the endothelial cell membrane to form a giant vesicle (Marchesi and Gowans, 1964). This route is probably more important than the movement of leukocytes across tight junctions.

The movement of sugars and proteins into CSF has been studied in a canine model of pneumococcal meningitis (Prockop and Fishman, 1968). 3-O-Methylglucose (3MG), mannitol, and albumin were used, and a non-specific increase in permeability was shown. The entry of albumin was affected less than that of the other two solutes, reflecting its greater molecular size. Meningitis also induced changes in CSF absorption; this was shown by studying the disappearance of inulin (MW 5000) and albumin (MW 69,000) following their intracisternal injection. In normal dogs both macromolecules disappeared from the cisternal fluid at the same rate but there was a discrepancy in their disappearance rates in the presence of meningitis. Meningitis slowed the absorption of the larger molecule, albumin, more than the absorption of the smaller molecule, inulin. This suggests that meningitis may interfere with the vesicular transport mechanism present in the arachnoid villi (Tripathi and Tripathi, 1974, 1977) that is considered responsible for the reabsorption of macromolecules (see CSF absorption, page 36.)

The carrier-mediated transport of sugars was also examined, using a nonmetabolized analogue, 3-O-methyl-glucose, to study the hypothesis that inhibition of carrier-mediated glucose transport might contribute to the low CSF glucose seen in meningitis (Fishman, 1965; Cooper *et al.*, 1968). Prockop and Fishman (1968) presented evidence which indicated the presence of bidirectional inhibition of the membrane carrier for hexoses present in the barrier. However, they concluded that this inhibition was not sufficient to account for the low CSF glucose characteristic of meningitis, because of the greater nonspecific increase in permeability to sugars, which resulted in a net increase in glucose entry. The increased concentrations of penicillin obtained in purulent CSF are further evidence of the nonspecific increase in barrier permeability in meningitis. Spector and Lorenzo (1976) have also shown that in bacterial meningitis the active removal of penicillin by the choroid plexus is inhibited.

There is uncertainty regarding the respective roles of vesicular transport, defective tight junctions, and transendothelial transport in the pathogenesis of the alterations in barrier permeability observed in meningitis. The mechanism whereby polymorphonuclear leukocytes might increase membrane permeability have been studied in an *in vitro* model of granulocytic brain edema (Fishman *et al.*, 1977). The factors responsible for such changes in membrane integrity probably include the effects of lysosomal enzymes, as well as the direct toxic effects of polyunsaturated fatty acids (PUFA's) derived from granulocytic membranes. The toxic effects of PUFA's on endothelial cell membranes may be mediated by the effects of free radicals upon membrane intregrity (Chan and Fishman, 1978). (See discussion of brain edema.)

The changes in the composition of the CSF characteristic of meningitis (to be discussed in Chapter 7) make it more closely resemble the plasma in composition, apart from the fall in CSF glucose (see Chapter 6). It should be noted that other forms of inflammation than purulent meningitis have been shown to increase barrier permeability including allergic encephalomyelitis and multiple sclerosis (Vulpe, *et al.*, 1960; Lumsden, 1972). In the latter instance, the relative importance of cells of the lymphocytic series compared with granulocytes in the pathogenesis of the changes in the barrier has not been determined.

Hormonal Effects

Adrenal glucocorticoids, thyroid hormone, and parathormone help to maintain the normal integrity of the blood-brain barrier. In each case, the mechanisms involved are poorly understood. Glucocorticoids have been shown to improve the increased endothelial cell permeability that characterizes various forms of vasogenic brain edema. The mechanism of this normalizing effect is not known. Despite the extraordinary interest in the fundamental basis for the anti-inflammatory and immunosuppressive effects of the glucocorticoids, their ability to stabilize the pathologically more permeable barrier is not understood. Although mineralocorticoids are known to influence cation flux across the barrier, they have no effect on permeability *per se* (Katzman and Pappius, 1973). The therapeutic effects of glucocorticoids are discussed later (see brain edema). It is noteworthy that patients with adrenal insufficiency (primary Addison's disease and following steroidal withdrawal) may develop intracranial hypertension. The mechanism in these cases is also obscure.

Thyroid deficiency may profoundly affect brain metabolism and function, as seen in cretinism and myxedema. In these conditions, the CSF protein may be dramatically elevated. The mechanism of the stabilizing effects of thyroid hormone upon barrier permeability to protein has not been explained. Parathormone also has a poorly understood effect on the barrier. Graziani *et al.* (1967) showed that the hormone influences the transport of calcium from blood to CSF. However, the curious occurrence of papilledema and intracranial hypertension as prominent manifestations of hypoparathyroidism is an enigma.

Immaturity and Kernicterus

The brain and CSF appear to be far more permeable to a variety of substances in immaturity than in maturity. Rapoport (1976) has reviewed the experimental literature and has shown the difficulty in interpreting this phenomenon as a consequence of the high metabolic rate and rapid cerebral blood flow observed in the fetal and neonatal nervous system. Perhaps the best evidence in human subjects of increased permeability of the immature barrier is the presence in normal infants below the age of 6 months, and particularly in premature infants, of an increased CSF protein content, in excess of 100 mg/dl (see Chapter 7). In immaturity, many factors operate in concert that may contribute to such findings. Immature capillaries may have more fenestrae similar to those found in the endothelial cells of brain tumors (Long, 1970; Hirano *et al.*, 1974). Immaturity of endothelial, choroidal, and arachnoidal tight junctions should also be considered. Finally, the efficiency of CSF protein absorption by the arachnoid villi may be reduced in immaturity.

The best defined clinical example of the role of the barrier in the pathogenesis of disease in infancy is kernicterus. In this condition the focal deposition of biliribin in the basal ganglia has been attributed to focal immaturity of the barrier (Diamond and Schmid, 1966). In high concentrations, bilirubin is probably toxic to neurons. Bilirubin is present in serum as unconjugated bilirubin, which is lipid soluble, and as bilirubin glucuronide, a water soluble conjugate. Both forms are bound to albumin unless the plasma concentration is elevated in excess of the binding capacity of albumin. Bilirubin glucuronide is readily dissociated and is excreted in the urine. Kernicterus has been attributed to the occurrence of hyperbilirubinemia with deficiency of glucuronyl transferase, the hepatic enzyme that conjugates bilirubin with glucuronic acid to form its water soluble metabolite. It is not clear whether the special staining of the basal ganglia in kernicterus is due to greater permeability of the endothelial cells in that region, which allow the entry of free and albumin-bound bilirubin, or whether there might be an increase in binding affinity for bilirubin by the cells of the basal ganglia. Thus, the regional vulnerability of the brain in kernicterus and the factors responsible for the immature blood-brain barrier to protein in the neonate require further elucidation.

CHAPTER 4

INTRACRANIAL PRESSURE: PHYSIOLOGY, PATHOPHYSIOLOGY, AND CLINICAL ASPECTS

This chapter deals with normal intracranial pressure and the pathophysiology of intracranial hypertension. The subjects to be covered include cerebrovascular autoregulation as it pertains to intracranial pressure-volume relationships, and the physiological consequences and systemic manifestations of intracranial hypertension. The effects of drugs and osmotic alterations upon the intracranial pressure are discussed. Finally, the pathophysiology and selected clinical aspects of hydrocephalus, brain edema, benign intracranial hypertension (pseudotumor), and intracranial hypotension are reviewed.

An extensive literature underlies these subjects. The reviews of Davson (1967), Milhorat (1972), Langfitt (1975), Lundberg (1975), Miller (1975), and Welch (1975) provide valuable summaries of the early and more recent literature. The publication of several symposia has also provided useful guides to recent laboratory and clinical investigations (Brock and Dietz, 1972; Reulen and Schurmann, 1972; Lundberg *et al.*, 1975; Berks *et al.*, 1976; Pappius and Feindel, 1976; McLaurin, 1976; Ingvar and Lassen, 1977).

NORMAL CEREBROSPINAL FLUID PRESSURE

Manometry

The measurement of the intracranial pressure is very much influenced by the physical characteristics of the manometer in use. The utility of the clinical manometer depends upon displacement of fluids into the bore of the tube. Early investigators found that large bore manometers gave erroneously low pressures because of the loss of fluid into the lumen and that very narrow bore manometers gave excessively high pressures because of capillarity (Becht, 1920; Masserman, 1935; Pollack and Boshes, 1936; Davson, 1956). The clinical manometer now in common use has a bore of 2 mm, which provides a fairly accurate measure of the mean CSF pressure. (Merritt and Fremont-Smith [1938] reported that capillarity accounted for an average overestimation of 8 mm by the clinical manometer compared with the pressure measured with a mercury manometer.) Isovolumetric pressure transducers, first applied by Goldensohn *et al.* (1951) to the study of CSF pressures, were a major technical improvement. Such strain gauge manometers permitted precise recordings of ventricular pressures; this was a major advance in the study of intracranial hypertension. In dealing with CSF pressure, the usual clinical convention is to express the pressure either in terms of mm CSF or mm water. Some investigators prefer mercurial units. Thus, the normal limits of the CSF pressure may be expressed as 5 to 15 mg Hg, which is equal to 65 to 195 mm CSF or water.

Normal CSF Mean Pressure

The pressure level within the right atrium represents the reference zero level in measuring the lumbar CSF pressure (Langfitt, 1975). The level of the CSF pressure is greatly affected by postural influences on central venous pressure; therefore, the patient should be positioned so that the craniovertebral axis is horizontal (see the method of lumbar puncture in Chapter 5). The normal lumbar CSF pressure has ranged between 50 and 200 mm CSF in most clinical reports, and the CSF pressure of experimental animals has been similar. Merritt and Fremont-Smith (1938) reported the distribution of initial lumbar CSF pressures in a group of 1033 patients; 94 per cent had pressures between 70 and 180 mm CSF. These patients had normal blood pressures and showed no evidence of inflammatory or expanding lesions. Patients with convulsive seizures, uremia, and congestive heart failure were also excluded. Pressures between 180 and 200 mm were considered doubtful, and pressures above 200 mm indicated intracranial hypertension.

Masserman (1934) reported that the average pressure in 284 apparently normal subjects was 148 mm CSF ± 2 mm (SEM). He also reported the average pressure, recorded in the same patients while seated, as 397 mm CSF ± 4 mm (SEM). Thus, the fluid rose in the manometer to the level of the cisterna magna, which measured about 400 mm above the site of insertion of the needle in the lumbar sac. The distance from the latter level to the cisterna magna is clearly quite variable in patients of different heights. The sitting position does not allow accurate measurement of lumbar CSF pressure because of uncertainty regarding the normal limits in that posture. (The effects of positional change on CSF pressure will be discussed later.)

Tourtellotte *et al.* (1964) examined the CSF pressure in 105 normal volunteers who had an average pressure of 150 mm ±33 (SD). After exactly 20 ml of fluid was removed, the closing pressure was 68 mm ±31 (SD). If twice the standard deviation is used to describe the normal limits (±62 mm), the data indicate that the initial pressure in these subjects ranged between 84 and 216 mm ±2.0 (SD), the upper limit being somewhat higher than that reported in other series. The major pitfall in obtaining a spuriously elevated lumbar CSF pressure is failure to position the patient properly and to ensure that muscular straining, which elevates central venous pressure, has been avoided (see Chapter 5).

Normal CSF Pulsations

In normal subjects, minor pulsations are usually seen with a clinical manometer unless the needle tip is partially obstructed or not completely within the subarachnoid space. Pulsations range between 2 and 5 mm and are synchronous with respiration. They vary with the depth of respiration, and with deep breathing they usually range between 5 and 10 mm. Pulsations synchronous with systole are also seen, ranging between 1 and 2 mm. O'Connell (1943) suggested that both the vascular and the respiratory pulsations were important in the flow and mixing of CSF, as subsequent work has demonstrated. The use of isovolumetric pressure transducers is essential for the study of CSF pulsations because the clinical manometer dampens and obscures their true size. With isovolumetric recording, the arterial pulsations observed in lumbar CSF with a normal mean CSF pressure are about 20 to 30 mm CSF in amplitude, and the respiratory pulsations range between 10 and 30 mm. The normal ranges have not been systematically studied or reported in the literature. The approximations given are derived from multiple sources (Lundberg *et al.*, 1968; Lakke, 1975; Miller, 1975).

There is a gradient in the height of the arterial pulsations recorded along the cranio-vertebral axis. Bering (1955) studied the pulsations in a patient with a normal mean CSF pressure by simultaneously recording the pressures in the ventricular, cisternal, and lumbar fluids, as indicated in Figure 4–1. The pulsatile pressures were about 60 mm in the ventricle, 50 mm in the cisterna magna, and 30 mm in the lumbar fluid. Note that the elevation of the pulse pressure occurred first in the ventricle and last in the lumbar fluid. This temporal sequence and the decreasing amplitude of the three pulse pressures indicates that they originate in part within the ventricular system. These regular fluctuations in pressure are considered to contribute to the normal mixing of the CSF and its flow from the ventricular system to the subarachnoid space (DuBoulay, 1966).

The absolute size of the arterial pressure pulsation is greatly influenced by the mean CSF pressure. Whenever the CSF pressure is elevated (whether by transient jugular venous compression, inspiration of carbon dioxide, injection of saline into the subarachnoid space, brain edema of diverse etiology, or intracranial mass lesions), the arterial pulsations are increased in magnitude (Langfitt, 1975). The physiological basis for this finding will be dealt with later in the discussion of intracranial compliance, elasticity, and pressure-volume regulation.

Bering (1955) showed that choroid plexectomy in experimental animals, substantially reduced the amplitude of the systolic pulsations, and he concluded that they were derived chiefly from pulsations of the choroid plexus. However, subsequent studies by Dunbar *et al.* (1966) and Adolph *et al.* (1967) contradicted this conclusion. They concluded that the systolic pulsations are derived chiefly

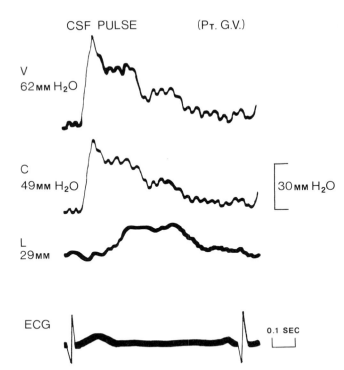

CSF PULSE   (Pᴛ. G.V.)

V
62ᴍᴍ H₂O

C
49ᴍᴍ H₂O

30ᴍᴍ H₂O

L
29ᴍᴍ

ECG

0.1 SEC

Figure 4-1 Simultaneous isovolumetric pressure recordings from the
lateral ventricles (V), cisterna magna
(C), and lumbar subarachnoid space (L)
of an 11 year old patient illustrating the
magnitude of the pulsations at the three
levels and their relation to heart. The
late occurrence of the systolic pressure
elevation in the lumbar sac illustrates
that the vascular pulsations arise within
the cranial cavity (from Bering, 1955).

from arterial pulsations of the circle of Willis and from within the parenchyma
of the brain. It is of interest that Wolff (D'Alessio, 1972) showed that the pulsations of the temporal artery and the CSF were increased in amplitude during experimental fever in patients and during migraine attacks. This presumably occurred because of increased pulsations of the arteries derived
from the circle of Willis. Similarly, *acute* elevations in systemic blood pressure due to epinephrine result in increased amplitude of the CSF pulsations,
although there is no evidence that this occurs in essential hypertension. The
vascular pulsations are probably exaggerated secondary to widening of the
systemic arterial pulse pressure in conditions such as thyrotoxicosis and aortic
insufficiency. The effect of heightened CSF pulsations (apart from the effect of
a sustained increase in mean pressure) on bone metabolism is not known, in the
pathogenesis of suture separation and decalcification of the skull that occur with
chronic intracranial hypertension. The possible role of pulsatile pressures in the
pathogenesis of the ventricular dilatation accompanying hydrocephalus also
requires elucidation.

Respiratory Pressure Waves

The amplitude of respiratory fluctuations varies considerably in normal
subjects. Antoni (1946) and Lakke (1975) systematically studied the effects of
respiration on CSF pressure. With normal inspiration there is a fall in CSF
pressure, and with expiration there is an increase in CSF pressure. These

changes reflect the dependency of the CSF pressure upon the intracranial venous pressure, both of which change in the same direction with respiration. In cases of complete spinal subarachnoid block, the CSF pressure changes that occur with respiration recorded below the block are reversed; with inspiration CSF pressure rises, and with expiration it falls. The explanation given by Lakke (1975) for this difference is that only the pressure in the inferior vena cava is reflected in the isolated CSF below a complete spinal block.

Plateau Waves and Other Abnormal Pulsations

The continuous recording of the intracranial pressure was initiated by Guillaume and Janny (1951) and further developed by Lundberg (1960) in the study of neurosurgical patients. The technique established that patients with intracranial hypertension frequently have rapid fluctuations in pressure. Three main variations have been described. First are rhythmic variations, related to periodic breathing of the Cheyne-Stokes type, with a frequency of 0.5 to 2 per minute. Second are B waves, rhythmic variations related to Traube-Hering-Breuer waves of the systemic blood pressure, which have a usual frequency of 6 per minute. Kjallquist *et al.* (1964) considered both types of pressure variation to arise from periodic fluctuations in pressure within the cerebral vascular bed, probably related to intrinsic rhythmic activity originating in the medulla. These rhythmic variations are generally of low amplitude, and they are not considered to have deleterious effects. Pressure waves of the third type were originally called Type A waves, but the term "plateau waves" was later adopted by Lundberg and colleagues (1968, 1975). These waves are of considerable importance in the pathophysiology of intracranial hypertension.

Plateau waves have commonly been recorded in patients with intracranial hypertension of diverse causes, most frequently tumor, trauma, or hydrocephalus. The plateau wave is an acute elevation in intracranial pressure, usually lasting 5 to 20 minutes. Then the pressure falls, usually rapidly, to its former level. The amplitude of the plateau is variable but often reaches very high levels, 600 to 1300 mm CSF (50 to 100 mm Hg). Figure 4–2 shows typical plateau waves in a patient with a glioblastoma, reported by Lundberg (1960). During each plateau wave episode, the patient gave evidence of increasing headache, restlessness, impaired consciousness, and increased rigidity of the limbs. Other transient, paroxysmal symptoms may also occur during the plateau wave, including nausea, vomiting, facial flush, confusion, forced breathing, and tonic or clonic movements of the limbs or both. The clinical signs have been interpreted as manifestations of acute brain stem dysfunction. However, such signs of decompensation need not occur, and at times there is no change in the patient's clinical status during a typical plateau wave. It is noteworthy that plateau waves have been reported to occur during sleep, concomitant with REM sleep in patients with normal-pressure hydrocephalus (Symon *et al.*, 1972; 1975). Increased cerebral blood flow has been reported in normal subjects during REM sleep (Towsend *et al.*, 1973). Plateau waves during REM sleep probably occur as a result of changes in the cerebral circulation with an acute increase in cerebral blood volume (Hulme and Cooper, 1968; Risberg *et al.*, 1969).

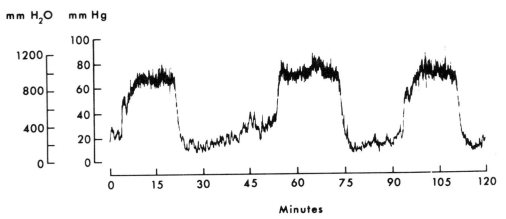

Figure 4–2 Plateau waves as visualized with an intracranial pressure transducer in a patient with a malignant brain tumor. During the waves a rapid increase in signs of cerebral dysfunction was noted (from Fishman, 1975, adapted from Lundberg, 1960).

The following observations were made by Lundberg and colleagues (1968) regarding the pathophysiology of plateau waves:

1. Plateau waves occurred with advanced stages of intracranial hypertension when the intracranial pressure was substantially elevated to over 260 mm CSF or 20 mm Hg. When the intracranial pressure was decreased by ventricular drainage or by the administration of hypertonic solutions, the plateau waves could be temporarily abolished.

2. Plateau waves were not observed in hydrocephalic infants with an open fontanelle and intracranial hypertension.

3. Plateau waves occurred at times without any appreciable change in systemic blood pressure. However, a rise in blood pressure concomitant with the plateau waves was commonly recorded.

4. At times, respiratory irregularities causing hypercarbia preceded the onset of plateau waves. Hyperventilation with hypocarbia also preceded the fall in pressure at the end of the plateau wave. Plateau waves also occurred during artificial ventilation at a constant rate, with a constant alveolar pCO_2 and a normal mean intrathoracic pressure.

5. In patients with spontaneous plateau waves, similar pressure waves could be provoked by inducing a relatively small rise in intracranial pressure by various measures such as injecting fluid into the ventricular cavity, compressing a cranial defect, breathing CO_2, or the intravenous injection of histamine.

6. Spontaneous plateau waves often occurred without visible cause. The initial rise in pressure at times appeared to coincide with bodily activity, emotional upset, or painful stimuli.

7. Angiograms performed during spontaneous plateau waves showed wider vessels in the arterial phase than those during the interval between waves, but the venous phase was not affected. It is noteworthy that Risberg et al. (1969) measured an increase in cerebral blood volume during episodes of plateau waves which occurred despite a reduction in cerebral blood flow during such periods (Lundberg et al., 1978).

The occurrence of plateau waves indicates a failure of the compensatory mechanisms for maintaining a normal intracranial pressure. When the clinical conditions are such that the patient is on the steeply rising slope of the pressure-volume curve, a relatively small further increase in intracranial blood (or CSF) volume gives rise to a critical increase in intracranial pressure. (Intracranial elastance will be discussed later.) Dilatation of pial arteries in response to intracranial hypertension was observed in the early experiments by Wolff and Forbes (1928). Kety *et al.* (1948) demonstrated a decrease in cerebral blood flow with intracranial hypertension in patients with brain tumor. Cerebral blood flow is decreased further during plateau waves (Lundberg *et al.*, 1968). More recently, Langfitt and colleagues (1975) presented evidence that intracranial hypertension in monkeys was associated with cerebral vasodilation, termed *cerebral vasomotor paralysis.* This apparently paradoxical occurrence of vasodilation with a concomitant decrease in cerebral blood flow supports the view that changes in cerebrovascular autoregulation are the basis for the appearance of plateau waves (Matsuda *et al.*, 1979).

There is an extensive literature about the monitoring of intracranial pressure in patients with head injury (Bruce *et al.*, 1973; Johnston and Jennett, 1973; Fieschi *et al.*, 1974; Rosner and Becker, 1976). Although much new information and insight have been obtained regarding the pathophysiology of intracranial hypertension, the precise role of pressure monitoring in clinical practice has not been clearly defined. Its advocates have stated that monitoring has helped to reduce the morbidity and mortality of severe head injury. Monitoring is considered of special value in the management of Reye's syndrome (Venes *et al.*, 1978).

Factors Influencing Intracranial Pressure

The intracranial cavity is closed by thick bone that is nondistensible (after closure of the sutures), and its contents are fixed in total volume. The intracranial cavity is vented through the foramen magnum into the spinal subarachnoid space, which has some degree of elasticity, particularly at the caudal end of the lumbosacral sac. There are three displaceable components within the cranium: blood, CSF, and brain tissue. (The last-named may undergo displacement by herniation or by pressure atrophy, as observed in hydrocephalus.) The brain volume is about 1400 ml; the CSF volume is about 150 ml, of which about 75 ml is within the cranial cavity; the intracranial vascular volume is about 75 ml of blood. This last figure is based on the determination of cerebral blood flow of about 750 ml/min and an angiographic transit time of 6 seconds for contrast media (Lassen, 1959; Sokoloff, 1959; Betz, 1972). Normally, the volumes of intracranial blood and CSF vary reciprocally, which helps maintain intracranial pressure within normal limits. The fact that the skull is a rigid sphere filled with non-compressible contents has been epitomized as the Monro-Kellie doctrine (Purves, 1972), whose history was summarized in Chapter 1. Two major factors that determine the level of the intracranial pressure in normal and pathological conditions are the arterial pressure and the intracranial venous pressure. Their respective roles will be considered next.

Arterial Blood Pressure

Early investigators appreciated that changes in blood pressure and venous return could influence the CSF pressure (Weed, 1935). However, O'Connell, in

1943, was apparently the first to question the previously accepted theory that the normal intracranial pressure was due chiefly to the balance between the processes of CSF formation and absorption. He showed that the CSF pressure obtained in cadavers in the horizontal position was never greater than atmospheric pressure, and he concluded that the fall in CSF pressure with cardiac arrest was due to the decrease in pressure within the intracranial vasculature. These observations regarding the primary dependence of the intracranial pressure on the cardiac output, rather than on the rate of CSF secretion, were widely supported thereafter (Ryder *et al.,* 1952; Lofgren, 1973; Langfitt, 1975).

However, there is substantial evidence that the level of the intracranial pressure normally is largely independent of wide ranges in the level of the arterial blood pressure. Thus, in a review of 1418 patients without evidence of any neurological disease that might elevate the intracranial pressure, Fremont-Smith and Merritt (1933) found that the average CSF pressure was not influenced by the level of the systolic or diastolic arterial pressure or even by arterial hypertension. However, some exceptions to this generalization can be readily reproduced in the laboratory and also occasionally observed in patients. Experimentally, an acute increase in arterial blood pressure induced by the administration of norepinephrine or vasopressin causes an acute elevation of the intracranial pressure with heightened arterial pulsations as well (Davson, 1967; Langfitt, 1975). This also occurs in patients with very acute elevations in blood pressure due to epinephrine. An analogous situation may be seen in patients with intracranial hypertension due to hypertensive encephalopathy or pheochromocytoma, a decrease in intracranial pressure and a disappearance of papilledema are obtained with the return of the blood pressure to normal following treatment.

Venous Pressure

The immediate dependence of the CSF pressure upon the intracranial venous pressure is illustrated by the jugular compression test (see Queckenstedt test in Chapter 5); rapid jugular compression and release induce simultaneous parallel changes in the CSF pressure. Patients with congestive heart failure and elevated venous pressures show increased CSF pressure, with a return to normal following therapeutic doses of digitalis (Harrison, 1933; Friedfield and Fishberg, 1934). By a similar mechanism, chronic obstruction of the superior vena cava by mediastinal tumors may cause intracranial hypertension (Fitz-Hugh *et al.,* 1966). These effects are generally attributed to the absence of valves in the jugular venous system; hence, increased venous pressures are directly transmitted to the intracranial cavity (Weed and Flexner, 1933; Bedford, 1936). However, jugular occlusion usually results in only transient increases in the intracranial pressure, in both animals and patients (Gius and Greer, 1950; Fitz-Hugh *et al.,* 1966).

In some cases, complete caval obstruction does not result in intracranial hypertension because of the capacity for collateral drainage provided by the paraspinous venous plexus (Batson's veins). Similarly, acute thrombosis of the superior longitudinal sinus results in severe intracranial hypertension; with gradual occlusion, compensatory increases in collateral drainage *via* emissary veins and other collateral veins at the base of the brain allow for the maintenance of normal intracranial pressure (Kalbag and Woolf, 1967).

It is important to note that simultaneous changes in arterial and venous pressure may have either parallel or opposing effects upon the intracranial pressure. Thus, Ryder *et al.* (1952) showed that inhalation of 5 per cent CO_2 simultaneously raised both arterial and venous pressures as well as the intracranial pressure. However, inhalation of amyl nitrate lowered the blood pressure while increasing the CSF pressure, the latter occurring because of the increase in venous pressure induced by the drug.

In summary, the following generalizations hold: (1) rapid changes in arterial pressure will produce rapid, parallel, but highly dampened changes in CSF pressure; (2) chronic increases in arterial pressure usually do not affect the CSF pressure; and (3) changes in venous pressure are also directly transmitted to the CSF and may take precedence over the arterial effects. The interdependence of the vascular pressures and the intracranial pressure will be discussed again later.

Thoracic Influences

Coughing, sneezing, and straining induce complex changes in intracranial pressure (Hamilton *et al.*, 1944). These changes are mediated largely by the circulatory effects associated with increased intrathoracic pressure. This is well illustrated by the changes associated with *Valsalva's maneuver,* which involves forced expiration with the glottis closed; this in turn causes increased intrathoracic and intra-abdominal pressure with elevation of the central venous pressure. The latter is transmitted to the jugular venous system and to the epidural venous plexus, because there are no valves between the azygos vein and the plexus or in the jugular system. In normal subjects, the CSF pressure rises with straining and then falls within the cessation of straining. Then, often, the CSF pressure is seen to rise again — a so-called "secondary overshoot" in pressure. This is considered to be an arterial phenomenon secondary to the transient increase in arterial blood pressure that may result with the sudden improvement in venous return and cardiac output.

Postural Effects

The dependence of CSF pressure upon posture was studied by Weed and Flexner (1933), Loman (1934, 1935), Pollack and Boshes (1936), and Carmichael *et al.* (1937), and critically reviewed by Davson (1967) and Langfitt (1975). Loman (1934, 1935) compared the cisternal and lumbar fluid pressures simultaneously in seated patients. The lumbar pressure in 14 patients varied between 375 and 565 mm CSF, while the cisternal pressure was between 40 and −85 mm CSF. In each case the difference in pressure was equal to the vertical distance between the two needles.

Masserman (1935) studied the effects of elevation from the horizontal to the vertical position. When the pressure was measured with the patient first in the horizontal position and then tilted to vertical, the pressure increase observed was only about 40 per cent of the expected increase based on the height of the hydrostatic column. Likewise, if the patient was tilted downward 30 degrees, the pressure decrease observed was only about 33 per cent of the expected decrease based on the height of the hydrostatic column. These discrepancies appear to be due to the elasticity of the subarachnoid space in the lumbar sac and to the collapse of the venous volume along the neuraxis. The changes in posture change the pressure in the intracranial venous sinuses parallel to the changes in CSF pressure. Davson (1967) concluded that the change in intracranial venous pressure is the major factor underlying the alterations in CSF pressure associated with postural change.

Blood Gases

The inhalation of 5 per cent carbon dioxide serves as a potent cerebral vasodilator. It increases cerebral blood flow by 75 per cent, along with increased arterial blood pressure and CSF pressure. In contrast, respiratory alkalosis obtained by hyperventilation is a cerebral vasoconstrictor which reduces cerebral blood flow and blood volume, resulting in a fall in intracranial pressure. An extensive literature documents these changes in various species and in patients (Sokoloff, 1959; Lassen, 1959; Purves, 1972; Reivich, 1974). The control mechanism involved appears to be located in the cerebral arteriole, where changes in tone are responsible for the alterations in cerebral blood flow and blood volume and in turn the CSF pressure. The key factor affecting arteriolar tone appears to be the local tissue hydrogen ion concentration. Chronic states of pulmonary insufficiency, whether paralytic or due to chronic obstructive pulmonary disease, may also result in sustained intracranial hypertension, papilledema, and pulmonary encephalopathy due to respiratory acidosis (Miller *et al.*, 1962).

Hypoxia also induces arteriolar vasodilatation and increased cerebral blood flow and volume with a secondary elevation in intracranial pressure. The separate effects of hypoxia and of hypercarbia upon the cerebral circulation were compared in human subjects by Kety (1948), who found that hypercarbia had a greater effect. The metabolic basis for the vasodilating effects of hypoxia is probably also dependent upon increased hydrogen ion concentration at the arterioles secondary to increased glycolysis and lactic acid production. In asphyxia, both hypercarbia and hypoxia act in concert to cause maximal increases in cerebral blood flow and secondary intracranial hypertension.

Hypothermia

The introduction of hypothermia during brain surgery and in the treatment of head injury was based on its ability to reduce the cerebral metabolic rate. Its protective effect on the blood-brain barrier was reviewed in detail by Jeppsson (1962). Rosomoff (1961, 1962) reported that hypothermia caused a reduction in cerebral blood flow and intracranial pressure, associated with a compensatory increase in the CSF volume within the cranial cavity. The latter observation was also documented in hyperosmotic dehydration of the brain. *These findings illustrate the dependency of the CSF pressure on circulatory factors, which often supersede the effects of changes in the volume of the CSF.*

CEREBRAL BLOOD FLOW AND AUTOREGULATION

The dependence of the intracranial pressure upon hydrostatic pressures in both the arterial and venous systems has been described earlier. In order to further clarify the physiological basis for this dependency, the physiology of the cerebral blood flow and its autoregulation will be reviewed with special reference to the pathogenesis of intracranial hypertension.

Regulation of Cerebral Blood Flow

The early history of investigation into the cerebral circulation in relation to the intracranial pressure has been well summarized by Purves (1972). The species variation in cerebrovascular control mechanisms led to uncertainty regarding the application of animal experiments to humans. The introduction of a quantitative method for estimating the cerebral blood flow in humans by Kety and Schmidt (1945) initiated major advances in the clinical investigation of the cerebral circulation and brain metabolism. The method utilized the Fick principle, with nitrous oxide as an inert diffusible marker, and required inhalation of a 15 per cent nitrous oxide mixture in air followed by serial sampling of arterial and jugular venous blood over the next 10 minutes to measure the time course with which nitrous oxide reached saturation in both compartments. It allowed the calculation of cerebral blood flow in terms of ml of blood per 100 grams of brain per minute; the blood flow in several series of normal subjects was between 50 and 60 ml (Lassen, 1959; Sokoloff, 1959). Assuming a normal brain weight of 1400 grams, the total cerebral blood flow falls between 700 and 840 ml of blood per minute, about 1/5 of the normal cardiac output. The simultaneous measurement of arterial and jugular venous oxygen and glucose levels allows the determination of cerebral oxygen and cerebral glucose consumption. The calculation is as follows: A-V oxygen (or glucose) difference × cerebral blood flow = cerebral oxygen (or glucose) consumption, i.e., the cerebral metabolic rate for oxygen or glucose. Thus, the normal A-V oxygen difference is about 6.0 vols per cent; therefore the cerebral oxygen consumption would be about 3.5 ml/min per 100 grams of brain. Similarly, the normal A-V glucose difference is about 8 mg/dl, therefore, the cerebral glucose consumption would be about 5 mg/min per 100 grams of brain. Thorough reviews of this method and its early applications have been provided by Lassen (1959), Sokoloff (1959), and Purves (1972).

Although the Kety-Schmidt technique provides data on blood flow and metabolism of the whole brain, it is not suited for the investigation of regional blood flow, which is of special relevance to the study of focal neurological disorders. Lassen *et al.* (1963) introduced a quantitative radioisotopic technique for the measurement of regional cerebral blood flow in patients, using the intracarotid injection of Xenon-133. A further modification introduced the Xenon-133 inhalation method, in which the subject inspires the gas, thus avoiding the need for intracarotid injection (Veall and Mallett, 1966; Obrist *et al.*, 1967). This noninvasive technique has the advantage of allowing repeated studies in acutely ill patients. Several reviews provide valuable source material regarding these techniques and their applications (Betz *et al.*, 1972, Lassen, 1975). These recent advances have made possible the study of the regional cerebral circulation in various neurological disorders.

Cerebral Blood Volume

The volume of blood in the human brain, estimated at about 75 ml, has proved difficult to measure with accuracy (Betz, 1972). However, qualitative changes have been appreciated in various conditions. Early experiments in cats with calvarial windows demonstrated that pial vessels *dilated* as the intracranial pressure was increased (Wolff and Forbes, 1928; Purves, 1972). Using the same technique, arterial hypertension was shown to cause vasoconstriction of pial arteries; a fall in blood pressure had the opposite effect. These experiments, confirmed and extended by more recent investigators, have led to the conclusion that intracranial hypertension of diverse etiology such as trauma or tumor alters vasomotor tone of cerebral blood vessels. When severe, it leads to progressive vasodilatation and to *cerebral vasomotor paralysis* (Langfitt *et al.*, 1965; Langfitt, 1975).

The effect of intracranial hypertension upon cerebral blood volume and oxygen consumption has been further studied with radioactive oxygen by Grubb *et al.* (1975). The production of intracranial hypertension by the intracisternal injection of artificial CSF was shown to cause a steady *increase* in cerebral blood volume. This appears to be a contradiction to the Monro-Kellie doctrine. However, the cerebral blood flow remained nearly normal, reflecting arteriolar vasodilatation, as long as the arterial blood pressure was maintained. With return of the intracranial pressure to normal, a transient period of reactive hyperemia was observed, presumably as a result of tissue acidosis.

There are few data available regarding cerebral blood volume in various diseases. Raichle *et al.* (1978) reported a minor increase in the volume of cerebral venous blood without an alteration in cerebral blood flow in patients with pseudotumor cerebri. The mechanism of this change and its functional significance await further clarification. The recent availability of improved methods measuring cerebral blood volume should help elucidate the pathophysiology of hydrocephalus and benign intracranial hypertension (pseudotumor cerebri).

Neurogenic Influences

There is substantial anatomical evidence of an extensive nerve supply, including vasoconstrictor (noradrenergic) and vasodilator (cholinergic) innervation, to the cerebral blood vessels (Purves, 1972). The larger vessels and the pial vessels appear more densely innervated, although unmyelinated fibers extending to the small cerebral arterioles have been observed.

The functional importance of the nerve supply has been a matter of dispute for many years. Sokoloff (1959) and Lassen (1959) dismissed the action of cerebral vasomotor nerves as negligible. More recently, Purves (1972) summarized the evidence supporting the hypothesis that there may be an integrated neural regulation of cerebrovascular responses. On the basis of changes in blood flow induced by atropine in baboons, Kawamura *et al.* (1975) suggested that the vasodilator tone of cerebral blood vessels is maintained by cholinergic neurons. Raichle *et al.* (1975) proposed that the central noradrenergic system is analogous to the peripheral sympathetic system, with the special function of regulating both brain vascular permeability and blood flow. While neurogenic effects have been demonstrated experimentally, their functional importance is conjectural. Lassen (1975) suggested that nervous control is related to cerebral vascular volume regulation, which is important for the regulation of the intracranial pressure. Neurogenic influences may provide some protection to the brain from sudden or perhaps massive changes in arterial and intracranial pressure. Further work in humans is needed to clarify the functional importance of the innervation of the cerebral vasculature.

Autoregulation

Prior to the human studies using the Kety-Schmidt technique, it was assumed that the cerebral blood flow varied directly with changes in systemic blood pressure. This proved *not* to be the case, for the cerebral blood flow was shown to be remarkably constant and independent of changes in arterial blood pressure as long as the latter was above shock levels. This regulatory mechanism, termed *autoregulation,* has been defined as the intrinsic capability of the brain to regulate its flow in accordance with its metabolic needs. There is much evidence to support a "blood flow metabolism couple" in normal brain (Brock *et al.,* 1969; Betz, 1972; Reivich, 1974; Lassen, 1975; Harper *et al.,* 1975). Autoregulation is achieved by the fine control of the cerebrovascular resistance. This is determined chiefly by the tone of the cerebral arteriole, which is governed by the local hydrogen ion concentration (Severinghaus *et al.,* 1966). The precise location of the major resistance in the cerebral vascular bed is still in doubt. Purves (1972) reviewed the literature regarding the respective roles of the large arterioles, the precapillary sphincters, and the terminal arterioles.

Loss of autoregulation means that the cerebral blood flow and blood volume change passively with changes in systemic blood pressure. Autoregulation helps in the maintenance of a normal intracranial pressure, because capillary pressures and tissue pressures are thereby protected from the higher hydrostatic pressures within the cerebral arteries. The presence of normal autoregulatory responses has been assessed by observing the effect of infusing a pressor agent, such as angiotensin or Aramine, upon cerebral blood flow (Harper, 1966; Zwetnow, 1968; Lofgren, 1973). *If cerebral blood flow and the intracranial pressure remain constant despite an acute rise in blood pressure, autoregulation is normal. However, if cerebral blood flow and the intracranial pressure are increased by the pressor agent, autoregulation is impaired.*

Impairment of autoregulation, in which cerebral blood flow develops a passive dependency upon blood pressure, occurs in various pathological conditions. The change is a general one with hypercarbia and hypoxia, although the time course of the impairment of autoregulation is variable. Thus, impairment may occur transiently with acute hypercarbia or hypoxia, or it may be persistent after the return of the blood gases to normal (Lassen, 1975). Intracranial hypertension and persistently impaired autoregulation have been attributed to the tissue acidosis that results from increased anaerobic metabolism with either hypercarbia or hypoxia. Impairment of autoregulation has also been shown to occur focally in the region of localized cerebral ischemia or of brain tumor and with severe head injury.

Hoedt-Rasmussen *et al.* (1967) found, during the first days following an acute stroke, localized regions of hyperperfusion. This correlated with angiographic evidence of early filling of veins and with impaired autoregulation of adjacent tissue. Such focal hyperemia, termed "luxury perfusion" by Lassen (1966, 1975) might result in intracranial hypertension when sufficiently large areas of brain are involved.

Dissociation between the responses of cerebral blood flow and intracranial pressure, assessed with angiotensin infusion and the responses to CO_2 inhalation, has been observed in very severe head injury (Enevoldsen and Jensen, 1978). These patients had a marked CSF lactic acidosis, with preservation of autoregulation. Cerebral blood flow was unaffected by angiotensin, despite the loss of CO_2 responsiveness, i.e., cerebral blood flow was not increased by CO_2 inhalation. It is uncertain whether the preservation of a pressor response to angiotensin is an example of preserved autoregulation by the arterioles in such very sick patients or whether it might be a result of increased intracranial pressure which was sufficiently elevated to prevent an increase in cerebral blood flow. This circumstance has been termed "false autoregulation" (Bruce *et al.*, 1973; Fieschi *et al.*, 1974). *The clinical implications of these observations indicate that an increase in blood pressure obtained with pressor drugs in patients with severe head injury may aggravate the severity of the intracranial hypertension because of impaired autoregulation.* This will be discussed further in the section on the Cushing response. Another major clinical inference is that since carbon dioxide accumulation and hypoxia have deleterious effects on cerebral autoregulation, both should be avoided in the management of intracranial hypertension.

PRESSURE-VOLUME RELATIONSHIPS: INTRACRANIAL COMPLIANCE AND ELASTANCE

There has been renewed interest in many laboratories in pressure-volume relationships within the cranial cavity. There have been efforts to quantify and better understand the factors that regulate the CSF pressure in normal states and to clarify the mechanisms underlying decompensation, defined as the progressive increase in intracranial pressure that finally occurs with expanding mass lesions.

Early investigators, most notably Ayala (1925), Weed (1932), and Masserman (1935), explored pressure-volume relationships in patients and animals with experiments which noted the change in pressure when CSF was either added or removed. Masserman (1935) observed that the pressure change induced with CSF removal was not a linear one, but Ryder *et al.* (1953) first systematically studied the change in CSF pressure obtained with fractional additions and removal of CSF. Ryder *et al.* (1953) considered that the pressure-volume curve resembled a hyperbolic function; they noted only minimal changes in dP/dV (the observed change in pressure divided by the induced change in volume) when the CSF pressure was low, close to the central venous pressure. As the CSF pressure increased, the dP/dV was increased hyperbolically.

More recently, Lofgren (1973), Langfitt (1975), Marmarou and Shulman (1975), Miller (1975), Sklar *et al.* (1977), Marmarou *et al.* (1978) and others have restudied the problem and have concluded that the CSF pressure-volume curve is an exponential function. Pressures increase logarithmically with stepped linear increases in CSF volume obtained by the injection of a bolus of CSF or by progressive inflation of an intracranial balloon. Marmarou *et al.* (1978) defined the *pressure-volume index* as the slope of the pressure-volume curve which had a linear function when pressure was graphed exponentially. Thus, the pressure-volume index was defined as the volume needed to raise the pressure by a factor of 10.

The theoretical intracranial pressure-volume curve is illustrated in Figure 4–3 (Miller, 1975). It shows that as volumes of CSF are added and intracranial pressure rises, uniform increments of volume (dV) cause progressively larger, logarithmic elevations in intracranial pressure (dP). The term *compliance*, dV/dP, is a measure of the volume distensibility of the intracranial cavity. The term *elastance*, dP/dV, is the reciprocal of compliance; it represents the change in intracranial pressure that results from alterations induced in the intracranial volume. The units of measurement of compliance are ml per mm Hg, and the units for elastance are mm Hg per ml. Compliance decreases and elastance increases as the intracranial pressure or the volume of the intracranial compartments (blood, CSF, or brain), or both, are increased.

The intracranial compliance has been studied extensively, using the injection of saline or artificial CSF (Elliott's solution) into the subarachnoid space or the ventricles of patients with hydrocephalus, brain tumor, head injury, or stroke. Intracranial elastance increases (compliance falls) in parallel with increases in the intracranial pressure, independently of the cause. This occurs normally in many pathological conditions. Thus, jugular compression in the Queckenstedt test increases the CSF pressure secondary to the increased intracranial venous pressure. When this occurs, the amplitude of the pulsatile pressure waves is increased (as illustrated in Chapter 5, Figure 5–1), reflecting the increased intracranial elastance (or decreased compliance) obtained with

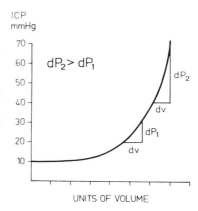

Figure 4–3 Theoretical intracranial volume-pressure curve. As intracranial volume and pressure (ICP) rise, uniform increments of volume (dV) cause larger and larger rises in intracranial pressure (dP). Intracranial elastance (dP/dV) thus increases in parallel with the intracranial pressure during progressive addition to the volume of the intracranial contents. Intracranial compliance is defined as dV/dP, and it changes in reciprocal fashion. Note that dV/dP$_2$ is less than dV/dP$_1$. Thus, the intracranial compliance falls as the intracranial pressure is elevated. See text (from Miller, 1975).

increasing pressure. Similar changes are seen with acute hypertension obtained by the injection of epinephrine, as well as with intracranial hypertension due to such conditions as brain tumor, head injury, or hydrocephalus. Lofgren and Zwetnow (1973) and Marmarou *et al.* (1978) have estimated the compliance of the cranial and spinal compartments separately, showing analogous changes in both. As a guide to management, several laboratories have measured the intracranial elastance in neurosurgical patients by injecting 1 ml of saline in one second into the lateral ventricle, via an intraventricular catheter, and measuring the immediate change in intracranial pressure. In head injury, for example, if the volume-pressure response is more than 3 mm Hg/ml, such a high elastance figure has been considered to indicate a need for surgical decompression (Miller *et al.*, 1973; Miller and Leech, 1975; Miller, 1975).

Several mathematical models have been designed to study the kinetics of the intracranial pressure responses with various changes in intracranial volume. Marmarou *et al.* (1975, 1978) considered four parameters necessary to adequately describe intracranial pressure-volume relationships: (1) the rate of CSF production; (2) the intracranial compliance (elastance) given by the exponential relationship of CSF pressure to volume following additions of artificial CSF; (3) the outflow resistance (chiefly determined by the arachnoid villi); and (4) the intradural venous sinus pressure. The papers of Marmarou *et al.* (1975, 1978) should be consulted for discussion of the proposed mathematical model.

Mann *et al.* (1978) studied intracranial pressure regulation in rats, dogs, and humans following brief, low volume infusions of artificial CSF into the subarachnoid space. They considered two factors to play a major part in maintaining the intracranial pressure within a narrow range: (1) a compliance (elastance) factor arising from distension of meningeal membranes and compression of vascular volume; and (2) a resistance factor that modulates reduction of CSF volume by venting fluid through the arachnoid villi into the venous circulation. In an unanesthetized patient with a normal CSF pressure, supracortical subarachnoid pressure was measured during infusions of artificial CSF into the lateral ventricle for 1 minute at rates of 0.62 to 5.92 ml/min. From the data, they calculated the rate of CSF production, CSF outflow resistance, and intracranial compliance. The authors concluded that *humans, compared with other species, have the highest rate of CSF formation, the greatest efflux capacity, and the lowest outflow resistance.* (The last-named is dependent upon both the arachnoid villi and the intracranial venous pressure.) They emphasized that the low outflow resistance is probably the major mechanism protecting the brain during sustained elevations in intracranial pressure.

With an expanding mass lesion or an increase in the volume of CSF or blood, the compensatory changes at first include increased CSF absorption, and collapse of the cerebral veins and dural sinuses. The intracranial presssure remains within normal limits, in a compensated state, despite changes in intracranial blood, CSF, or tissue volume, because of several compensatory mechanisms. These include: (a) change in CSF volume, (b) change in intracranial blood volume (chiefly venous volume), (c) slight distensibility of the dura, and (d) plasticity of the brain. In both normal and pathological states, reciprocal changes in intracranial blood and CSF volumes play a key role in the avoidance of intracranial hypertension. The fall in CSF volume depends chiefly upon the low outflow resistance of the arachnoid villi. In pathological conditions, brain plasticity becomes increasingly important because the tissue may be displaced with mass lesions and because hydrocephalus may develop as a compensatory response to intracranial hypertension.

The most labile component is the intracranial blood volume, its modification greatly influences the level of the intracranial pressure. Thus, factors which increase the intracranial blood volume and blood flow will increase the intracranial pressure; these include hypercarbia, hypoxia, REM sleep, and volatile anesthetics. Furthermore, factors which decrease the intracranial blood volume and blood flow will decrease the intracranial pressure; these include hypocarbia, hyperoxia, and hypothermia. The therapeutic implications of the dependency of the intracranial pressure upon cerebral blood volume and blood flow will be discussed later.

At present, there is uncertainty about the value of measuring intracranial elastance (compliance) in clinical practice. The data summarized above support the suggestion that the measure of elastance serves as a better indicator of a patient's clinical state than does the level of the mean intracranial pressure. Thus, it appears likely that the therapeutic value of hyperosmolal solutions depends more on their ability to shift the pressure-volume curve to the left rather than on the reduction obtained in mean CSF pressure *per se* (Miller and Leech, 1975). Rather than speculate about a patient's position on the pressure-volume curve, some investigators have reported that measurement of intracranial elastance provides valuable information useful in the management of patients with intracranial hypertension (Miller *et al.*, 1977). However, despite its usefulness in clinical investigation, the role of this technique and of the monitoring of intracranial pressure in clinical practice have not yet been firmly established (see discussion of brain edema).

INTRACRANIAL HYPERTENSION

Intracranial Pressure Gradients

While significant pressure gradients are lacking along the normal CSF pathways (apart from the pulsations secondary to systole and respiration, which are greatest in the ventricles), this is clearly not the case in pathological conditions associated with mass lesions and displacement of brain tissue. The presence of tissue pressure gradients is clearly evident in various types of cerebral herniation, in the development of obstructive hydrocephalus, and in the movement of edema fluid through the white matter. Such tissue pressure gradients may be present without a measurable increase in intracranial pressure. For example, clinicians have long observed that extensive displacement of brain tissue may occur with slowly expanding tumors, at times sufficient to shift the pineal or even expand the middle fossa of the skull, without evidence of intracranial hypertension (although reduced intracranial compliance would be demonstrable in such a patient). The presence of intercompartmental pressure gradients with expanding lesions has been documented in animals, using transducers placed in the supratentorial, infratentorial, subarachnoid, and spinal spaces (Johnston and Rowan, 1974, Langfitt, 1975).

The role of brain tissue pressure has been studied, using the technique of cotton wick pressure recording (Schettini *et al.*, 1971). The wick-catheter pressure technique minimizes the tissue damage done by implanted capsules and balloons, while it enables the recording of analogous data. By use of the wick-catheter, brain tissue pressure gradients from 1 to 2 mm Hg were measured in the areas surrounding experimental cryogenic lesions. Such pressure gradients were seen in expanding areas of edema, although the gradients were finally reduced when the pressure reached high levels. Several investigators have observed similar transient pressure gradients in regions of cerebral ischemia. However, Brock *et al.* (1975) were not able to demonstrate that tissue pressures were significantly altered by ischemic infarction, hypercarbia, or hypertension. Reulen and Kreysch (1973) considered that pressure gradients occurred chiefly within the interstitial fluid, where they would facilitate the bulk flow of edema fluid into the surrounding area from a focal region of vasogenic edema. The effects of such tissue pressure gradients on the microcirculation and on cellular metabolism require further study. This subject will be considered further in the discussion of the pathogenesis of hydrocephalus.

Intracranial Hypertension Due to Mass Lesions

Tumors and other mass lesions cause a generalized increase in intracranial pressure (1) when they reach a critical mass because of the fixed volume of the cranial cavity, (2) by obstruction of the intracranial venous system, or (3) by obstruction of the CSF pathways. In terms of the factors that determine critical mass, intracranial hypertension is often more closely correlated with the *rate* of tumor growth than with the absolute size of the tumor. Thus, slowly growing tumors, like meningioma, may become very large, filling the middle fossa and causing several centimeters of shift of midline structures, without evidence of intracranial hypertension, despite a reduced intracranial compliance. In contrast, rapidly growing gliomas and metastatic tumors, relatively small in size, may be accompanied by evidence of severe intracranial hypertension. This occurs because rapidly growing tumors are more likely to evoke severe peritumoral edema, brain infiltration, and necrosis. In addition, the brain is sufficiently plastic to undergo pressure atrophy with the slowly growing extra-axial tumors, whereas this does not occur with rapidly expanding infiltrative tumors. The factors underlying pressure atrophy of the cerebrum, whether due to extra-axial compression or to pressure atrophy of the periventricular white matter in hydrocephalus, are poorly understood.

As noted, brain tumors cause intracranial hypertension for reasons other than their mass *per se*. Tumors which obstruct the ventricular system or subarachnoid spaces at the tentorium, over the convexities, at the arachnoid villi, or in more than one of these locations, cause intracranial hypertension and hydrocephalus due to impaired CSF absorption. These include the gamut of intraventricular tumors as well as the heterogenous tumors responsible for diffuse meningeal neoplasia (carcinomatous meningitis). Tumors which invade the intracranial venous sinuses may also cause intracranial hypertension; such tumors include meningiomas as well as metastatic neoplasms.

Mass lesions may be responsible for several kinds of cerebral herniation: transtentorial, cingulate, cerebellar, and transcalvarial. These are illustrated in Figure 4–4. *Transtentorial herniation* includes both *central herniation* and *uncal herniation.* In *central herniation,* the hemispheres and basal nuclei compress the midbrain rostro-caudally through the tentorial notch, giving rise to a reduced state of consciousness, sighs, and yawns, followed by periodic respirations of the Cheyne-Stokes type, small pupils, and "doll's head" ocular signs. In *uncal herniation,* the uncus, the most medial gyrus of the temporal lobe, is displaced inferiorly by a hemispheric mass through the tentorial notch, thus causing compression of the midbrain, which results in depression of consciousness and ipsilateral, contralateral, or bilateral dilated and fixed pupils secondary to third nerve compression. *Cerebellar herniation* most often results in *downward herniation* of the cerebellar tonsils through the foramen magnum by a posterior fossa mass, causing compression of the medulla and respiratory arrest. *Upward herniation* of the cerebellum occurs with superior displacement of the cerebellum through the tentorial notch, causing midbrain compression (Cuneo *et al.,* 1979). This is caused by pontine hemorrhage or posterior fossa tumors, and it may also occur with the Dandy-Walker syndrome, i.e., hydrocephalus due to obstruction of the outflow of the fourth ventricle. *Cingulate herniation* occurs when the cingulate gyrus is displaced contralaterally beneath the falx by a hemispheric mass lesion. *Transcalvarial herniation* is the displacement of the brain through a bony defect as

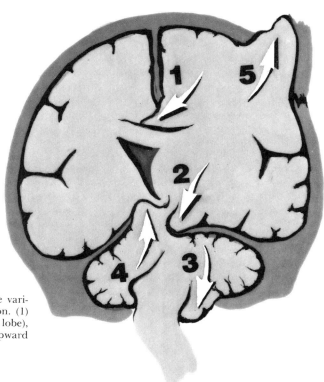

Figure 4-4 Schema of the various forms of cerebral herniation. (1) Cingulate, (2) uncal (temporal lobe), (3) cerebellar tonsillar, (4) upward cerebellar, (5) transcalvarial.

a result of surgery or head trauma. The pathophysiology and clinical manifestations of the various herniation syndromes have been thoroughly reviewed by Plum and Posner (1972) and by Zulch *et al.* (1974).

THE CUSHING RESPONSE (VASOPRESSOR REACTION)

The elevation in arterial blood pressure that often follows increased intracranial pressure was observed and recorded by several investigators (including Spencer and Horsley, 1892) prior to the observations of Harvey Cushing (1902). However, Cushing first analyzed the changes quantitatively, and his name has generally been identified with the circulatory and respiratory responses to severe intracranial hypertension. He infused saline into the subdural space of dogs and noted that the arterial pressure increased when exceeded by the intracranial pressure in association with bradycardia and slowing of respiration. He found that (1) section of the descending sympathetic pathways prevented the arterial hypertension, (2) section of the vagus blocked the appearance of the bradycardia, and (3) cocainization of the medulla abolished both reactions. Cushing postulated that the pressor effects were due to medullary ischemia and that the hypertension served to improve the blood flow to the brain stem.

While the Cushing triad of hypertension, bradycardia, and respiratory slowing is present in some patients with increased intracranial pressure, clinical studies have shown a variable relationship between the intracranial pressure and changes in vital signs. Using the nitrous oxide technique in patients with brain tumors, Kety *et al.* (1948) studied the relationship between cerebral blood flow and intracranial pressure. They observed a critical CSF pressure of about 450 mm CSF, above which there was a progressive decrease in cerebral blood flow associated with a gradual increase in arterial pressure, thus confirming the occurrence of Cushing response in patients with brain tumors. They also noted a decrease in cerebral oxygen consumption that paralleled the depression in the patients' states of consciousness. In contrast to these observations, Browder and Myers (1938), Evans *et al.* (1951), and others have reported that rather abrupt elevation of the intracranial pressure for brief periods to levels between 700 and 1000 mm water by the intrathecal injection of saline, in patients without mass lesions, did not have an immediate effect on pulse, respiration, or blood pressure, nor did the subjects report any awareness of having received the injection. In similar experiments, Wolff (D'Alessio, 1972) reported that patients complained of low back pain as the major manifestation of an acute increase in pressure obtained by lumbar sac infusions. However, Fay (1940) reported the occurrence of headache with similar spinal injections, although he observed great variation in the threshold for headache induction by this technique. It is also noteworthy that many patients with benign intracranial pressure are often headache-free despite CSF pressures greater than 400 mm. *Thus, headache and the Cushing triad are likely to occur with a shift or displacement of cerebral structures in association with mass lesions that cause intracranial hypertension. Their occurrence is not directly dependent upon the level of the intracranial pressure* per se.

The pathophysiology of the Cushing response has been the subject of controversy, and various mechanisms are considered to be of primary importance. These include: (1) ischemia or hypoxia of the medullary centers, proposed by Cushing; (2) stimulation of intracranial baroreceptors in response to changes in cerebral perfusion pressure, proposed by Rodbard and Saiki (1952); (3) distortion of the brain stem, proposed by Thompson and Malina (1959); and (4) local pressure on discrete areas of the floor of the fourth ventricle adjacent to the vasomotor nuclei, proposed by Hoff and Reis (1970) and by Rowan and Johnston (1975).

Recently, McGillicuddy *et al.* (1978) restudied the Cushing response in monkeys, comparing separately the effects of intracranial hypertension, hypoxia, and hypercarbia upon the arterial blood pressure. Efforts were made to exclude the role of peripheral baroreceptors and chemoreceptors by carotid-to-carotid cross perfusion experiments in order to obtain a purely cerebral hypoxia and hypercarbia. Both intracranial hypertension and hypoxia produced a similar degree of arterial hypertension, but hypercarbia alone did not elicit a Cushing response. However, carbon dioxide retention was considered to contribute to the latter's intensity because of the increase in intracranial pressure induced by hypercarbia. These data indicate that anoxia and intracranial hypertension have common effects on brain stem function which are independent of the purely mechanical effects of increased intracranial pressure upon the brain.

Zwetnow (1970) correlated the appearance of the vasopressor reaction with an increase in brain lactate and pyruvate and a fall in brain ATP and phosphocreatine, findings indicative of brain ischemia. Thus, Cushing's generalization regarding the mechanism of the vascular responses to intracranial hypertension appears to hold true, namely, that the vasopressor response is an adaptation to maintain sufficient perfusion of the brain stem. However, Shalit and Cotev (1974) have questioned the conclusion that the pressor responses must necessarily have a beneficial effect in maintaining cerebral perfusion in the face of intracranial hypertension; their data indicate that the arterial hypertension may have a deleterious effect in the presence of intracranial hypertension! It seems likely that the blood flow to the medulla is a major determinant of the response, and this factor has proved difficult to quantify in various animal experiments and clinical studies.

Thus, uncertainty persists regarding the mechanism and the biological role of the Cushing response. Although the triad of arterial hypertension, bradycardia, and respiratory irregularity can easily be reproduced in animals by injection of saline into the subarachnoid space, the Cushing signs correlate irregularly with the other clinical findings in patients. Some patients with rapidly progressive intracranial hypertension, such as that due to cerebral hemorrahge, seem to replicate the animal experiment, but in other cases the signs may not be seen despite marked intracranial hypertension. If the intracranial hypertension is diffuse and there are no pressure gradients within the cranial cavity, the pressor response is unlikely to occur until the intracranial pressure reaches or exceeds the diastolic blood pressure. However, with compression or displacement of the brain stem due to a mass lesion, the pressor response may occur at relatively low levels of intracranial pressure.

SYSTEMIC EFFECTS OF INCREASED
INTRACRANIAL PRESSURE

There are other systemic effects of intracranial hypertension to be considered besides the vasopressor response described above. These include: (1) cardiac effects, (2) respiratory effects, and (3) gastrointestinal hemorrhage.

Cardiac Effects

Cardiac arrhythmias occur in animals and patients with increased intracranial pressure in a variety of experimental and clinical settings. Experimentally, arrhythmias have been induced with electrical stimulation applied to different regions of the brain, including the hypothalamus, the midbrain, the orbital surface of the frontal lobe, and the insula. Stretching the vessels of the circle of Willis, inflating an intracranial balloon, and experimental subarachnoid hemorrhage also have produced cardiac arrhythmia (Weintraub and McHenry, 1974).

The arrhythmias and electrocardiographic changes reported have included auricular fibrillation; atrial, nodal and ventricular bradycardia; large T waves; prolonged QT intervals; and changes in the ST segment. These findings probably explain the high incidence of unexplained sudden death in patients with subarachnoid hemorrhage. The occurrence of subendocardial hemorrhages in such cases has been attributed to excessive sympathetic stimulation. In support of such a mechanism, Offerhaus and Van Gool (1969) have found increased tissue catecholamines in the heart following intracranial hemorrhage. Estanol and Marin (1975) showed that the cardiac arrhythmias in dogs could be produced by direct autonomic stimulation of the heart. Similar arrhythmias were obtained following the intrathecal injection of blood or saline. These experimental observations appear to explain the cardiac effects of intracranial hypertension which contribute to the death rate in acute stroke and subarachnoid hemorrhage.

With acute increases in intracranial pressure that elicit systemic hypertension, there is experimental evidence of reduction in renal blood flow, which when severe may result in a falling glomerular filtration rate and reduced urinary flow. Less severe increases in intracranial pressure have not been shown to affect glomerular filtration rate or sodium excretion in anesthetized animals (Fishman, 1953). Such changes have not been documented in the clinical setting. Whether the innervation of the kidney is important in the Cushing response is not clear (Di Bona, 1978).

The Effects of Intracranial
Hypertension upon Pulmonary Function

An extensive clinical literature has documented that a variety of central nervous system disorders may result in pulmonary edema in the absence of underlying cardiopulmonary disease (Simmons et al., 1969; Theodore and Robin, 1976). Central neurogenic pulmonary edema has been reported in cases of cerebral hemorrhage, seizures, subarachnoid hemorrahge, cervical cord injury, head trauma, bulbar poliomyelitis, cerebral embolus, vertebral artery ligation, and brain tumor. The frequency of neurogenic pulmonary edema in these disorders is uncertain; it is probably an uncommon complication. It probably occurs chiefly as a manifestation of the Cushing response with systemic hypertension and sympathetic discharge (see discussion in McLaurin, 1976). In Ducker's (1968) report of 11 patients with diverse central nervous system lesions associated with pulmonary edema, increased intracranial pressure was considered the unifying factor. Transtentorial herniation was a frequent complication, and postmortem examination revealed varying degrees of cerebral edema. The precise mechanism of the changes in pulmonary function responsible for central neurogenic pulmonary edema is still poorly understood.

Gastrointestinal Hemorrhage

The occurrence of upper gastrointestinal hemorrhage as a complication of intracranial disease was recognized for a century before Cushing's (1932) report, which focused attention on the problem. Acute gastrointestinal ulceration developing after intracranial trauma or operation often consists of deeply penetrating lesions involving the full thickness of the esophagus, stomach, or duodenum. Gordon *et al.* (1973) have reported increases in gastric mucosal permeability and gastric acid and pepsin secretion in neurosurgical patients. Serum gastrin levels, perhaps related to increased vagal activity, were higher in patients with head injury than in those with other bodily injuries (Bowen *et al.*, 1974). The specific role of the intracranial pressure in the pathogenesis of a Cushing's ulcer is not clear, although intracranial hypertension is probably present in many neurosurgical patients who develop gastrointestinal hemorrhage.

Karch (1972) reported the occurrence of hemorrhagic ulceration of the gastrointestinal tract in 7.2 per cent of 2206 consecutive autopsies. The incidence in patients dying with intracranial disorders was twice that in those dying from all other causes (12.5 per cent *vs.* 6.0 per cent). Esophageal ulceration was more common in the neurological than in the nonneurological patients. The intracranial disorders associated with hemorrhagic ulceration included brain tumor, cerebral hemorrhage, and subarachnoid hemorrhage. Other disorders listed included sinus thrombosis, brain laceration, encephalitis, embolism, subdural hematoma, and cerebral edema. The data in this series were deliberately derived from a time before steroid therapy, with its well-known increased risk of ulceration, was commonly used in neurosurgical management (Karch, 1972).

EFFECTS OF DRUGS ON INTRACRANIAL PRESSURE

Theoretically, the effects of various drugs on the intracranial pressure might be mediated by (1) changes induced in the rates of CSF formation and absorption, (2) changes in the circulation of the brain, or (3) changes in the permeability of the blood-brain barrier. The effect of drugs on CSF formation and absorption have been discussed in Chapter 3.

The only drugs which have been shown to depress the rate of CSF formation *in vivo* in animals are acetazolamide and furosemide (McCarthy and Reed, 1974). Dexamethasone has no effect on CSF formation or absorption in normal dogs (Vela, 1979). The cardiac glycosides, such as digitalis, probably do not alter CSF formation or the intracranial pressure when given systemically, although there is a single clinical report in support of such an effect that has not been further substantiated (Neblett *et al.*, 1972; Schott and Holt, 1974). The rate of CSF formation rarely appears to play a primary role in the genesis of pathological increases in the intracranial pressure (choroid plexus papilloma is the rare exception); therefore, drugs like acetazolamide and furosemide have only a limited place in the therapy of conditions such as benign intracranial hypertension and brain edema. Brain edema fluid is cleared in part by the sink action of the ventricular fluid; that is, it enters the ventricular system and is removed by bulk flow reabsorption (Hochwald *et al.*, 1976; Reulen *et al.*, 1978). There are experimental data that reduction of CSF formation by the choroid plexus with acetazolamide or furosemide facilitates the clearance of edema fluid from the hemispheres. This effect may occur solely because of a reduction in the rate of choroidal CSF formation; some data suggest that furosemide may affect extrachoroidal CSF formation as well (Clasen *et al.*, 1974; McCarthy and Reed, 1974, Vela *et al.*, 1979).

The role of the adrenal steroids in the treatment of brain edema is discussed later. Their therapeutic effects on the intracranial pressure are considered to be secondary to their anti-edema effects rather than to direct effects on the CSF pressure or turnover. However, it is possible that glucocorticoids facilitate bulk flow reabsorption that has been impaired by inflammatory changes in the subarachnoid space or arachnoidal villi. This possibility has not yet been clearly established, although the favorable response to steroid therapy sometimes observed in patients with intracranial hypertension due to pseudotumor and granulomatous meningitis (sarcoidosis and meningeal cysticerosis) suggests that this does, in fact, occur.

Drugs that increase cerebral blood flow usually have parallel effects on the intracranial pressure (Sokoloff, 1959; Shapiro *et al.*, 1974). The volatile anesthetic agents, halothane, trichloroethylene, and methoxyflurane increase the intracranial pressure because of their vasodilating effects. Nitrous oxide and ketamine have similar effects (Fitch *et al.*, 1969, 1971). Morphine, diazepam, and pentazocine raise the intracranial pressure because they inhibit the CO_2 responsiveness of the brain stem sufficiently to inhibit respiration and thereby elevate the arterial pCO_2 and the cerebral blood flow (Keats and Mithoefer, 1955). This is most likely to occur with high doses, although the presence of pre-existing neurological disease may also inhibit the CO_2 responsiveness of the brain stem and enhance the clinical effects of hypercarbia upon the intracranial pressure.

A number of pharmacological effects on the intracranial pressure have not been explained. These include the occurrence of benign intracranial pressure in patients receiving tetracycline, nalidixic acid, or vitamin A (Maroon *et al.*, 1971, Deonna *et al.*, 1974, Lombaert and Carton, 1976). It is noteworthy that both vitamin A deficiency and intoxication have been reported to cause increased intracranial pressure. The mechanisms in these cases have not been elucidated.

EFFECTS OF OSMOTIC ALTERATIONS ON INTRACRANIAL PRESSURE

The osmotic properties of the brain were first systematically studied by Weed and McKibben (1919), who realized that the brain behaved like a crude osmometer. They observed that opposing changes in the intracranial pressure followed acutely the systemic administration of sufficiently large volumes of hypotonic or hypertonic fluid. An extensive literature, well summarized by Katzman and Pappius (1973) and Rapoport (1976) has shown that such pressure effects reflect changes in brain volume that are usually transient because complex mechanisms operate to restore cellular volumes to normal. The latter occurs because the intracellular osmolality changes to equal the plasma osmolality, and water moves passively in accordance with the laws of diffusion (Rapoport, 1976, MacKnight and Leaf, 1977, Andreoli *et al.*, 1977). The processes involved whereby the brain reaches a new osmotic equilibrium, termed "isosmotic intracellular regulation," have been studied *in vivo* and *in vitro,* using brain slices (Fishman, 1974). The data have elucidated the changes in intracranial pressure associated with osmotic derangement as well as the concomitant changes in cerebral function occurring with severe deviations in plasma and tissue osmolality (Fishman *et al.*, 1977, Chan and Fishman, 1979).

Effects of Hypo-osmolality

Hypo-osmolality results from dilution or depletion of plasma sodium. An extensive literature deals with the effects of hyponatremia caused by salt depletion, water intoxication, or both (Katzman and Pappius, 1973, Arieff *et al.*, 1976; Fishman, 1976). These experiments may be categorized into two groups: (1) very acute studies of the brain edema associated with water intoxication, and (2) longer-term studies analyzing the changes in the ionic composition of brain that accompany chronic hypo-osmolality. The brain edema obtained is usually transient. Dodge *et al.* (1960) showed that the increase in intracranial pressure *per se* was not responsible for changes in cerebral function but that the latter resulted from changes in brain metabolism. With acute water intoxication, brain volume is increased because of an increase in brain water. However, the latter change is temporary because the intracellular potassium falls as the brain adapts to reach a new equilibrium with the hypotonic plasma (Rymer and Fishman, 1973). This allows the restoration of normal cellular volume, and the intracranial pressure falls to normal. Rymer and Fishman (1973) considered the encephalopathy of water intoxication to reflect the increase in brain intracellular water, whereas Dila and Pappius (1972) considered depletion of brain intracellular potassium to be the critical event. This issue requires further study.

The brain is relatively protected from water intoxication, compared with other tissues such as muscle and liver. The brain's adaptation reflects its ability to reduce intracellular osmolality rapidly in the face of acute hypo-osmolality of the plasma. The sink action of the CSF is also important in the resolution of hypotonic brain edema in that, with recovery, the brain water moves to the cerebral ventricles to be removed by bulk flow reabsorption (DiMatteo *et al.*, 1975). This mechanism probably also plays a role in the resolution of other types of brain edema.

Effects of Hyperosmolality

The effects of hyperosmolality upon the intracranial pressure have long been recognized in the clinical setting; children with severe dehydration have sunken fontanelles. An extensive literature shows that the parenteral administration of hypertonic solutions will acutely reduce both brain volume and the intracranial pressure when the blood-brain barrier is intact. Pappius and Dayes (1965) showed that the administration of hypertonic urea could "shrink" the normal hemisphere but fail to reduce the volume of the edematous hemisphere. The rapid entry of the urea into the pathological region erased the osmotic gradient between blood and brain, which is essential to induce the efflux of water and a reduction in brain volume. These important experiments showed that osmotherapy would be most effective in reducing brain volume in normal subjects and least effective in the presence of a defective blood-brain barrier.

Hyperosmolal Therapy

The introduction of osmotic agents in the treatment of intracranial hypertension was initiated by the experiments of Weed and McKibben (1919) which showed the ability of intravenous hypertonic solutions to acutely lower intracranial pressure. Hypertonic glucose (50 ml of 50 gm/dl) given intravenously was first used in clinical practice, but it was soon recognized that after an initial drop in intracranial pressure, a secondary rise or *rebound* in intracranial pressure occurred as the solute rapidly reached equilibrium in CSF and brain. Hypertonic (50 per cent) sucrose had a brief vogue in clinical practice during the 1930's (Bullock *et al.*, 1935), but the occurrence of hematuria and crystalluria ended its use. The intravenous administration of concentrated human serum albumin, a hyperoncotic solution, does not significantly reduce the intracranial pressure, and it has no clinical usefulness in this regard (Fender and MacKenzie, 1948). In recent years, the major hypertonic solutes in use have been hypertonic urea, mannitol, and glycerol.

Urea

The ability of hypertonic urea to reduce the intracranial pressure was first studied by Fremont-Smith and Forbes (1927), but urea was not introduced into clinical practice until the studies of Javid and Settlage (1956). Urea is a potent dehydrating agent because of its low molecular weight (MW 60), its slow elimination from the blood, and its relatively slow penetration of the blood-brain and blood-CSF barriers (Reed and Woodbury, 1962). Sterile lyophilized urea in 10 per cent invert sugar or 5 or 10 per cent dextrose has been given intravenously as a 30 per cent weight-volume solution to reduce intracranial pressure, using 1.5 grams per kilogram of body weight; in elderly patients, dosages of 0.5 grams per kilogram have been recommended. Doses of 1.5 grams per kilogram administered at 20 to 60 drops per minute will reduce the CSF pressure for 3 to 8 hours. Subsequently, 1 gram per kilogram of body weight may be given intravenously during the next 24 hours.

Special attention must be paid to the measure of fluid intake, urinary output, electrolytes, and water replacement because of the diuretic effect of the solute load. In the presence of severe renal insufficiency, urea must be administered with caution. Potential side effects include pain and thrombosis at the injection site and skin slough if subcutaneous infiltration is extensive. Headaches secondary to intracranial hypotension may occur.

Following therapy, a rebound of CSF intracranial pressure to above the initial level may occur when urea has reached equilibrium in the CSF and brain (McQueen and Jeanes, 1964). The frequency and severity of rebound have not been defined with any degree of certainty; to minimize its development excessive hydration should be avoided. Administration of urea at a rate in excess of its urinary excretion favors the occurrence of rebound. Furthermore, urea is not inert; it has been shown to have epileptogenic properties, apparently independently of its osmotic effects, and to have a direct neurotoxicity in high concentration (Glaser, 1974). For these reasons, it is now little used in clinical practice, having been largely replaced by mannitol.

Mannitol

This hexatol, with a molecular weight of 182, was first used in neurosurgical practice by Wise and Chater in 1962. It has an osmotic disadvantage compared to urea because of its three-fold greater molecular weight; however, this is counterbalanced by the fact that mannitol is excluded from the CSF and brain to a greater degree. While this relative exclusion tends to minimize a rebound in intracranial pressure, rebound does occur in clinical practice (McGraw et al., 1978). Rebound occurs when large doses of mannitol are given at a frequency that exceeds its urinary excretion. If sustained hyperosmolality of the brain is obtained, rebound is likely to occur when the plasma osmolality falls more rapidly than the brain level. Although mannitol is a less potent osmotic diuretic than urea, it is also probably less toxic to the nervous system.

Mannitol, 1 gram per kilogram of body weight, given intravenously in a period of 10 to 15 minutes, causes a rise in serum osmolality of approximately 20 to 30 mOsm/l, with return to control levels in about three hours. A dose of 1.5 to 2 grams per kilogram lowers CSF pressure significantly for three to eight hours (Wise and Chater, 1962). Lower dosages of mannitol (0.5 mg/kg or less) are desirable if repeated administration is likely, e.g., in the treatment of Reye's syndrome to avoid excessive hyperosmolality and rebound (McGraw et al., 1978; Trauner et al., 1978). Twenty per cent or 25 per cent solutions have been used usually, higher concentrations will crystallize at room temperature.

Miller and Leech (1975) reported 8 patients studied before and after the administration of mannitol. The ventricular fluid pressure, the intracranial pressure-volume response (intracranial elastance), and the arterial pressure were determined before and after the intravenous infusion of 0.5 gm per kilogram over 10 minutes. The ventricular fluid pressure was reduced in all 8 patients; the maximum ventricular fluid pressure reduction of 35 per cent occurred 15 minutes after mannitol administration, and it remained at this level for 45 minutes. The pressure-volume response was tested by injecting 1 ml of saline in one second into the ventricular fluid and recording the pressure change thereafter. The maximum reduction in the pressure-volume response was attained at 15 minutes. The authors concluded that mannitol not only influenced the intracranial pressure but also favorably influenced intracranial pressure-volume relationships; thus, an improvement in the patient's neurological status may occur with osmotherapy even when there is little measurable effect on the intracranial pressure *per se.*

The clinical studies of McGraw *et al.* (1978) emphasize the need for individualizing therapy in the treatment of intracranial hypertension with mannitol. To avoid rebound, the smallest effective dosage should be used. Smaller dosages (100 ml of 20 per cent mannitol) were often as effective as larger doses. Osmolality, electrolytes, urinary flow, and intracranial pressure should be monitored when repeated doses of mannitol are given.

Glycerol

Glycerol (1,2,3-propanetriol) is a trivalent alcohol that has been used both systemically and orally in the treatment of glaucoma and intracranial hypertension since its introduction by Cantore *et al.* (1964). Unlike mannitol, glycerol is not metabolically inert; it is partially metabolized to carbon dioxide and water, producing 4.3 calories per gram. Glycerol is present in animal tissues as an integral part of fats (triglycerides and phosphatides) in amounts of approximately 1 per cent of body weight.

When large amounts of glycerol are given, the drug is not metabolized completely, being excreted in part unchanged in the urine (Tourtellote *et al.,* 1972). While therapeutic doses produce a diuresis, glycerol also reduces intracranial pressure in nephrectomized animals. Glycerol may be given orally by nasogastric tube in doses of 0.5 gm/kg, and it may reduce the intracranial pressure within 30 to 60 minutes; 1.2 gm/kg may be administered initially with maintenance therapy of 0.5 to 1.0 gm/kg every 3 to 4 hours. When the glycerol is administered intravenously, a dilute solution of not greater than 10 per cent glycerol in 0.4 normal saline is needed, because higher concentrations result in the hemolysis of red cells. Ten per cent glycerol should not be given at a rate greater than 4.5 ml/min for the same reason.

Cantore *et al.* (1964) reported their use of glycerol in doses of 1 to 2 grams per kilogram of body weight in 258 patients on a neurosurgical service. The patients received glycerol orally, 1.5 gm/kg, and some patients received additional doses of 1 gm/kg 2 hours later with maintenance therapy of 0.5 to 0.7 gm/kg of glycerol every 3 to 4 hours until surgical intervention was carried out. The authors did not comment on the possible incidence of symptomatic hyperosmolality or hyperosmolar coma, which has been reported as a complication of glycerol therapy (Sears, 1976).

Many workers reporting the chronic use of glycerol did not monitor the serum osmolality. Rottenberg *et al.* (1977) have described the difficulties in planning the timing and dosage of glycerol administration when it is used for long periods of time. They concluded that an osmotic gradient of only 10 mOsm between blood and CSF could be effective in lowering the intracranial pressure. Tourtellotte *et al.* (1972) reviewed the complications and toxicity of glycerol therapy, which include hemolysis, hemoglobinuria, renal failure, and hyperosmolal coma. Another problem in the use of oral glycerol is that nausea and vomiting may be induced by the very sweet taste of glycerol in solution.

Mathew *et al.* (1972) reported significant benefit with glycerol in the treatment of acute cerebral infarction, although these authors did not monitor the serum osmolality in their patients. The beneficial effect of glycerol in stroke patients was *not* confirmed in a double-blind trial by Larsson *et al.* (1976). It is possible that glycerol has beneficial effects in brain edema apart from inducing hyperosmolality. The metabolic effects of glycerol therapy require further exploration.

The Mechanism of Pressure Reduction

To discuss the mechanism whereby osmotic loads result in a reduction in intracranial pressure and brain volume, it is necessary to consider the osmotically active constituents of the brain. The osmolality of brain, CSF, and blood is the same in normal subjects, about 300 mOsm per l. The major ions in mmol per kg wet weight in the cerebral cortex of mammalian brain (rats, cats, dogs, humans) have been reported as follows: Na^+/50 to 60, K^+ 88 to 100, Cl^- 36 to 42, Ca^{2+} 2 to 4, MG^{2+} 5 to 6, HCO_3^- 10 to 12, and glucose about 18 mmol/kg wet weight (Katzman and Pappius, 1973). It is clear that the sum of the inorganic cations present is greater than that of the inorganic anions. The total brain cation concentration is about 170 mmol/kg wet weight, and the anions, including chloride, bicarbonate sulfate, phosphate, and organic acids (including lactate, pyruvate, glutamine, glutamate, etc.), are about 85 mmol/kg wet weight. The remaining intracellular anions are lipids and proteins. The precise osmotic activity of each intracellular solute is not known.

Most of the intracellular calcium and magnesium are probably bound and hence are not osmotically active as free ions. The intracellular sodium is probably largely free and osmotically active, because it varies directly with changes in the plasma (extracellular) fluid sodium. There is considerable uncertainty about the osmotic activity of the intracellular potassium, some of which is bound and osmotically inactive (Katzman and Pappius, 1973). However, a substantial part of the intracellular potassium is free and readily influenced by osmotic gradients. This is supported by the observation that the intracellular potassium falls as the brain adapts to hypo-osmolality in experimental water intoxication (Rymer and Fishman, 1973). The data suggest that the reversible binding and release of intracellular potassium may be a control mechanism for varying the intracellular osmolality in response to acute variations in plasma osmolality (Fishman, 1974). Such a mechanism for adjusting intracellular osmolality would minimize changes in brain cell volume that are favored by an osmotic gradient between the intracellular and extracellular compartments. It is possible that a reduction in the degree of binding of intracellular potassium contributes a portion of the idiogenic osmoles, discussed later, that appear transiently in brain in hyperosmolar states (Holliday *et al.*, 1968; Arieff and Kleeman, 1973, Fishman *et al.*, 1977, Chan and Fishman, 1979).

The physiological principles that determine the pressure-lowering effects of any hypertonic solution, independent of the solute, are much the same. The solute must be relatively restricted in its entry across the blood-brain barrier. An osmotic gradient is necessary to drive the movement of water from the brain cell to the site of higher osmolality, the plasma. It is not clear whether the drop in brain water induced by hypertonic loads is due only to a decrease in intracellular water or also to a decrease in interstitial fluid volume. It seems likely that both compartments are affected with severe dehydration, but there are no data available regarding the changes induced by conventional doses of hypertonic fluids.

The water that leaves brain cells in response to hyperosmolality flows into the ventricular system; this is an example of the sink action of CSF volume flow (Hochwald *et al.*, 1976). Once the solute has reached equilibrium in both plasma and brain so that the osmolalities of both compartments are equal, the intracellular volume returns to its initial state and the intracranial pressure returns to its initial level. DiMattei *et al.* (1975) showed that in cats a minimum change of 10 per cent in serum osmolality, about 30 mOsm/l, was needed to increase or decrease the water content of brain. However, smaller osmotic gradients have been shown to be effective in humans. In a clinical study of glycerol therapy, Rottenberg *et al.* (1977) reported that an osmotic gradient of only 10 mOsm/l appeared to effectively reduce the intracranial pressure.

In addition to its complex effects on brain volume and brain metabolism, hyperosmolality has also been shown to inhibit the formation of CSF within the ventricular system (DiMattio *et al.*, 1975; Hochwald *et al.*, 1976). Although there are no data regarding the quantitative importance of this effect in patients, it appears more likely that with the usual dosage schedule the major factors responsible for the reduction in intracranial pressure with osmotherapy are the reductions in brain volume and intracranial compliance rather than a reduction in the rate of CSF formation.

Idiogenic Osmoles

Osmotic gradients between brain and plasma are sustained for only brief periods of time, for two reasons: (1) the solute administered (whether urea, mannitol, or glycerol) crosses the blood-brain barrier to enter both the extracellular and intracellular fluid spaces of the brain so that the osmotic gradient is dissipated; (2) additional osmotically active solutes appear within brain to increase intracellular osmolality as an adaptive response to equal the increased osmolality of the serum. These unidentified intracellular osmoles have been termed, *idiogenic osmoles*, i.e., osmoles of undetermined origin (McDowell *et al.*, 1955). Their appearance has been demonstrated both *in vivo* and *in vitro*, using cortical brain slices (Holliday *et al.*, 1968; Arieff and Kleeman, 1973; Fishman *et al.*, 1977; MacKnight and Leaf, 1977; Chan and Fishman, 1979). They are transient in nature, that is, they appear rapidly in response to a steep osmotic gradient, but subsequently they are no longer detected as the intracellular and extracellular osmolalities approach equality.

While some of the unidentified osmoles can be attributed to an increase in the intracellular concentration of the free amino acids, the latter are probably insufficient to account for more than a small part of the total idiogenic osmoles that appear (Chan and Fishman, 1979). It has been suggested earlier than an increase in the ionic dissociation of intracellular potassium from a bound to a free state may account for the transient appearance of idiogenic osmoles. The fact that acute hyperosmolality alters the concentration and release of some free amino acids will be discussed further in the section on the dialysis dysequilibrium syndrome.

Dose Response Curve

The efficacy of osmotherapy in reducing the intracranial pressure depends upon the presence of an osmotic gradient between blood and CSF and brain. Once the osmotic gradient has been obliterated by the entry of the solute into the CSF and brain compartments and by the transient appearance of idiogenic osmoles, the therapeutic effectiveness is lost, and rebound in the intracranial pressure may develop. There is uncertainty in the literature regarding the magnitude of the osmotic gradient needed for therapeutic effectiveness. While several authors (Stern and Coxon, 1964; Guisado et al., 1976) concluded that an acute increase in plasma osmolality of 30 to 35 mOsm per l water would be required to induce a net movement of water from brain to blood, Rottenberg et al. (1977) pointed out that there is no theoretical reason to expect that a "critical" osmotic threshold must be exceeded before changes in intracranial volume occur. Thus, with the use of oral glycerol, the latter investigators noted that smaller increases in serum osmolality significantly lowered intraventricular pressure; the changes in serum osmolality varied between 14 and 26 mOsm per l water in 9 of 11 studies.

However, there are insufficient data on the ranges of osmolality obtained with various intravenous doses of mannitol or of other osmotic agents. The time courses of various osmotic loads cannot be predicted with any degree of accuracy because of the many factors influencing the rate of urinary excretion of the solute and the diuresis obtained. A wide range of responses should be expected in heterogeneous patients with intracranial hypertension. *It is essential that the serum osmolality be monitored as a guide to therapy if repeated doses of hypertonic mannitol or glycerol are intended.* Serum osmolalities of about 350 mOsm/l commonly cause coma, and higher osmolalities have caused death, often with intracerebral venous hemorrhages (Sotos et al., 1960; Loeb, 1974; Swanson, 1976).

The Mechanism of Rebound

A secondary increase or rebound in intracranial pressure takes place following the administration of each of the solutes used clinically (Rottenberg et al., 1977). The available experimental and clinical data suggest that several factors contribute to the pathophysiology of rebound.

First, the progressive entry of the administered solute from the plasma into brain cells not only obliterates the osmotic gradient but also increases the total osmolality of the brain. Thereafter, there is a delay in the disappearance of the solute from brain cells. This accounts in part for a reversal in the osmotic gradient, which fosters an increase in intracellular water.

Second, the solute also reaches equilibrium in CSF, following which its exit from the CSF is slower than its disappearnce from the plasma. Such a delay would be responsible for greater osmolality of the CSF than of the plasma; the greater osmolality could account for water flux into the CSF and a higher CSF pressure. Increased absorption of CSF compensates for increased CSF pressure. CSF osmolality is probably of little importance in the pathogenesis of rebound.

Third, new idiogenic osmoles, described earlier, appear within brain cells; this is the normal adaptive response of brain to the acute increase in plasma osmolality just described. While idiogenic osmoles are considered to be transient, they increase intracellular osmolality and favor water retention (McDowell *et al.*, 1955; Arieff and Kleeman, 1973; Arieff *et al.*, 1977). The quantitative role of this mechanism in the genesis of rebound is difficult to assess, but it is probably an important factor.

Fourth, there may be a defective blood-brain barrier. Thus, Pappius and Dayes (1965) have shown that while hypertonic urea reduced the volume and water content of normal brain tissue, it had no effect on focal areas of vasogenic brain edema because the solute entered the pathologically permeable tissue so rapidly. Thus, with extensive damage to the barrier; rebound is more likely to occur; as a result, osmotherapy may have little or no effect on extensive vasogenic edema because of the ready entry of the solute into the pathological tissue. Thus, the more normal the brain, the greater the effect osmotherapy would have on intracranial hypertension, and the more abnormal the brain, the lesser the effect. The factors underlying the occurrence of rebound also are considered to contribute to the pathogenesis of the *dialysis disequilibrium syndrome*.

Dialysis Disequilibrium Syndrome

Disordered osmotic regulation underlies the major features of the dialysis disequilibrium syndrome, which occurs during or immediately after hemodialysis or peritoneal dialysis. The clinical features include headache, intracranial hypertension, and papilledema, as well as irritability, delirium, obtundation, coma, and seizures (Raskin and Fishman, 1976). An intracellular shift of water, due to a higher intracellular osmolality, appears to be responsible for the manifestations of the syndrome, which is akin to a water intoxication syndrome. The syndrome occurs with very rapid hemodialysis but can be averted with slow dialysis.

In an animal model of the syndrome, Arieff *et al.* (1973) demonstrated the presence within the brain of osmotically active solutes (osmoles) which exceeded the osmolality of the plasma or CSF. Their precise composition was not established, and they were considered to include idiogenic osmoles. There was an insufficient increase in the concentrations of urea or creatinine to make them quantitatively important. Similarly, the increase in the concentrations of the amino acids and ammonia in brain that also occurs in hyperosmolal states was also insufficient to account for the increased brain osmolality. However, changes in the metabolism of neurotransmitter amino acids probably underlie the vulnerability to seizures seen in the dysequilibrium syndromes. Changes in the reversible dissociation of intracellular potassium from a free to a bound state may serve as a control mechanism for the release and uptake of intracellular osmoles in response to osmotic gradients. This mechanism, suggested earlier to have a role in isosmotic regulation, may also be involved in the pathogenesis and resolution of the dysequilibrium state. (See page 91.)

In the cerebral edema associated with the treatment of diabetic ketoacidosis, the intracranial hypertension and the encephalopathy are probably also related to the presence of excessive intracellular glucose and other solutes which occurs with hyperglycemia (Arieff and Kleeman, 1973). The edema represents a form of osmotically determined cellular swelling that is analogous to the dialysis dysequilibrium syndrome. The increased polyols in the brain in hyperglycemia, discussed by Prockop (1971), are not present in sufficient concentration to be important osmotically; they may have other metabolic effects related to the encephalopathy.

HYDROCEPHALUS

Hydrocephalus is characterized by an increase in the volume of CSF associated with dilatation of the cerebral ventricles. Hydrocephalus is termed *active* when it is progressive and associated with increased intraventricular pressure, or *arrested* when intraventricular pressure has returned to normal and is no longer a stimulus for ventricular enlargement. *Normal pressure hydrocephalus* refers to hydrocephalus without apparent evidence of intracranial hypertension associated with inadequacy of the subarachnoid spaces. These forms of hydrocephalus are distinguished from *hydrocephalus ex vacuo*, which is characterized by an increase in the volume of CSF under normal pressure that is compensatory to the loss of brain tissue. In children, prior to the fusion of the cranial sutures, hydrocephalus causes enlargement of the skull. Hydrocephalus is termed *occult* when there are no signs or symptoms of intracranial hypertension. Hydrocephalus must be distinguished from other causes of macrocephaly in infancy, including subdural hematoma. The terms internal and external hydrocephalus are obsolete and no longer considered useful. The syndromes associated with benign intracranial hypertension (pseudotumor) will be discussed separately.

The terms *communicating* and *noncommunicating* hydrocephalus were introduced by Dandy and Blackfan (1914), based on the phenolsulfonphthalein (PSP) test, in which 1 ml of dye was injected into the lateral ventricle. In communicating hydrocephalus, the dye was detected in lumbar CSF 20 minutes later, but if the fluid was colorless then the hydrocephalus was termed noncommunicating in type. This functional classification has been accepted widely because it proved useful in the appropriate surgical placement of a shunt.

A heterogeneous group of neurological disorders underlies the pathogenesis of hydrocephalus (MacNab, 1966; Milhorat, 1972; De Lange, 1977). The pathological studies of Dorothy Russell (1949) emphasized that obstruction of the cerebrospinal fluid pathways was responsible for most forms of hydrocephalus. Obstruction secondary to congenital and acquired lesions could be responsible for either communicating or noncommunicating hydrocephalus.

The patency and capacity of the subarachnoid spaces in normal subjects and in the various forms of hydrocephalus are difficult to evaluate. With advanced communicating hydrocephalus, the cortical gyri are flattened and the sulci are grossly narrowed. In such cases, pneumoencephalography and isotope cisternography demonstrate variable degrees of obstruction of the basal cisterns as well as incisural block. Similar changes have also been seen in advanced cases of noncommunicating hydrocephalus. Table 4–1 provides a classification of the various forms of hydrocephalus based on etiology.

TABLE 4–1 Pathogenesis of Hydrocephalus

OBSTRUCTION OF CSF PATHWAYS: Intraventricular (noncommunicating) or extraventricular
    (communicating or noncommunicating)
        Postinflammatory or posthemorrhagic obstruction
        Congenital malformations:
           Arnold-Chiari malformations, meningomyelocele
           Occlusion of outlets of 4th ventricle (Dandy-Walker syndrome)
        Neoplasms obstructing the ventricular system
OVERPRODUCTION OF CSF:
        Choroid plexus papilloma (may also cause ventricular obstruction)
DEFECTIVE ABSORPTION OF CSF:
        Impaired venous drainage
        Defective arachnoid villi (congenital or acquired)

Pathophysiology of Hydrocephalus

Four possible mechanisms are considered to underlie the development of hydrocephalus: (1) oversecretion of CSF, (2) venous insufficiency, (3) impaired CSF absorption at the arachnoid villi, and (4) obstruction of the CSF pathways.

OVERSECRETION. The relative constancy of the rate of CSF formation and absorption in the face of various physiological and pharmacological manipulations has been described in Chapter 3. The data regarding the absorptive capacity of the subarachnoid space in normal subjects indicate that the intracranial pressure remains within normal limits with lumbar infusion rates of about 1.0 ml/min, three times the normal rate of CSF formation of 0.35 ml/min (Hussey and Katzman, 1970, Mann *et al.*, 1978). Thus, for oversecretion of CSF formation to induce intracranial hypertension, formation rates well in excess of 1.0 ml/min would be required.

There is no convincing evidence that increased CSF formation sufficient to cause intracranial hypertension occurs in any condition apart from choroid plexus papilloma. The literature about this rare tumor has been reviewed by Milhorat (1972) and by Welch (1977). In several case reports, hydrocephalus has been attributed either to ventricular obstruction due to the mass effect of the tumor or to the intraventricular hemorrhage that this tumor may precipitate. However, oversecretion of CSF by the tumor has been implicated in many cases because of the presence of marked hydrocephalus associated with small nonobstructive tumors.

Recently, Eisenberg *et al.* (1974) measured the rate of CSF production by the method of ventriculo-lumbar perfusion, both preoperatively and postoperatively, in a child with choroid plexus papilloma. The preoperative formation rate was greatly increased, about four times the normal rate, and it fell to a normal level following surgical removal. This observation supports earlier suggestions that the tumor may induce hydrocephalus by oversecretion of CSF, although this is only one of several mechanisms that may be responsible for the occurrence of hydrocephalus with such intraventricular tumors.

As discussed in Chapter 3, the rate of CSF production in normal subjects is relatively constant and is not affected by acute changes in intraventricular pressure. The data regarding the changes that occur in the presence of hydrocephalus are complex. Atrophy of the choroid plexus has been reported in patients with chronic hydrocephalus. Hochwald *et al.* (1969) reported a moderate reduction in CSF formation in hydrocephalic cats. Lorenzo *et al.* (1970) studied CSF formation in hydrocephalic patients by using ventriculo-cisternal perfusion and found an average formation rate of 0.30 ml/min, slightly lower than the rate of their normal patients. Welch (1975), in a detailed review of the subject, concluded that despite some contradictions in various experimental models, CSF formation probably occurs at normal or nearly normal rates in hydrocephalus, unless a choroid plexus papilloma is present. Regrettably, there are insufficient data available in patients to document this conclusion.

VENOUS INSUFFICIENCY.   Impaired cerebral venous drainage due to venous hypertension or thrombosis of the intracranial venous sinuses is generally not an important factor in the pathogenesis of hydrocephalus. Dural sinus thrombosis commonly leads to intracranial hypertension, but its role in the development of hydrocephalus is less well defined. As discussed earlier, the dural sinus pressure is normally lower than the intracranial pressure; this facilitates the normal absorption of CSF. In many clinical reports, intracranial hypertension has been documented with venous sinus thrombosis, either idiopathic or due to infection, trauma, tumor, or dehydration (see benign intracranial hypertension). The clinical syndromes vary, depending upon the precise location and extent of the venous occlusion and particularly upon the latter's rate of development, whether acute or chronic (Silbermann and Fishman, 1951). Focal neurological deficits occur when thrombosis extends into the hemispheric veins to cause venous infarction. However, whether or not venous sinus occlusion *per se* is responsible for ventricular dilatation has been a subject of some controversy.

Experimental studies designed to produce ventricular enlargement secondary to increased intracranial venous pressure have been inconsistent. Bering and Salibi (1959) reported success in obtaining ventricular dilatation by occlusion of all accessible intracranial venous structures in dogs, but Guthrie *et al.* (1970) were unsuccessful in obtaining dilatation by blocking the torcular. Radical neck dissection, superior vena cava obstruction, and dural sinus thrombosis have produced variable degrees of intracranial hypertension in patients, but ventricular enlargement has been reported only rarely (Symonds, 1937; Gius and Grier, 1950; Kinal, 1962; Kalbag and Woolf, 1967).

The various features responsible for the development of ventricular enlargement with venous obstruction require further elucidation. Under normal conditions, the CSF pressure exceeds the saggital sinus pressure; this facilitates the bulk flow reabsorption of CSF, as described before. However, in hydrocephalic children, Shulman and Ransohoff (1965) showed the sagittal sinus pressure to be equal to or to exceed the intracranial pressure. They attributed this to distortion and collapse of the dural venous sinuses, and they concluded that in hydrocephalus the CSF pressure becomes a determinant of the dural sinus pressure. Moreover, such an increase in venous outflow resistance serves further to inhibit bulk CSF absorption, thus favoring a vicious cycle. There are complex adjustments in such circumstances, and the degree of ventricular enlargement depends upon the compliance of the CSF spaces as well as on the compliance of the cerebrum and its vascular compartment. Another factor is the capacity for CSF absorption into the radicular veins that takes place in the spinal subarachnoid space. The quantitative importance of spinal absorption in humans is unknown.

In summary, while under some circumstances venous insufficiency plays a role in the pathogenesis of hydrocephalus, impaired CSF absorption by the arachnoid villi and obstruction of the CSF pathways are considered to be of much greater importance.

IMPAIRED CSF ABSORPTION BY THE ARACHNOID VILLI.   The unique ultrastructural features of the arachnoid villi have been described in Chapter 2. They include the presence of giant intracellular vesicles which, Tripathi (1977) suggested, are responsible for bulk CSF absorption. The arachnoid villi are difficult to study *post mortem*, and the literature regarding changes in the arachnoid villi in disease is sparse. Some case reports have attributed the occurrence of communicating hydrocephalus in infancy to the congenital agenesis of the villi (Gilles and Davidson, 1971; Gutierrez *et al.*, 1975). This defect may be a good deal more common than is realized, but it goes unrecognized because detailed pathological study of the number of villi present and their structural characteristics is a difficult task that is rarely performed.

The possibility of impaired function of the villi was suggested by Russell (1949) and other investigators to be responsible for some forms of communicating hydrocephalus. Bagley (1929) observed in dogs that intracisternal injections of blood resulted in hydrocephalus. Foltz and Ward (1956) and Kibler *et al.* (1961). defined the clinical syndrome that is now recognized as a frequent complication of subarachnoid hemorrhage. Ellington and Margolis (1969) provided a detailed pathological study of the morphological changes induced by blood in six cases of subarachnoid hemorrhage. They found a variable degree of distension of the arachnoid villi with packed red cells and suggested that this might lead to an acute disturbance of CSF absorption and to persistent scarring and impairment of function.

Denny-Brown (1952) described a patient with "external hydrocephalus" associated with polyneuritis and an elevated CSF protein. In his discussion of the pathogenesis of the syndrome, he mentioned "amorphous" material plugging the pacchionian granulations. Such a possible mechanism has been mentioned in subsequent case reports describing the occurrence of intracranial hypertension associated with papilledema and headache in patients with elevated CSF protein due to polyneuritis and spinal cord tumors. In these reports the ventricular size generally has not been described, and the frequency of the occurrence of ventricular dilatation in such cases is not known. The presence of normally sized ventricles has been observed in several such cases.

The most common cord tumor has been ependymoma, and in some reports the possibility of seeding of the tumor to the arachnoid villi has not been excluded (Teng *et al.*, 1960; Glasauer, 1964; Morley and Reynolds, 1966; Arseni and Maretsis, 1967; Buchsbaum and Gallo, 1969; Mittal *et al.*, 1970; Ridsdale and Moseley, 1978). However, the occurrence of papilledema, with or without hydrocephalus, in patients with spinal neurofibroma or meningioma, as well as the apparent cure of the intracranial hypertension following excision of either benign or malignant tumors, provides support for the hypothesis that substances derived from the spinal tumor (presumably cellular elements, including proteins and lipids) have blocked normal CSF absorption in an as yet undetermined fashion.

Prockop and Fishman (1968) showed that elevation of the spinal fluid protein in dogs by the intracisternal injection of homologous serum acutely slowed the clearance of inulin and iodinated albumin from the CSF, an observation that supports the existence of such a mechanism. On the other hand, there is a poor correlation in patients between the occurrence of the syndrome and the degree of protein elevation as measured in the lumbar sac. In no case has the concentration of protein in the subarachnoid space adjacent to the venous sinuses been reported, so this point is uncertain. It is possible that variations in the number of arachnoid villi and in their functional activity may be a major determinant in the rare development of intracranial hypertension with spinal tumors. The available data indicate that in some as yet unknown way, cellular products, proteins, lipids or all these, interfere with the vesicular transport of CSF by the villi to the venous system.

OBSTRUCTION OF THE CSF PATHWAYS. The best characterized and most common form of hydrocephalus is that following obstruction of either the intraventricular or the extraventricular CSF pathways. The site of obstruction determines the occurrence of hydrocephalic dilatation of the ventricle proximally, with preservation of normal ventricular size distally. The reviews of Milhorat (1972) and Welch (1975) have critically assessed the experimental literature, which will be referred to only briefly.

In noncommunicating hydrocephalus, the obstruction may be found at the foramen of Monro, the third ventricle, the aqueduct, the fourth ventricle, or the outflow of the foramina of Luschka and Magendie. In the latter instance, the fourth ventricle is expanded, and in early life there is expansion of the posterior fossa of the skull, i.e., the Dandy-Walker syndrome (Taggart and Walker, 1942; Welch, 1977). A variety of congenital malformations and acquired lesions, including neoplasms and inflammatory scarring following meningitis, may be responsible for noncommunicating hydrocephalus. Johnson and Johnson (1969) demonstrated that intrauterine viral infection may be responsible for the subsequent development of gliosis of the periaqueductal gray. These observations suggest that many obstructive lesions of the aqueduct, such as gliosis and forking, that were considered to be developmental by Russell (1949) may in fact be the residue of prior inflammatory lesions of viral origin occurring *in utero* or in early life.

Various developmental and acquired lesions are resonsible for the CSF obstructions that underlie the development of communicating hydrocephalus. The most common developmental lesion is the Arnold-Chiari malformation; the most common cause of communicating hydrocephalus is inflammation of the leptomeninges due to prior infection or hemorrhage. In the latter case, the subarachnoid spaces at the base of the brain, at the level of the tentorium, and over the convexities of the hemisphere, are narrowed and obstructed by gliosis and fibrosis. In addition, it seems likely that some patients with communicating hydrocephalus also have an absorptive defect at the level of the arachnoid villi, or that such a defect may be the major etiologic factor. It has often been difficult to determine the precise location of the absorptive block in communicating hydrocephalus because of the inherent limitations of pneumoencephalography and cisternography. Nevertheless, the question can be answered best in the clinical setting, because the artificial distortions of the post mortem state still make it very difficult to evaluate the patency and the capacity of the subarachnoid space after death.

The Pathogenesis of Ventricular Dilatation

The degree of ventricular enlargement that occurs at the expense of the adjacent cerebral tissue varies greatly, depending on the heterogeneous pathological processes that underlie both communicating and noncommunicating hydrocephalus. Active hydrocephalus is characterized by progressive ventricular dilatation, whereas in arrested or compensated hydrocephalus the ventricular size does not further increase and actually may decrease following a surgical shunt if done early enough, before the development of irreversible changes. Figure 4–5 reveals the striking increase in the thickness of the cerebral mantle (decrease in ventricular size) following a successful shunt. A reduction in the hydrocephalic edema affecting the periventricular white matter was also obtained. Ventricular enlargement is not a uniform process; it occurs chiefly at the expense of the periventricular white matter. The gray matter, including the cortex and basal ganglia, is relatively spared and little reduced in size.

The relative preservation of gray matter has not been satisfactorily explained. Gray matter normally has a greater blood supply and metabolic rate than does white matter (Purves, 1972). Grietz *et al*. (1969) reported, in hydrocephalus, a further reduction in the regional blood flow to the periventricular white matter. In advanced hydrocephalus, some of the changes in the mantle may be secondary to ischemia, but in the presence of mild or moderate degrees of ventricular dilatation there is evidence only of thinning of the white matter without any more specific pathological change. The role of changes in the microcirculation of the periventricular white matter in the pathogenesis of ventricular dilatation remains to be clarified.

The pathogenesis of ventricular dilatation has been studied in various laboratory models of obstructive hydrocephalus obtained following the intracisternal injection of foreign materials like kaolin or silicone oil, or by the inflation of a balloon in the posterior fossa (Welch, 1975). The first event in the subsequent development of ventricular enalrgement appears to be transependymal movement of ventricular fluid into the periventricular white matter, causing *interstitial* or *hydrocephalic* edema (*q.v.*). This was documented by Fishman and Greer (1963) in dogs made hydrocephalic with intracisternal kaolin. After 24 hours, there was an increase in water and sodium content in the periventricular white matter, despite the reduction in the thickness of the white matter and in its lipid content. These findings indicate that increased hydrostatic pressures in the periventricular white matter are responsible for a rapid disappearance of myelin lipids, which apparently may be a reversible process with therapy. Analogous findings were observed by Weller and Wisniewski (1969), who observed stretching of the ependyma and extracellular edema of the subependymal white matter in rabbits made hydrocephalic with intracisternal silicone oil.

Milhorat (1972, 1975) has documented the occurrence of ventricular enlargement within 4 hours following a thalamic hemorrhage from an ar-

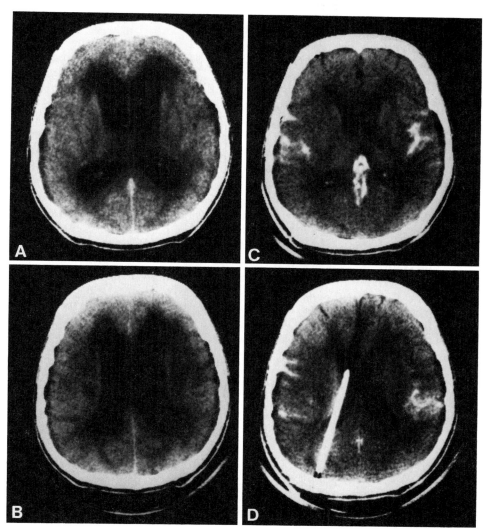

Figure 4-5 Computed tomograms. The effect of a ventriculoatrial shunt on obstructive hydrocephalus due to coccidioidal meningitis. Scans *A* and *B* were performed before the shunt. They reveal ventricular dilatation and a very striking hydrocephalic (interstitial) brain edema of the periventricular white matter, particularly at the frontal poles. Scans *C* and *D* were performed 7 days after placement of the shunt, which is visible. Note the striking reduction in ventricular size and the partial resolution of the interstitial edema of the periventricular white matter. (The areas of heightened contrast seen in the subarachnoid spaces and in the fourth ventricle are caused by the presence of metrizamide following its lumbar injection for cisternography.) (Courtesy of Dr. Edward M. Miller, San Francisco General Hospital.)

teriovenous malformation. Milhorat (1972, 1975) also studied the time course of ventricular enlargement in monkeys following obstruction of the fourth ventricle with an inflated balloon. Ventricular enlargement began immediately, and within 3 hours the hydrocephalic changes were pronounced. Thereafter, the rate of enlargement slowed, but persisted for 48 to 72 hours and longer. The rapid expansion of the ventricular cavities was associated with hemispheric enlargement and obliteration of the cerebral sulci, the cerebral fissures, and the basal cisterns. At 3 hours, acutely stretched and flattened ependymal cells were noted, and there were breaks in their continuity, beginning first at the lateral angles of the lateral ventricles. Within 24 to 48 hours, the white matter became spongy and edematous with a loss of white matter volume. The changes in the white matter indicate that increased hydrostatic tissue pressures have a major effect on the function of oligodendroglial cells, which are the parent cells for the formation of the multilamellated structure of myelin. However, Milhorat (1972) considered the astrocytes to be the most vulnerable cells because they appeared to be reduced in numbers.

It is of special interest that there was no evidence of axonal swelling, demyelinization, or neuronal change. With regard to the reversibility of hydrocephalus, Milhorat (1972) reported that the thickness of the mantle could be returned to normal if the ventricular obstruction was removed during the first three weeks. Thereafter, the changes became irreversible, with persistent loss of glial cells and the presence of lipid-laden macrophages.

In summary, the precise mechanism whereby hydrocephalic (interstitial) edema leads to pressure atrophy of the white matter is not understood, nor are the factors known which determine reversibility of hydrocephalus. While it has been often assumed, as noted earlier, that the changes are largely ischemic in origin (Greitz et al., 1969), the pathological findings are in many ways different, and, at present, the biological basis of hydrostatic pressure-induced atrophy of the white matter (ventricular dilatation) is not known.

Normal Pressure Hydrocephalus

The recognition of normal pressure hydrocephalus (NPH) as a potentially treatable dementia has captured wide attention. Although the occurrence of the delayed onset of hydrocephalus following subarachnoid hemorrhage had been reported earlier (Foltz and Ward, 1956; Kibler et al., 1961), the syndrome was first delineated by Hakim (1964), and by Adams et al. (1965) as an occult form of communicating hydrocephalus, wherein the occurrence of intracranial hypertension was either absent or not recognized.

Typically, there is a gradual development, over weeks or months, of a mild impairment of memory and intellect with mental and physical slowness (psychomotor retardation), which progresses insidiously to a severe dementia with an apraxic gait and finally urinary incontinence. Patients are free of headache and have no obvious signs of increased intracranial pressure, that is, they have normal fundi and normal CSF pressure at the time of routine diagnostic lumbar puncture. Pneumoencephalography has revealed large ventricles, a widening of the callosal angle, and a lack of filling of the subarachnoid space over the hemispheres. Computed tomography reveals analogous findings and has become a most useful screening test. There have been efforts to use the size of the callosal angle in differentiating NPH from Alzheimer's disease (Sjaastad and Nordvik, 1973), but the diagnostic reliability of the size of the callosal angle is limited. Clinical deterioration following pneumoencephalography has been commonly observed in NPH. Isotope cisternography following lumbar injections has often (but not invariably) revealed pathological reflux of the isotope into the ventricular system with delayed and inadequate visualization of the cortical subarachnoid spaces (Harbert, 1972). Greitz (1969) reported the angiographic findings to include delayed emptying of the cerebral veins, narrowing of the cerebral arteries, and prolongation of the circulation time — radiographic features not seen with cerebral atrophy. However, these features have not been sufficiently definitive to make them diagnostic in the clinical analysis of such cases.

In a few patients, the occurrence of NPH has also been attributed to ectasia of the basilar artery, which apparently interferes with CSF flow through the aqueduct (Ekbom et al., 1969). The syndrome is termed "symptomatic NPH" when it develops following subarachnoid hemorrhage or meningoencephalitis; however, in primary NPH the cause is obscure. The true incidence of primary and symptomatic NPH is not known, nor is the natural history of the disorder well defined in terms of either its rate of progression or the temporal factors that underlie reversibility of the process spontaneously or with a surgical shunt.

Pathophysiology

The results of pneumoencephalography and isotope cisternography indicate that NPH represents a form of communicating hydrocephalus with obliteration or insufficiency of the subarachnoid spaces over the hemispheric convexities, resulting in a block to the circulation and absorption of the CSF. The absence of papilledema and increased intracranial pressure led to the use of the term "normal pressure" hydrocephalus. However, the likelihood that intracranial hypertension occurs intermittently has been supported by the observations of Symon et al. (1972) obtained while monitoring the intracranial pressure in suspected cases. Patients with NPH had episodic intracranial hypertension, with plateau waves, which occurred only during REM sleep; these authors have depended upon this finding as a guide to the selection of patients for a surgical shunt. They concluded that clinical improvement following shunting occurs in those patients who demonstrated episodic intracranial hypertension during sleep. However, Nornes et al. (1973) reported that this correlation was not an invariable one.

There has been considerable speculation about the pathophysiology of NPH. Hakim (1972, 1977) emphasized the relevance of Pascal's law (force = pressure × area) to the viscoelastic properties of the brain in the pathogenesis of ventricular dilatation. He suggested that NPH occurs as a result of high pressure hydrocephalus, which induces ventricular enlargment, and that the latter is perpetuated by the greater force directed to the ventricular surface when its surface area is increased, despite the return of the intraventricular pressure to the normal range. While Pascal's law regarding a perfect sphere is not in question, its relevance to the pathophysiology of NPH has not been established. The viscoelastic properties of the cerebrum are complex. The metabolic basis of hydrostatic pressure-induced atrophy of the periventricular white matter is poorly understood. The biological basis for ventricular enlargement and its return toward normal after shunting remains largely unexplained.

I have suggested that the transmural pressure gradient between the ventricles and the subarachnoid space might be more important than the actual level of intraventricular pressure (Fishman, 1965) in the pathogenesis of ventricular dilatation. Thus, if the pressure in the cortical subarachnoid space was lower — for example, 50 mm less than the intraventricular pressure — then this transmural pressure gradient could serve as a factor underlying ventricular enlargement, despite a normal intraventricular pressure.

Hoff and Barber (1974) tested this hypothesis in 4 patients with post-traumatic NPH. They recorded, under anesthesia, the intraventricular and the cerebral subdural pressures while infusing normal saline into the lumbar sac at a rate of 0.76 ml/min to elevate the CSF pressure (see the flush test). The baseline intraventricular pressure was 1 to 2 mm Hg (13 to 26 mm water) higher than the subdural pressure, which represented the initial transmural pressure gradient. After lumbar infusion for 30 minutes, the pressure had risen in both sites with an average peak pressure of 34 mm Hg (440 mm water), and the transmural

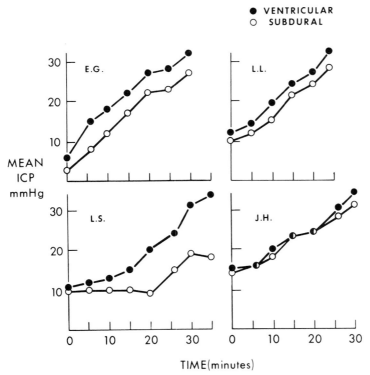

● VENTRICULAR
○ SUBDURAL

MEAN
ICP
mmHg

TIME(minutes)

Figure 4–6 The intracranial pressure recorded in the lateral ventricle and subdural space during lumbar saline infusion (0.76 ml/min). Note the progressive increase in the pressure gradient across the cerebral mantle in patient L. S. See text (from Hoff and Barber, 1974).

pressure gradient was maintained, rising to 2 to 4 mm Hg (26 to 52 mm water). The peak gradient obtained was 16 mm Hg (208 mm water). The findings are illustrated in Figure 4–6. Only 1 patient was clinically improved after shunting, the patient who showed the highest transmural pressure gradient.

This study supports the hypothesis that obliteration or inadequacy of the cortical subarachnoid space results in a pressure gradient across the cerebral mantle which contributes to the process of ventricular dilatation despite normal ventricular pressures. Perhaps a key factor is the degree of transependymal movement of CSF which induces the pressure atrophy of the periventricular white matter. This possible mechanism needs further study with regard to the effects of transcerebral pressure gradients upon the microcirculation and the metabolism of the cerebral mantle.

Lorenzo and associates (1974) studied CSF absorption in 5 patients with NPH, using ventriculo-cisternal perfusion. The average rate of CSF formation was 0.31 ml/min, somewhat less than the rates of 0.37 ml/min in patients with brain tumor and 0.35 ml/min in children with meningeal leukemia and subacute sclerosing panencephalitis. It is possible that this minor decrease in formation reflected a reduction in choroid plexus function. The 5 patients showed three different abnormal patterns of CSF absorption. In Type I, absorption occurred at a normal rate, but the pressure at which CSF absorption appeared to begin was increased from 68 mm to 164 mm, and the equilibrium pressure (the pressure at which CSF formation equals absorption) was increased from 112 mm to 208 mm. In Type II, absorption increased linearly with pressure, as expected, but at a much slower rate. In Type III, absorption increased with pressure at an apparently normal rate at low pressure levels, but when pressures of 120 to 160 mm were reached, the rate of absorption was very much reduced.

The three types of absorptive defects and the normal patterns are illustrated in Figure 4–7. The pathological changes that underlie each type of absorptive defect are not clear. Whether a defect in arachnoid villus function, rather than obliteration of the subarachnoid spaces, is associated with a specific type of absorptive defect is not known. Further use of this kind of functional analysis of the absorptive defects in NPH is needed to elucidate its mechanism as well as the factors that underlie progressive and compensated forms of hydrocephalus.

Isotope Cisternography in the
Evaluation of Normal Pressure
Hydrocephalus

The introduction of isotope (radionuclide) encephalography by DiChiro and others in 1962 led to its application to various clinical problems, including the elucidation of the CSF pathways in hydrocephalus, the demonstration of CSF rhinorrhea and other fistulas, and the assessment of shunt function (Harbert, 1972). A wide variety of radioactive agents, in both colloidal and soluble forms, have been used to evaluate the CSF spaces following intrathecal injection, using external detectors to measure the gamma radiation. An ideal agent would be metabolically inert in the nervous system, lipid insoluble, non-irritant, non-antigenic, non-pyrogenic, easily sterilized, and easily labelled

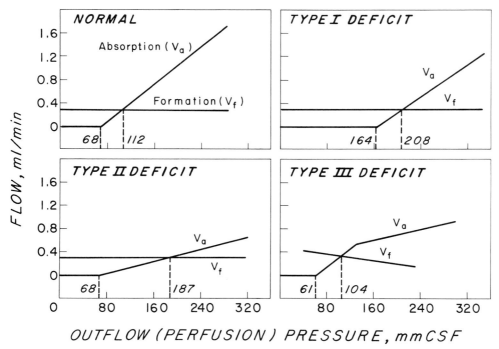

Figure 4-7   Pressure-absorption relationship observed in patients with and without obstruction to CSF pathways. Opening pressures and pressures at which formation equals absorption are designated in italic numbers. See text (from Lorenzo, Bresnan, and Barlow, 1974).

with a suitable gamma-emitting isotope. It would also have rapid blood clearance and a high rate of molecular diffusion, and it would disappear from the CSF by bulk flow absorption. Radioiodinated serum albumin, technetium-labelled serum albumin, and technetium-labelled EDTA have been the most widely used preparations. The technique is subject to technical error and misinterpretation when the isotope is injected unknowingly into the subdural space instead of the subarachnoid space.

When the tracer is injected into the lumbar sac, it is detected in the basal cisterns in about an hour, and thereafter it rises over the hemispheric convexities toward the parasagittal region. There have been several classifications of the distribution of the tracer (Harbert, 1972). Reflux of the isotope into the ventricular system had been demonstrated in patients with communicating hydrocephalus, including normal pressure hydrocephalus (Bannister *et al.*, 1967; Benson *et al.*, 1970; Harbert, 1972). However, the presence of ventricular reflux has not proved to determine reliably which patients are likely to improve following a surgical shunt (Wolinsky *et al.*, 1973; Stein *et al.*, 1974).

The occurrence of frequent false positive and false negative tests with cisternography is perplexing. False positive tests appear to indicate that the hydrocephalus is in a compensated or new steady state, and shunting is unable to reverse the process. With false negative tests, it seems likely that local anatomical variations at the foramina of Luschka and Magendie prevent entry of the isotope into the ventricular system, despite relative insufficiency of the subarachnoid spaces. Despite the limitations of cisternography, it continues to be used by many clinicians in the diagnosis of normal pressure hydrocephalus.

Water soluble contrast media (metrizamide) used with computed tomography shows promise as a means of visualizing the CSF pathways in normal subjects and in patients with various forms of hydrocephalus. Its patterns of distribution are likely to be similar to those observed with isotope cisternography.

Treatment of Hydrocephalus

A discussion of the treatment of hydrocephalus, including indications, methods, and results, is not within the scope of this volume. Pharmacological approaches to therapy have been limited (Milhorat, 1972). There have been a few favorable reports regarding the use of acetazolamide; the rationale for its use is based on its ability to reduce CSF formation about 50 per cent in animals, as discussed earlier. Rubin *et al.* (1966) reported a similar effect in patients. It is not known whether the acute effects of the drug are sustained for a long time. Huttenlocher (1965) treated 15 children for 6 months to 2½ years with an apparent arrest of the hydrocephalus in 8 of them. The spontaneous rate of arrest in such patients is conjectural. Other reports indicate that carbonic anhydrase inhibitors are ineffective in the management of hydrocephalus (Schain, 1969). Further clinical studies are needed to determine the role of the drug in clinical practice.

The major approach to therapy has been surgical. Many different procedures have been advocated in various neurosurgical centers in the last 50 years. They serve as a testament to the ingenuity of neurosurgeons in their efforts to empty the CSF pathways more efficiently. The procedures are indicated schematically in Figure 4–8. The reader is referred to Milhorat's (1972) review of the various approaches to surgical therapy for further discussion. Shurtleff *et al.* (1975) studied the effects of shunting on infantile hydrocephalus. After 15 years the survival rate was about 50 per cent, and about 15 per cent of these survivors were retarded. With regard to the treatment of normal pressure hydrocephalus, Messert and Wannamaker (1974) concluded that 51 per cent of 142 cases reported in the literature were improved by operation. The success rate was greater in patients having the characteristic syndrome of mild dementia, gait disorder, and incontinence as well as a history of *recent* progression. In chronic cases, the pathological process was unlikely to be reversed.

BRAIN EDEMA

Cerebral edema accompanies a wide variety of pathological processes in the brain, and it contributes to the morbidity and mortality of many neurological diseases. It plays a major role in head injury, stroke, and brain tumor, as well as in cerebral infections, including brain abscess, encephalitis and meningitis, lead encephalopathy, hypoxia, hypo-osmolality, the disequilibrium syndromes associated with dialysis and diabetic keto-acidosis, and the various forms of obstruc-

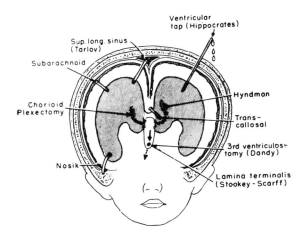

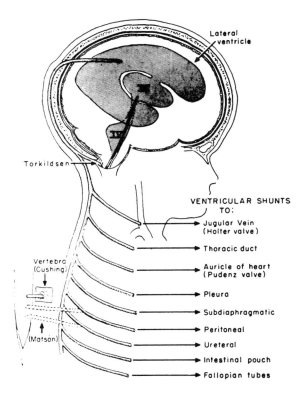

Figure 4-8 Hydrocephalic shunts. This figure illustrates the many surgical shunting procedures that have been used in the past to reduce CSF volume by facilitating CSF removal from the craniospinal space (from Ransohoff, Shulman, and Fishman, 1960).

tive hydrocephalus. In the last 15 years, clinical investigation and laboratory studies of brain edema using neurochemical, physiological, and ultrastructural techniques have clarified many pathological and clinical uncertainties. Cerebral edema may occur in several different forms; it is inappropriate to view brain edema as a single pathological or clinical entity.

This section summarizes current views of the biochemistry and pathophysiology of brain edema and their clinical and therapeutic implications. Several monographs and symposia deal with various aspects of the problem (Reulen and Schurmann, 1972; Katzman and Pappius, 1973; Pappius and Feindel, 1976; Beks *et al.*, 1976; Katzman *et al.*, 1977).

Definitions

In the early literature, brain edema and brain swelling were considered to be different processes, but these terms are now used synonymously. Brain edema is best defined as an increase in brain volume due to an increase in its water and sodium content. Brain edema, when well localized or mild in degree, is associated with little or no clinical evidence of brain dysfunction, but when severe it causes major focal or generalized signs of brain dysfunction, including the various types of cerebral herniation described earlier and medullary failure of respiration and circulation.

Brain edema and brain engorgement are different processes. *Brain engorgement* is an increase in the blood volume of the brain caused by obstruction of the cerebral veins and venous sinuses, or by arterial vasodilatation such as that caused by hypercarbia. Brain engorgement may result in a major increase in brain volume during craniotomy because of the absence of the rigid restriction of the bone skull; such vasodilatation may coexist with brain edema. Intracranial hypertension and brain edema commonly occur together, but they do not necessarily coexist. For example, brain edema may affect one hemisphere and cause focal signs of neurological dysfunction with preservation of normal intracranial pressure, and intracranial hypertension may occur without brain edema, as happens when 5 per cent carbon dioxide is inhaled by normal subjects.

Measurement of Edema

The usual procedure for the definition of edema *in vivo* involves sampling the edematous area of brain (or spinal cord) and a control area (preferably the homologous contralateral area) and determining the respective dry weight percentages. This is most conveniently done by weighing each fresh tissue sample (wet weight) in a tared container, drying the sample at approximately 100° C to constant weight (usually within 12 to 14 hours), and reweighing to obtain the weight of the residue (dry weight). The percentage is simply calculated as:

$$\text{(dry weight/wet weight)} \times 100 = \% \text{ dry weight (P)}$$

The percentage of swelling or edema (or of shrinkage) can then be calculated by the formula of Elliott and Jasper (1949):

$$(P_{control} - P_{exptl})/P_{exptl} \times 100 = \% \text{ swelling (or shrinkage)}$$

The same techniques are suitable for measuring edema in *in vitro* studies.

Biochemistry of Brain Edema

The chemical basis of brain edema was first established by Stewart-Wallace (1939) in terms of the changes in water and electrolyte content of the edematous tissue surrounding brain tumors. He showed that the cortex surrounding tumors had only a minor increase in swelling, less than 5 per cent, compared with the white matter where the swelling was increased 77 per cent. These data verified in chemical terms the neuropathological observation that white matter is far more vulnerable to edema formation than gray matter.

These clinical observations were later confirmed in various experimental models, including freezing lesions, stab wounds, implanted tumors, and compressive lesions due to intracranial balloons and foreign materials like psyllium seeds (Katzman and Pappius, 1973). With these disruptive lesions, the edema fluid was shown to have the features of a plasma exudate, a high sodium and plasma protein content and an increased volume of the extracellular fluid space. The most commonly studied lesion has been a freezing lesion of the cortex, but the data obtained with the gamut of disruptive lesions have been quite similar. Laboratory models of hypoxia and water intoxication showed increased brain water and sodium, but the extracellular fluid space was decreased in volume, as opposed to the findings in the models just described. These changes were the basis for the delineation of the vasogenic and cytotoxic brain edemas by Klatzo (1967). (The methods used for measurement of the extracellular fluid volume were discussed in Chapter 3.) There has also been special interest in the ability of various toxins to induce brain edema, most notably triethyl tin and lead.

Triethyl tin induces severe brain edema affecting both the white and gray matter in humans and animals (Katzman *et al.*, 1963; Hirano *et al.*, 1968). The major accumulation of water and sodium is intracellular, with astrocytic swelling being more marked than neuronal swelling. There is a striking abnormality of the white matter with accumulation of fluid within the myelin sheath; the myelin lamellae split at the interperiod line to form large blebs. Thus, triethyl tin appears to have special effects on the integrity of the oligodendroglia, from whose cellular membranes myelin is derived. The water and sodium content of the white matter is increased, but the integrity of the blood-brain barrier is preserved, measured by radioiodinated albumin or vital dyes. Thus, unlike the findings in lead encephalopathy, the integrity of cerebral capillary endothelial cells is preserved in triethyl tin poisoning. The biochemical basis for the toxic effects of triethyl tin is not specifically known. The activity of sodium-activated ATPase, the enzyme that functions as the ion pump in cellular membranes, is not affected. While morphological changes in brain mitochondria as well as inhibition of oxidative phosphorylation have been described, the relationships of these changes to edema formation are not clear. It is of interest that a surgical biopsy performed on a patient with the brain edema of Reye's syndrome revealed a splitting of the myelin lamellae reminiscent of triethyl tin intoxication, so that such changes are not unique to this toxin (Partin *et al.*, 1975).

Using an animal model of lead encephalopathy, Goldstein *et al.* (1977) demonstrated that the capillary endothelial cell is selectively poisoned by lead, giving rise to massive vasogenic edema, particularly in infancy. The special vulnerability of the immature brain to lead intoxication has not been explained.

In Vitro *Studies of Brain Edema*

The extensive literature about the factors influencing the swelling of brain slices *in vitro* was summarized by Katzman and Pappius (1973). These studies are relevant chiefly to cellular (cytotoxic) edema as opposed to vasogenic edema, because the blood-brain barrier is absent in such preparations. Hypoxia and the addition of chemical inhibitors of glycolysis to the incubating medium cause cellular swelling, in each case attributable to a failure of the energy-dependent active transport of sodium and water from the cell, with a fall in brain ATP levels. Increases in the water and sodium content of rat cortex associated with a decreased inulin space have been used as an *in vitro* bioassay for the analysis of factors responsible for tissue swelling (Fishman *et al.*, 1977a, 1977b).

The cardiac glycoside ouabain has been identified as a specific inhibitor of sodium and potassium transport. Its effect is mediated by its binding to and inhibition of the enzyme sodium-potassium activated ATPase, present in cellular membranes. Ouabain causes cellular edema when used in both *in vitro* with brain slices and *in vivo* studies. Local application of ouabain to the cortex results in convulsions and the morphological and biochemical changes of edema (Lewin, 1971). Thus, with light microscopy status spongiosus was observed, and with electron microscopy there was evidence of cellular swelling. Both neuronal and glial elements are probably affected by the topical application of ouabain in both *in vivo* and *in vitro* studies, but there are possible differences in the vulnerability of the two cell types to ouabain and to other edema-producing agents (Towfighi and Gonatas, 1973).

Free Radicals

The experimental literature supports a role for free radicals in the genesis of the permeability changes underlying brain edema (Demopoulos *et al.*, 1972, 1977). Free radicals are ions with a lone electron, possessing unusual chemical reactivity, including an ability to alter and to fragment membrane lipids. Free radicals are short-lived because they are rapidly inactivated by either direct chemical transmutation or specific enzymes. Three free radicals studied in various biological systems are *superoxide ions, hydroxyl radicals,* and *singlet oxygen.* Specific enzymes rapidly convert the free radicals to less reactive metabolites; they include superoxide dismutase and catalase (Fridovich, 1975). An extensive literature suggests that free radicals are involved in the peroxidation of membrane lipids (Michelson *et al.*, 1977). The role of free radicals in the pathogenesis of the various types of brain edema is under active study. Experimentally, protective effects of barbiturates on the development of hypoxic edema may be related to the drugs' protective action against the effects of free radicals, apart from the protective effects of depressing brain metabolism (Flamm *et al.*, 1978).

Free radicals have a role in the process of phagocytosis by polymorphonuclear granulocytes. This role is of special interest because granulocytes and their products constitute pus, which is associated with *granulocytic brain edema*, a condition occurring with purulent meningitis and brain abscess. The presence in pus of polyunsaturated fatty acids like arachidonic and linolenic acids has been considered to contribute to the induction of edema (Chan and Fishman, 1978). Recent data indicate that polyunsaturated fatty acid–induced brain edema is associated with increased superoxide formation in the cortex (Fishman *et al.*, 1979).

Polyunsaturated Fatty Acids

The ability of the membranes of polymorphonuclear leukocytes (WBC's) to induce cortical swelling has provided an *in vitro* model of granulocytic brain edema (Fishman *et al.*, 1977; Chan and Fishman, 1978). Analysis of the granulocytic membranes revealed that only lipid soluble components were responsible for edema formation. Further analysis of the membrane lipids demonstrated that several polyunsaturated acids (PUFA's), including arachidonic acid (C20:4) and linoleic acid (C18:2), produced edema, whereas saturated fatty acids like palmitic acid (C16:0) had no such effects.

Arachidonic acid is of special interest because it is a major constituent of the cellular and subcellular membranes of normal brain tissue and brain tumors, as well as of granulocytic leukocytes (Bazan, 1976). The fact that arachidonic acid is a precursor of the prostaglandins was *not* considered relevant to edema production. First, other PUFA's were equal to arachidonic acid in their edema-producing effects, although they were not precursors of the prostaglandins. Second, the prostaglandins were shown to lack edema-producing effects in the bioassay system (Chan and Fishman, 1978).

It is probably only the free polyunsaturated fatty acids that produce edema, i.e., protein-bound PUFA's are inactive in this regard. We have suggested that the special vulnerability of the brain to swelling from various injuries and malignant tumors might depend upon the local release of intrinsic arachidonic acid and other PUFA's from a bound to a free form. As noted earlier, the superoxide free radical may mediate the deleterious effects of PUFA's on cell membranes, a process manifested by the increased formation of lipid peroxides. Furthermore, adrenal glucocorticoids inhibit the release of arachidonic acid from cell membranes; this may be an important factor in the antiedema effects of such steroids (Hong and Levine, 1976). This hypothesis requires further substantiation in various models of brain edema.

Neurotransmitters, Kinins, and Lysosomal Enzymes

Preliminary data suggest that various chemical agents may be factors in the induction of brain edema. Several neurotransmitters and biogenic amines have been shown to induce brain edema *in vivo* and *in vitro*. Intracerebral injection of serotonin (5-hydroxytryptamine) causes vasogenic edema associated with stimulation of pinocytosis in capillary endothelial cells (Westergaard, 1975). The excitatory neurotransmitter amino acids, glutamate and aspartate, and their structural analogs and isomers induce brain edema *in vitro* (Chan *et al.*, 1979). On the other hand, inhibitory neurotransmitter amino acids, such as gamma aminobutyric acid (GABA), acetylcholine, and choline, have no such effect. Whether the effects of the excitatory neurotransmitters, demonstrated experimentally, also contribute to edema formation in concussion or states of osmotic disequilibrium requires elucidation.

Study of the edema-promoting effects of the plasma kallikrein-kinin system was initiated because plasma constituents make direct contact with the cerebral parenchyma in vasogenic edema (Baethmann *et al.*, 1979). Sicuteri *et al.* (1970) showed that the dilution of plasma with CSF leads to activation of the kallikrein-kinin system. Kallikrein is the activating enzyme in tissues, including brain. Kinogens, the precursors of kinins, are constituents of the alpha globulin plasma fraction. Preliminary data of Baethmann *et al.* (1979) showed that ventriculo-cisternal perfusion with plasma induced brain edema concomitantly with kinin formation. The role of the kallikrein-kinin system in the development of vasogenic brain edema requires further study.

The role of lysosomal enzymes, the proteolytic enzymes contained within membrane-bound intracytoplasmic units, in the response to cord trauma was studied by Clendenon *et al.* (1978). They concluded that the release of these enzymes into the cytoplasm or extracellular fluid does not play a role in the early response to injury. Bingham *et al.* (1971) suggested that the protective effects of steroids on cold-induced vasogenic edema were related to a stabilizing influence on lysosomal enzymes. The possible place of these proteolytic enzymes in the pathogenesis of vasogenic edema requires substantiation.

Pathophysiology of Brain Edema

Klatzo (1967) classified brain edema into two major categories, *vasogenic* edema and *cytotoxic* edema, based on both neuropathological and experimental observations. To these has been added a third general category, termed *interstitial* or *hydrocephalic* edema (Manz, 1974; Fishman, 1975), which refers to the increase in brain water that characterizes hydrocephalus. The features of the three forms of cerebral edema are summarized in Table 4–2 in terms of pathogenesis, location and composition of the edema fluid, and changes in capillary permeability. The term *vasogenic edema* appropriately indicates the importance of the capillary endothelial cell in the pathogenesis of this type of edema. The term *cellular edema* is preferable to that of cytotoxic edema because it focuses on the importance of increased cellular volume as the basis for the edema, and it avoids assuming that toxic states are necessarily the cause, i.e., it may arise from energy depletion *per se*.

Vasogenic Edema

Vasogenic edema is the most common form of brain edema observed in clinical practice. It is characterized by increased permeability of brain capillary endothelial cells to macromolecules, such as albumin and various other molecules, whose entry is limited by the capillary endothelial cells. The special anatomical features and permeability characteristics of brain capillaries and the blood-brain barrier have been described in Chapters 2 and 3. In the vasogenic edemas, the functional integrity of the endothelial cells is altered. Increased endothelial permeability has been found in various experimental models, including freezing lesions, stab wounds, brain compression, anoxia, experimental brain tumors, and allergic encephalomyelitis (Katzman *et al.*, 1977; Rapoport, 1976). The increase in permeability varies inversely with the molecular weight of various markers, with a greater increase in the entry of inulin (MW 5000) than in that of albumin (MW 69,000).

There is ultrastructural evidence for defects in the tight endothelial cell junctions of the blood-brain barrier as well as for an increase in the number of vesicles in the endothelial cells responsible for the vesicular transport of macromolecules (see Chapter 3). There is increasing evidence that increased vesicular transport is characteristic of the vasogenic edemas (Westergaard, 1978; Petito,

TABLE 4–2   Classification of Brain Edema

	VASOGENIC	CELLULAR (*Cytotoxic*)	INTERSTITIAL (*Hydrocephalic*)
Pathogenesis	Increased capillary permeability	Cellular swelling – glial, neuronal, endothelial	Increased brain fluid due to block of CSF absorption
Location of edema	Chiefly white matter	Gray and white matter	Chiefly periventricular white matter in hydrocephalus
Edema fluid composition	Plasma filtrate including plasma proteins	Increased intracellular water and sodium	Cerebrospinal fluid
Extracellular fluid volume	Increased	Decreased	Increased
Capillary permeability to large molecules (RISA, insulin)	Increased	Normal	Normal
Clinical disorders	Brain tumor, abscess, infarction, trauma, hemorrhage, lead encephalopathy Ischemia Purulent meningitis (granulocytic edema)	Hypoxia, hypo-osmolality due to water intoxication, etc. Disequilibrium syndromes Ischemia Purulent meningitis (granulocytic edema) Reye's syndrome	Obstructive hydrocephalus Pseudotumor (?) Purulent meningitis (granulocytic edema)
EEG changes	Focal slowing common	Generalized slowing	EEG often normal
THERAPEUTIC EFFECTS			
Steroids	Beneficial in brain tumor, abscess	Not effective (? Reye's syndrome)	Uncertain effectiveness (? Pseudotumor, ? meningitis)
Osmotherapy	Reduces volume of normal brain tissue only, *acutely*	Reduces brain volume *acutely* in hypo-osmolality	Rarely useful
Acetazolamide	? Effect	No direct effect	Minor usefulness
Furosemide	? Effect	No direct effect	Minor usefulness

(After Klatzo, 1967; Manz, 1974; Fishman, 1975)

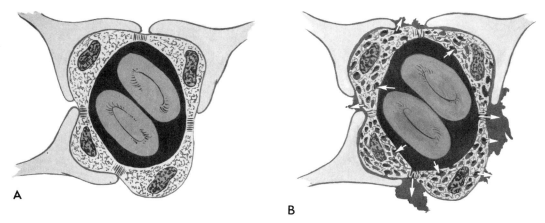

Figure 4–9A and B   On the left, A, the normal capillary is shown enclosing two red cells. The tight intercellular junctions are indicated. The capillary is surrounded by the feet of astrocytes. On the right, B, the alterations associated with vasogenic brain edema are shown schematically. There are increased numbers of pinocytic vesicles, which are probably responsible for the increased passage of macromolecules as noted in Figure 3–10. The passage of plasma solutes across tight intercellular junctions is also shown schematically. The quantitative importance of the two routes, increased vesicular transport and increased junctional leakage, is not known.

1979). The changes characteristic of vasogenic edema are shown in Figure 4–9. The quantitative importance of each of these two changes is not known. The cerebral white matter is far more vulnerable than the gray matter to vasogenic edema, but this vulnerability is not well understood; it may be related to the lower capillary density and blood flow in normal white matter than in the cortical and subcortical gray matter. The extracellular fluid volume is increased by the edema fluid, which is a plasma filtrate containing plasma proteins.

Vasogenic edema is associated with those clinical disorders in which there is frequently a positive contrast enhanced computed tomogram, including brain tumor, abscess, hemorrhage, infarction, and contusion. It also occurs with lead encephalopathy (Goldstein *et al.*, 1977) and with purulent meningitis (Prockop and Fishman, 1968). An increase in endothelial cell permeability is responsible for the characteristic increase in CSF protein observed in these disorders. Vasogenic edema can displace the hemisphere and be responsible for the various types of cerebral herniation described earlier in this chapter. The functional manifestations of vasogenic edema include focal neurological deficits, focal electroencephalographic slowing, disturbances of consciousness, and severe intracranial hypertension. In patients with brain tumor, whether primary or metastatic, the clinical deficits are often caused more by the peritumoral edema than by the tumor mass itself.

Cellular (Cytotoxic) Edema

Cellular edema is characterized by swelling of all the cellular elements of the brain (neurons, glia, and endothelial cells), with a concomitant reduction in the volume of the brain's extracellular fluid space. These changes are shown in

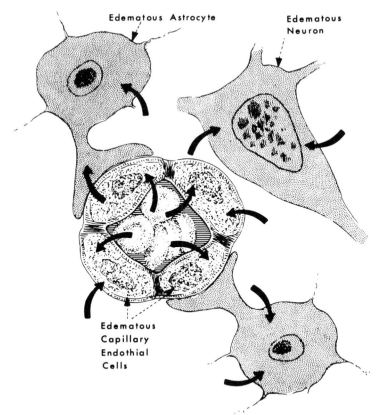

Edematous Astrocyte

Edematous
Neuron

Figure 4–10 Cellular (cytotoxic) edema. Neurons, glia, and endothelial cells swell as a result of the intracellular movement of the extracellular fluid (from Fishman, 1975).

Edematous
Capillary
Endothial
Cells

Figure 4–10. Their occurrence in acute ischemia was described by Van Harreveld (1966), who used a rapid increase in electrical impedance as an index of such changes. Hossmann (1976) studied such changes in cats subjected to 30 minutes of clamping of the middle cerebral artery. This resulted in a rapid increase in the electrical resistance of the tissue, indicating an acute reduction in the volume of the extracellular fluid space. Brain cells swell within seconds of hypoxia because of failure of the ATP-dependent sodium pump within cells; sodium rapidly accumulates within cells, and water follows to maintain osmotic equilibrium (MacKnight and Leaf, 1977). These changes are illustrated in Figure 4–11, as are their reversibility following removal of the arterial clamp. (When endothelial cells are particularly affected, the capillary lumen may be encroached upon, perhaps contributing to an increased resistance to arterial perfusion, the "no-reflow" phenomenon. The occurrence of "no-reflow" has been a controversial issue in the laboratory; its importance in disease states is not known.) Capillary permeability is usually not affected in the various cellular edemas; patients so affected have a normal CSF protein, isotopic brain scan, and computed tomogram.

There are several causes of cellular edema. (1) Hypoxia after cardiac arrest or asphyxia results in cerebral energy depletion. The cellular swelling is osmotically determined by the appearance of increased intracellular osmoles (especially sodium, lactate, and hydrogen ions), which induce the rapid entry of water into cells (Siesjo, 1978). (2) Acute hypo-osmolality of the plasma and extracellular fluid is due to acute dilutional hyponatremia, inappropriate secretion of antidiuretic hormone, or acute sodium depletion (Dila and Pappius, 1972; Rymer and Fishman, 1973; Grantham, 1977). (3) Osmotic disequilibrium syndromes occur with hemodialysis or diabetic ketoacidosis, wherein excessive intracellular solutes result in excessive hydration when the plasma osmolality is rapidly reduced with therapy (Arieff and Kleeman, 1973). The precise composition of the osmotically active intracellular solutes responsible for cellular swelling in the disequilibrium syndromes associated with hemodialysis and diabetic ketoacidosis is not known. In uremia, the intracellular solutes presumably include a number of organic acids which have been recovered in the dialysis bath. In diabetic ketoacidosis, the intracellular solutes include glucose and ketone bodies. However, there are also unidentified osmotically active intracellular solutes, termed idiogenic osmoles. Increased intracellular osmolality in excess of the plasma level not only causes cellular swelling but also is responsible for complex changes in brain metabolism affecting the concentra-

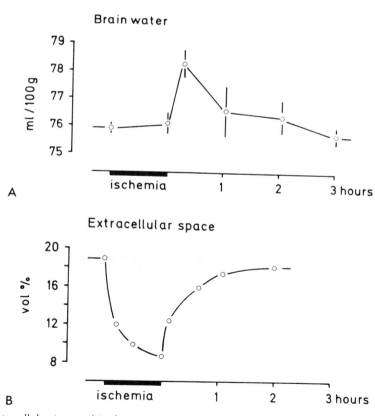

Figure 4–11 Acute cellular (cytotoxic) edema due to ischemia. In this experiment, the middle cerebral artery of the cat was occluded for 30 minutes. In *A* the brain water was acutely elevated after the circulation was restored. In *B* the extracellular space, measured by the impedance method, fell from a normal level of about 19 per cent to about 9 per cent at the end of 30 minutes, and it returned to normal within 2 hours of restoration of the circulation.

Continued on following page

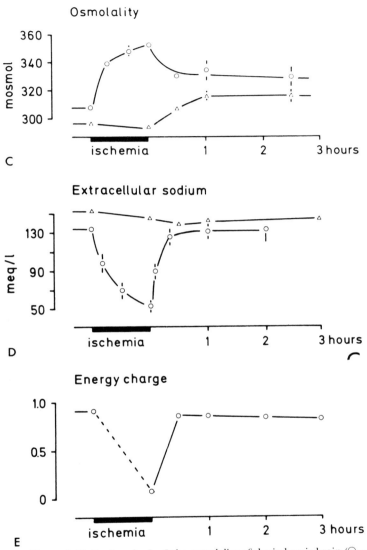

Figure 4–11 *Continued.* In *C* the osmolality of the ischemic brain (O——O) rose from about 305 mOsm to 350 mOsm and it returned toward normal one hour after circulation was restored. The contralateral hemisphere (△——△) was unaffected. In *D* the extracellular sodium fell promptly with the onset of ischemia and was rapidly restored to normal with removal of the arterial clamp. In *E* the energy charge, which reflects the ATP content of the tissue, fell from a normal level of about 0.95 to about 0.15 after 30 minutes of ischemia. It returned to normal 30 minutes after restoration of the circulation (from Hossman, 1976).

tion of the neurotransmitter amino acids, ammonia, and other metabolites (Chan and Fishman, 1979).

There is no evidence of cerebral edema in uremic encephalopathy (Olsen, 1961; Fishman and Raskin, 1967) in the form of an increase in brain water content. However, impedance studies of uremic encephalopathy have not been done. These might provide evidence of cellular edema despite lack of evidence of a change in the total brain water content. There is also an extensive literature regarding experimental cellular brain edema induced by toxic metabolic inhibitors, such as dinitrophenol, 3-acetylpyridine, 6-aminonicotinamide, and triethyl tin, which cause variable degrees of cellular swelling (Katzman and Pappius, 1973). The biochemical basis for these changes is not known.

Major changes in cerebral function (stupor, coma, decreased seizure threshold, and diffuse electroencephalographic slowing) occur with the cellular edemas. The encephalopathy is often severe with acute hypo-osmolality, but, in sustained states of hypo-osmolality of the same severity, neurological function may be spared. The brain adapts to hyponatremia by losing intracellular osmoles, chiefly potassium, thereby preserving cellular volume (Fishman, 1974). Acute hypoxia causes cellular edema, which is followed by vasogenic edema as infarction develops. Vasogenic edema usually occurs several days after an acute arterial occlusion. The delay in obtaining a positive isotopic scan following an ischemic stroke illustrates that the passage of time is needed for defects in endothelial cell function to develop and mature. Verhas et al. (1975) found that the greatest intensity of isotopic uptake in 84 patients with cerebral infarction took place between 10 and 30 days after onset, with an average half-life of 17 days. The delayed appearance of positive scans may depend upon the appearance of newly formed capillaries, which are more permeable than mature blood vessels (Rapoport, 1976).

Ischemic Brain Edema

Most patients with arterial occlusion have a combination of first cellular and then vasogenic edema, together termed *ischemic brain edema*. The two phases of ischemic brain edema overlap. The cellular phase takes place over minutes to hours and may be reversible. The vasogenic phase takes place over hours to days and results in infarction, a largely irreversible process, although the increased endothelial cell permeability usually reverts to normal within weeks. The factors that determine the reversibility of ischemic edema at the cellular level are poorly understood (Katzman et al., 1977).

Reye's Syndrome

Reye's syndrome, a neurological disorder of children, is characterized by fulminant hepatic failure, a rapidly progressive encephalopathy, and severe intracranial hypertension, with brain edema as a major and often fatal complication (De Vivo and Keating, 1976). The brain has features of cellular (cytotoxic) edema in which, characteristically, the CSF protein content is normal. There are electron microscopic findings of astrocytic swelling and the appearance of intralamellar blebs in the myelin, analogous to the findings described in triethyl tin intoxication (Partin *et al.*, 1975). However, these changes have not been described in other forms of fulminant hepatic failure. The monitoring of intracranial pressure has been considered to be a valuable guide to the use of osmotherapy in patients with Reye's syndrome. However, the mortality in about 30 monitored cases reported from five centers approached 40 to 50 per cent (De Vivo, 1978). (This high mortality rate may reflect the fact that only the sickest patients with Reye's syndrome were selected for monitoring.)

Interstitial (Hydrocephalic) Edema

Interstitial edema is the third type of edema, best characterized in obstructive hydrocephalus, in which there is an increase in the water and sodium content of the periventricular white matter due to the movement of CSF across the ventricular walls (Fishman and Greer, 1963; Milhorat, 1972). Obstruction of the circulation of the CSF within the ventricular system (or of CSF absorption in the subarachnoid space) results in the transependymal movement of cerebrospinal fluid and thereby an absolute increase in the volume of the brain's extracellular fluid. The chemical changes are those of edema, with one exception: the periventricular white matter is rapidly reduced rather than increased in volume, because of the rapid disappearance of myelin lipids as the hydrostatic pressures within the white matter increase. The pathogenesis of ventricular enlargement has been discussed earlier. Figure 4–5 (page 101) illustrates the computed tomograms performed before and 8 days after a ventriculo-atrial shunt. The presence of interstitial edema in the periventricular white matter is striking. Its reduction, occurring along with partial restoration of the thickness of the mantle, is apparent following the shunt.

The factors (physiological, biochemical, and temporal) that determine the restoration of the cerebral mantle edema require elucidation. There are usually relatively minor functional manifestations of interstitial edema in chronic hydrocephalus unless the changes are advanced, when dementia and gait disorder become prominent. The electroencephalogram is often normal in interstitial edema. This indicates that the accumulation of CSF in the periventricular extracellular fluid space is much better tolerated than is the presence of plasma in the extracellular fluid space, as seen with vasogenic edema, which is characterized by focal neurological signs and EEG slowing. The differences in the ionic and protein composition of plasma and CSF may be a factor in explaining the disparate functional responses.

The pathophysiology of the syndromes associated with benign intracranial pressure (pseudotumor cerebri) will be discussed later. The mechanism in most patients, except in those with obstruction of the intracranial venous sinuses, is not well defined. Brain edema has been documented by brain biopsy during subtemporal decompression (Sahs and Joynt, 1956), but it is noteworthy that there are a few, if any, clinical signs of encephalopathy associated with the syndrome; the electroencephalogram is characteristically normal, and consciousness is preserved. The brain edema of pseudotumor appears to have the features of an interstitial (hydrocephalic) edema compatible with defective cerebrospinal fluid absorption at the arachnoid villi.

Granulocytic Brain Edema

Severe brain edema occurs with brain abscess and purulent meningitis due to collections of pus, which are often sterile as a result of antibiotic treatment. As mentioned earlier, such edema, associated with membranous products of granulocytes (pus), has been termed granulocytic brain edema (Fishman *et al.*, 1977). The features of cellular and vasogenic edema occur concurrently in purulent meningitis, and in severe cases interstitial (hydrocephalic) edema also develops, so that granulocytic brain edema may include the features of all three types. The vasogenic edema that occurs in purulent meningitis is associated with a marked increase in endothelial cell permeability, as evidenced by the increased CSF protein and by positive scans using radioisotopes or contrast-enhanced computed tomography. In a canine model of pneumococcal meningitis, there were graded changes in membrane permeability affecting the entry into and exit from CSF of macromolecules of increasing size (Prockop and Fishman, 1968). In purulent meningitis, the membranes of capillaries, brain cells, and arachnoid villi are adversely affected. It is possible that in each case the presence of free radicals may underlie the membrane damage.

Therapeutic Considerations

The therapy of brain edema is dependent upon the cause. Appropriate and early treatment of intracranial infections is essential. Surgical therapy is directed toward alleviating the cause by excision or decompression of intracranial mass lesions as well as by a variety of shunting procedures (see discussion of the treatment of hydrocephalus). A patent airway, maintenance of an adequate blood pressure, and the avoidance of hypoxia are fundamental requirements in the care of such patients. The administration of parenteral fluids to meet the needs of the patient is also essential. However, caution is necessary in the choice of isotonic parenteral fluids. The administration of salt-free fluids should be avoided. Intravenous infusion of 5 per cent glucose solution results in a significant increase in intracranial pressure that may be avoided with use of normal saline or 5 per cent glucose in saline (Fishman, 1953; Bakay *et al.*, 1954). If the excessive administration of salt is to be avoided, the use of 2.5 per cent or 5 per cent glucose in half-normal (0.42 per cent) saline is satisfactory. In patients with cerebral edema, serum hypo-osmolality has deleterious effects and should be avoided.

The pharmacological treatment of brain edema is based on the use of (1) glucocorticoids, (2) osmotherapy, and (3) drugs which reduce CSF formation. Hyperventilation, hypothermia, and barbiturate therapy have also been tested experimentally and in clinical practice. Each of these treatments will be reviewed briefly.

Glucocorticoids

The adrenal glucocorticoids were introduced in the treatment of peritumoral brain edema by Kofman *et al.* (1957), Galicich *et al.* (1961), and Rasmussen and Gulati (1962). The rationale for the use of steroids was largely empirical. Prompted by Menkin's (1940) work, Prados *et al.* (1945) showed that crude adrenal cortical extract protected capillary integrity in physiological studies of the cat cerebral cortex. Since 1961, various high potency glucocorticoids, chiefly dexamethasone, have been used widely in the management of intracranial hypertension and brain edema. There is widespread conviction among neurologists and neurosurgeons that these steroids dramatically and rapidly (in hours) begin to reduce the focal and general signs of brain tumor. The mechanism of such beneficial effects is poorly understood. There has been much interest in the anti-inflammatory, immunosuppressive, and antiedema activities of glucocorticoids (Reulen and Schurmann, 1972; Pappius and Feindel, 1976; Axelrod, 1976; Fauci, 1976). The major mechanism suggested to explain their usefulness in vasogenic brain edema is a direct effect on endothelial cell function that restores normal permeability.

The action of adrenal steroids on inflammation and immune mechanisms is a fundamental issue in biology. A review of the huge literature is beyond the scope of this book. It is difficult to relate much of the basic information to the beneficial effects of steroids in brain edema. It is of special interest that glucocorticoids were shown to inhibit the release of arachidonic acid from cellular membranes (Hong and Levine, 1976). In view of the ability of arachidonic acid to induce both vasogenic and cellular edema, discussed earlier, it is possible that one of the beneficial effects of steroids may be related to inhibition of release of edema-producing polyunsaturated fatty acids from cellular membranes. A specific effect of glucocorticoids on free radical metabolism has not been shown.

The favorable responses of brain tumor to steroids indicate that the clinical manifestations of tumor may be due more to peritumoral edema than to the tumor mass itself. Dramatic responses have been seen with metastatic tumors as well as primary intracerebral tumors. There is experimental evidence that some tumors are steroid responsive and may undergo a reduction in size, apart from the reduction of peritumoral edema (Shapiro and Posner, 1974). Unfortunately, the response to steroid therapy is often short lived, although some patients have benefited from long term, high dose therapy over many months.

Long-acting, high potency glucocorticoids like dexamethasone have been used most widely. The usual dosages of dexamethasone are a starting dose of 10 mg and 4 mg four times a day thereafter — a dose equivalent in potency of 400 mg of cortisol daily. These large doses are about 20 times the normal rate of human endogenous cortisol production. In experimental trials, both conventional and high dosages of dexamethasone have been used to treat severe closed head injury. The high dose group received 200 mg in the first 6 hours and then 4 mg every 6 hours for 8 days. The high dose group revealed improved therapeutic effects compared with those receiving conventional doses. These results were based on a small number of patients, and the conclusions are considered tentative (Faupel *et al.*, 1976). At present, since insufficient data are available to establish a formal dose-response curve for steroids in the treatment of brain edema, the dosage schedules remain empirical.

Although all the complications of steroid therapy are to be expected, gastric hemorrhage is usually the most troublesome. Fortunately, convulsive seizures apparently have not been increased in frequency by high dosages of the glucocorticoids. The risks of increased wound infection and impaired wound healing appear to be outweighed by the therapeutic effects in most patients receiving short-term therapy (Axelrod, 1976; Fauci, 1976).

I have previously suggested that steroid psychosis is relatively uncommon in patients on high doses of dexamethasone, and that psychosis may be more likely to occur in patients receiving cortisol or prednisone (Fishman, 1975). There are no formal data to support this suggestion. The relationship between the adrenal corticoids and psychosis is complex. Mental changes occur often in the primary forms of Cushing's disease; major psychiatric symptoms have been reported in 25 per cent of patients (Plotz *et al.*, 1952). The major glucocorticoid secreted by the human adrenal in primary Cushing's disease is cortisol. It is my impression that mental effects (varying between moderate changes in mood to a full blown psychosis) have been seen less often and less severely with dexamethasone, the high potency long-acting glucocorticoid, than with prednisone, a steroid with intermediate potency and duration of action. Similarly, psychosis with prednisone therapy appears to be less frequent than with primary Cushing's disease.

It is possible that these clinical impressions result from differences in the diseases under treatment, because prednisone is used more often for treatment of lupus or arteritis, and dexamethasone is likely to be used for treatment in brain or spinal cord edema. Despite this reservation, it seems probable that the behavioral effects and anti-inflammatory effects of glucocorticoids have independent modes of action. The dosage of high-potency dexamethasone provides about 1/25 and 1/5 of the number of steroid rings obtained with equivalent dosages of cortisol and prednisone, respectively. This fact may be responsible for the apparently low incidence of steroid psychosis in patients treated with dexamethasone compared with its more common occurrence in patients receiving lower potency steroids or with primary Cushing's disease. This hypothesis requires substantiation.

Although published data indicate that dexamethasone has therapeutic value in the treatment of vasogenic edema associated with brain tumor, brain abscess, and head injury, its effectiveness with acute cerebral infarction has not been established (Mulley *et al.*, 1978). The literature recommending its use in stroke has, in general, been poorly documented and is controversial (Katzman *et al.*, 1977). Steroids may be useful in the treatment of intracerebral hematoma with extensive vasogenic edema due to the mass effect of the clot. In head injury, steroid therapy has been used frequently. While its effectiveness following trauma has been documented (Schuermann and Reulen, 1972; Faupel *et al.*, 1976), reduced morbidity and mortality attributable to steroids is not great.

Although the literature is difficult to assess, there are no convincing data, clinical or experimental, that glucocorticoids have beneficial effects in the cellular (cytotoxic) edema associated with hypo-osmolality, asphyxia, or hypoxia in the absence of infarction with mass effects. There is little basis for recommending steroids in the treatment of the cerebral edema associated with cardiac arrest or asphyxia. Mulley *et al.* (1978) made a double-blind study of the effects of dexamethasone in acute stroke which led them to conclude that there is no indication for the routine administration of dexamethasone to a heterogeneous group of patients with stroke.

The use of steroids in the management of Reye's syndrome is controversial. Some investigators have discontinued their use (De Vivo and Keating, 1976; De

Vivo, 1978; Schubert, 1979), whereas other groups continue to advocate steroid therapy. It is my view that steroid therapy benefits chiefly the vasogenic edemas and would not be expected to be useful in the management of Reye's syndrome. However, there are no controlled data which support either conclusion.

When intracranial hypertension and obstructive hydrocephalus occur because of inflammatory changes in the subarachnoid space or at the arachnoid villi, whether attributable to leukocytes or to blood, there is a reasonable rationale for the use of steroids. However, despite the frequent use of steroids in purulent or tuberculous meningitis, there are few data available to document their effectiveness against the brain edema associated with the acute disease. There are conflicting reports regarding the efficacy of steroids in acute bacterial meningitis (Harris *et al.*, 1978; Levin *et al.*, 1978) and in tuberculous meningitis (O'Toole *et al.*, 1969; Tandon, 1978). The use of steroids has not been shown to affect the subsequent incidence of chronic sequelae such as obstructive hydrocephalus or seizures. In my experience, steroids appear useful in the management of conditions characterized by an inflammatory CSF, such as chemical meningitis following intrathecal RISA, meningeal sarcoidosis, and cysticercosis.

The management of idiopathic pseudotumor cerebri (*q.v.*) is difficult to evaluate because spontaneous remission and cure are to be expected. Glucocorticoids are used in pseudotumor, and some patients appear to benefit from the treatment. It is possible that the anti-inflammatory steroids improve CSF absorption at the arachnoid villi; steroids have not been shown to reduce CSF formation (Vela *et al.*, 1979).

Osmotherapy

The effects of a variety of hypertonic solutions (including urea, mannitol, and glycerol) on CSF formation and the intracranial pressure have been discussed earlier. The various solutes have been difficult to compare because a large variety of laboratory models, dosages, time intervals, and pathological processes were used. Few data are available regarding the level of plasma osmolality achieved with the use of various solutions and dosage schedules (Rottenberg *et al.*, 1977; McGraw *et al.*, 1978).

A few principles seem certain. First, the brain volume will fall only as long as an osmotic gradient exists between blood and brain to allow the water shift that results in decreased brain volume and lowered intracranial pressure. Second, osmotic gradients obtained with hypertonic parenteral fluids are short-lived because each of the solutes in use reaches an equilibrium concentration in the brain after a delay of only a few hours. Third, the parts of the brain most likely to "shrink" are those areas which have normal endothelial cell permeability; thus, with focal vasogenic edema the normal regions of the hemisphere shrink, but the edematous regions with increased capillary permeability do not. Fourth, a rebound in the severity of the edema may follow use of any of the suggested hypertonic solutions because the solute is not excluded from the edematous tissue, and if tissue osmolality rises the tissue water is increased. Finally, there is a poor rationale for the chronic use of hypertonic fluids, either orally or parenterally, because the brain adapts to sustained hyperosmolality of the plasma with an increase in intracellular osmolality due to entry of the added solute.

To recapitulate, in response to hyperosmolality of the plasma, brain volume is relatively preserved because brain osmolality increases to reach equilibrium with the plasma because of the entry into brain of the added solute and the appearance of idiogenic osmoles. Thus, hypertonic solutions have a limited place in the treatment of brain edema. Often, no more than one or two intravenous loads are generally necessary to obtain time for more definitive treatment such as surgical decompression of an intracranial mass, hematoma, or abscess. Additional doses should be given with caution in conditions like post-traumatic and postoperative edema and Reye's syndrome. An increasing number of reports advocate intracranial pressure monitoring as an essential guide to therapy in these disorders (Fourth International Symposium on Intracranial Pressure, 1979). If additional osmotherapy is intended, then careful monitoring of the plasma osmolality and electrolytes is necessary as a guide to the frequency of administration of additional solute.

There is some uncertainty about the size of an increase in plasma osmolality that causes a therapeutically significant decrease in brain volume and intracranial pressure in humans. Several workers (Guisado *et al.*, 1974; Di Mattio *et al.*, 1975) suggested that increases in plasma osmolality in the range of 30 mOsm per l are needed to reduce brain volume in the presence of normal intracranial pressure; however, with intracranial hypertension, smaller osmotic gradients may prove more useful. Rottenberg *et al.* (1977) suggested that increases as little as 10 mOsm per l may be therapeutically effective. The value of frequent small increments in serum osmolality in the management of intracranial hypertension has also been reported by McGraw *et al.* (1978). It should be emphasized that accurate dose-response relationships in different clinical situations have not been well defined with any of the hypertonic agents.

In the choice of a specific agent, the laws of diffusion remind the clinician that the osmotic pressure of a given solution is dependent upon the number of molecules present and not upon their size. Solutions of 25 per cent urea and 25 per cent mannitol have been used to reduce the intracranial pressure; neither compound is metabolized, and both are excreted unchanged in the urine (Wise and Chater, 1961; Wise, 1963; Shenkin *et al.*, 1962). However, the osmolality of urea (MW 60) is about three times the same concentration of mannitol (MW 180). Thus, *in vitro*, the osmolality of 25 per cent urea would be about 3 times greater than that of 25 per cent mannitol. The apparent advantage of using the smaller molecule, urea, is counterbalanced because it has the disadvantage of entering the brain and CSF more rapidly than mannitol, thus dissipating its *in vitro* advantage. Urea also has toxic effects on the brain (Glaser, 1974). Currently, 25 per cent mannitol is the preferred osmotic solute in clinical practice in most American hospitals. Although some investigators have suggested that both oral and intravenous administration of hypertonic glycerol (MW 92) may be useful (Tourtellotte *et al.*, 1972; Rottenberg *et al.*, 1977), it has the disadvantage of being metabolized rapidly and having high caloric effects, as discussed earlier. Whether glycerol has therapeutic usefulness other than its osmotic effects is not known. If continued use of oral glycerol is intended, the guidelines regarding its use described by Rottenberg *et al.* (1977) should be followed.

Despite the widespread use of hypertonic mannitol in clinical practice, there are relatively few detailed analyses of its therapeutic effectiveness. James *et al.*

(1977) summarized their experience with the use of 25 per cent mannitol administered as a bolus (0.18 to 2.5 gm/kg) over 2 to 10 minutes in patients being monitored for intracranial hypertension. In 38 patients, treated 67 times, intracranial pressure reduction ranging from 10 to 98 per cent (mean 52 per cent) was obtained. Maximal pressure reduction was obtained from 20 to 360 minutes after injection, with the average reached after 88 minutes. The intracranial pressure returned to control levels after 45 minutes to 11 hours (average 210 minutes) following the intravenous bolus. The elevations of plasma osmolality and the degree of water diuresis obtained with those dosages were not recorded. However, the authors noted a rebound in intracranial pressure in only 3 patients. Thus, the ability of hypertonic mannitol to acutely lower the intracranial pressure was again confirmed, using rather empirical dosage schedules.

Acetazolamide and Furosemide

Evidence that the diuretic drugs acetazolamide and furosemide affect choroidal formation of CSF and ion exchange within the hemisphere has already been summarized. Acetazolamide has been used in the treatment of hydrocephalus for about 20 years. There is recent interest in the use of furosemide in the treatment of brain edema. The effects of acetazolamide on CSF formation were discussed in Chapter 3. As an inhibitor of carbonic anhydrase (the enzyme that catalyzes the formation of carbonic acid from carbon dioxide and water), acetazolamide causes about 50 per cent reduction in the rate of CSF formation within the ventricles, presumably by reducing the availability of hydrogen ions to exchange with sodium ions within the cells of the choroid plexus. Bulk formation of cerebrospinal fluid, normally about 500 ml per day, is directly dependent upon the rate of sodium transport, with rapid diffusion of water to maintain iso-osmolality with the plasma.

Acetazolamide may have a limited role in the treatment of the interstitial edema of obstructive hydrocephalus and pseudotumor because it reduces the bulk formation of cerebrospinal fluid and thereby would reduce the transependymal movement of CSF into the adjacent hemisphere (Huttenlocher, 1965; Rubin *et al.*, 1966). Preliminary data indicate that acetazolamide and furosemide may be useful in the treatment of vasogenic edema because the induction of reduced CSF formation might facilitate the drainage of edema fluid from the edematous cerebrum to the ventricular system (Long *et al.*, 1976; Meinig *et al.*, 1976). Furosemide also inhibits the formation of cerebrospinal fluid by about 25 per cent, independently of the action of carbonic anhydrase (Sahar and Tsipstein, 1978). Using both drugs together experimentally in rabbits reduced CSF formation by about 75 per cent (see Chapter 3). These drugs appear worthy of further clinical assessment in the treatment of cerebral edema and benign intracranial pressure. Further support for their effectiveness was presented at the Fourth International Symposium on Intracranial Pressure, 1979. Ethacrynic acid, an inhibitor of chloride transport in the renal tubule and in astrocytes, is a new agent that may prove useful in the management of brain edema. Initial reports describe its effectiveness in head injury (Yen *et al.*, 1979).

Hyperventilation Therapy

Controlled hyperventilation has been in widespread use by anesthesiologists during intracranial surgery to acutely reduce brain volume in order to facilitate the neurosurgical procedure. The therapeutic effectiveness of hyperventilation is based on the vasoconstrictor effects of respiratory alkalosis, which is responsible for a reduced cerebral blood flow and blood volume.

James *et al.* (1977) reviewed their experience with 50 trials in 34 patients in whom intracranial pressure was reduced by 10 to 80 per cent, with a mean reduction of 47 per cent. The time from initiation of hyperventilation to maximum reduction in pressure ranged from 2 to 30 minutes, with a mean of 7.6 minutes. The intracranial pressure returned to control levels in less than 5 minutes following cessation of hyperventilation. However, they reported that hyperventilation failed to reduce intracranial pressure with severe brain insults caused by cerebral vasomotor paralysis. At present, hyperventilation appears to be useful chiefly in the operating room under careful supervision by the anesthesiologist.

Hypothermia and Barbiturates

Hypothermia has been used to treat brain injury and brain edema both in the operating room and in critical care units. Its use is based on the reduction in cerebral metabolism, cerebral blood flow, and brain volume obtained with experimental hypothermia, which has been shown to protect animals from a variety of acute cerebral injuries. Its role in clinical practice is not well defined. James *et al.* (1977) reviewed their experience with 40 trials in 40 patients with intracranial hypertension. Mild hypothermia (32° to 36° C) decreased intracranial pressure by an average of 50 per cent from 240 to 720 minutes. In moderate hypothermia (27° to 31° C), similar pressure reductions were obtained but in lesser time intervals, the average being 150 minutes. The investigators found the data regarding the therapeutic efficacy of hypothermia to be difficult to evaluate; its place in the management of the various kinds of brain edema is conjectural.

Experimentally, barbiturates have been shown to partially protect animals from ischemic infarction (Hoff *et al.*, 1975). Several preliminary reports suggest that barbiturates may be useful clinically. It is not clear whether the protective effects require anesthetic doses to suppress brain metabolism or whether lesser doses may prove effective by interfering with the ability of free radicals to induce lipid peroxidation. Whether barbiturates will be validated in the therapy of brain edema awaits further study (Flamm *et al.*, 1979; Marshall *et al.*, 1979).

Unsolved Problems

Many unsolved problems remain in the study of the various forms of brain edema. The factors responsible for the resolution of the various kinds of edema are not well defined, nor are the relationships between blood flow, plateau waves, and interstitial pressure clearly understood. The possible roles of biogenic amines, excitatory neurotransmitter amino acids, free radicals, polyunsaturated fatty acids, and lipid peroxidation in the pathogenesis of vasogenic, cellular, and interstitial brain edema require further study. The preliminary evidence that barbiturates may have protective effects against cerebral edema requires elucidation.

There are many other questions. What is the basis of the alterations in membrane integrity that underlie the vasogenic edemas? How do glucocorticoids interact with membrane components to stabilize membrane structure and function? What are the effects of hyperosmolal agents on brain metabolism? What are the factors that control cellular volume? What is the pathogenesis of brain edema in Reye's syndrome? What are the mobile constituents of the periventricular white matter that disappear because of transependymal hydrostatic pressures and then return with ventricular decompression following a surgical shunt? Answers to these questions should yield a better insight into the pathophysiology of the various forms of brain edema and their treatment.

BENIGN INTRACRANIAL HYPERTENSION (PSEUDOTUMOR CEREBRI) AND RELATED DISORDERS

The syndrome of *benign intracranial hypertension* (BIH) is characterized by increased intracranial pressure without focal signs of neurological dysfunction (Greer, 1968; Boddie *et al.,* 1974; Johnston and Paterson, 1974; Weisberg, 1975). Many disorders give evidence of papilledema due to intracranial hypertension without localizing signs; they include mass lesions, obstructive hydrocephalus, chronic meningitis, hypertensive encephalopathy, and pulmonary encephalopathy. These disorders must be ruled out in order to establish the diagnosis of BIH. BIH includes a heterogeneous group of disorders in which several different causes have been identified, although in most cases the cause and pathogenesis are poorly understood (see Table 4–3). The terms "benign intracranial pressure" and "pseudotumor cerebri" have been used synonymously by most workers (Foley, 1955; Greer, 1968; Johnston and Paterson, 1974). Older terms no longer in use include "serous meningitis" and "otitic hydrocephalus." The latter was used to describe intracranial hypertension due to thrombosis or thrombophlebitis of the lateral dural venous sinus, which was a common complication of mastoiditis in the pre-antibiotic era (Symonds, 1937). The term "benign" is used because spontaneous recovery generally occurs; however, serious threats to vision also may develop, and the term "benign" in such cases seems inappropriate.

Clinical Manifestations

The presenting symptoms are usually headache, disturbance of vision, or both. The headache is often worse on awakening and aggravated by cough and strain. It is often relatively mild and may be entirely *absent*. The most common ocular complaint is visual blurring, a manifestation of papilledema observed in most patients. Some patients complain of brief, fleeting moments of dimming or complete loss of vision, occurring many times during the day (amaurosis fugax), at times accentuated or precipitated by coughing and straining. This

TABLE 4–3   Differential Diagnosis of Benign Intracranial Hypertension: Etiologic Factors and Related Disorders

1. Endocrine and metabolic disorders
    Obesity and menstrual irregularities
    Pregnancy and postpartum (without sinus thrombosis)
    Menarche
    Female sex hormones
    Addison's disease
    Adrenal steroid withdrawal
    Hypoparathyroidism

2. Intracranial venous sinus thrombosis
    Mastoiditis and lateral sinus thrombosis
    After head trauma
    Pregnancy and post partum
    Oral progestational drugs
    "Marantic" sinus thrombosis
    Cryofibrinogenemia
    Primary (idiopathic) sinus thrombosis

3. Drugs and Toxins
    Vitamin A
    Tetracycline
    Nalidixic acid
    Chlordane (Kepone)

4. Hematological disorders
    Iron deficiency anemia
    Infectious mononucleosis
    Wiskott-Aldrich syndrome

5. High cerebrospinal fluid protein
    Spinal cord tumors
    Polyneuritis

6. "Meningism" with systemic bacterial or viral infections

7. Empty sella syndrome

8. Miscellaneous
    Sydenham's chorea
    Familial
    Lupus erythematosus
    Rapid growth in infancy

9. Idiopathic

10. Symptomatic intracranial hypertension without localizing neurological signs simulating BIH
    Mass lesions
    Obstructive hydrocephalus
    Chronic meningitis (sarcoid, fungal, or meningeal neoplasia)
    Hypertensive encephalopathy
    Pulmonary encephalopathy due to
      paralytic hypoventilation, chronic
      obstructive pulmonary disease or
      pickwickian syndrome

ominous symptom indicates that the patient's vision may be in serious jeopardy. However, visual loss may be minimal, despite severe chronic papilledema with retinal hemorrhages, although blindness rarely may develop very rapidly — in less than 24 hours. Visual fields characteristically show enlargement of the blind spots, and may show constriction of the peripheral fields and central or paracentral scotomas. Diplopia secondary to unilateral or bilateral sixth nerve palsy may develop as a result of increased intracranial pressure. The neurological examination is otherwise normal. Occasionally, the physician notes the appearance of apparent papilledema on routine funduscopy in asymptomatic patients. The appearance of true papilledema may simulate pseudo-papilledema.

A major clinical point is that patients with BIH commonly look well, that is, their appearance and apparent well-being belie the ominous appearance of the papilledema. There are usually no sequelae following recovery. Recurrent episodes have been noted in about 5 per cent of cases (Lysak and Svien, 1966). The illness may last two years and more, although often it is self-limited in several months.

Radiological Features

BIH has been considered responsible for the development of the "empty sella" syndrome, in which radiological examination shows enlargement of the sella simulating a pituitary tumor, although pituitary function is not affected. The enlarged sella is filled with CSF because of a defect in the diaphragm of the sella. The precise mechanism is obscure whereby localized hydrostatic pressures induce pressure atrophy and enlargement of the bony sella (Foley and Posner, 1975). Whereas the "empty" sella may be an unexplained incidental finding, its presence suggests that the patient may have had BIH sometime in the past.

Many clinicians have noted that the ventricular system, when visualized with pneumoencephalography or ventriculography, appeared small or "slit-like" in patients with BIH. However, this finding was not confirmed with computed tomography; Huckman *et al.* (1976) have found the ventricular size to be normal in BIH. The divergence in the appearance of ventricular size with the two radiographic techniques has not been explained. Wyper *et al.* (1979) reported that there is a 20 to 30 per cent error in estimating ventricular volume with computed tomography, and it seems likely that ventricular volume is commonly reduced in BIH, an event compatible with the pressure of brain edema.

Pathophysiology

The signs and symptoms of BIH are due to the effects of increased intracranial pressure; pressures between 300 and 600 mm CSF are frequent. To rationalize the pathophysiology of BIH, these factors should be considered: (1) alterations in the intracranial venous and arterial pressures, and (2) alterations in the cerebral blood, CSF, and brain volumes.

The direct dependency of the CSF pressure upon the intracranial venous pressure has been discussed earlier. Changes in the latter pressure are readily transmitted to the CSF, and thus a sustained increase in intracranial venous pressure may result in the syndrome of chronically increased intracranial pressure. This has been well documented in patients with occlusion of the superior longitudinal sinus or the lateral sinuses or both, whether due to thrombosis, thrombophlebitis, or metastatic tumor. However, arterial hypertension of diverse etiology is not associated with intracranial hypertension except in the rare syndrome of hypertensive encephalopathy. This syndrome is readily distinguished by the presence of hypertensive retinopathy and by evidence of an encephalopathy (alterations in mental state and seizures) which is not seen in BIH.

Chronic CO_2 retention due to chronic obstructive pulmonary disease or paralytic pulmonary insufficiency results in intracranial hypertension with papilledema and variable degrees of encephalopathy, including alterations in mental state, asterixis, and electroencephalographic slowing (Miller *et al.*, 1962). This syndrome is attributable to sustained cerebral vasodilatation with increased cerebral blood flow and blood volume due to respiratory acidosis. In such cases, the associated clinical signs of encephalopathy with pulmonary insufficiency will usually exclude idiopathic BIH as the basis for papilledema and intracranial hypertension.

Limited data are available regarding the cerebral circulation in the idiopathic forms of BIH (Johnston and Paterson, 1974). Foley (1955) reported a significant increase in cerebral blood flow in 3 patients with BIH, using the nitrous oxide technique, and Mathew *et al.* (1975) calculated an increase in cerebral blood volume. Foley's (1955) observations were not confirmed by Raichle and colleagues (1978), who reported a minor *decrease* in cerebral blood flow in BIH, using an isotopic modification of the Kety method. They also reported a small but significant increase in cerebral blood volume in BIH, suggesting that a segment of the vascular bed was dilated. This was presumed to occur distal to the cerebral arterioles, the site of autoregulation of the cerebral blood flow, because cerebral autoregulation was considered to be normal. There was no apparent explanation for such a segmental increase in blood volume, and its importance in the pathogenesis of BIH is not clear.

The question of whether the CSF volume is altered in BIH has not been resolved because of the difficulty in its measurement. Greer (1968) suggested that the occurrence of a high Ayala index favored the presence of a large CSF volume in many patients. In view of the unreliability of the Ayala index, this conclusion may not be warranted. Bercaw and Greer (1970) also reported the occurrence in 3 patients with BIH of a delay in the disappearance of radioiodinated serum albumin along the superior longitudinal sinus visualized with isotope cisternography. More recently, Calabrese *et al.* (1978) reported abnormal responses in 9 of 10 patients with BIH studied with a spinal infusion test, indicating impairment of CSF absorption. Mann *et al.* (1979) confirmed this finding, using a similar technique. These observations suggest the presence of defective CSF absorption analogous to the occurrence of papilledema and intracranial hypertension, in association with benign spinal cord tumors or polyneuritis.

Prockop and Fishman (1968) showed that elevation of the CSF protein in dogs slowed the clearance of inulin and iodinated albumin from CSF, which indicates that the transport properties of the arachnoid villi (see Chapters 2 and 3) are altered by endogenous proteins, although the cellular mechanisms involved are obscure. While this observation might be relevant to the occurrence of intracranial hypertension with high CSF protein, Greer (1968) reported that most patients with BIH have normal or even lower than normal lumbar CSF protein levels (5 to 20 mg/dl). If inhibition of bulk flow reabsorption of CSF underlies the development of BIH, then it is difficult to explain the characteristic maintenance of a normal or reduced CSF protein level. The mechanism of the presumed alterations in function of the arachnoid villi in BIH requires further elucidation. There is no evidence to support an increase in CSF formation in BIH.

That the brain volume is increased in BIH was suggested by the frequent pneumoencephalographic findings of small or "slit-like" ventricles, although this has not been confirmed with computed tomography (Huckman *et al.,* 1976). Subtemporal decompression was a frequent treatment for BIH until the 1960's, and a bulging temporal lobe was commonly found at operation, although in some patients large lakes of CSF overlying the cerebral hemispheres were also found (Dr. Joseph Ransohoff, personal communication). Sahs and Joynt (1956) reported the occurrence of "brain edema" in temporal lobe biopsies obtained at the time of subtemporal decompression. Their techniques were limited to light microscopy, which did not indicate the specific location of the increase in water content. It is of special interest that Raichle *et al.* (1978) calculated a possible increase in brain water content from a normal level of 79 per cent to 83 per cent, based on the prolongation of the mean transit time for water. They concluded that this increase in brain water was responsible for the increase in intracranial pressure. I would assume that the water accumulates in the interstitial (extracellular) fluid space.

Thus, clinical and experimental evidence supports the hypothesis that BIH is associated with an increase in brain volume due to an increase in water content and is therefore a form of brain edema. What kind of brain edema does this represent? There is no evidence for vasogenic edema, that is, there is no evidence of increased capillary permeability assessed by isotope encephalography or by contrast-enhanced computed tomography. Similarly, the CSF protein is not increased — further evidence against the presence of vasogenic edema. There is also no evidence of cellular (cytotoxic) edema, in that neurological function is not affected and the EEG is normal in BIH. Thus, assuming that the increase in brain volume and brain water associated with BIH represent edema, then the findings would be best explained as a form of interstitial (hydrocephalic) edema. Such a mechanism is supported by the evidence, noted earlier, for the association of BIH with impaired CSF absorption.

The fact that ventricular dilatation does not develop is quite consistent with the proposed mechanism. Patients with spinal cord tumors or polyneuritis associated with intracranial hypertension do not necessarily develop hydrocephalus. Ridsdale and Moseley (1978) reported that ventricular dilatation occurred in only 23 of 40 reported such cases. Hoff and Barber (1974) obtained some data which support the hypothesis that a transmural pressure difference (from ventricular system to cortical subarachnoid space) is required to develop ventricular dilatation. (See discussion of normal pressure hydrocephalus.) Thus, the presence of free communication between the ventricular system and the cortical subarachnoid spaces in BIH would protect the periventricular white matter from the pressure atrophy that characterizes hydrocephalus.

In summary, the evidence favors the occurrence of increased extracellular fluid volume characteristic of interstitial brain edema in both obstructive hydrocephalus and BIH. The fundamental defect may be a block to CSF absorption. Such a mechanism appears to underlie the development of BIH, whether due to occlusive venous disease or associated with the other multiple factors, although the precise pathophysiology is obscure.

Ventricular Size in BIH

That the ventricular size was commonly reduced in BIH was first emphasized by Davidoff and Dyke (1936). However, there is uncertainty regarding the actual frequency of such a change. With pneumoencephalography, Guidetti *et al.* (1968) observed normal ventricular size in 69 per cent of cases, smaller ventricles in 20 per cent, and slight enlargement in 11 per cent. Boddie *et al.* (1974) concluded that small ventricles with sharp superior lateral angles, defined by pneumoencephalography, were not reliable diagnostic features of BIH; 76 per cent of their patients had ventricular volumes which were larger than normal. Huckman *et al.* (1976) evaluated ventricular size in 17 patients, using computed tomography. The quantitative comparison of ventricular size by computer analysis failed to detect any significant change, although many of the patients had small ventricles with prominent concavities in the area of the basal ganglia.

Thus, the data indicate that BIH may be present with normal, slightly reduced, or even slightly enlarged ventricles and that the appearance of ventricular narrowing may not be confirmed by radiographic or tomographic techniques. The factors responsible for the variation in ventricular size observed with pneumoencephalography are obscure.

Etiologic Factors and Related Disorders

In the evaluation of patients with the clinical findings of BIH, it is necessary to systematically search for the multiple factors and disorders associated with the syndrome. Most often, no specific cause is established. However, it is hazardous to make a diagnosis of idiopathic BIH without considering the various factors outlined in Table 4–3 (page 129). It is of special importance to exclude the other causes of intracranial hypertension without localizing signs.

Endocrine and Metabolic Disorders

In the differential diagnosis of BIH, the syndrome most commonly occurs in women with a history of menstrual dysfunction. Such patients are frequently moderately to markedly overweight (without evidence of alveolar hypoventilation). Menstrual irregularity is common, and galactorrhea is a rare associated symptom. There is often a history of excessive premenstrual weight gain. Endocrine studies thus far have not revealed any abnormalities of urinary gonadotropins or estrogens, and the pathogenesis of the syndrome is unknown. Occasionally, BIH has been observed during early pregnancy or the postpartum state. The syndrome has occurred without evidence of dural sinus thrombosis. Greer (1968) has reported a series of cases occurring during menarche and menopause.

The other endocrine disorders are uncommon or rare. BIH has been reported as a complication of Addison's disease, with improvement following steroid replacement therapy (Jefferson, 1956). Hypoparathyroidism may give evidence of increased intracranial pressure which disappears with replacement therapy (Sugar, 1953). The presence of hypocalcemic seizures and cerebral calcifications may further complicate the clinical picture in such cases. BIH has been found in women taking oral progestational drugs, in which cases angiography has ruled out sinus thrombosis (Weisberg, 1975). BIH has been reported in patients treated with adrenal corticosteroids for prolonged periods of time, usually months to years. Many of the patients have been children with allergic skin disorders or asthma. The syndrome has been more frequent when the steroid dosage was reduced, suggesting that relative adrenal insufficiency might have been present, but this has not been substantiated (Walker and Adamkiewicz, 1964; Neville and Wilson, 1970). It is noteworthy that BIH has not been reported with primary Cushing's disease.

In cases associated with any of the endocrine disorders, the mechanism of the intracranial hypertension remains an enigma. The effects of the various hormones on the function of the arachnoid villi require systematic study. It is of interest also that pseudotumor has occurred in infancy as an apparent consequence of rapid growth and weight gain (Sondheimer *et al.,* 1970; Bray *et al.,* 1973).

Intracranial Venous Sinus Thrombosis

Thrombophlebitis of the intracranial venous sinuses secondary to otitis media occurs with extension of the infection into the petrous bone and to the wall of the lateral sinus. Its occurrence was far more common before the introduction of antibiotic therapy, when the term "otitic hydrocephalus" was introduced (Symonds, 1931; 1937). Sinus thrombosis is still an uncommon complication of both acute and chronic infection; at times, the evidence for mastoiditis or petrositis is minimal and easily overlooked. The sixth cranial nerve may also be affected, giving rise to diplopia on lateral gaze as a result either of intracranial hypertension *per se* or of petrositis and thrombophlebitis of the lateral petrosal sinus. Thrombosis of the superior longitudinal sinus may occur as a consequence of relatively mild closed head injury and may give rise to a pseudotumor syndrome. Severe occlusion of this sinus, which drains both cerebral hemispheres, is likely to result in hemorrhagic infarction of the cerebrum as thrombosis extends into the cerebral veins, giving rise to bilateral signs. In such cases, the course is frequently fulminant and the prognosis guarded, although occasionally complete recovery may occur. Thrombosis of the superior longitudinal sinus may develop as a complication of pregnancy and be responsible for a pseudotumor syndrome. This has been reported to occur with the use of oral contraceptive drugs, at the end of the first trimester of pregnancy, and during the first two to three weeks post partum. A disorder of the blood clotting mechanism has been suggested as a basis for these events, although this has not been substantiated (Weisberg, 1975). Sinus thrombosis occurs as a complication of cachexia (marantic thrombosis). This was more common in the past; it occurred most often in infants with severe dehydration (Bell and McCormick, 1978). Rarely, cryofibrinogenemia is also responsible for sinus thrombosis (Dunsker *et al.,* 1970).

Finally, primary or idiopathic sinus thrombosis should be considered as a cause of BIH, although acute and chronic cases of sinus thrombosis often give signs of focal hemispheric dysfunction rather than BIH. The clinical manifestations of sinus thrombosis are protean (Silbermann *et al.*, 1951, Kalbag and Woolf, 1967). It has been difficult to explain the mechanism of primary thrombosis in such cases.

Drugs and Toxins

Vitamin A, tetracycline, and nalidixic acid have been implicated as causative agents. BIH has been found in otherwise healthy adolescents taking excessive doses of vitamin A for the treatment of acne. Ingestion of doses as low as 25,000 units per day has caused headache and papilledema. Rapid improvement occurs within a few weeks after cessation of the therapy. The syndrome is said to have occurred in Artic explorers who consumed polar bear liver, a great source of the vitamin (Lombaert and Carton, 1976). Curiously BIH is also rarely associated with vitamin A deficiency as well. A few cases of BIH, manifested by a bulging fontanelle and papilledema, have been found in children after the administration of tetracycline or nalidixic acid (Maroon *et al.*, 1971; Deonna *et al.*, 1974). Tetracycline has induced the syndrome in an adult as well (Koch-Weser and Gilmore, 1967). Spontaneous rapid recovery occurred when the drugs were stopped. Rechallenge of a patient with nalidixic acid recreated the syndrome, demonstrating that the occurrence was not a coincidence. Intoxication with chlordane (Kepone) has also caused BIH (Sanborn *et al.*, 1979). The mechanisms whereby these drugs and toxins cause BIH are obscure.

Hematologic Disorders

Papilledema and increased intracranial pressure have been attributed to severe iron deficiency anemia, with striking improvement after treatment of the anemia (Stoebner *et al.*, 1970). The mechanism presumably is dependent upon the marked increase in cerebral blood flow and blood volume that accompanies profound anemia. BIH has occurred with infectious mononucleosis and the Wiskott-Aldrich syndrome, but the mechanism in these cases is not known.

High Spinal Fluid Protein

Rarely BIH occurs secondary to a spinal cord tumor or polyneuritis, without any evidence of pulmonary insufficiency. As discussed earlier, a normal ventricular size has been found in about half the patients reported to have cranial hypertension secondary to a spinal tumor (Ridsdale and Moseley, 1978). The papilledema and headache have disappeared with treatment of the spinal tumor or with recovery from the polyneuritis. Morley and Reynolds (1966) reviewed the literature regarding the association of papilledema and polyneuritis. They concluded that a block to CSF absorption because of an elevated protein could not be substantiated. An alteration in the function of the arachnoid villi affecting vesicular transport and bulk absorption of CSF may be important in the pathophysiology, despite the absence of a close correlation with the protein level in lumbar CSF.

"Meningism" With Systemic Bacterial or Viral Infections

"Meningism" is a term used in the older literature (Merritt and Fremont-Smith, 1938) to describe the occurrence of an acute syndrome of headache and mild meningeal signs in children or young adults without meningitis. The syndrome occurs with various acute systemic viral or bacterial infections, including gastroenteritis, streptococcal pharyngitis, upper respiratory infections, chickenpox, and roseola infantum. The symptoms generally have been noted with the onset of the acute infection, although at times the onset has been delayed for a week or more thereafter (Rose and Matson, 1967).

The CSF in such patients is characteristically normal with regard to protein and glucose levels and cell count, but the CSF pressure is elevated to levels between 200 and 400 mm. In some patients, the spinal tap appears to relieve the symptoms. While papilledema was observed in some patients (Rose and Matson, 1967), the fundi usually have been normal. The differentiation of such cases from early bacterial or viral meningitis, epidural abscess, sinus thrombosis, and so on may prove difficult. A normal computed tomogram would help exclude such disorders. The diagnostic importance of accurate CSF cytology cannot be overemphasized. The pathogenesis of "meningism" is obscure. Merritt and Fremont-Smith (1938) suggested that acute hypo-osmolality of the blood might be responsible. However, data in support of the hypothesis were not reported. It is possible that the transient occurrence of inappropriate secretion of antidiuretic hormone might account for some cases, but usually the etiology of the syndrome is obscure.

Idiopathic BIH

BIH is also not uncommon in otherwise healthy subjects in the absence of any of the causes just described. On rare occasions, the familial occurrence of pseudotumor has been reported (Rothner and Brust, 1974). Both sexes may be involved, and the patients are most often between 10 and 50 years of age. These cases represent the idiopathic form of BIH; its pathogenesis is a mystery like that of all the other cases except for those with venous sinus occlusion. There are rare case reports of BIH with Sydenham's chorea (Rose and Matson, 1967), in which the mechanism is also unknown.

Symptomatic Intracranial Hypertension Without Localizing Signs

Many disorders are associated with the syndrome of intracranial hypertension without localized neurological signs, which must be differentiated from BIH. These include mass lesions, obstructive hydrocephalus, chronic meningitis (due to sarcoid or meningeal neoplasia or fungi), hypertensive encephalopathy, and pulmonary encephalopathy. Intracranial hypertension can be a major complication of chronic hypoxic hypercarbia caused by paralytic hypoventilation, whether due to muscular dystrophy, polyneuropathy, cervical myelopathy, chronic obstructive pulmonary disease, or the pickwickian syndrome. The mechanism is dependent upon the chronic increase in cerebral blood flow and blood volume induced by hypoxia and carbon dioxide retention. The clinical signs of encephalopathy (alteration in consciousness and asterixis) differentiate such cases from idiopathic forms of BIH (Miller *et al.*, 1962). Any clouding of the sensorium speaks against BIH and favors symptomatic intracranial hypertension. Lupus erythematosus has been associated with BIH in the absence of evidence of lupus encephalopathy (Silberberg and Laties, 1973).

Diagnosis

The patient with headache and papilledema without other neurological signs must be considered to have an intracranial mass, ventricular obstruction, or intracranial infection until proved otherwise. Although the diagnosis of BIH may be suspected by the appearance of apparent well-being and by the history of some of the associated features listed above, the diagnosis is essentially dependent on ruling out the various causes of increased intracranial pressure. Brain tumor, particularly when located in relatively silent areas such as the frontal lobes or right temporal lobe or when obstructing the ventricular system, may be manifest only by headache and papilledema. Patients with chronic subdural hematoma, without a history of significant trauma, may have the same symptoms. Berg *et al.* (1955) did a retrospective analysis of 238 patients with intracranial hypertension without localizing signs. Of these, 30 per cent had a midline obstructive lesion, 57 per cent had a lateralized mass lesion, and 13 per cent had a pseudotumor syndrome. Weisberg (1975) provided a similar appraisal of 100 consecutive patients who also had intracranial hypertension without localizing signs. The final diagnosis of idiopathic BIH was made in 71 per cent of the patients, of whom 61 per cent were women and 10 per cent men. In the 29 remaining cases, the intracranial hypertension was due to a mass lesion or chronic meningitis. It is clear that the diagnosis of BIH is one of exclusion!

In the past, diagnostic evaluation depended upon skull films, electroencephalography, arteriography, air studies, or a combination of these methods, as well as studies of the CSF pressure and composition. The availability of computed tomography has negated the need for angiography or air studies in many cases, although angiography may be needed to exclude dural sinus thrombosis. *Lumbar puncture is essential to confirm the presence of intracranial hypertension, to exclude the ophthalmological diagnosis of pseudopapilledema, and to exclude evidence of a chronic meningitis.* This is generally deferred until computed tomography has revealed that the ventricular system is not enlarged nor displaced. Laboratory studies regarding possible hypoadrenalism or hypoparathyroidism would be rewarding in the rare cases of these disorders that are associated with the pseudotumor syndrome.

In patients with BIH, the cerebrospinal fluid pressure is elevated, usually between 250 and 600 mm, but the fluid is otherwise normal except in patients with venous occlusive disease. The protein content is generally low normal, and lumbar CSF protein levels below 15 mg/dl are common (Greer, 1968). This finding suggests that such patients have increased rates of CSF absorption due to the intracranial hypertension (see discussion of low CSF protein syndromes). The electroencephalogram is typically normal in BIH (Sidell and Daly, 1961).

However, mild generalized slowing has been reported to occur, particularly in children (Bell and McCormick, 1978).

Pseudopapilledema may be a source of diagnostic confusion. It is a developmental anomaly of the fundus wherein the opthalmological appearance may be indistinguishable from that of the true papilledema; there is no elevation of the optic disk, but neither are there exudates or hemorrhages. The visual acuity is normal, although visual fields may show some enlargement of the blind spots in both BIH and pseudopapilledema. The unchanging appearance of the fundus with subsequent examinations favors the diagnosis of pseudopapilledema, as does the finding of normal CSF pressure on lumbar puncture.

Therapeutic Considerations

The management of BIH depends upon the results of the search for a specific cause. In patients with lateral sinus thrombosis caused by chronic infection of the petrous bone, surgical decompression and antibiotic therapy are often indicated. When the pseudotumor syndrome is a manifestation of hypoadrenalism or hypoparathyroidism, replacement therapy is indicated. Vitamin A intoxication disappears when administration of the vitamin is stopped, and patients respond to withdrawal of nalidixic acid and tetracycline when those are the etiologic agents. Anticoagulation therapy has been recommended for patients with dural sinus thrombosis; however, for patients with extension of the clot into cerebral veins causing infarction of tissue, anticoagulation is hazardous or may be contraindicated because it increases the likelihood of hemorrhagic infarction.

For cases secondary to steroid withdrawal, Neville and Wilson (1970) have made some specific recommendations. After prolonged corticosteroid administration, withdrawal should be gradual for at least one month; sudden reduction of the dosage by more than 50 per cent should be avoided. When reducing the steroid dosage, the physician should be alert to the possibility of irritability and headache as a manifestation of the syndrome, particularly in young children. In symptomatic cases, particularly when there is a threat to vision, reintroduction of the corticosteroid at a dosage of two-thirds to one-half the original dosage is indicated, with gradual tapering over a period of two to three months. If vision is deteriorating, large therapeutic dosages of high-potency glucocorticoids like dexamethasone may be necessary.

The idiopathic form of BIH and its occurrence in patients with menstrual disorders and obesity require individualized management. The syndrome is self-limited in most cases, and after some weeks or months spontaneous remission occur, making evaluation of therapy difficult. Recurrent episodes have been noted in about 5 per cent of cases (Lysak and Svien, 1966). In rare instances, the illness may last two years or longer. The major threat to the patient is progressive visual failure, which may be very rapid.

In the very obese, weight reduction is recommended. In the past, the use of daily lumbar punctures has been advocated to lower pressure to normal levels by removing sufficient fluid (Grant, 1971; Greer, 1968); drainage of 15 to 30 ml of fluid might be required to reach a normal pressure, but the value of CSF drainage is dubious. In my experience, most patients rebelled against the treatment, and the pressure usually returned to its initial high level within 24 or 48 hours.

Acetazolamide is the initial drug of choice in the management of BIH, with the addition of furosemide if needed. These drugs act independently to reduce CSF formation and have proved effective in some patients. Careful monitoring of the visual acuity, the fundi, and the CSF pressure and composition is essential. When these drugs fail, then steroid therapy is indicated. Dexamethasone has been used empirically because it minimizes cerebral edema of diverse causes. It has been speculated that its effects may be related to improvement in CSF absorption by the arachnoid villi.

Subtemporal decompression was widely used, and suboccipital decompression to a lesser degree, before 1960. Rarely, surgical decompression may still be necessary for patients with serious threats to vision caused by pressure. A CSF shunting procedure, such as the lumbar-peritoneal shunt, is probably the surgical procedure of choice in the treatment of failing vision due to papilledema (Vander Ark *et al.*, 1971). This seems more logical than surgical decompression of the sheath of the optic nerves (Galbraith and Sullivan, 1973) because it directly lowers the intracranial pressure that is responsible for the papilledema.

Hypertonic intravenous solutions (25 per cent mannitol) to lower intracranial pressure can be used in acute situations in which there is rapidly failing vision, while one awaits neurosurgical intervention; however, prolonged dehydration therapy has limitations because of its deleterious systemic effects discussed earlier. The prolonged use of oral glycerol for obese patients has the disadvantage of high caloric intake. In view of the adaption of the brain and CSF to chronic hyperosmolality, the effectiveness of oral glycerol may be questioned on theoretical grounds, although it has been considered useful in some reports (Tourtellotte *et al.*, 1972). Further data are needed to establish the advantages and disadvantages of hyperosmolal therapy in BIH. Management of these patients may be difficult; it requires the careful attention of experienced neurologists and neurosurgeons. (See therapy of brain edema, pages 121–128.)

INTRACRANIAL HYPOTENSION

As noted, the normal intracranial pressure is 70 to 200 mm water (or 5 to 15 mm Hg). Symptoms of intracranial hypotension occur with pressures between 50 and 90 mm water or lower. At times the CSF pressure is not measurable, and the fluid can be obtained only by aspiration with a syringe. The symptoms of intracranial hypotension are discussed in Chapter 5 (see complications of lumbar puncture). They include severe headaches precipitated by the erect position and relieved by the supine position, which are aggravated by cough or strain. There also may be nausea, vomiting, and dizziness precipitated by similar postural changes. A unilateral or bilateral 6th nerve palsy may accompany low pressure syndromes.

The most common cause is previous lumbar puncture with persistent CSF leakage into the subdural or epidural spaces. Low pressure syndromes also occur secondary to spinal fluid rhinorrhea, either spontaneous or post-traumatic, or because of a pituitary tumor (MacGee, 1976). Bacterial meningitis may complicate such cases. Traumatic avulsions of spinal roots may also result in a CSF leak (Bell *et al.*, 1960). Severe dehydration also results in intracranial hypotension, as exemplified by the sunken fontanelle observed in dehydrated infants. An erroneously low CSF pressure may be recorded in the presence of spinal block or when there are technical difficulties in placing the needle in the subarachnoid space.

Cerebrospinal Fluid Rhinorrhea

The diagnosis of CSF rhinorrhea is established when a nasal discharge is shown to have the composition of CSF. The analysis of the nasal secretion for glucose content is misleading in this regard. Specifically, glucose-oxidase test papers are often falsely positive when used to test nasal secretions and tears in the absence of a CSF leak (Hull and Morrow, 1975). Probably the best test for CSF rhinorrhea is analysis of the nasal discharge for chloride content. The CSF chloride of 120 meq/l is 15 to 20 meq greater than the chloride level in plasma. The chloride level of nasal secretions is about 5 to 10 meq/l. The stability of chloride and its high concentration in CSF are advantageous when a nasal discharge is tested to determine whether it is of intracranial origin.

CHAPTER 5

CLINICAL EXAMINATION OF CEREBROSPINAL FLUID

This chapter deals with the techniques of lumbar puncture in adults and children, cisternal and lateral cervical puncture, manometric tests for spinal block, spinal infusion tests, and CSF lavage and barbotage. The complications of lumbar puncture and their avoidance and treatment are also discussed.

LUMBAR PUNCTURE: INDICATIONS AND CONTRAINDICATIONS

Lumbar puncture should be performed only after thorough clinical evaluation of the patient and serious consideration of the potential value and hazards of the procedure. It is difficult to give all-inclusive guidelines regarding the indications for lumbar puncture. Many neurological disorders are associated with changes in the composition of the fluid, and the experienced clinician has learned to depend upon the CSF findings as an important guide to diagnosis and management. A few clinical problems usually demand a very early, if not an emergency, lumbar puncture. The procedure clearly is indicated in cases of suspected bacterial or fungal meningitis; in many patients with a fever of unknown origin, an early lumbar puncture is essential as a guide to both diagnosis and treatment. Spinal fluid examination is usually necessary in patients with suspected acute subarachnoid hemorrhage in order to establish the diagnosis, although with the increasing availability of computed tomography, this noninvasive radiological procedure may be preferred in some cases. For example, blood in the cerebellum due to a primary cerebellar hemorrhage may be visualized with computed tomography; this finding would make diagnostic lumbar puncture an unnecessary hazard. Similarly, the finding by computed tomography of hemorrhagic regions in the brain parenchyma resulting from closed head injury also obviates the need for lumbar puncture in many patients.

On the other hand, the CSF findings prove invaluable in the definition of many clinical problems. For example, lumbar puncture often provides the essential data in determining whether an apparently confusional state is due to a viral encephalitis, neurosyphilis, or tuberculous meningitis. The CSF should be examined in patients with unexplained seizures. The CSF findings are very valuable in establishing the diagnosis of multiple sclerosis, neurosyphilis, and the gamut of inflammatory diseases of the central nervous system and meninges. Lumbar puncture is used to ascertain that the CSF is free of blood before anticoagulant therapy is begun. However, the physician should be aware of a rare complication of anticoagulation instituted shortly after a traumatic spinal puncture. A traumatic bloody tap may be severely aggravated by heparin anticoagulation begun 4 hours after the puncture. This has resulted in a major subarachnoid hemorrhage associated with extradural bleeding and signs of root compression (personal communication from Dr. Paul Altrocchi).

When the CSF is made available at the time of myelography the fluid should usually be removed for analysis before the injection of the radiopaque substance or air. Failure to do so often confuses the physician should subsequent lumbar punctures become necessary, because of the inflammatory changes induced by the injected material. Suspected complete spinal block is an exception to this recommendation, because spinal fluid drainage may aggravate cord compression in such a case.

A substantial portion of this book deals with the CSF changes associated with various neurological disorders. While many diseases are associated with the relatively nonspecific abnormality of an elevated CSF protein level, this finding indicates a pathological process in the nervous system which requires elucidation.

Although the major role of lumbar puncture in clinical practice is a diagnostic one, the technique may prove useful in therapy as well. In the pre-antibiotic era, CSF drainage was used in the treatment of meningitis with the concomitant administration of intravenous fluids to establish "forced drainage of the CSF" (Levinson, 1929). This method was abandoned with the advent of chemotherapy. However, lumbar puncture, with the slow removal of CSF to lower the pressure to the normal range, is still useful for the relief of headache and backache in the treatment of patients with chronic meningitis due to lymphoma, sarcoidosis, and so on. Repeated lumbar puncture has been used in the treatment of benign intracranial hypertension (see Chapter 4), although it has a very limited role in the treatment of this disorder. Intrathecal therapy will be discussed further.

Contraindications

Lumbar puncture is contraindicated if there is suppuration in the skin and deeper tissues overlying the spinal canal, because of the hazard of inducing purulent meningitis. While experimental lumbar puncture in dogs with bacteremia has been responsible for the induction of bacterial meningitis (Petersdorf *et al.*, 1962), in clinical practice such a remote possibility should not discourage use of the procedure when it is indicated. The major precaution in performing lumbar puncture is to avoid the various complications of the procedure.

The most serious complication is the possibility of aggravating a pre-existing, often unrecognized herniation syndrome (Korein *et al.*, 1959; Duffy,

1969; Menkes and Byers, 1973). This hazard is the basis for considering papilledema to be a relative contraindication to lumbar puncture. The procedure is dangerous when papilledema is due to an intracranial mass, although lumbar puncture is safe (indeed has often been used as a treatment) in patients with benign intracranial hypertension (pseudotumor cerebri). A key factor appears to be the degree of obstruction and displacement of the ventricular system. In the past, angiography was often performed as the initial diagnostic procedure before lumbar puncture, to exclude the possibility of an intracranial mass in patients suspected of having intracranial hypertension. The availability of computed tomography has simplified the management of patients with papilledema due to a mass lesion in the absence of localizing signs. When computed tomography reveals no evidence of a mass lesion, obstruction, or displacement of the ventricular system, lumbar puncture is considered a necessary and appropriate procedure in the evaluation of a patient with papilledema and suspected intracranial hypertension. It is needed to document the presence of intracranial hypertension and to determine whether the CSF gives evidence of inflammatory or neoplastic disease.

The Method of Lumbar Puncture

The procedure is best carried out with the patient in the lateral recumbent position, with the craniospinal axis parallel to the floor and the flat of the back perpendicular to the plane of the bed or table. Any degree of elevation of the head above the level of the spinal needle will spuriously elevate the pressure. Patients should be reassured and their anxiety allayed by informing them about each step of the procedure.

An assistant is usually needed to help maintain the patient as comfortably as possible in a flexed knee-chest position. The spinal processes and interspaces are palpated and identified; the line connecting the tops of the two iliac crests usually crosses the L3-L4 interspace. The L3-L4, L4-L5, or L5-S1 interspaces are usable. Needle insertion at higher levels should be avoided because the conus medullaris extends to the L1-L2 interspace in 94 per cent of patients and to L2-L3 in the rest. Particularly in infants, the lowest possible interspace should be used because the infantile conus extends even lower in the spinal canal (Reimann and Anson, 1944; Brown, 1976).

Sterile technique is essential. Gloves should be used, and the skin should be cleaned with antiseptic solution and alcohol before needle insertion. Local anesthesia is necessary in conscious patients; the skin is injected intradermally and the deeper tissues infiltrated with a small amount (2 to 3 ml) of procaine. After the local anesthetic has taken effect, a 20 or 22 gauge needle with a well-fitted stylet is inserted in the midline. A 25 or 26 gauge needle, often used by anesthesiologists, is suitable for injection of anesthetic agents. However, small gauge needles are more difficult to insert and are unsatisfactory for measuring the intracranial pressure.

The midline position facilitates entry into the subarachnoid space, and it avoids injury of the roots, which are fixed laterally as they exit from the lumbar sac. The use of the stylet is considered necessary during insertion of the needle to avoid implantation of an epidermoid tumor in the subarachnoid space (Shaywitz, 1972; Batnitsky *et al.,* 1977); it is probably necessary on withdrawal of the needle to avoid entrapment of a spinal root in the extradural space (Trupp, 1977). (Divergent opinions about the need to reinsert the stylet before withdrawal will be discussed.)

When the needle has passed the resistance of the longitudinal ligament and there is a slight "give," the needle usually has reached the subarachnoid space, and fluid appears when the stylet is removed. If this fails, replacement of the stylet and rotation of the needle about 90 degrees is often effective in obtaining fluid. If not, the needle is inserted a few millimeters further, and usually a second sensation of "give" is experienced when the dura is pierced. If this fails, redirection of the needle is necessary, and the needle must be withdrawn almost to the skin because redirection of the needle is not possible when the point is deep in the tissue.

When fluid appears at the needle hub, a 3-way stopcock and the clinical CSF manometer are rapidly attached to minimize any loss of fluid that would falsely lower the initial pressure. A very slow and minimal rise of fluid in the manometer reflects either partial obstruction of the needle tip by meningeal membrane or a truly low CSF pressure. Minor rotation of the needle may solve the former problem. To ascertain that the needle is properly placed, the response to abdominal pressure should be determined. Firm abdominal pressure applied with two hands by the assistant normally results in a prompt rise in pressure; with release, a rapid fall to the initial level occurs within seconds. If this fails to happen, the physician should assume that the needle is not properly placed to obtain a free flow of fluid.

The clinical manometer records the mean intracranial pressure; normally it also shows the dampened pulsations synchronous with the pulse of 2 to 5 mm and with respiration of 4 to 10 mm. The initial pressure usually reaches a steady state within a minute or two, if the patient is at ease and is neither moving nor straining. The patient should be assisted to relax, because movement or straining will result in spurious elevation of the pressure. If the pressure is abnormally elevated, above 200 mm, the physician should wait for a minute or two to make sure that the patient is not straining, thereby increasing the intra-abdominal pressure. The patient must be cautioned not to hyperventilate, because hyperventilation sufficient to lower the arterial CO_2 pressure will spuriously lower the intracranial pressure.

If the CSF pressure is clearly elevated, the physician should allow CSF to drain very slowly to obtain sufficient fluid for essential diagnostic tests. The stopcock should be turned frequently to monitor the falling CSF pressure. The major factor whereby CSF removal aggravates cerebral herniation is the hole in the dura which allows persistent leakage of fluid from the subaranchoid space. Some clinicians suggest removing no more fluid when the CSF pressure has fallen to one-half of the initial pressure. The closing pressure should be determined just before removal of the needle. The drop from the initial pressure gives a rough measure of pressure-volume relationships. Sterile gauze is generally applied to the puncture site, because a small amount of fluid may continue to drain from the needle tract.

Lumbar Puncture in Infants

The most frequent indication for lumbar puncture in infants is to exclude meningitis. The technique of spinal puncture in infants may require some modification (Margolis and Cook, 1973). The sitting position may be desirable because the midline is more easily identified. Some authors have recommended the use of a non-styleted needle (butterfly scalp vein needle) in small infants because it allows the pressure to be estimated as the needle enters the sac, and if bleeding occurs a length of clear CSF can be seen in the tubing and cut off for culture (Greensher *et al.,* 1971). Naidoo (1968) used a scalp vein needle for lumbar punctures in 136 newborn infants without apparent complications. The failure to use a stylet may make the infant more vulnerable to the later development of an intraspinally transplanted epidermoid tumor (Shaywitz, 1972). However, this complication is probably rare. The position of the head is often critical; if the child is held very tightly flexed, CSF may not be obtained. However, if the head is held in midflexion, a brisk flow often results. If the correct position is not used, multiple punctures and a bloody tap are the usual consequences. An unsuccessful tap is more often due to a poor assistant than a poor operator (Brown, 1976)!

If CSF fails to flow after the child's position is adjusted, very gentle suction with a 1.0 ml syringe is permissable to exclude the possibility of a low CSF pressure. Unusual complications of lumbar puncture in infants have been reported, including the precipitation of tonic fits in the asphyxiated newborn and vagal cardiac arrest in children with cardiopulmonary disease. These complications were thought to be due to excessive physical restraint during the procedure (Margolis and Cook, 1973). Brown (1976) stated that leukemic meningitis may occur because of seeding after a traumatic lumbar puncture in patients with acute leukemia. He suggested that lumbar puncture should be avoided until the peripheral blood is cleared of blast cells. He has not provided the data to substantiate this view, and whether such cases represent needle-induced seeding of the meninges is conjectural.

Fontanelle Pressure

There has been considerable interest in measuring the intracranial pressure in infants with a noninvasive technique. This would avoid the complications of infection, hemorrhage, or local injury which may result from needle trauma. It would also allow the repeated or continuous measurement of intracranial pressure, which would be particularly valuable in the assessment of infants with hydrocephalus, without the hazards of invasive techniques which depend upon intraventricular catheters or subdural or epidural transducers. Clinicians often estimate the level of the intracranial pressure by palpation of the anterior fontanelle, but this method is subject to error. Several noninvasive techniques have been used and compared by Wealthall and Smallwood (1974). The measurement of the pulsations over the fontanelle with a tambour "fontanometer" proved unsuitable for routine use. Another method was to measure the tension of the anterior fontanelle to assess intracranial pressure, analogous to the use of the Schiøtz's tonometer to measure intraocular pressure. It also proved unsuitable for routine clinical use. A new technique, introduced by Wealthall and Smallwood (1974), uses an "aplanation transducer" as a "fontanometer." It shows promise as a noninvasive device for monitoring intracranial pressure over the anterior fontanelle.

Method of Cisternal Puncture

Puncture of the cisterna magna was introduced by Ayer (1920, 1923). The method was used widely in the past in some countries, because a lower incidence of postspinal headache resulted than with the usual lumbar technnique. (Presumably, the meningeal hole following cisternal puncture closes more readily because the CSF pressure at the level of the cistern is much lower than in the lumbar sac when the patient is in the erect position.) The technique has been seldom used in the United States. Before the introduction of myelography, it was often used with simultaneous lumbar puncture to allow comparison of the composition of the fluid and the pressures at both levels in suspected cases of spinal block due to spinal cord compression. Recently, cervical puncture has been introduced as an alternative procedure to cisternal puncture. At present, the use of cisternal or cervical puncture is limited to the following circumstances:

(1) Cisternal or cervical fluid is sampled when lumbar fluid cannot be obtained for technical reasons and when examination of the fluid is essential — for example, in patients suspected of having meningitis. Difficulties in obtaining lumbar fluid may arise in patients with rheumatoid spondylitis (Marie-Strümpell disease), previous spinal surgery (e.g., spinal fusion), spinal arachnoiditis of diverse origin, or cord tumor. At times there is no obvious explanation for a "dry tap."
(2) When complete spinal block has been revealed by a lumbar myelogram, injection of additional contrast medium into the cisterna magna is often needed to identify the upper level of the spinal block.
(3) Local suppuration in the lumbar region is a contraindication to lumbar tap.
(4) In patients with a lumbar peritoneal shunt for hydrocephalus, the cistern may be the preferred site for injection of a radioisotope to determine shunt patency.

Both the sitting position and the lateral recumbent position are used for cisternal puncture. The latter position is preferred because of the low cisternal fluid pressure obtained in the sitting position. The shoulders are placed in the vertical plane and the head is slightly flexed. A small pillow placed under the head helps keep the head and cervical vertebrae on the same horizontal plane. The skin of the suboccipital triangle is shaved and cleaned with antiseptic solutions. The usual spinal puncture needle is used, preferably one with a short bevel. The shaft should be marked precisely 7.5 cm from the point. The skin and subcutaneous tissues are infiltrated with procaine.

The puncture needle is inserted in the midline just above the spine of the atlas. It is directed forward and upward toward the plane of the external auditory meatus and the glabella, until the needle strikes the base of the occiput. It is then withdrawn a bit and depressed slightly to allow penetration of the dura just below the base of the occiput. The distance from the skin to the cisterna magna varies but is usually between 4.0 and 6.0 cm. There is usually a distance in the midline of 2.5 cm between the dura and the medulla, and the cistern contains about 25 ml of fluid. It is hazardous to insert the needle beyond the 7.5 cm mark on the shaft of the needle. Reported complications have included injury to the medulla (Levinson, 1929).

Bloody taps due to needle trauma are less frequent than in the lumbar region, presumably because the dural veins overlying the cistern are less extensive. Fluid can be removed for analysis and contrast medium injected in the usual way. Any solutions to be injected into the cisterna magna should be close to body temperature. Cisternal puncture is *contraindicated* in patients suspected of having an Arnold-Chiari malformation or posterior fossa tumor, which would fill the cisterna magna.

Method of Lateral Cervical Puncture

The lateral cervical puncture (LCP) is a useful alternative method to cisternal puncture. The technique was derived from a method for percutaneous cordotomy, in which a needle was inserted through the skin into the C1-C2 interspace under fluoroscopic control. The needle was advanced through the subarachnoid space into the spinal cord in order to interrupt spinothalamic fibers.

In recent years, lateral cervical puncture has been introduced as a bedside procedure without fluoroscopic control (Zivin, 1978). The C1-C2 interspace is used because there is no overlap of the cervical vertebrae laterally at the atlantoaxial joint and because there is a fairly wide intervertebral space at this level.

The patient is placed in the supine position in bed, without a pillow, and with the neck placed as straight as possible. The landmark for needle insertion is 1 cm caudal and 1 cm posterior to the tip of the mastoid process. The skin is then prepared in sterile fashion and local anesthetic is injected at the site. A standard lumbar puncture needle (usually 20 gauge) is inserted parallel to the plane of the bed and perpendicular to the neck. As the needle is inserted, a number of tissue planes are crossed and several "pops" are usually felt, so that it is sometimes impossible to tell by feel alone when the subarachnoid space has been entered. Therefore, the stylet is removed and replaced frequently to check whether CSF is flowing out of the needle. This method of slow advancement prevents too deep penetration into the subarachnoid space or spinal cord. The CSF pressure can be measured and fluid collected as in performing a lumbar tap, but the needle must be supported more carefully since it is not as deeply seated in surrounding tissue and moves quite easily.

After the procedure, the needle is rapidly removed without special precautions. The most common problems during needle insertion are due to malpositioning of the needle. If it is inserted too far posteriorly, the subarachnoid space will be missed and the needle will enter the paraspinal muscles. If the needle penetrates too deeply without encountering either bone or CSF, it has probably been positioned too far posteriorly or it is being angled toward the bed. If bone is encountered, reposition of the needle in the rostrocaudal plane is indicated. Lateral movements of the needle should be avoided. If anatomical anomalies are encountered or the patient is not completely co-operative, fluoroscopic control is advisable!

The contraindications for this procedure are the same as those for lumbar puncture: local infection, increased intracranial pressure with impending herniation and so on. The LCP engenders several additional risks. The vertebral artery runs near the puncture site and may be punctured. Experience with percutaneous cannulation of this vessel for arteriography indicates that significant injury is unlikely if the needle is removed and local pressure applied. Puncture of the spinal cord is said to cause the patient some pain; if this happens the needle should be removed and repositioned. The detrimental effects of inserting a relatively small needle into the spinal cord are probably minor because even when surgical lesions of the cord were intended (Rosomoff *et al.*, 1969) no major complications were reported when the surgery was unilateral (in patients with normal respiratory functions).

As in lumbar puncture, a traumatic tap may occur with its attendant consequences; a nerve root may be injured, producing local pain; and postspinal puncture headache may develop. While the technique is not difficult, the inexperienced physician is advised to observe the technique before putting it to use and then to obtain supervision from one familiar with the method.

Manometric Tests for Spinal Block

The Queckenstedt (1916) test was introduced to determine the absence or presence of spinal subarachnoid block. With the widespread use of contrast myelography to study patients suspected of having cord compression or a swollen cord, the test is now little employed. However, in a few special circumstances the test is particularly useful. In patients with chronic meningitis, periodically repeated diagnostic lumbar punctures are necessary to evaluate the response to treatment and to find out whether patients are developing a partial or complete spinal block. This is the case with patients receiving chemotherapy for tuberculous and fungal meningitis, sarcoidosis, meningeal lymphoma and carcinoma, and arachnoiditis of diverse causes.

Repeated myelograms are generally not appropriate, but serial jugular compression tests, coupled with cellular and chemical analyses of the fluid, provide a useful guide to the progress of meningeal disease and its response to therapy. The jugular compression test is particularly useful in the management of the patient with signs of a myelopathy, when it is uncertain whether a myelogram is essential. For example, it is desirable to avoid the stress of myelography in a patient with respiratory insufficiency or with an unstable cardiac status. If the jugular compression test is completely normal, a neurosurgical emergency is unlikely and the myelogram may be deferred. *However, if the test indicates either a partial or a complete block, Pantopaque should be injected before the removal of the needle in order to facilitate performance of a subsequent myelogram.* (In this instance, a water soluble contrast medium is not advantageous because of its rapid disappearance from the CSF.) The immediate injection is usually necessary because it may be impossible to re-enter the lumbar canal with a needle in patients with spinal block after an initial tap has resulted in loss of lumbar fluid.

Unilateral jugular compression, or the Tobey-Ayer test (1925), to be discussed later, has been used to verify the patency of the lateral dural venous sinuses when thrombosis was suspected. Except in this circumstance, jugular compression is usually contraindicated in suspected intracranial disease, particularly when there is increased intracranial pressure. Jugular compression causes an acute increase in intracranial venous pressure which is transmitted to the cranial subarachnoid space. The elevated pressure wave moves down the craniospinal axis and is recorded in the lumbar sac if there is no obstruction in the spinal subarachnoid space. Gilland (1964, 1966) systematically studied the dynamics of spinal block, devising an equation to describe the relationship between the degree of obstruction and the pressure responses recorded after jugular compression. Gilland also re-examined the data to be obtained by simultaneous cisternal and lumbar puncture in the diagnosis of spinal block. This technique was used widely in the pre-myelographic era. Cisternal or cervical injection of contrast media is now customary in cases of spinal block when the lumbar injection fails to delineate the block.

Jugular Compression Test (Cuff Manometrics)

Jugular compression may be done manually or with a blood pressure cuff. In the Queckenstedt test, the jugular veins are compressed manually by an assistant, first with light pressure and then with firm pressure, first unilaterally and then bilaterally. There should be a rapid rise in CSF pressure during 10 seconds of firm bilateral jugular compression. The peak pressure is normally 100 mm to 300 mm above the initial pressure, with a fall to the initial pressure within 10 seconds following release. Lack of such a pressure increase is an abnormal response, assuming the needle is properly placed in the lumbar sac. If the lumbar pressure rises and falls rapidly with abdominal pressure, it may be assumed that the needle is within the lumbar sac. Manual pressure must be sufficient to compress the veins but not firm enough to compress the carotid arteries.

The technique of cuff manometrics was introduced by Grant and Cone (1934). It is very much preferred to manual compression, particularly in eliciting evidence of partial block and in the circumstances just described in which repeated tests might be needed for the evaluation of chronic meningeal disorders. Cuff manometrics provides a quantitative assessment of the lumbar pressure response to a standardized, measured, and graded degree of jugular compression that cannot be obtained with manual compression.

First, the pressure response to 10 seconds of firm abdominal compression, manually applied by an assistant, is recorded to ascertain that a 20 gauge needle has been properly placed within the lumbar subarachnoid space. A narrow sphygmomanometer cuff (pediatric size) wrapped about the neck is inflated rapidly to 20 mm Hg for 10 seconds, and then the cuff pressure is abruptly released to zero. This should be demonstrated to the patient before the lumbar

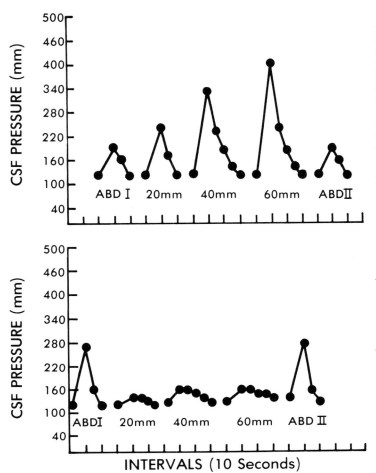

Figure 5–1 Cuff manometrics (quantitative Queckenstedt test). The upper figure shows normal cuff manometrics. The prompt response to abdominal pressure before and after the study indicates that the needle is properly placed. The graded responses to precisely 10 seconds of neck compression at 20, 40, and 60 mm Hg with a pediatric size blood pressure cuff indicate free transmission of increased intracranial venous pressure to the lumbar sac where the pressure is recorded. The lower figure illustrates the findings in a patient with complete spinal block caused by a thoracic meningioma. Note the excellent pressure responses to abdominal compression, I and II, performed before and after jugular compression. These responses verify that the lumbar needle is properly placed in the lumbar sac. The absence of any transmission of pressure to the lumbar sac, despite 10 seconds of jugular compression at 20, 40, and 60 mm, indicates complete spinal block. With partial degrees of block, partial responses are observed with minor elevations and a slow fall toward normal with jugular release. This test is often useful in following the course of patients receiving treatment for chronic meningitis.

tap, so that the patient may appreciate that the cuff pressures are not painful nor do they interfere with breathing. The inflated cuff feels like nothing more than a tight collar.

The spinal fluid pressure is recorded at the end of the 10 second period of neck compression; following release, its subsequent fall is recorded at 5 second intervals until the resting pressure is reached. The same procedure is repeated, using 40 mm and then 60 mm Hg pressure in the cuff. In patients with complete spinal block, there is no rise in lumbar pressure with jugular compression. With partial block, there may be a slight rise, perhaps only with 40 to 60 mm Hg compression, followed by a very slow fall after the release of the cuff pressure. If such blunted responses are noted, abdominal compression should be repeated to make certain that the needle has not become displaced from the lumbar sac to cause a simulated spinal block.

The normal response and the findings in a patient with complete spinal block due to a thoracic cord tumor are recorded in Figure 5–1. Note that the magnitude of the response to abdominal compression is increased if there is a block. This increase reflects the reduced compliance of a small, loculated volume of fluid in response to increasing hydrostatic pressure. The latter is transmitted directly to the lumbar sac from the paraspinal venous plexus when the abdominal compression has increased the abdominal vena cava pressure.

There are no available data defining the range of changes in pressure seen in normal subjects. Manual abdominal compression, depending upon its intensity and duration, may elevate the lumbar pressure over a wide range in normal subjects. Pressure elevations of 50 mm to 150 mm CSF above the resting level are readily elicited. The degree of lumbar pressure elevation normally obtained with 20, 40, and 60 mm Hg pressures in the cuff is also variable. The peak lumbar pressure elevations reached at 10 seconds are approximately 2, 3, and 4 times the initial pressure respectively with the use of the increasing cuff pressures described above. The peak levels reached are greater when a 19 gauge needle is used than with the usual 20 gauge needle. (Smaller gauge needles are unsatisfactory because the pressure responses are blunted.)

The time needed for the lumbar pressure to fall from its peak to its initial level varies between 10 and 15 seconds, if the patient remains relaxed and does not move or otherwise elevate the intra-abdominal pressure.

(The presence of a partial spinal block, in some cases, was demonstrated by manual jugular compression with the neck placed in marked flexion or extension [Kaplan and Kennedy, 1950]. This was interpreted to indicate inadequacy of the cervical subarachnoid space. The findings in such instances must be interpreted with caution, because false positive results have been obtained in normal subjects. The test has fallen into disuse.)

The initial CSF pressure is often very low or unobtainable when there is a complete spinal block, particularly when in the lumbar region. In such cases, there is usually a marked fall in pressure after removal of a small amount of fluid. (See Ayala index.) A minimal amount of fluid should be removed when spinal block is suspected, to minimize the risk of increasing the degree of cord compression which may result from cord impaction. In such instances it is often advisable to immediately inject a contrast medium for myelography. Patients with complete spinal block may develop a rapidly progressive increase in neurological deficit after myelography even when CSF is not removed, because of the aggravation of cord compression by subsequent spinal fluid leakage through the dural hole.

Tobey-Ayer Test (Unilateral Jugular Compression)

This test was developed to determine the patency of the lateral venous sinus in patients suspected of having sinus thrombophlebitis (Tobey and Ayer, 1925). The pressure response in the lumbar fluid is recorded after 10 seconds of unilateral compression of the jugular vein and again after similar compression of the other side. While no response or a reduced response suggests ipsilateral sinus occlusion, false positive responses also are observed. The right lateral sinus is often much larger than the left lateral sinus, resulting in a blunted response to compression of the left jugular vein.

*Pressure-Volume Relationships: The
Closing Pressure*

The relative degree of fall in the CSF pressure following removal of lumbar fluid is a rough index of the volume of the CSF reservoir. Thus, in complete spinal block the initial pressure, often low, perhaps 80 mm CSF, may fall to zero after removal of only 1 ml of fluid, indicating the presence of only a small reservoir. In contrast, a small fall in pressure after the removal of a rather large volume of fluid indicates a large reservoir. In hydrocephalus, for instance, the initial pressure may fall from 180 to 160 mm after removal of 10 ml. Such changes are the basis for recommending the routine measurement of the final pressure at the end of the spinal puncture, after the fluid has been removed for laboratory study.

Ayala (1923) devised an equation for estimating the size of the reservoir, as follows: quantity of fluid removed (precisely 10 ml) × final pressure divided by the initial pressure = the "rachidian quotient" or Ayala index. Values between 5.5 and 6.5 were considered normal. A value below 5 would suggest a small reservoir that might occur with spinal block or with increased brain volume due to a mass lesion or tonsillar herniation. A value above 7 would suggest a large reservoir that might occur with cerebral atrophy, hydrocephalus, or some forms of pseudotumor. While these generalizations hold, the Ayala index is little used because its normal limits are not well defined and because there are frequent exceptions with both falsely positive and falsely negative indices. The precise volume of fluid removed is critical, because there is not a simple linear relationship between changes in pressure and volume. The physician is advised to note these generalizations, but to have no confidence that the quantitative index provides specific or reliable information.

Tourtellotte and co-workers (1964) reported the initial pressure and the final pressure in 105 normal volunteers. The mean initial pressure was 150 mm ± 33 (SD) and the final pressure was 68 mm ± 31 (SD), after precisely 20 ml was removed. The average calculated Ayala index was 9.06, far in excess of the normal index calculated when 10 ml is removed, thus illustrating the critical dependence of the index on the volume of CSF removal. Thus, the Ayala index as orginally described is unreliable and subject to error. The physiology of pressure-volume regulation and the methods used in its assessment are discussed in Chapter IV.

Constant Infusion Manometric Test ("Flush" Test) and Other Spinal Infusion Tests

The application to patients of the technique of ventriculo-cisternal perfusion, developed in goats by Pappenheimer *et al.* (1961) indicated that the normal rate of CSF formation and reabsorption in humans is about 0.35 ml/min (see Chapter 3). With these data in mind, Katzman and Hussey (1970) developed a simple bedside test, the constant infusion manometric test ("flush" test) to assess the adequacy of spinal fluid absorption. The method has been used in the diagnosis and evaluation of "occult" hydrocephalus in adults and of communicating hydrocephalus in children.

The test is a refinement of a test proposed by Foldes and Arrowood in 1948. It is based on the infusion of normal saline at a constant rate into the lumbar subarachnoid space, with serial measurement of subarachnoid pressures during the period of infusion. The pressures obtained depend initially upon the distensibility of the subarachnoid space (a function of its compliance or elastance) and then upon the rate of bulk flow reabsorption of CSF into the venous system. The authors recommended infusion of normal saline at the rate of 0.76 ml/min over a 30 to 60 minute period. This rate is approximately two times the average normal rate of spinal fluid formation, 0.35 ml/min, so that maintenance of a normal CSF pressure would require absorption of a total volume of about 1.1 ml/min by bulk flow into the venous system.

Figure 5–2 reveals the average manometric response during a one-hour infusion of normal saline at 0.76 ml/min, in 21 control patients. In the control group a relatively steady state was observed within 30 minutes of infusion, with little change in pressure thereafter. Thus, an upper limit of 295 mm H_2O is the maximal pressure to be expected in control subjects. The test is technically simple to perform, and no serious adverse reactions to the procedure have been reported.

Abnormal tests are characterized by pressure elevations to levels above 300 mm H_2O during the period of infusion. Such abnormal responses have usually been noted within the first 20 minutes of an infusion. Abnormal curves were obtained in infants with progressive communicating hydrocephalus and in adults with invasion of the subarachnoid space by tumor. Similarly, Hussey *et al.* (1970) noted impaired CSF absorption in 2 adult patients with chronic polyra-

Figure 5–2 Constant infusion test ("flush test"). The mean lumbar CSF pressures during a one-hour period of infusion of 0.76 ml/min were recorded in 21 control patients. The confidence limits (dotted lines) indicate the normal range. The almost vertical line indicates an abnormal elevation in pressure in one patient with communicating hydrocephalus caused by malignant melanoma. This abnormal response may be artificially simulated by faulty placement of the needle in the subdural space (from Hussey, Schanzer, and Katzman, 1970).

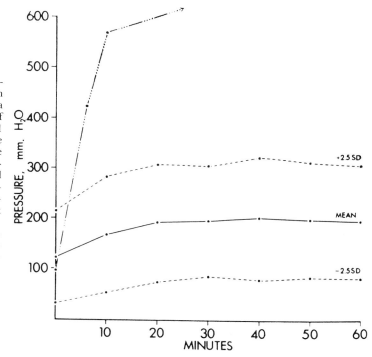

diculopathy and pseudomotor cerebri. (The latter finding has been confirmed by Calabrese *et al.* [1978] and Mann *et al.* [1979].)

Theoretically, this simple test should provide quantitative data regarding the adequacy of the mechanism for CSF absorption. However, the test is subject to the same technical difficulty experienced with isotope cisternography, namely, subdural injection of the saline solution. In Figure 5–2, the findings in a patient with an apparent block to CSF absorption are superimposed upon the data obtained in control patients. A pressure in excess of 550 mm was obtained in 10 minutes after injection of only 7.6 ml. This finding would be simulated if the saline was injected into the subdural space rather than the subarachnoid space. The occurrence of such false positive tests is a limitation of the technique. Wolinsky *et al.*, (1973) reported that the test was unreliable for the evaluation of patients suspected of having normal pressure hydrocephalus, because the results were abnormal in only 4 of 13 patients in whom pneumoencephalography and cisternography had indicated communicating hydrocephalus, and the results were also normal in 2 patients with normal pressure hydrocephalus who later improved following a surgical shunt. (Similarly, isotope cisternography also failed to reliably distinguish those patients who would be benefited by a surgical shunt.)

Nelson and Goodman (1971) modified the test by injecting larger amounts of normal saline at different rates. Using an isovolumetric strain gauge manometer instead of a clinical manometer, they recorded the slope of the change in pressure with time. They indicated that this would more clearly differentiate between normal and abnormal subjects. When they injected larger volumes of isotonic saline solution (which has a pH of 4.5 and differs in ionic composition from CSF), patients became restless, agitated, and tremulous.

Braham *et al.* (1971) reported another modification of the spinal infusion technique. They measured the initial lumbar pressure, allowed 5 ml to flow into a syringe, and waited for the pressure to return to its initial level, which took 30 minutes in some instances. Then the 5 ml was reinjected, raising the intracranial pressure, and the pressure was followed until it fell to its original level. The diagnostic specificity of this procedure has not been established.

Borgesen and associates (1978) have used a lumbo-ventricular perfusion test with the lumbar infusion of lactated Ringer's solution at rates between 0.5 and 4.0 ml per minute while recording the ventricular pressure with a strain gauge. They graphically analyzed the relationship between intraventricular pressure and absorption rate. Considerable variation in the calculated resistance to absorption was found in relation to the clinical findings in patients with normal pressure hydrocephalus. They concluded that the technique did not appear useful in the selection of patients for shunting procedures. However, Caldarelli *et al.* (1979) reached the opposite conclusion in a study of 59 children with hydrocephalus. They found the infusion test, performed as described by Hussey *et al.* (1970), to be useful as an adjunct to neuroradiological studies in determining indications for surgery.

In summary, various spinal infusion tests have demonstrated the presence of an absorption block in some patients with the pseudotumor syndrome and normal pressure hydrocephalus. However, the reliability of the infusion tests in identifying those patients with normal pressure hydrocephalus who might be benefited by a surgical shunt is uncertain. The underlying principle, namely, the direct measurement of the absorptive capacity of the subarachnoid space, seems to be a very logical way to establish the presence of absorptive defects. Perhaps, with great attention to technique, the manometric infusion test may prove to be of special value in serial studies of a single patient.

Cerebrospinal Fluid Lavage and Barbotage

Lavage of the subarachnoid space with normal saline was used as a treatment for patients with purulent meningitis in the pre-antibiotic era. It was sometimes recommended as a prelude to the injection of immune serum in the treatment of meningococcal meningitis (Levinson, 1929). When the CSF was very thick, the lavage technique sometimes made use of two needles, a cisternal needle for the introduction of saline and a lumbar needle for drainage. There are side effects with the injection of large volumes of normal saline, described by Nelson and Goodman (1971); 100 ml injected over 40 to 50 minutes caused mild headache, root pain, and restlessness in some patients. Normal saline has a pH of about 4.5 to 5, and it induces an inflammatory response when injected into the subarachnoid space. Elliott's solution has an ionic composition which is quite similar to that of normal CSF, and it would be better tolerated.

In the 1930's and 1940's, there was an interest in the method of CSF barbotage developed by Speranski in Russia and described by Savage in England. Speranski reported that the technique was beneficial in the treatment of rheumatoid arthritis, malaria, and typhus! The method involved lumbar puncture with the removal of 20 ml of CSF into a syringe followed by slow reinjection of the fluid (Savage, 1948). This procedure, termed "spinal pumping," was repeated twenty times over an hour. While Speranski minimized the hazards of the procedure, it is noteworthy that Bunge *et al.* (1961) used a technique of spinal barbotage to induce demyelination in cats. A few case reports have described flushing of the skin and sweating as a response to the Speranski treatment and the death of a patient from a brainstem hemorrhage (Savage, 1948).

More recently, spinal fluid lavage was suggested by Di Chiro (1974) as an emergency treatment for the acute paraparesis that may develop as a complication of abdominal aortography. This complication was attributed to a direct toxic effect of iodine in the contrast media on the spinal cord. In an effort to treat such a patient, Morariu (1978) reported the rapid withdrawal of 70 ml of CSF in 10 ml aliquots and replacement of a similar volume of normal saline, about 25 minutes after the onset of paraplegia. Substantial concentrations of iodine were detected in the fluid. Although the patient improved rapidly, it is not clear whether the suggested cause of the paraparesis, and the therapeutic rationale, are correct. The possibility that injection of the contrast media induced vasoconstriction of the radicular arteries, with secondary transient spinal ischemia, would be a good alternative explanation. Whether spinal drainage to remove iodine derived from the contrast media is of therapeutic benefit is still to be determined.

COMPLICATIONS OF LUMBAR PUNCTURE

Upon proper indications, the performance of a lumbar puncture (LP) by a skillful physician is normally well tolerated by patients. There are, however, several potential hazards and complications of the procedure which are of importance. These include the worsening of brain herniation or cord compression, headache, diplopia, subarachnoid bleeding, backache, radicular symptoms, either localized inflammation or a diffuse meningitis, and implantation of an epidermoid tumor. In addition, spinal anesthesia, intrathecal therapy, and the injection of diagnostic agents such as air, contrast media, and isotopes offer the additional hazards of the toxic effects of the material injected. These complications of lumbar puncture are now considered in detail.

Brain Herniation

The potential hazards of lumbar puncture in patients with papilledema were recognized soon after its introduction (Mestrezat, 1912). The occurrence of both uncal and cerebellar tonsillar herniation in patients with expanding lesions was noted in patients who showed almost immediate clinical deterioration after removal of fluid by the lumbar route. The mechanism of herniation, simply stated, is this: when the brain volume is sufficiently increased because of a mass lesion or edema, rostrocaudal displacement will occur if the skull is intact. As the brain volume is pathologically increased, there is a compensatory decrease in CSF volume attributed to the increased rate of CSF absorption that occurs with intracranial hypertension (see Chapter 4). It appears likely that herniation following the removal of spinal fluid occurs only in the presence of some degree of pre-existing obstruction in the CSF pathways. When there is free communication between the CSF pathways of the cranial cavity and of the spinal subarachnoid space, the fall in CSF pressure obtained with spinal puncture reaches equilibrium along the CSF pathways without tissue displacement.

It is noteworthy that lumbar puncture in the past has been used as a routine treatment of patients with benign intracranial hypertension (pseudomotor cerebri) without deleterious effects, despite very elevated CSF pressures. On the other hand, lumbar puncture may aggravate a pre-existing herniation which has caused blockage of the subarachnoid space, although symptoms and signs of herniation may first appear only after the puncture has been performed. The clinical manifestations of the several herniation syndromes have been well described by Plum and Posner (1972).

The frequency with which lumbar puncture was reported to have deleterious effects on patients with papilledema and intracranial hypertension has varied. Korein *et al.* (1959) reviewed the results of spinal puncture performed on 70 patients with papilledema and on 59 patients with intracranial hypertension in the absence of papilledema. A wide variety of diagnostic categories, including tumor and subdural hematoma, was included in both groups. Any unfavorable change during the following 48 hours was noted. The authors also compiled the data from 6 previously published reports and concluded that the incidence of complications in their cases and in the literature was less than 1.2 per cent.

Swartz and Dodge (1965) reported fatal cerebral herniation in 3 of 175 children with purulent meningitis. Duffy (1969) reported that of 30 patients with intracranial hypertension who appeared to worsen following lumbar puncture, 5 deteriorated within 12 hours of the procedure. All the patients were critically ill, with progressive headache, mental changes, and focal signs. Duffy concluded that the patients had already formed a tentorial or cerebellar pressure cone before the procedure.

When there is a strong indication for lumbar puncture, such as the need for bacterial cultures if meningitis is suspected, lumbar puncture should be performed despite the possible risks of the procedure. The availability of computed tomography has simplified the management of patients with papilledema and suspected intracranial hypertension. The technique establishes the absence or presence of distortion or displacement of the ventricular system, thus facilitating the physician's decision about the appropriateness of spinal puncture.

Headache

Headache is the most common complication of lumbar puncture, whether performed for diagnostic purposes or for spinal anesthesia. The precise incidence has been variously reported. The monograph of Tourtellotte and associates (1964) provides a meticulous review of the world literature about spinal headache, beginning with Quincke's report in 1891 and continuing through 1960, and involving over 21,000 patients! Individual reports of the incidence of headache have varied considerably, but the average incidence of headache, whether mild or severe, was a surprising 32 per cent. This figure remained constant in various reports over the intervening decades, despite the heterogeneous nature of the patient population and variations in the performance of the physicians and in their techniques.

Nevertheless, my clinical impression is that a much lower incidence, perhaps 10 to 15 per cent, is observed in neurological inpatients and outpatients. The high incidence before 1960 may have reflected the repeated use of lumbar puncture needles, many of which were blunted or fish-hooked. The modern LP needle is much sharper and easier to use. A tabulation of reports of over 79,000 patients who were given spinal anesthesia revealed an average incidence of headache of about 10 per cent, the figure being higher (18 per cent) in obstetrical patients than in general surgical patients (Tourtellotte et al., 1964). (The lower incidence following spinal anesthesia may reflect the prolonged period of time during which post-operative patients remain in bed.)

The symptoms of postspinal headache are characteristic. Tourtellotte and colleagues (1964) systematically studied headache after lumbar puncture in normal subjects. They described the clinical features in 24 normal volunteers as follows. The time of onset of the headache varied from 15 minutes to 4 days after the tap. Headache persisted for 2 to 14 days, in most cases lasting 4 to 8 days. The headaches were usually localized in the frontal region, often in the retro-orbital area, and were characterized by aching, pounding sensations. (In some patients, the headache is chiefly occipital in location.) The characteristic and most diagnostic feature of the headache was its onset with the patient in the upright position and its prompt relief when the patient lay flat. Generally, the headache was mild at first and became more severe in the following hours or days; it came on sooner after arising and left only after long periods of reclining.

The headache stayed at a plateau of severity for several days before it waned. Postural nausea occurred less often than headache and was shorter in duration. It was occasionally associated with vomiting, "cold sweats," and rarely vertigo and light headaches. Aching of the neck and particularly of the lower back were also common.

Dripps and Vandam (1954) summarized the complication of spinal anesthesia in 6000 patients. They considered postspinal headache to be due to low CSF pressure rather than to the anesthetic agent. They described the delay in onset of headache to be as long as 7 to 10 days (the number of days the postoperative patients remained in bed was not given), and in some cases headache lasted for months. The symptoms of neck pain and stiffness predominated and were more disturbing than the headache to some patients.

Etiology of Spinal Headache

It has been widely held that postspinal headache is due to low CSF pressure that results from the persistent leakage of fluid through a hole in the arachnoid and dural membranes. Pickering (1948) observed that repeated lumbar puncture in patients with postspinal headache revealed the pressure to be very low or atmospheric; fluid did not drip from the needle and could be obtained only with gentle aspiration with a syringe. After lumbar puncture, a dural hole and subdural collection of CSF have been observed in patients, at the time of subsequent laminectomy or at autopsy (Tourtellotte et al., 1964). Postspinal headache is less likely to occur in patients with inflammatory changes in the fluid due to meningitis. This probably means that the hole is more readily closed when there is cellular infiltration of the meninges.

Kunkle et al. (1943) explored the pathophysiology of postspinal headache by acutely inducing spinal drainage headaches in normal subjects. Headache appeared when pressures were reduced by the removal of about 20 ml of CSF, an amount close to 15 per cent of the estimated CSF volume. The estimated vertex pressure fell to between -220 and -290 mm from a normal level of about -100 mm (relative to the right atrium) in the sitting position. It was concluded that pain was evoked by displacement or stretching, or both, of the pain-sensitive structures, blood vessels and meninges. Kunkle et al. (1943) also studied spinal drainage headache induced in a patient who previously had undergone section of the roots of the 5th and 9th cranial nerves and the upper 4 cervical nerves, all on the left side, with analgesia in the regions to which these nerves project. Induced drainage headache produced pain in the right forehead but none in the left. This result was interpreted to support the view that traction displacement of structures innervated by the 5th nerve are responsible for the referred pain of frontal headache induced by drainage.

It is noteworthy that the intravenous injection of hypotonic solutions transiently reduces puncture headache, whereas hypertonic solutions augment the headache (Tourtellotte et al., 1964). Such fluid loads have opposite effects on brain volume and intracranial pressure, and such changes are probably responsible for the opposite effects on the headache. The fact that jugular compression acutely increases postspinal headache despite the transient increase in intracranial pressure induced by the procedure supports the conclusion that the headache is due not to low CSF pressure *per se* but to displacement and stretching of pain-sensitive structures, such as meninges and vessels, induced by intracranial hypotension (Pickering, 1948; Wolff, 1972).

Some patients with postspinal headaches complain of tinnitus, decrease in hearing, and "blocking" of the ears, which disappear as the headache improves. This was attributed by Vandam and Dripps (1956) to a concomitant reduction in intralabyrinthine pressure. There is an anatomical connection between the subarachnoid space and the cochlea in animals; Hughson (1932) demonstrated that with reduction in CSF pressure there is impaired hearing for high tones. Both relief of headache and improvement in hearing apparently occurred after injection of fluid into the subarachnoid space (Vandam and Dripps, 1956).

Factors Influencing Postspinal Headache

Many factors that might influence the incidence of postspinal headache have been considered by various authors. These include: age, sex, psychological state, hydration, position during the puncture, needle size and shape, technique and anesthetic agent, number of perforations of the meninges, initial pressure, rapidity of CSF removal, volume removed, and position or activity after the tap. The various factors are considered here. The data have been annotated in detail in the monograph by Tourtellotte *et al.* (1964).

AGE. According to most reports, the incidence of headache has been higher in younger than in older patients, but the reasons for this difference have not been ascertained. Presumably, the holes in the arachnoid and dura close more readily in older subjects.

SEX. There is a significant increase $(p < 0.05)$ in the frequency of headache in women that has not been explained, according to many reports.

PSYCHOLOGICAL STATE. While the role of psychological factors in the pathogenesis of the headache has been stressed by some authors in the past, Tourtellotte *et al.* (1964) concluded that these factors play no important role. Certainly, the stereotyped syndrome, its constancy for seven decades, and its characteristic response to treatment argue in favor of an organic cause in most cases. Torrey (1979) and Ballenger *et al.* (1979) have reported a much lower incidence in schizophrenic patients than in control subjects, perhaps reflecting decreased sensitivity to pain in schizophrenia.

POSITION DURING LP. Several reports indicate that headache is lessly likely to occur when the puncture is performed with the patient in the horizontal position rather than in the sitting position. This was not confirmed by Tourtellotte *et al.* (1964). However, it is clear that the horizontal position is needed to accurately measure the CSF pressure.

SIZE OF NEEDLE. Although there are some inconsistencies in the published reports, most authors agree that the smaller the needle, the milder and/or the less prolonged the post-LP headache; the incidence after use of an 18 gauge needle is greater than after use of a 20 or 22 gauge needle. Anesthesiologists sometimes favor 25 or 26 gauge needles. While such small needles are suitable for the injection of anesthetic agents, they are not as suitable for recording the CSF pressure or for the drainage of CSF. A short beveled needle is preferred, because a long bevel is more likely to result in insertion of the needle's point into both the subdural and subarachnoid spaces. This would result in a poor flow of fluid, and in cases when contrast media or medications are injected, a subdural injection of the material would be more likely to occur.

TECHNIQUE.   The midline approach is usual for spinal puncture because it best allows the physician to use the spinous processes as anatomical landmarks. Recently, Hatfalvi (1977) advocated the lateral approach, in which the needle is introduced 2 to 3 cm from the midline. The author reported that more than 600 spinal anesthetics were given with a 20 gauge needle without a single case of postspinal headache! His explanation for these results is that lateral punctures produce holes in the dura and arachnoid that do not overlap, and thus spinal fluid leakage is minimized following the procedure.

QUANTITY OF CSF REMOVED.   There have been some inconsistencies in various reports. However, Sciarra and Carter (1952) found no difference in the incidence of postspinal headache in a group of patients from whom 7 to 12 ml of fluid was removed, compared to a group on which LP's were done without any removal of fluid. If 20 to 30 ml is removed rapidly, with an immediate fall in pressure, a mild transient postural headache may occur, but removing large amounts of fluid will not cause a persistent postspinal headache unless there is a continual CSF leak through a dural hole. Large volumes of CSF are more likely to yield positive bacteriological and cytological findings.

ACTIVITY OR POSITION AFTER LUMBAR PRESSURE.   This has been a controversial issue. Tourtellotte *et al.* (1964) statistically analyzed five major studies and summarized the very contradictory results. These included a worsening, an improvement, and no effect on headaches when patients were immediately mobilized after puncture. The reasons for such discrepancies are obscure. Brocker's (1958) study is of special interest. Several hundred patients were instructed to stay in either the prone or the supine position for 3 hours following lumbar puncture performed with an 18 gauge needle. A 36 per cent incidence of headache was noted in the supine group and 0.5 per cent incidence in the prone group! Presumably, the prone position caused hyperextension of the spine which favored closure of the meningeal hole. However, the striking advantage of the prone position in reducing the incidence of headache was not confirmed by the studies of Tourtellotte *et al.* (1964), in which 20 gauge needles were used, and no difference in incidence was found in a group of several hundred patients. The basis for the discrepancy in these two studies is not apparent.

HYDRATION.   Although there are several reports that intravenous fluids, either saline or 5 per cent glucose, may be of benefit in the prevention of headache, Tourtellotte *et al.* (1964) criticized this conclusion on statistical grounds. The rate of CSF formation has been shown to be relatively constant in the face of various physiological stresses (see Chapter 3) and, almost surely, it is unaffected by intravenous infusion of isotonic fluids. Whereas dehydration would be undesirable in the management of spinal headache because it would lower the intracranial pressure and might therefore aggravate headache, there is little rationale for inducing a water diuresis either for prevention or for treatment.

EFFECTS OF MEDICATIONS IN PREVENTION AND TREATMENT.   The use of many medications and other preparations has been advocated — barbiturates, codeine, neostigmine, ergot derivatives, Benadryl, Dramamine, Benzedrine, caffeine, ephedrine, intravenous fluids, magnesium sulfate, vitamins, and so on. There are no convincing data that any of these agents has a specific effect on the headache syndrome. Most clinical studies have not been adequately controlled for the placebo effects of the medication in question.

The Avoidance and Treatment of Post-LP Headache

The voluminous literature, summarized by Tourtellotte *et al.* (1964), indicates much uncertainty over the prevention of headache and other complications. There is general consensus among most clinicians regarding the following points:

(1) Use as small a styleted needle as possible. For routine diagnostic purposes, except in infants, a 20 gauge needle is usually preferred to a 22 gauge because its greater stiffness makes it easier to use. A 22 gauge needle is rather unsatisfactory for the jugular compression (Queckenstedt) test because the small bore excessively dampens the pressure responses. Fluid flow through a 22 gauge needle is slow; this prolongs the routine tap, which is a disadvantage in a restless patient. A 22 gauge or smaller needle can be used for spinal anesthesia.

(2) Multiple puncture holes of the meninges should be avoided to minimize the possibility of headache.

(3) There is uncertainty over the best position after puncture. Most patients tolerate well the prone position; I usually recommend that they remain in it for about an hour post puncture. This practice is a modification of Brocker's (1958) use of 3 hours, although Tourtellotte *et al.* (1964) did not confirm the protective value of the prone position.

(4) In the management of postspinal headache, strict bed rest in the horizontal position is recommended. Simple analgesics are used. The use of parenteral fluids to obtain diuresis is not recommended. If symptoms are severe and do not respond to bed rest, use of the "blood patch" is recommended. (This has been a rare occurrence in our inpatient and outpatient services.)

The incidence of postspinal headache does not appear to be influenced by hospitalization, and therefore lumbar puncture can often be done as an outpatient office procedure, to rule out such diseases as neurosyphilis. If spinal block is suspected, hospitalization is usually necessary to permit an emergency myelogram if one is indicated.

Blood Patch Treatment of Postspinal Headache

The use of a "blood patch" has proved to be very useful in the treatment of persistent postspinal headache (Ostheimer *et al.*, 1974; Abouleish *et al.*, 1975). It is not useful for treatment of brief minor headaches; rather, it should be applied to only those few patients with intractable headaches that fail to respond to a period of strict bed rest. The technique utilizes the epidural injection of autologous blood at the site of the dural puncture to form a thrombotic tamponade which seals the dural opening. The technique has been used widely by anesthesiologists in the treatment of postanesthetic spinal headache. A two-year follow-up of 118 patients so treated revealed no serious complications of the epidural blood patch (Abouleish *et al.*, 1975). No cases of infection, arachnoiditis, or cauda equina injury have been reported.

The technique requires an assistant to facilitate the almost simultaneous withdrawal of the patient's venous blood and its injection into the epidural space. The patient is placed in the lateral position, the skin is prepared antiseptically, and the same interspace previously used for lumbar puncture is re-entered. A 16 gauge needle is placed epidurally, using the loss of resistance technique to identify the epidural space (Ostheimer *et al.*, 1974). Once the needle is properly placed in the epidural space, an assistant draws 10 ml of blood from a suitable vein using a strictly sterile technique; the use of gloves, cap, and mask is recommended. The 10 ml volume of blood is slowly injected into the epidural space. Entry of blood into the subarachnoid space must be avoided. The needle is then removed and the patient returned to the supine position for about an hour. The patient should be advised that discomfort in the back with some radiation to the legs may be experienced. This is usually transient, but there are reports of discomfort lasting up to three days. Improvement in the headache begins within a few hours and is usually complete by the following day. A success rate of 80 to 95 per cent for the procedure has been reported (Abouleish *et al.*, 1975).

Other Complications of Lumbar Puncture

Diplopia

An uncommon complication of lumbar puncture is the development of diplopia due to unilateral or bilateral 6th nerve palsy (Dattner and Thomas, 1941). This has been seen in patients concurrently with symptoms of post-LP headache, usually a few days after diagnostic lumbar puncture or spinal anesthesia. Dripps and Vandam (1951) found diplopia in 5 of 140 patients with postspinal headache. By 1950, more than 500 cases following spinal anesthesia had been reported. The 6th nerve palsy is attributable to low CSF pressure secondary to a persistent CSF leak into the subdural space which results in stretching or displacement of the 6th nerve as it passes over the petrous ridge of the temporal bone. The palsy may be partial or complete. The diplopia is usually transient, clearing in days or weeks, although it may last as long as 9 months. The onset of diplopia with spinal headache usually requires reassurance of both the patient and the physician by the neurological consultant.

Subarachnoid Bleeding and Spinal Subdural Hematoma

Trauma to the arachnoid and dural vessels, usually venules, by the spinal needle generally causes only an asymptomatic "bloody tap." Occasionally, extensive subarachnoid bleeding may be induced by the needle, simulating a primary subarachnoid hemorrhage with the subsequent appearance of meningeal signs as well as the usual spinal fluid changes, xanthochromia and pleocytosis. This probably results most often from direct injury to the small

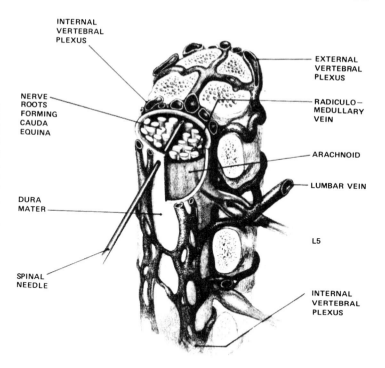

Figure 5–3 Spinal contents at the fourth and fifth lumbar vertebrae to show relationship of a lumbar puncture needle to the major vessels at this level. The major radiculomedullary vein, shown accompanying the L5 nerve root, is situated far laterally to a needle correctly positioned in the midline of the dural sac. Note the avascular subdural space (from Edelson, Chernik, and Posner, 1974).

radicular vessels of the cauda equina (Masdeu *et al.,* 1979). Subarachnoid bleeding is particularly likely to occur in patients with a bleeding diathesis or in those on anticoagulant drugs (Edelson *et al.,* 1974). The administration of heparin four hours after a traumatic lumbar puncture has resulted in this complication (Dr. Paul Altrocchi, personal communication). Injury to spinal radicular arteries may also occur, giving rise to a spinal subdural hematoma or epidural hematoma. Spinal subdural hematoma is much rarer than spinal epidural hematoma. Figure 5–3 illustrates the relationship of a lumbar puncture needle to the major vessels at the L4-L5 level.

Hazards of Thrombocytopenia and Anticoagulation

The presence of thrombocytopenia or other bleeding diatheses demands special consideration. They serve as relative contraindications to lumbar puncture because of the hazard of needle-induced subarachnoid hemorrhage or spinal subdural or epidural hematomas. The prothrombin, bleeding, and clotting times, and platelet count should be evaluated before lumbar puncture in vulnerable patients. There is often a lack of an obvious relationship between the platelet count and bleeding manifestations. Thus, in severe idiopathic thrombocytopenic purpura, some patients will have no bleeding, while others with a less severe decrease in the number of platelets may have marked bleeding. This variation is probably attributable to the better correlation of the bleeding time with the number of young platelets present than with the absolute platelet count.

The standardized bleeding time is therefore of special importance in evaluating the hazard of lumbar puncture in patients with low platelet counts (Harker and Slichter, 1972).

It should be emphasized that lumbar puncture should be undertaken only for pressing clinical indications when the platelet count is depressed to levels of about 50,000 or below. Edelson *et al.* (1974) recommended the administration of a platelet transfusion just before the puncture, if the count is below 20,000 or dropping rapidly. They advised the use of a 22 gauge needle and careful observation following the puncture; if pain or abnormal neurological signs develop, additional platelet transfusions are indicated.

Anticoagulant therapy also increases the hazard of lumbar puncture, which may then result in both symptomatic subarachnoid hemorrhage and epidural spinal hematoma with compression of the cauda equina. Thus, the administration of protamine to patients receiving heparin, and vitamin K or fresh frozen plasma to those receiving coumadin, should be considered before lumbar puncture to minimize the hazard of the procedure.

Backache and Radicular Symptoms

The traumatic effects of the needle are commonly responsible for minor local back discomfort. However, the needle may pass beyond the subarachnoid space and damage the annulus fibrosus. Rarely, frank disc herniation has been reported (Gellman, 1940). Gelatinous material from the nucleus was seen to drip from the needle when the patient moved inadvertently during spinal anesthesia. Dripps and Vandam (1951) also reported that irritation of the roots of the cauda equina during the lumbar puncture occurred in 13 per cent of cases, resulting in acute radicular pain or dysesthesias. More persistent sensory symptoms have been noted. Rarely, the spinal cord itself may be injured by the needle. Studies of 129 adult cadavers indicated that the cord ended at the level of the 1st or 2nd lumbar vertebrae in 94 per cent of them. In the others, however, the cord ended as low as the middle of the third lumbar vertebral body (Reimann and Anson, 1944). It is clear that lumbar puncture above the L3-L4 interspace should be performed with great caution. This is particularly important in infancy or early childhood, when the cord descends more caudally within the spinal canal than it does after maturity (Brown, 1976).

Implantation of Epidermoid Tumor: The Need for the Stylet

The introduction of a plug of epidermis into the subarachnoid space has been attributed to the use of a non-styleted needle (Batnitsky *et al.*, 1977). As a result, slowly growing implantation epidermoid tumors have developed, giving rise to signs of a spinal tumor years later. This emphasizes the need for the use of a stylet when the lumbar puncture needle is inserted through the skin. Similarly, the history of patients with spinal epidermoid tumors should be scrutinized for a previous spinal anesthetic or diagnostic puncture.

Another complication of failure to properly use the stylet when withdrawing the spinal needle is the trapping of a lumbar nerve root and adjacent arachnoid within the needle lumen. This has resulted in aspiration of the nerve into the epidural space. Such root fixation was reported to cause a painful syndrome that required laminectomy and replacement of the nerve root within the subarachnoid space (Trupp, 1977). On the other hand, Young and Burney (1971) reported the transection of a nerve filament which was then fixed to the needle wall with the insertion of the stylet. As the needle was withdrawn, the trapped nerve was also pulled along the needle tract and out the lumbar puncture site.

Thus, while it is essential to use the stylet with insertion, there is some controversy over whether the stylet should be reinserted before removal. It is difficult to resolve this because it is not clear which technique is less hazardous.

Infection

Lumbar puncture is contraindicated if there is evidence of infection in the region of the puncture site (for instance, cellulitis, furunculosis, or epidural abscess) because of the hazard of inducing meningitis with the needle. After lumbar puncture, infections may occur because of failure to use an aseptic technique or because local tissue injury has fostered a metastatic hematogenous infection. The complications of vertebral osteomyelitis, disc infection, epidural abscess, and bacterial meningitis as a result of errors in technique have been reported (Findlay and Kemp, 1943; Rangell and Glassman, 1945; Bromley et al., 1949).

There is a theory that diagnostic puncture, used in patients with bacteremia, might be responsible for the induction of meningitis. This has been shown experimentally in dogs by Petersdorf et al. (1962); several analogous clinical reports suggest that this may have occurred in humans (Fischer et al., 1975). Shinefield (1975), in a thoughtful comment, emphasizes that this potential hazard is not a reason to withhold lumbar puncture when meningitis is suspected. It has been suggested that patients with acute leukemia and multiple circulating blast cells may also risk developing leukemic meningitis from the introduction of malignant cells into the CSF by the spinal puncture. However, there are no convincing data available indicating that this has actually taken place.

Subdural Injections

Another complication of lumbar puncture is the creation of a subdural collection of CSF which is slowly absorbed. There may or may not be evidence of a CSF leak and a postspinal headache due to low CSF pressure. Such a pool of CSF has been considered responsible for the occurrence of a subdural injection of contrast medium during a myelogram or of air during a pneumoencephalogram. How often a previous lumbar puncture has proved to be responsible is not clear. Jones and Newton (1963) reported a 10 per cent incidence of accidental extra-arachnoidal injection of contrast medium (Pantopaque) in 244 myelograms. However, only 1 of 20 patients with this complication had received a diagnostic lumbar puncture within the week preceding the myelogram. Furthermore, there was a 10 per cent incidence of subdural injection of Pantopaque in the *absence* of a recent tap!

I believe that the role of previous lumbar punctures in causing subdural injections has not been established; it is less important than the technical skill of the physician performing the myelogram. There is no evidence that a recent lumbar puncture makes deferral of either myelography or pneumoencephalography necessary. This conclusion is further supported by the observations of Larson *et al.* (1972), who examined the influence of a previous lumbar puncture or pneumoencephalogram (PEG) upon the injection of radioisotope into the lumbar sac for cisternography. In 271 cases, the failure rate of cisternograms was 11 per cent, and this figure was not affected by previous lumbar puncture or PEG done 2 days, 1 week, or 2 weeks before the cisternogram.

Arachnoiditis Due to Spinal Anesthesia and Other Injections

Much has been written about the neurological sequelae of spinal anesthesia and intrathecal therapy and their relationship to the pathogenesis of acute and chronic spinal arachnoiditis (Whisler, 1978). The apparent complications of intrathecal injections have included (1) acute chemical meningitis, (2) chronic adhesive arachnoiditis, (3) convulsive seizures, and (4) aggravation of a pre-existing neurologic disorder. Agents responsible for the acute and chronic meningitides have included the inadvertent or inapparent injection into the subarachnoid space of talcum powder, alcohol, bits of cotton, and antiseptic solutions used for sterilization of the patient's skin and the anesthetic vials. Older anesthetics such as Cinchocaine or Stovaine were incriminated in the past, as were excessively high concentrations of procaine or tetracaine (usually in epidural injections that penetrated the subarachnoid space).

Acute chemical meningitis usually develops within the first 24 hours following the puncture. Headache, meningeal signs, and low grade or spiking fever are the usual manifestations. Examination of the spinal fluid at this time may reveal a pleocytosis (at times eosinophilic), elevated protein, and normal or low glucose. The symptoms are usually short lived, disappearing over a few days. The main diagnostic problem is to ascertain that the syndrome is an aseptic meningeal reaction and not the result of bacterial infection. The clinical manifestations of chronic adhesive arachnoiditis are attributable to a chronic leptomeningitis with the formation of adhesions causing spinal block, thick cicatricial bands, and an ischemic radiculopathy and myelopathy. A slowly progressive paraparesis with sensory loss, radicular pain, and loss of sphincter function has been observed. The occurrence of chronic adhesive arachnoiditis after Pantopaque myelography is greater when there is subarachnoid blood (Whisler, 1978). *Therefore, the occurrence of a bloody tap should serve to postpone myelography, unless there are grave indications for an immediate study.*

Aggravation of pre-existing neurological disorders by spinal anesthesia also has been reported. (The aggravation of spinal block after spinal fluid drainage has been noted earlier.) In addition, the toxic effects of the injected agent may be greater below the level of a spinal block. The presence of a myelopathy due to multiple sclerosis, amyotrophic lateral sclerosis, or other diseases should serve as a general contraindication to spinal anesthesia. The abnormal spinal cord is considered to be more vulnerable to damage when the inflammatory effects of a chemical meningitis are added. Although this view is difficult to substantiate in the literature, it represents the consensus of many experienced clinicians. Banford *et al.* (1978) reviewed the occurrence of relapse after spinal anesthesia in patients with multiple sclerosis; they concluded that spinal anesthesia should probably be avoided in patients with this disease.

False Laboratory Data

An important but seldom considered complication of lumbar puncture is the acquisition of false laboratory data and its adverse implications for therapy (Levin *et al.*, 1978). False positive Gram stains have been caused by (1) failure to clean the slide with alcohol before the smear, (2) failure to filter the Gram stain, and (3) contaminated collection tubes (Musher and Schell, 1973; Weinstein *et al.*, 1975). Failure to record the CSF pressure correctly with a manometer often results in erroneous reports of normal or increased intracranial pressure based on how the fluid dripped from the needle! Finally, clinicians are at the mercy of the clinical laboratories upon which they depend, some of which fail to meet a high standard of performance for the chemical, bacteriological, serological, and cytological study of the CSF.

CHAPTER 6

COMPOSITION OF CEREBROSPINAL FLUID

This chapter deals with the physical characteristics of the CSF, including its cellular elements and chemical composition. Few of the numerous laboratory tests in routine clinical use for the study of blood and other biological fluids have proved of diagnostic value when applied to the CSF. In clinical practice, valuable information is derived chiefly from the study of the composition of the CSF with attention to these features: the appearance of the fluid, cellular elements, protein content and composition, glucose content, bacterial cultures, and serological reactions. These aspects will be reviewed first, followed by discussion of the many other chemical constituents that are of limited value in neurological diagnosis. The pathophysiology of the various changes in composition of the fluid, and their interpretation in the differential diagnosis of neurological disease, will also be summarized. The major constituents of the normal CSF and plasma are summarized in Table 6–1.

Appearance

The appearance of the CSF is normally crystal-clear and colorless. In pathological conditions, the CSF may appear cloudy, frankly purulent, bloody, or pigment-tinged. Its consistency may be increased so that it becomes viscous, and it may coagulate or form a thin pellicle of variable size and shape, either at room temperature or in a refrigerator. To ascertain that the fluid is crystal-clear, a volume of *at least* 1 ml of fluid is required, preferably in a clear glass test tube because many plastic tubes are not sufficiently clear. Minor degrees of color change can be best detected by comparing the fluid to an equal volume of clear water in an identical tube, in white light, viewed down the long axis of the tube. Larger volumes of CSF, 3 to 10 ml, provide a better opportunity to detect slight degrees of color change. Any degree of coloration of the fluid is pathological and should be explained.

The Tyndall Effect

Spinal fluid appears clear and colorless until there are approximately 400 cells per mm^3, when a turbid (ground-glass or cloudy) quality to the fluid will

TABLE 6-1 Composition of Normal Lumbar Cerebrospinal Fluid and Serum*

	CEREBROSPINAL FLUID		SERUM	
Osmolarity	295	mOsm/l	295	mOsm/l
Water content	99	%	93	%
Sodium	138.0	mEq/l	138.0	mEq/l
Potassium	2.8	mEq/l	4.5	mEq/l
Calcium	2.1	mEq/l	4.8	mEq/l
Magnesium	2.3	mEq/l	1.7	mEq/l
Chloride	119.0	mEq/l	102.0	mEq/l
Bicarbonate	22.0	mEq/l	24.0	mEq/l (arterial)
CO_2 tension	47.0	mm Hg	41.0	mm Hg (arterial)
pH	7.33		7.41	(arterial)
Oxygen	43.0	mm Hg	104.0	mm Hg (arterial)
Glucose	60.0	mg/dl	90.0	mg/dl
Lactate	1.6	mEq/l	1.0	mEq/l (arterial)
Pyruvate	0.08	mEq/l	0.11	mEq/l (arterial)
Lactate/pyruvate ratio	26.0		17.6	(arterial)
Fructose	4.0	mg/dl	2.0	mg/dl
Polyols	340	μmole/l	148	μmole/l
Myoinositol	2.6	mg/dl	1.0	mg/dl
Total protein	35.0	mg/dl	7.0	gm/dl
prealbumin	4	%	trace	
albumin	65	%	60	%
alpha$_1$ globulin	4	%	5	%
alpha$_2$ globulin	8	%	9	%
beta globulin (beta$_1$ + tau)	12	%	12	%
gamma globulin	7	%	14	%
IgG	1.2	mg/dl	987	mg/dl
IgA	0.2	mg/dl	175	mg/dl
IgM	0.06	mg/dl	70	mg/dl
kappa/lambda ratio	1.0		1.0	
beta-trace protein	2.0	mg/dl	0.5	mg/dl
fibronectin	3.0	μg/ml	300	μgm/ml
Total free amino acids	80.9	μmole/dl	228.0	μmole/dl
Ammonia	24.0	μg/dl	37.0	μg/dl (arterial)
Urea	4.7	mmole/l	5.4	mmole/l
Creatinine	1.2	mg/dl	1.8	mg/dl
Uric acid	0.25	mg/dl	5.50	mg/dl
Putrescine	184.0	pmole/ml		
Spermidine	150.0	pmole/ml		
Total lipids	1.5	mg/dl	750.0	mg/dl
free cholesterol	0.4	mg/dl	180.0	mg/dl
cholesterol esters	0.3	mg/dl	126.0	mg/dl
cAMP	20.0	nmole/l		
cGMP	0.68	nmole/l		
HVA	60.0	μg/ml		
5-HIAA	0.04	μg/ml		
Norepinephrine	200.0	pg/ml	350.0	pg/ml
MHGP	15.0	mg/ml		
Acetylcholine	1.8	mg/dl		
Choline	2.5	mM/ml		
Prostaglandin PGF$_2$ alpha	92.0	pg/ml		
Insulin	3.7	mμ/ml	36.0	mμ/ml
Gastrin	3.4	pmole/l		
Cholecystokinin	14.0	pmole/l		
Beta endorphin	145.0	pmole/l	10.0	pmole/l
Phosphorus	1.6	mg/dl	4.0	mg/dl
Iron	1.5	μg/dl	15.0	mg/dl

*Average or representative values are given, see text for other compounds, references, and discussion. See Table 6-8B, page 193, for additional proteins.

gradually appear. However, CSF cell counts well below the number necessary to produce turbidity can be readily detected with the unaided eye by use of the Tyndall effect, which is the physical ability of suspended particles to scatter ambient light. When such spinal fluid is observed in *direct sunlight,* the suspended cells cause light scatter that imparts a characteristic "snowy" or "sparkling" appearance to the tube. This snowy appearance is unmistakably different from that of either clear (acellular) or turbid specimens. Simon and Abele (1978) have recently studied the sensitivity of the Tyndall effect in the estimation of a CSF pleocytosis by the bedside.

The Tyndall effect is best seen by holding the top of a clean glass test tube containing the CSF sample with one hand and briskly flicking or snapping the bottom of the tube with a finger of the other hand. Observations should be made using direct sunlight (fluorescent and incandescent light sources are inadequate) with the tube viewed against a darker background. The specimen is held so that the observer's line of gaze is at right angles to the direction of incident sunlight. Frequent flicking of the sample and comparison with a cell-free tube accentuate the "snowy" appearance. At less than 400 cells per mm^3 the fluid is clear and colorless, but the presence of cells can still be detected by using the Tyndall effect. Pleocytosis can be recognized when there are fewer than 50 RBC per mm^3.

Although the literature suggests that erythrocytes produce turbidity at lower concentrations than do leukocytes and that polymorphonuclear cells produce turbidity at concentrations lower than do lymphocytes (Simon and Abele, 1978), equal sensitivity of the Tyndall effect for both erythrocytes and leukocytes has been found. The Tyndall effect thus does not distinguish between the pleocytosis of meningitis and traumatically introduced erythrocytes. Also, protein (albumin) added to the specimens in concentrations simulating purulent fluid (150 mg/dl) does not alter the sensitivity of the Tyndall effect.

Accurate observation requires practice, perfectly clean dust-free glass tubes, and direct sunlight; then minimal CSF pleocytosis may be reliably detected by unaided visual inspection of the specimen, using the Tyndall effect of light scatter by suspended particles.

Cloudy Fluid

Some authors grade turbidity from 0 to 4+, as follows: 0, crystal clear fluid; 1+, faintly hazy; 2+, turbidity present but newsprint can be read through the tube; 3+, newsprint not easily read through tube; 4+, newsprint cannot be seen through tube (Krieg, 1979).

With the use of artificial light, the CSF is easily perceived as being grossly bloody when the red cell count is greater than 6000 per mm^3. At concentrations between 500 and 6000 per mm^3, the color is generally perceived as cloudy, xanthochromic, or pink-tinged (Lee *et al.,* 1975). The visual judgment depends upon the observer, the use of bright light, the availability of at least 1 ml of CSF, and finally the use of clear glass tubes rather than plastic tubes.

A cloudy, opalescent, or turbid fluid is usually due to a pleocytosis; at least 200 white cells per mm^3 must be present for such a change to be detected, although fewer cells may be detected with the naked eye by the Tyndall effect. A greenish tinge is sometimes observed in grossly purulent fluid. An oily emulsion may be seen after the intrathecal injection of contrast media such as iophendylate (Pantopaque). A cloudy, fatty emulsion has resulted from the release of the semiliquid contents of a lobule of epidural fat during lumbar puncture (Mealey, 1962). After fat embolism to the brain, large and small sudanophilic globules have been found in the sediment after centrifugation of the CSF (Cross, 1965). However, Tedeschi *et al.* (1969) found sudanophilic fat globules in the sediment of 16 of 60 cases without fat embolism. Thus, the earlier observation has not been confirmed.

Viscous Fluid

Rarely, I have observed the CSF to have increased viscosity, dripping like glycerine from the lumbar puncture needle. This was due to large amounts of mucin secreted by metastatic mucinous adenocarcinoma of the colon which had diffusely infiltrated the meninges. Mucin may be readily identified by staining the dried residue of the fluid with mucicarmine stain. One case report describes the presence in a youngster of a viscous material in the CSF attributed to needle injury of the annulus fibrosus with release of the liquid nucleus pulposus into the fluid (Dripps and Vandam, 1951). A more common cause of increased viscosity is the presence of large numbers of cryptococci. The polysaccharide capsules of the yeast are responsible for the viscous quality of the fluid.

Clot and Pellicle Formation

The formation of a clot and a surface pellicle occurs when sufficient serum proteins, including fibrinogen, are present in the CSF. This may occur within a few minutes after fluid is obtained, although pellicle formation is more often noted after the specimen is refrigerated. When fluid is bloody, clot formation is not usually seen unless there are over a million red blood cells present. In Froin's syndrome (Froin and Foy, 1908) there is clot formation of CSF after removal. This is characteristically observed with a complete spinal block, most often due to a cord tumor. The CSF protein level is usually in excess of 1.5 gm per dl in such patients. Pellicle formation, which looks like a surface scum or a spider web, is most often seen with a high protein content and in the presence of inflammatory cells. Clots and pellicles may decompose to form a sediment after standing overnight. Cellular elements in the fluid, particularly polymorphonuclear granulocytes, also are subject to cytolysis, and such fragments contribute to sediment formation. This occurs much more rapidly at room temperature than at 4°C in the refrigerator.

Blood in the CSF: Differential Diagnosis and the Three-Tube Test

Several observations are required to differentiate between a traumatic spinal puncture and pre-existing subarachnoid hemorrhage (see Table 6–2). At the time of puncture, the fluid should be collected in at least three separate tubes (the "three-tube test"). In traumatic punctures, the fluid generally clears between

TABLE 6–2   Differential Features of Subarachnoid Hemorrhage and Traumatic Puncture: the Three-Tube Test

CSF FINDING	SUBARACHNOID HEMORRHAGE	TRAUMATIC PUNCTURE
Pressure	Increased or normal	Normal
Appearance	Equal blood in all tubes	First or last tube is bloodier, others are clearer
Supernatant fluid color	Pigment in excess of protein level	Clear
RBC count and hematocrit	Essentially similar in all tubes	Variable in different tubes
WBC count	Proportional to RBC count in earliest stages, relatively increased later	Proportional to RBC count
Clot formation	Absent	Occurs rarely
Repeat puncture at higher interspace	Findings similar to those at initial tap	Usually clear

the first and the third collections. This is detectable by the naked eye and should be confirmed by cell count. In subarachnoid bleeding, the blood is generally evenly admixed in the three tubes. A sample of the bloody fluid should be centrifuged and the supernatant fluid compared with tap water as described earlier.

In a sample from a traumatic puncture, the supernatant fluid is crystal-clear, while in subarachnoid bleeding the supernatant fluid is pigmented, indicating that the blood has been present for sufficient time to permit lysis of red cells. This probably requires at least 2 to 4 hours, although the average life of the red cell in the peripheral blood is about 120 days. The rapid lysis of red cells in CSF has not been well explained (Dupont *et al.*, 1961; Tourtellotte *et al.*, 1964; Tourtellotte *et al.*, 1965). It is not due to any osmotic difference between plasma and CSF, for the osmolarity of both fluids is essentially the same. It appears likely that the absence from the CSF of sufficient plasma proteins, which stabilize the red cell membrane, is largely responsible for the rapid lysis of red cells. The supernatant fluid may be faintly yellow in a traumatic puncture if sufficient serum has entered. This usually requires at least 100,000 red blood cells per mm^3 and enough serum to raise the protein concentration about 100 mg/dl above the initial level. Crenation of the red blood cells is of no value in differentiating between traumatic and subarachnoid bleeding, for it occurs in both circumstances (Matthews and Frommeyer, 1955).

It is important to note that the supernatant fluid usually remains clear for two to four hours after the onset of subarachnoid bleeding (Walton, 1956). (This may mislead the physician to erroneously conclude that the observed blood is due to needle trauma in patients who have received a lumbar puncture within four hours of aneurysmal rupture.) Walton (1956) reviewed the CSF findings in 286 cases of subarachnoid hemorrhage and found that 10 per cent of patients with bloody fluid had clear supernatant fluid 12 hours after the presumed onset, while all the fluids were xanthochromic thereafter. After an especially traumatic puncture, some blood and xanthochromia may be present for as long as two to five days following the initial puncture. In pathological states associated with a CSF protein greater than 150 mg/dl, and in the absence of bleeding, a faint degree of xanthochromia may be detected. When the protein is elevated to much higher levels, as in spinal block, polyneuritis, and meningitis, the xanthochromia may be considerable. *A xanthochromic fluid with a normal protein level or an elevation to less than 150 mg per dl usually indicates a previous subarachnoid or intracerebral hemorrhage* (although rarely the xanthochromia is due to severe jaundice).

Xanthochromia due to carotenoids has been observed in food faddists with dietary hypercarotenemia, whose CSF actually looks orange in color. A faintly brown or darker color of the fluid has been noted rarely in malignant melanomatosis of the meninges (Lups and Haan, 1953)

Pigments

Three major pigments derived from red cells may be detected in the fluid: oxyhemoglobin, bilirubin, and methemoglobin. These have been identified quantitatively by absorption spectrophotometry and by calculations based on absorbance at specific wave lengths (Barrows *et al.*, 1955; Van Der Meulen, 1969; Kjellin and Soderstrom, 1974). However, the eye can usually readily differentiate the color changes.

Oxyhemoglobin is red in color, but after dilution it appears pink or orange. It is released with lysis of red cells and may be detected in the supernatant fluid within about 2 hours after the release of blood in the subarachnoid space. It reaches a maximum in about the first 36 hours and gradually disappears over the next 7 to 10 days. Its presence may also be detected with the benzidine test.

Bilirubin is yellow in color; it is an iron-free derivative of hemoglobin produced *in vivo* following the hemolysis of red cells. Free bilirubin is conjugated with glucuronic acid in the liver to form bilirubin glucuronide. Both free and conjugated bilirubin are albumin-bound, although conjugated bilirubin dissociates readily to enter the urine. With severe jaundice, both free and conjugated bilirubin are detected in the CSF, and the degree of bilirubin pigmentation is increased when the CSF protein is elevated. Xanthochromia, by definition, means yellow color, but it has been customary to use the term for pink or yellow coloration of the fluid. In view of the significance of the different pigments, it is more useful to describe the color as yellow, pink, or orange.

Bilirubin formation in the CSF is considered to depend on the ability of macrophages and other cells in the leptomeninges to degrade hemoglobin. Roost *et al.* (1972) studied the conversion of hemoglobin heme to bilirubin in a rat model of subarachnoid hemorrhage. The enzyme responsible for the conversion, heme oxygenase, was found in the choroid plexus, arachnoid, and cortex. Its activity was increased fourfold after a delay of about 12 hours, analogous to the delay in the appearance of bilirubin observed in patients. The delay may depend upon the migration of sufficient macrophages into the leptomeninges.

Bilirubin is first detected about 10 hours after the onset of subarachnoid bleeding. It reaches a maximum at 48 hours and may persist for two to four weeks after extensive bleeding (Walton, 1956). The severity of the meningeal signs associated with subarachnoid bleeding may be roughly correlated with the level of bilirubin in the spinal fluid, although bilirubin itself does not cause

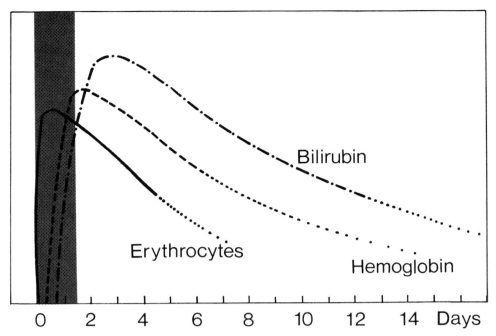

0 2 4 6 8 10 12 14 Days

Figure 6–1 Subarachnoid bleeding. The pigmentary changes in CSF following a single sub-arachnoid hemorrhage. The red blood cell count is usually maximal within the first 24 hours, and the cells disappear in 7 to 10 or more days depending upon the size of the initial bleed. Hemoglobin is usually apparent in the supernatant CSF within the first 4 to 10 hours after bleeding. The pink color is usually maximal within the first 24 to 48 hours, then gradually disappears. Bilirubin appears after the detection of hemoglobin. Its yellow color usually appears 9 to 15 hours after bleeding (excluding the bilirubin that enters from the serum) as hemoglobin is degraded by the leptomeningeal cellular infiltrates. The meningeal signs are usually maximal at about the same time that the CSF bilirubin is at its height. The bilirubin disappears slowly from the CSF, often being present for 10 to 14 or more days (see text).

meningeal irritation (in severe jaundice, the CSF is bilirubin stained without a pleocytosis). The usual temporal pattern of these changes following subarachnoid hemorrhage is shown in Figure 6–1. Bilirubin is also the major pigment responsible for the xanthochromia associated with a high spinal fluid protein level. The presence of bilirubin may be also determined with the van den Bergh reaction.

Methemoglobin, a brown pigment that is dark yellow in dilution, is a reduction product of hemoglobin characteristically found in encapsulated subdural hematomas and in old loculated intracerebral hemorrhages. It may be detected by spectrophotometry of the spinal fluid in patients with such encapsulations of large size, but the pigment is not generally observed in other xanthochromic spinal fluids. The presence of methemoglobin may be confirmed by a potassium cyanide test.

Xanthochromic spinal fluid may also occur with jaundice (Amatuzio *et al.,* 1953; Berman *et al.,* 1954). In jaundice secondary to liver disease, the spinal fluid may contain both free bilirubin and conjugated bilirubin in the presence of a normal or elevated spinal fluid protein level. The amount of bilirubin in the spinal fluid is not well correlated with the degree of hyperbilirubinemia. The

CSF is usually not stained until the total plasma bilirubin level is 10 to 15 mg/dl. When the CSF protein level is elevated, CSF pigmentation may be observed with somewhat lower plasma bilirubin levels. Furthermore, the level of CSF bilirubin is not consistently related to the color of the CSF. This discrepancy is best explained by another pigment or pigments, as yet unidentified; for example, in some jaundiced patients the spinal fluid rarely appears slightly green, probably because it contains biliverdin, but is otherwise normal in composition.

The concentration of bilirubin may vary between one tenth and one hundredth of the serum value, depending in part upon the duration of the jaundice, the presence or absence of hepatic coma, and the protein content of the fluid. Lumbar fluid will be more deeply stained than ventricular fluid, which parallels the usual difference in protein concentration in both locations. In hemolytic disease of the newborn, xanthochromia commonly occurs owing to elevation of the conjugated bilirubin in the spinal fluid and serum (see "CSF in Infancy," Chapter 7). In children so affected, the spinal fluid level correlates well with the serum level and with the amount of protein present in the spinal fluid.

It is useful to note the degree of pigmentation in relation to the protein level. *The presence of xanthochromic spinal fluid out of proportion to the total protein content (under 150 mg/dl), and in the absence of jaundice or hypercarotenemia, is a reliable index of previous bleeding into the CSF or into the brain or spinal cord adjacent to the CSF.*

Cellular Elements

Soon after the introduction of lumbar puncture, counting chambers (hemocytometers) were developed which, with minor modification, are still used in counting the cells in the fluid. The Fuchs-Rosenthal chamber in common use has a volume of 3.2 mm^3. The technical details are well summarized in such standard texts as the reviews by Alami and Affifi (1976) and Krieg (1979). CSF cell counts should be performed promptly because red and white cells begin to lyse within about an hour at room temperature. Normal CSF contains no more than 4 lymphocytes or mononuclear cells per mm^3. (In the Continental literature, normal values are often expressed as up to $^{12}/_3$ cells per mm^3. This notation uses 3 as the denominator because it is the volume of fluid within the counting chamber.) According to Merritt and Fremont-Smith (1938), a count between 5 and 10 cells per mm^3 should arouse suspicion, and a count greater than 10 is pathognomonic of disease in the central nervous system or meninges. I consider white cell counts between 5 and 10 per mm^3 to signify a pathological condition. A pleocytosis of 5 to 50, 50 to 200, or more than 200 white cells is graded as mild, moderate, or marked, respectively.

Precise enumeration and identification of the cells are important to neurological diagnosis. Red cells may be present because of a traumatic puncture or because of subarachnoid bleeding. A useful approximation of the white cell count is obtainable despite a traumatic puncture, using the following correction for the presence of the added blood. Assuming a normal hemogram, the number of white cells in the fluid before the addition of the blood may be obtained as follows: 1 white cell per mm³ for every 700 red blood cells per mm³ is subtracted from the total white count. Thus, if a bloody fluid reveals 7000 red blood cells and 100 white cells, 10 white cells could be accounted for by the blood present, and before contamination there would have been about 90 white cells present.

If there is a significant anemia or leukocytosis, the following formula may be used:

$$W = WBC_F - \frac{WBC_B \times RBC_F}{RBC_B}$$

W is the white count of the fluid before the blood was added; WBC_F is the total white count in the bloody fluid; WBC_B is the white count in the blood; RBC_F and RBC_B are the number of red cells per mm³ in the fluid and in the blood respectively. For example, if a bloody fluid contains 7000 red blood cells and 100 white cells, and the peripheral blood contains 3.0 million red cells and 15,000 white cells, the calculation reveals that 35 white cells are due to the added blood and that the white count of the fluid before contamination was 65.

An accurate cell count also permits calculation of the true total protein content despite a traumatic puncture. This assumes a normal hemogram and serum protein level. (Krieg [1979] provides formulas that may be used to correct for an abnormal peripheral blood count.) The correction is as follows: 1 mg per 100 ml of protein for every 1000 red blood cells per mm³ is subtracted. Thus, if the red cell count is 10,000 and the total protein is 110 mg/dl, the corrected protein would be 100 mg/dl. *This correction is valid only if the cell count and the total protein content are determined in the same tube of spinal fluid!*

Cytology

The identification of the specific cell types in the CSF is done routinely with samples obtained by lumbar, cisternal, or ventricular puncture. The use of the clinical counting chamber (hemocytometer) provides reliable information about the total number of cells present, but it does not allow an accurate differential count of the white cells present. For the latter purpose, the traditional technique is the centrifugation of CSF in a conical tube followed by smear preparation of the sediment. This technique is subject to some error because of distortion and fragmentation of cells. There is controversy over the optimal techniques for cellular identification (Kolar and Zeman, 1968; Schmidt, 1969; Den Hartog Jager, 1969; Baringer, 1970; Krentz and Dyken, 1972; Sornas, 1972; Drewinko *et al.*, 1973; Dyken, 1975; Oehmichen, 1976; Barrett and King, 1976; Gondos and King, 1976; Kolmel, 1976).

The Shandon cytocentrifuge, developed by Watson (1966) and marketed by the Shandon Scientific Company, has proved to be a useful technical device suitable for routine clinical use. Morphological identification of cells is possible with CSF leukocyte counts ranging from 0 to 5 per mm³ as well as with a pleocytosis. The cytocentrifuge accumulates all the cells in a volume of 0.5 to 1.0 ml of CSF, in comparison to the clinical hemocytometer which has a volume of only 3.2 mm³. Thus, cytocentrifugation of 1.0 ml of CSF traps about 300 times the number of cells observable in the counting chamber. Several reports indicate its usefulness in routine diagnosis and in meningeal leukemia (Drewinko et al., 1973; Woodruff, 1973; Evans *et al.,* 1974; Hansen, 1974). However, a large number of leukocytes are destroyed by cytocentrifugation (Barrett and King, 1976), and this fact limits it as a technique for measuring the total number of cells. It also has limitations in the cytological identification of malignant cells because the cytocentrifuge extensively alters cell structure despite low speed centrifugation (500 RPM for 10 minutes). The preferred techniques for the preservation of cellular morphology — filtration and sedimentation — will be discussed later (see Tumor Cells).

Increasing the oncotic pressure of the CSF samples by the addition of albumin either to the sediment or before cytocentrifugation improves the quality of staining with Wright's stain (Tourtellotte, 1967). This confirms the old clinical observation that the cellular structure of granulocytes in purulent fluid was much improved compared with that in fluids containing normal levels of protein. Most American centers use the Wright stain for differential counts and the Papanicolaou stain for tumor cytomorphological study; many European authorities prefer to use the May-Grünwald/Giemsa stain (Oehmichen, 1976).

Immunofluorescent Techniques

There has been interest in the application of immunofluorescent techniques to the study of CSF cells with regard to the diagnosis of various inflammatory disorders, including meningitis, encephalitis, and radiculitis, associated with the production of immunoglobulins or with evidence of delayed hypersensitivity. The lymphoid and plasma cells in CSF were partially stained selectively with fluorescein-labelled specific antiglobulin sera and then stained further for immunoglobulins (IgG and IgM). These techniques were used to establish the specific viral agent in patients with viral meningitis and encephalitis and to diagnose cryptococcal meningitis (Dayan and Stokes, 1973; Lindeman *et al.,* 1974; Wolf *et al.,* 1974). There are also reports of identifying the number of B and T cells in CSF by similar techniques (Allen *et al.,* 1975; Kam-Hansen *et al.,* 1978). To date, these techniques have been used chiefly in clinical investigation. The immunofluorescent techniques appear to be a major advance in laboratory diagnosis, and their increasing application in clinical practice is expected.

Cytogenesis of CSF Cells

It is generally agreed that the various leukocytes in CSF, including round cells, mononuclear phagocytes, plasma cells, polymorphonuclear granulocytes, eosinophils, and basophils, are derived chiefly from the circulating blood. These cells are shown in Figure 6–2. Normal CSF may also rarely contain cells derived from the choroidal epithelium, the ependyma, or the arachnoid (Oehmichen, 1976). There has been some uncertainty in the past about whether the mononuclear phagocytes are derived from the proliferation of leptomeningeal cells. With the use of tritiated thymidine autoradiography, however, mononuclear phagocytes, including microglial and perivascular cells associated with inflammatory lesions, have been shown to be derived from the blood; i.e., they are transformed circulating monocytes.

B Cells and T Cells

Most of the round cells in normal CSF are lymphocytes, representing both B cells (antibody-forming cells derived from the bone marrow) and T cells (thymus-derived cells involved in cell-mediated immune responses). There are only limited data regarding the precise number of each type of lymphocyte in normal subjects and in pathological conditions.

Allen *et al.* (1975) reported an increase in the number of T cells during the first week of an exacerbation of multiple sclerosis, with little change in the B cell number. Kam-Hansen *et al.* (1978) enumerated B cells and T cells in CSF and blood in patients with multiple sclerosis, optic neuritis, and mumps meningitis, and also in control subjects (blood donors). Patients with MS and mumps meningitis had significantly higher T cell values in CSF compared to blood, while the B cell values in CSF were significantly lower in mumps meningitis only. No significant differences were observed between multiple sclerosis patients in exacerbation and those in remission.

More recently, Kam-Hansen (1979), using another technique, found that the percentages of active T cells were significantly *lower* in the CSF of multiple sclerosis patients than in blood obtained simultaneously. These results suggest that there may be a depression or deficiency of a functional subpopulation of T lymphocytes confined to the central nervous system in multiple sclerosis. The pathophysiological significance and the clinical implications of changes in B and T cells in CSF require further study.

Figure 6-2   Cerebrospinal fluid cytology with Papanicolaou staining. Magnification 400×. Papanicolaou-stained sediment from cerebrospinal fluid. Courtesy of Eileen B. King, M. D., Lois Kromhourt, CT(ASCP), and Paul Harra, San Francisco.

Upper left, polymorphonuclear neutrophil with four lobes in focus does not show specific neutrophilic granulation in Papanicolaou-stained preparations. A small mature lymphocyte has a minimal amount of cytoplasm. *Upper center,* polymorphonuclear neutrophil has the plane of focus on two of the lobes. Wet fixation of cells preserves the spherical shape, and thus the third lobe of this cell's nucleus is at a different level and out of the plane of focus. The larger cell with indented nucleus is interpreted as histiocytic in origin. *Upper right,* the bilobed cell with distinct, uniform, yellow-orange granules is a typical eosinophil. Next to it is a large histiocyte with abundant, irregularly shaped, and unevenly staining cytoplasm.

Middle left, an eccentrically located, deeply indented, and folded nucleus is seen in a histiocyte. Chromatin is dispersed in fine granules. The cytoplasm is characteristically cyanophilic and has a poorly defined border. *Middle center,* another histiocyte has a more centrally located reniform nucleus. *Middle right,* this histiocyte shows an "active" appearance of the nucleus and has a prominent nucleolus. The cytoplasm contains engulfed erythrocytes situated within vacuoles.

Lower left, in this collection of five cells from a fluid associated with chronic meningitis, the central cell is a neutrophil which has some degenerative changes. In the lower left part of the group is a cell exhibiting mitosis. This is probably part of the continuum of immature lymphocytic and plasmocytoid variety that is represented by the remaining three cells depicted here. These cells are associated with an immunoblastic reaction. *Lower right,* there are two lymphocytes showing extremes in their morphological features. A small mature cell has densely distributed chromatin. The larger immature cell shows characteristics of both nucleus and cytoplasm that suggest a very different functional capacity. However, accuracy in classification of T and B cell types requires serological and special techniques.

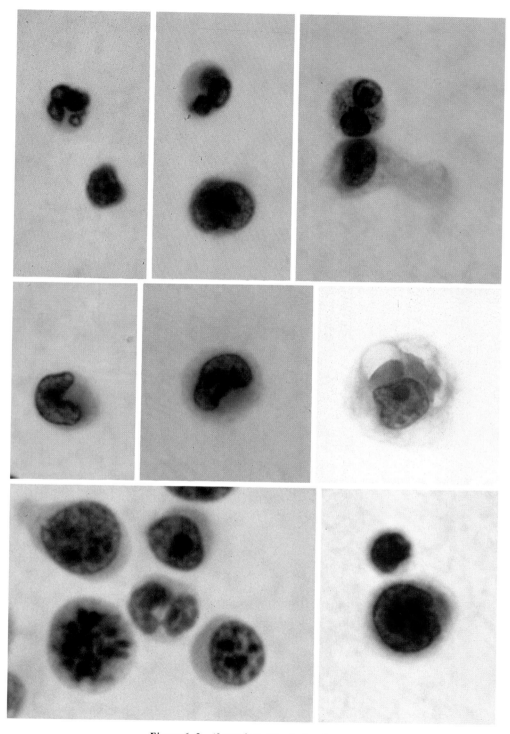

Figure 6–2   (*Legend on opposite page.*)

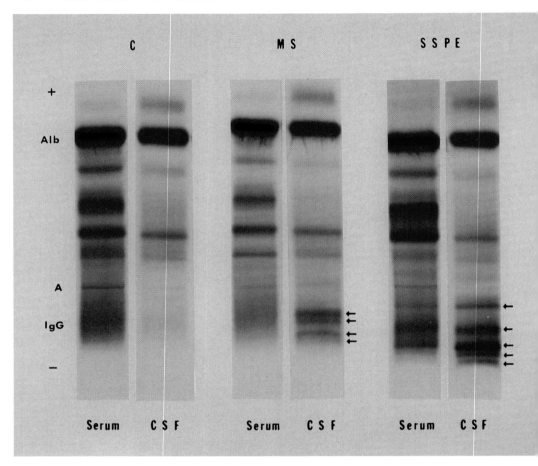

Figure 6–4 Agar gel electrophoresis of CSF (concentration × 50) and serum from a control patient, a patient with multiple sclerosis (MS), and a patient with subacute sclerosing panencephalitis (SSPE). The + and − poles of the electrophoresis are indicated. A is the site of application. Alb is the albumin area, and IgG is the immunoglobulin zone. Note the discrete oligoclonal IgG bands (arrows) in the IgG zone of the MS and SSPE CSF samples. The prominent prealbumin in the CSF samples is also seen (courtesy of Dr. K. P. Johnson, San Francisco).

Disappearance of CSF Cells

Red and white cells disappear from the CSF by lysis as well as by macrovesicular transport across the arachnoid villi, as discussed in Chapter 3. Oehmichen (1976) summarized the literature in support of the conclusion that leukocytes disappear from both normal and pathological fluids by cellular degeneration or cytolysis within the CSF as well as by migration into the blood. There is some evidence in animals that radioactive-labelled macrophages may enter the cervical lymph nodes after subarachnoid injection (Oehmichen, 1976). However, the existence in humans of such a mechanism for cellular removal has not been established. It is important to note that cytolysis of cells occurs rapidly after puncture; therefore, the CSF should be fixed as quickly as possible for optimal cytological examination. Cytolysis depends also upon the temperature at which the CSF is stored. At room temperature there is a significant decrease in cell count; after 24 hours, the cells are no longer vital; that is, they no longer exclude trypan blue. Refrigeration helps cellular preservation, and cell structure can be relatively preserved for 48 hours after puncture by storage at 4° C

TABLE 6–3   Cell Types Present in Normal and Pathological Fluids

Round (Immunocompetent) Cells
    Small lymphocytes (B cells, marrow derived, and T cells, thymus derived)
    Lymphoid cells (large stimulated lymphocytes)
    Plasma cells
Mononuclear Phagocytes
    Monocytes
    Activated monocytes (histiocytes)
    Macrophages (lipophages, erythrophages, siderophages, leukocytophages, giant cells)
Polymorphonuclear Granulocytes
    Neutrophils
    Eosinophils
    Basophils
Erythrocytes
Cells Lining the CSF Spaces
    Choroid plexus cells, ependymal cells, arachnoid cover cells
Other Cellular Elements
    Cartilage cells
    Bone marrow cells
    Lupus erythematosus cells
Tumor Cells

(Modified after Oehmichen, 1976)

Neutrophils and eosinophils are most vulnerable to cytolysis, probably reflecting the high lysosomal enzyme content of granulocytes. *Cytological studies should be done soon after spinal puncture for accuracy, and the fluids must be refrigerated promptly to avoid cytolysis.*

Cell Types in Normal and Pathological Fluids

Many cells have been identified in normal and pathological fluids. The terminology used in the extensive, mostly Continental, literature has been complex. Oehmichen's (1976) atlas reviewed this subject in detail and described the histological features of the various cellular elements found in normal and pathological conditions. Table 6–3 is largely derived from his classification. (This detailed classification was established by using sedimentation techniques, which probably best preserve the cell structure.)

Round Immunocompetent Cells

Small round cells are the predominant leukocyte found in normal and many pathological fluids. These small lymphocytes have a diameter of 6 to 10 microns and are approximately the size of red blood cells. Larger *lymphoid cells* (large stimulated lymphocytes), 10 to 20 microns in diameter, are seen occasionally in normal fluids but are found chiefly in pathological conditions. An increase in the number of lymphoid cells may be an indication of a local cell-mediated or humoral antigen-antibody reaction, or it may occur as a nonspecific response to tissue injury. The appearance of such lymphoid cells in CSF is associated with a wide variety of bacterial, viral, fungal, granulomatous, and spirochetal diseases. These cells also increase in number following subarachnoid hemorrhage or brain infarction as well as with primary and metastatic neoplasms infiltrating the brain, spinal cord, or meninges.

Plasma cells, according to Oehmichen (1976), are not seen in normal CSF. They appear in the various inflammatory conditions along with small and large lymphocytes, and in cases of malignant brain tumor and carcinomatous cerebral degeneration. There are no data yet available regarding the correlation of their presence with the appearance of oligoclonal bands or with any specific proteins in CSF. There is uncertainty about the frequency of occurrence of plasma cells and small and large lymphoid cells in many pathological conditions. Since most clinical laboratories do not usually differentiate between the various types of mononuclear cells in routine reports of round cells, they are most often identified simply as lymphocytes or mononuclear cells.

Mononuclear Phagocytes

Various terms have been used for the different forms of mononuclear phagocytic cells observed in pathological fluids. In the past, three cell types were identified: monocytes, histiocytes, and macrophages. Recently, the techniques of electron microscopy, phase microscopy, cell culture, and histochemistry have led to the conclusion that monocytes may be transformed into histiocytes (activated monocytes) and various forms of macrophages (Kölmel, 1976; Oehmichen, 1976).

Monocytes, 15 to 30 microns in diameter, are generally readily distinguished from lymphoid cells on the basis of size, nuclear shape, and the staining characteristics of the cytoplasm. They are present in normal CSF with a relatively constant ratio to round cells, approximately 3:7. They increase in a wide variety of inflammatory, ischemic, and neoplastic disorders.

Activated monocytes are larger than their parent cells and have cytoplasmic alterations, including vacuoles. These cells differ from macrophages only in the absence of any phagocytosed material in their cytoplasmic vacuoles. Their chief diagnostic value is as a nonspecific sign of an inflammatory disorder; they also appear after the meningeal irritation induced by pneumoencephalography, myelography, or the injection of drugs.

Macrophages are structurally similar to activated monocytes; they are distinguished further by the specific material that has been phagocytosed. The most common types are phagocytes containing lipids, erythrocytes, hemosiderin, or leukocytes. Lipid-containing phagocytes, *lipophages,* appear vacuolated after exposure to organic solvents used in staining. They are found in association with brain infarction of various causes. Lipophages have also been found in cases of Tay-Sachs disease. *Erythrophages,* containing one or more red cells, are large, distended macrophages, characteristically associated with subarachnoid hemorrhage. They are often found during the first week following the bleeding as well as within a few hours after a traumatic lumbar puncture.

Siderophages are phagocytes that contain hemosiderin; they develop following red cell lysis with the degradation of hemoglobin to form hemosiderin (an iron-containing pigment) and hematoidin (an iron-free pigment) by the phagocyte. Siderophages have not been detected during the first three days after subarachnoid hemorrhage. They may persist in the CSF for many weeks or months after intracerebral hemorrhage. Phagocytes containing hematoidin are usually found only 10 to 14 days after a hemorrhage. *Leukocytophages,* which contain phagocytosed leukocytes, vary in appearance depending upon the cell type engulfed, whether granulocyte, monocyte, or macrophage. They are found in all the inflammatory and traumatic conditions that elicit a pleocytosis. They have been observed in the last volume of CSF obtained with pneumoencephalography.

Giant cells, either mononuclear or polynuclear, are never found in normal CSF, although they may appear following a pneumoencephalogram or a myelogram. They lack diagnostic specificity and have been observed in various forms of inflammation and brain tumor and with contusion (Oehmichen, 1976).

Polymorphonuclear Leukocytes

While it is generally stated that *granulocytes* are never seen in normal CSF, this statement must be qualified. With the use of the cytocentrifuge, an occasional granulocyte is seen in a small percentage of normal fluids with a normal total white cell count. This is presumed to be derived from the blood at the time of puncture. Thus, an isolated granulocyte in the CSF is not necessarily pathological if the WBC count is normal, less than 5 WBC per mm^3. A granulocytic pleocytosis is associated with the gamut of bacterial infections of the brain and meninges; its presence should alert the clinician first to this possibility. A few or moderate numbers of granulocytes, usually 5 to 10 per mm^3, also may occur following spinal anesthesia, myelography, and other intrathecal injections, or with trauma, hemorrhage, or infarction, in the absence of infection. A similar increase also may be seen in some patients with malignant brain tumors, most notably glioblastoma associated with tissue necrosis. A granulocytic phase at the onset of viral meningitis, prior to the development of a purely mononuclear reaction, is also common (see Chapter 7).

Eosinophils

Eosinophils are not seen in normal fluids, although a single cell may be rarely seen with a normal total cell count by use of the cytocentrifuge. Diseases accompanied by eosinophilia of the CSF are listed in Table 6–4. The most common causes of a prominent eosinophilic reaction (5 to 10 per cent) are the parasitic diseases, including cysticercosis and trichinosis, as well as the involvement of the nervous system by *Toxocara cati, Angiostrongylus cantonensis, Gnathostoma spinigerum,* and larva migrans. In addition, eosinophilia, usually of minor degree (2 to 4 per cent), has been observed in other inflammatory diseases, including tuberculous meningitis, symptomatic neurosyphilis, subacute sclerosing panencephalitis, and some cases of viral meningitis due to Coxsackie virus. An increase in eosinophils has also been observed in cases of meningeal inflammation due to myelography, pneumoencephalography, subarachnoid hemorrhage, or intrathecal administration of radioiodinated serum albumin and penicillin, and in the presence of a surgical shunt. In some cases of brain tumor, malignant lymphoma, and Hodgkin's disease, CSF eosinophilia has also been observed. (The precise incidence of CSF eosinophilia in these disorders is not certain because many clinical laboratories fail to report it.)

Bosch and Oehmichen (1978) reported CSF eosinophilia in 94 patients in a series of 10,000 qualitative cytological examinations; all patients with confirmed parasitic diseases were excluded from the study because of the known relation-

TABLE 6–4   Diseases Accompanied by Eosinophilia of the CSF

PARASITIC INFESTATIONS OF THE CNS
  Trichinella and Ascaris (Kolar *et al.*, 1969)
  Toxoplasma (Oehmichen, 1976)
  Cysticercus (Obrador, 1962; Spina-Franca, 1962)
  Toxocara cati (Nye *et al.*, 1970)
  Toxocara canis (Anderson *et al.*, 1975)
  Angiostrongylus cantonensis (Punyagupta *et al.*, 1975)
  Gnathostoma spinigerum (Bunnag *et al.*, 1970)

INFLAMMATORY DISEASES OF THE NERVOUS SYSTEM
  Tuberculous meningitis (Bosch and Oehmichen, 1978)
  Cerebrospinal syphilis (Merritt *et al.*, 1946)
  Subacute sclerosing panencephalitis (Kolar *et al.*, 1969)
  Granulomatous meningitis (Oehmichen, 1976)
  Viral meningitis (King *et al.*, 1975)
  Fungal infections (Dufresne, 1973)
  Idiopathic eosinophilic meningitis (Bosch and Oehmichen, 1978)

OTHER DISEASES AND CONDITIONS OF THE NERVOUS SYSTEM
  Malignant lymphoma (King *et al.*, 1975)
  Hodgkin's disease (Strayer and Bender, 1977)
  Leukemia (Budka *et al.*, 1976)
  Multiple sclerosis (Kolar *et al.*, 1969)
  Penicillin therapy (Oehmichen, 1976)
  Hemorrhage (Bosch and Oehmichen, 1978)
  Myelography (Summer and Traugott, 1975)
  Pneumoencephalography (Oehmichen, 1976)
  Obstructive hydrocephalus with shunt (Kessler and Cheek, 1959)
  Experimental injection of atheromatous matter (Bosch and Oehmichen, 1978)

ship of parasitic disease to eosinophilia. They found that only 10 per cent of the 94 patients had a blood eosinophilia. The degree of CSF eosinophilia varied between 2 per cent and 34 per cent; one fourth of the patients had 5 per cent eosinophilia or more. The eosinophilia was most often attributed to inflammatory disease of the nervous system due to bacteria or of unknown cause; it was seen also with stroke and tumors. Children were observed to have eosinophilia in a relatively high per cent of cases. It is clear that a mild degree of eosinophilia, 1 to 4 per cent, lacks diagnostic specificity. However, its correlation with parasitic infection and with chemical meningitis is often very useful diagnostically.

Other Cells

Basophils have been rarely reported in pathological fluids; their diagnostic significance has not been established. *Cells lining the CSF spaces* include *choroidal cells, ependymal cells* and *arachnoid cover cells.* They have been observed after pneumoencephalography or ventriculography but not considered of diagnostic significance. Increased numbers have been found in hydrocephalic infants (Wilkins and Odom, 1974). Arachnoid cover cells are large mesothelial cells which are constituents of the arachnoid membrane. Their presence has been reported by Oehmichen (1976), using a sedimentation chamber.

Cellular elements derived from the bone marrow and cartilage have been described in the CSF following needle trauma (Oehmichen, 1976). *Lupus erythematosus cells* in the CSF as a result of subarachnoid hemorrhage in systemic lupus have been reported (Nosanchuk and Kim, 1976), but not in patients with central nervous system lupus. *Atypical lymphocytes* similar to those observed in the blood in infectious mononucleosis have been seen in the CSF.

Tumor Cells

Tumor cells may be found in the CSF with the gamut of neoplasms that affect the brain or meninges. In clinical practice, their identification is the major goal of the cytological laboratory. The chances of tumor cell identification are greatly enhanced when large volumes of fluid are available for analysis; 20 ml or more is far more likely to provide a cellular diagnosis than are smaller volumes. Often serial lumbar punctures, six or more, may prove necessary before a cytological diagnosis can be made with certainty in patients with carcinomatous meningitis.

Several techniques have been developed which provide much better preservation of cellular structure and improve diagnostic accuracy. These include techniques for obtaining cells using a sedimentation chamber, accumulation in fibrin, and filtration with various membranes (Simon and Schroer, 1963; Sayak, 1966; Baringer, 1970; Sornas, 1972; Dyken, 1975). Two recent atlases by Oehmichen (1976) and by Kolmel (1976) review the technical aspects of several of these methods for cellular isolation and the various staining methods available. The sedimentation chamber developed by Sayk (1966) probably preserves cellular structure best, but it has not been used commonly in the United States, where membrane filtration is more widely used. The major disadvantage of the sedimentation chamber is a low cell yield (30 to 90 per cent loss), according to Oehmichen (1976).

The various membrane filters available for cellular recovery were compared by Barrett and King (1976) and Gondos and King (1976). They used Millipore (cellulose ester), Gelman Metricel (cellulose triacetate), and Nucleopore (Lexan polycarbonate resin) as well as cytocentrifugation in order to compare the numbers of cells recovered as well as the structural details obtained by use of the Papanicolaou stain. They concluded that Millipore filtration consistently recovered the highest percentage of cells and best preserved their structural details. These data are summarized in Table 6–5. The performance of the cytocentrifuge was least satisfactory in this study because of cellular loss and distortion, although its value for cytological studies, particularly in cases of meningeal leukemia, was supported by Woodruff (1973), Drewinko *et al.* (1973), Evans *et al.* (1974), and Hansen (1974). Ducos *et al.* (1979) considered cytocentrifugation to be about equally useful as a sedimentation method in the evaluation of leukemia and lymphoma. Thus, reports differ over the choice of the optimal technique. The literature regarding the cytological findings associated with various primary and secondary neoplasms is summarized in Chapter 7.

The significance of positive CSF cytological findings was studied by Glass *et al.* (1979) with regard to the correlation between the presence of malignant cells in CSF and the pathological findings at autopsy. They found that 26 per cent of 117 patients with brain tumors (chiefly metastatic) had positive cytological

TABLE 6–5 Cell Filtration Methods: Comparisons of Recovery Rates and Preservation of Cell Morphology

METHOD	PERCENTAGE OF CELLS RECOVERED FROM A PREPARATION (AVERAGE)	PERCENTAGE OF PREPARATION		
		Good Preservation	*Poor Preservation*	*Unsatisfactory Preservation*
Millipore	81 ± 3	82.1	10.7	7.1
Gelman	64 ± 3	46.1	26.7	26.7
Nucleopore	69 ± 3	32.1	21.4	46.4
Cytocentrifuge	11 ± 1	13.0	22.2	64.8

(From Barrett and King, 1976)

findings. Their data point out that such a result is a reliable indication of CNS malignancy, reflecting leptomeningeal or ependymal involvement by tumor.

Cerebrospinal Fluid Proteins

Almost all the proteins normally present in CSF are derived from the serum with the probable exception of the trace proteins, which appear to originate in brain, and some of the beta globulins, which appear to be modified in brain. The analytic and experimental data in support of this generalization will be summarized here. According to current views of the blood-brain barrier to proteins, summarized in Chapter 3, protein entry into CSF from the serum is probably dependent upon pinocytosis across the capillary endothelial cells of the brain and spinal cord.

The kinetics of protein exchange was studied with iodinated albumin (Fishman, 1953) and iodinated gamma globulin (Frick and Scheid-Seydel, 1958; Cutler *et al.*, 1970). The other serum proteins probably have similar exchange rates. Following intravenous injection, it took 20 hours for albumin to reach equilibrium in the cisternal fluid of dogs and 3 to 6 days for gamma globulin to reach equilibrium in the lumbar fluid of patients. The CSF proteins normally leave the CSF by passage across the arachnoid villi into venous blood, presumably by macrovesicular transport as discussed in Chapter 3 (Tripathi, 1977). In view of the 200-fold difference in the steady-state concentration between the two compartments (i.e., CSF protein concentration is 35 mg/dl and that of serum protein is 7.0 gm/dl), the exit rate of protein is about 200 times the entry rate. The steady-state concentration in the CSF of a substance derived solely from the serum is proportional to the net entry rate, K_{in}, divided by the net exit rate, K_{out} (concentration ratio = K_{in}/K_{out}).

Increased concentration of the CSF total protein was recognized as an indicator of neurological disease soon after the introduction of lumbar puncture. In the early years, the total protein was generally measured qualitatively until the sulfosalicyclic acid turbidity test was introduced. A variety of empirical tests was developed to assess qualitative changes in the CSF proteins; these included the Lange-colloidal gold test, the Nonne-Apelt test, and others (Levinson, 1929; Lups and Haan, 1954; Schmidt, 1968). These qualitative tests have largely disappeared from clinical practice since the introduction of quantitative methods that measure more specifically the various proteins in the fluid.

The modern era began with the application by Kabat *et al.* (1942) of the Tiselius method for electrophoresis of proteins to the study of the CSF. This showed that CSF and serum, so different in total protein content, were quite similar in the composition of their individualized proteins, although some differences were also recognized. Many techniques have been developed for the quantitative measurement of CSF total protein. These have included the use of the ultraviolet spectrophotometer, a variety of quantitative turbidimetric methods, biuret procedures, and the Lowry method. The technical aspects of the various laboratory methods have been summarized by Lumsden (1972). The accuracy of the methods used in many clinical laboratories is no better than ± 5 per cent.

Several techniques for the fractionation of the CSF proteins have also been developed. These include electrophoresis, using paper or cellulose acetate, agar, agarose, polyacrylamide, and starch gels. Immunoelectrophoresis, electroimmunodiffusion, radioimmunoassay techniques, and isoelectric focusing are more recent techniques. The newest of these, isoelectric focusing on polyacrylamide gel, provides high resolutions of the multiple proteins present. However, the patterns obtained are different from those obtained with the earlier electrophoretic methods. They are difficult to interpret, and Nilsson and Olsson (1978) have concluded that the technique is excellent for a research laboratory but not yet suitable for a routine clinical laboratory.

Most of the fractionation techniques have required a preliminary concentration of the fluid in order to raise its usually low protein content to the same range as that of plasma. CSF may be concentrated a hundred times or more, without apparent damage to the proteins, by ultrafiltration using positive pressure obtained by nitrogen or centrifugation. However, the dependency upon the various membranes needed to concentrate the fluid also gives rise to technical artifacts due to the absorption of some proteins by the membrane or to denaturation of some proteins.

A clinically useful technique that does not require concentration of the CSF is electroimmunodiffusion with commercially available prepared plates that measure CSF IgG and albumin simultaneously. The techniques described by Tourtellotte *et al.* (1971) and Laurell (1972) employ an agarose gel impregnated with antihuman IgG and albumin antibodies. When small amounts of unconcentrated CSF or diluted serum are placed in a central well and then subjected to electrophoresis, the IgG and albumin migrate in opposite directions and form rocket-shaped precipitant lines with their antibodies in the gel. With the use of appropriate standards, precise concentrations of both proteins can be measured. The published data obtained with the wide variety of techniques in use will be reviewed briefly.

Lumbar CSF Protein: Normal Values

The normal values reported for the lumbar CSF total protein have varied, reflecting differences in chemical methods. Representative values, given in Table 6–6, are derived from patients presumed to be normal as well as from

TABLE 6–6   Normal Lumbar CSF Total Protein

REFERENCE	SUBJECTS	NUMBER	MEAN (mg/dl)	RANGE (±2.0 SD) (mg/dl)
Widell (1958)	Patients	31	31	15–47
Tourtellotte *et al.* (1964)	Volunteers	105	38	18–58
Dencker (1962)	Patients (males)	850	29	23–25
	Patients (females)	758	23	17–29
Laterre (1965)	Patients	60	29	9–49
Cosgrove and Agius (1966)	Patients	35	31	9–53
Gilland (1967)	Volunteers	15	36	17–55

normal volunteers. The mean values range between 23 and 38 mg/dl and the upper and lower limits (mean ± 2.0 SD) range between 9 and 58 mg/dl. It is essential that the clinician know the range of normal values of the particular laboratory in use. The factors responsible for *increased* and *decreased* total protein values, the concentration of protein along the neuraxis, and the differences in the protein concentration in immaturity will be discussed later. A discussion of the individual proteins present in CSF and the changes therein associated with various diseases will follow.

Increased CSF Protein in Disease

An increase in the total protein content of the CSF is the single most useful change in the chemical composition of the fluid that serves as an indicator of disease. Merritt and Fremont-Smith (1938) classified the fluids according to their total protein content as follows: normal (20 mg to 45 mg/dl), slightly increased (45 mg to 75 mg/dl), moderately increased (75 mg to 100 mg/dl), greatly increased (100 mg to 500 mg/dl), and very greatly increased (500 mg to 3500 mg/dl).

Table 6–7 illustrates the range and distribution of increased CSF protein content with relation to the clinical diagnosis in 4157 patients. The data support several generalizations. A slight increase in protein content is common in many diseases, but increases to more than 500 mg/dl are infrequent, occurring chiefly in meningitis, cord tumor with spinal block, or bloody fluids. Such high levels are also seen occasionally in cases of polyneuritis and brain tumor.

The frequent occurrence of very high protein levels in patients with cord tumor reflects a subarachnoid block in addition to a local increase in endothelial cell permeability. Complete spinal block is responsible for *Froin's syndrome* (1903), in which the loculated fluid below the block clots when the fluid is drained. This reflects the entry of sufficient serum fibrinogen across capillary endothelial cells to allow clot formation. The protein concentration is generally greater than 1000 mg/dl. With complete block, the lower the level of a cord tumor, the higher the protein concentration and the more likely the occurrence of Froin's syndrome. Complete block at the cervical or high thoracic level, as revealed by myelographic or manometric techniques, is unlikely to result in clot formation because the protein elevations are much lower, in contrast to lesions at the lumbar level.

TABLE 6–7   The Total Protein Content of the Lumbar Cerebrospinal Fluid from 4157 Patients

DIAGNOSIS	TOTAL	NORMAL (45 mg/dl or less)	SLIGHTLY (45–75 mg/dl)	MODER-ATELY (75–100 mg/dl)	GREATLY (100-500 mg/dl)	VERY GREATLY (500–3600 mg/dl)	HIGHEST	LOWEST (mg/dl)	AVERAGE
				INCREASED					
Purulent meningitis	157	3	7	12	100	35	2220	21	418
Tuberculous meningitis	253	2	30	37	172	12	1142	25	200
Poliomyelitis	158	74	44	16	24	0	366	12	70
Neurosyphilis	890	412	258	102	117	1	4200	15	68
Brain tumor	182	56	45	22	57	2	1920	15	115
Cord tumor	36	5	4	3	14	10	3600	40	425
Brain abscess	33	9	15	3	6	0	288	16	69
Aseptic meningitis	81	37	20	7	17	0	400	11	77
Multiple sclerosis	151	102	36	9	4	0	133	13	43
Polyneuritis	211	107	33	17	44	10	1430	15	74
Epilepsy (idiopathic)	793	710	80	2	1	0	200	7	31
Cerebral thrombosis	300	199	78	13	10	0	267	17	46
Cerebral hemorrhage*	247	34	41	32	95	45	2110	19	270
Uremia	53	31	13	8	1	0	143	19	57
Myxedema	51	12	28	3	8	0	242	30	71
Cerebral trauma†	474	255	84	43	73	19	1820	10	100
Acute alcoholism	87	80	5	2	0	0	88	13	32
Total	4157	2128	821	331	743	134			

*Only the results from fluids removed at first puncture are used in most instances.
†Increase of protein is usually due to presence of admixed blood serum.
(After Merritt and Fremont-Smith, 1938)

Any lesion causing complete spinal block, such as intramedullary or extramedullary tumor, meningitis, arachnoiditis, or epidural abscess, may be responsible for Froin's syndrome.

While an elevated protein lacks specificity, it is usually a reliable index of a pathological process that increases endothelial cell permeability. In some conditions a defect in protein absorption may contribute to an increase in CSF protein. Experimentally, an elevation of the CSF total protein obtained by the injection of serum resulted in a decreased rate of absorption of CSF albumin. Thus, a vicious cycle resulted whereby an increase in protein further slowed protein absorption (Prockop and Fishman, 1968). This may be a factor in purulent meningitis and other pathological conditions associated with a very high CSF protein. Metabolic disorders may elevate the protein level. It is noteworthy that myxedema was associated with an elevated protein in 25 per cent of cases, with levels between 100 and 242 mg/dl in 8 of 51 patients (Merritt and Fremont-Smith, 1938; Nickel and Frame, 1958). The pathophysiology of this increase is not known, although an increase in the permeability of the barrier was shown in myxedematous rats (Raskin and Fishman, 1966).

Low CSF Total Protein

Two mechanisms might theoretically explain the occurrence of an unusually low CSF protein, e.g., lumbar fluid protein levels ranging between 3 and 20 mg/dl: (1) a decreased entry of serum protein, or (2) an increased rate of protein removal to the venous system. There is no evidence that the former mechanism, decreased entry of serum protein, ever occurs. However, an increased rate of removal of CSF proteins occurs when the intracranial pressure is increased, because the higher pressure facilitates more rapid bulk flow reabsorption of CSF. This was demonstrated in dogs when the rate of inulin clearance was increased in response to intracranial hypertension obtained with an acute water load (Prockop and Fishman, 1968). This phenomenon is seen in a few clinical situations wherein the permeability of the barrier to serum proteins is normal and the intracranial pressure is increased.

A low lumbar spinal fluid protein, ranging between 3 and 20 mg/dl, occurs in several circumstances: (1) It is normal in young children between the ages of 6 months and 2 years (see Chapter 7). (2) Removal of large volumes of fluid may result in a low level, as during a pneumoencephalogram when the lumbar fluid is diluted with fluid from the cisterna magna, which normally has a lower protein level. Low proteins also occur with CSF extradural leaks following lumbar puncture and are frequent in the post-lumbar puncture headache syndrome, reflecting a similar mechanism. (3) A low protein has been noted in about one-third of patients with benign intracranial hypertension (Greer, 1968). (4) Some patients with acute water intoxication associated with increased intracranial pressure have a lumbar CSF protein between 8 and 15 mg/dl (Fishman, unpublished observations). The low protein in the latter two conditions probably results from an increased rate of bulk flow removal of CSF due to increased intracranial pressure in the presence of a normal rate of protein entry into the CSF from blood. The latter mechanism for this finding is essentially the same as that for the normal concentration difference between CSF and plasma, i.e., 35 mg/dl and 7 gm/dl, respectively. The normal concentration ratio of 1:200 means that the entry rate of protein (Kin) exceeds the exit rate (Kout) by a factor of 200. Thus, if the Kin is increased by disease, the concentration of protein is increased. If the Kout is increased by intracranial hypertension and the Kin is unchanged, the protein concentration must decrease.

A low spinal fluid protein also occurs in hyperthyroidism, with return to average normal levels after therapy. The mechanism of this change in hyperthyroidism is uncertain but may be attributable to increased spinal fluid pulsatile pressures despite normal mean intracranial pressures.

Low protein levels have also been reported in leukemic patients, without obvious explanation (Paulson, 1968). Perhaps severe anemia caused increased cerebral blood flow and increased intracranial pressure, which in turn was responsible for an increased rate of bulk flow reabsorption.

CSF Proteins: Electrophoretic Studies

The development of electrophoresis enabled the separation of the serum proteins to form characteristic patterns that were dependent upon molecular weight and electrical charge. These proteins were identified at first as the albumin, alpha, beta, and gamma globulin fractions.

Electrophoretic analyses, using first paper and then cellulose acetate, revealed the similarities and differences between the proteins of normal CSF

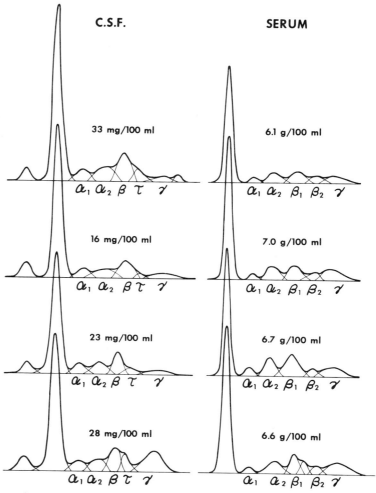

C.S.F.   SERUM

33 mg/100 ml   6.1 g/100 ml

α_1 α_2 β τ γ α_1 α_2 β_1 β_2 γ

16 mg/100 ml   7.0 g/100 ml

α_1 α_2 $\beta\tau$ γ α_1 α_2 β_1 β_2 γ

23 mg/100 ml   6.7 g/100 ml

α_1 α_2 β τ γ α_1 α_2 β_1 β_2 γ

28 mg/100 ml   6.6 g/100 ml

α_1 α_2 $\beta\tau$ γ α_1 α_2 β_1 β_2 γ

Figure 6–3 Electrophoresis on cellulose acetate of CSF (concentrated by ultrafiltration) and serum from three patients without neurological disease and one patient with multiple sclerosis (bottom). The CSF specimen at the top shows a post-gamma globulin band of unknown significance. Total protein concentrations are indicated. Note the prominent prealbumin band in the CSF. The tau fraction is separated insufficiently from the beta₁ fraction to be quantified separately (from Werner, 1969).

and plasma. Typical patterns (pherograms) are shown in Figure 6–3. The following differences between CSF and plasma are noteworthy. (1) CSF samples invariably show a prominent prealbumin fraction, which accounts for about 5 per cent of the lumbar fluid protein and which is not seen, or seen only faintly, in the serum electrophoresis using cellulose acetate. Prealbumin is present in serum and is observed with gel electrophoresis, although its concentration is substantially less than in CSF compared with the concentration of albumin or total protein. (2) Most normal CSF samples have a clear-cut electrophoretic fraction, the tau fraction, which moves with beta₂ globulin. The tau fraction is not seen in the serum. It is probably a degraded serum transferrin, according to

Verheecke (1975). The alpha$_2$ globulins, prominent in serum, are relatively lower in the CSF. When concentrated CSF and the corresponding serum are subjected to electrophoresis together at the same time protein concentrations, the albumin, alpha$_1$ and alpha$_2$ globulins, and the beta and gamma globulin peaks of the two fluids are superimposed, while the prealbumin and tau fractions remain distinct. (3) The gamma globulin is proportionately lower in CSF than in serum; it constitutes less than 12 per cent of the total CSF proteins and about 18 per cent of the serum protein, as shown by most electrophoretic methods. (4) CSF contains only small amounts of glycoprotein, about 1 to 2 mg/dl, which are associated with the beta, alpha$_1$, and alpha$_2$ globulins (Lumsden, 1972). There is also only a very small amount of lipoprotein in CSF, largely associated with the alpha$_1$ globulins; this is markedly different from the findings in serum (see Lipids, later in this chapter).

CSF Proteins: Immunoelectrophoretic Studies

The technique of immunoelectrophoresis utilizes electrophoresis for the separation of the proteins and an immune precipitation reaction to identify and make visible the multiple proteins present. These methods have established the presence of many more proteins in normal CSF than is suggested by simple electrophoretic separation (Lumsden, 1972). Many separate proteins have been identified within each major electrophoretic peak. The following serum proteins have been identified in normal CSF: prealbumin, albumin, alpha$_1$ globulin, alpha$_2$ globulin, glycoprotein, alpha$_1$ antitrypsin, haptoglobins, ceruloplasmin, hemopexin, transferrin, beta$_1$ globulin, and gamma-A (IgA), gamma-M (IgM), and gamma-G (IgG) immunoglobulins. Whereas 75 per cent of the gamma globulin in serum is IgG, almost all the gamma globulin in normal CSF is IgG. The major proteins identified with electrophoresis and immunoelectrophoresis are listed in Table 6–8A. If the blood-brain barrier is normal, serum proteins with a molecular weight greater than 160,000 (fibrinogen, alpha-macroglobulin,

TABLE 6–8A   Proteins Identified in CSF with Electrophoresis and Immunoelectrophoresis

Electrophoretic Fraction	Prealbumin	Albumin	Alpha$_1$ Globulin	Alpha$_2$ Globulin	Beta Globulin	Gamma Globulin
Immunoelectrophoretic proteins	prealbumin	albumin	alpha$_1$ antitrypsin	alpha$_2$ macroglobulin	beta lipoprotein	IgG
			alpha$_1$ lipoprotein	alpha$_2$ lipoprotein	transferrin	IgA
			alpha$_1$ glycoprotein (orosomucoid)	haptoglobulin	tau fraction (modified transferrin) plasminogen	IgM
			alpha$_1$ antitrypsin	ceruloplasmin	complement	IgD
				erythropoietin	hemopexin beta-trace	IgF gamma-trace

Data derived from Laterre, 1965; Schultze and Heremans, 1966; Dencker, 1969; Link and Olsson, 1972; Lumsden, 1972; Nerenberg *et al.*, 1978; Williams *et al.*, 1978.

TABLE 6–8B Concentrations of Proteins in Plasma and Cerebrospinal Fluid

Protein	Molecular Weight	Hydrodynamic Radius (Å)	Plasma Concentration (mg/l)	CSF Concentration (mg/l)	Plasma/CSF Ratio
Prealbumin	61,000	32.5	238	17.3	14
Albumin	69,000	35.8	36,600	155.0	236
Transferrin	81,000	36.7	2040	14.4	142
Ceruloplasmin	152,000	46.8	366	1.0	366
IgG	150,000	53.4	9870	12.3	802
IgA	150,000	56.8	1750	1.3	1346
α_2 Macro-globulin	798,000	93.5	2220	2.0	1111
Fibrinogen	340,000	108.0	2964	0.6	4940
IgM	800,000	121.0	700	0.6	1167
β Lipoprotein	2,239,000	124.0	3728	0.6	6213

(From Felgenhauer, 1974)

and beta$_2$ lipoprotein) are largely excluded from the CSF (Felgenhauer, 1974). (See Table 6–8B.) However, when the barrier is abnormal, as evidenced by an increased CSF total protein and albumin content, the various macromolecules in serum may be readily detected in the CSF. The major proteins present in CSF will be discussed separately.

Prealbumin

Prealbumin is a plasma protein, molecular weight about 55,000, with an electrophoretic mobility greater than that of serum albumin. Recent studies show that it has an important role in the plasma transport of vitamin A and thyroid hormones (Navab *et al.*, 1977). Prealbumin is one of three plasma proteins involved in the transport of the thyroid hormones in human blood, of which thyroxine-binding globulin is the most important. Prealbumin also forms a protein complex with retinol-binding protein, the specific plasma transport protein for vitamin A. While its presence in serum is observed with gel electrophoresis (see Fig. 6–4), prealbumin constitutes a much smaller fraction of the total protein in serum than in CSF, where it is seen prominently ahead of the albumin peak.

Prealbumin constitutes about 5 per cent of the total protein in lumbar fluid, but the relative concentration in ventricular fluid is much greater, composing about 10 per cent of the total protein therein (Fishman *et al.*, 1957). In view of the two to threefold greater concentration of total protein in lumbar fluid than in ventricular fluid, the absolute concentration of prealbumin is about the same along the neuraxis. The relatively increased concentration of prealbumin within the ventricles has been explained by Laterre (1965) as a consequence of concentration by the choroidal cells of the protein derived from serum. Others have suggested that this concentration in ventricular fluid implies that the protein is derived from the brain. However, there are no data to support this hypothesis. There are no known correlations between the prealbumin content of either ventricular or lumbar CSF and neurological disease. In view of the ability of vitamin A intoxication to cause the pseudotumor syndrome, it is possible that the interaction between vitamin A and prealbumin influences choroid plexus function and the rate of CSF production; no data are available to support this speculation.

Albumin

The relative concentration of albumin to the total protein content in normal lumbar fluid has been reported to be slightly greater than or the same as that in serum. Albumin constitutes between 56 and 76 per cent of the total CSF protein and 52 to 67 per cent of the total serum protein (Schultze and Heremans, 1966). The variation may be related to the gradient in albumin concentration along the CSF pathways and to the variable amounts of fluid removed for analysis. Study of the kinetics of albumin exchange between plasma and CSF, using radioiodinated serum albumin, established that the CSF albumin originates from the plasma (Fishman, 1953; Cutler *et al.*, 1970); it is synthesized only in the liver. The limited entry of albumin, like that of other macromolecules into the CSF, is probably dependent upon vesicular transport across endothelial cells. The exit of albumin from the CSF probably depends upon the macrovesicular transport system responsible for bulk flow reabsorption across the arachnoid villi. Transport of albumin and other macromolecules in the reverse direction, from the brain's interstitial fluid to the capillary lumen, might play a role in the resolution of an intracerebral hematoma. That is, in pathological states vesicular transport in the capillary endothelial cells might occur from the albuminal side to the capillary lumen.

There is a relatively greater per cent increase in albumin when the total protein is increased; the albumin to total protein ratio generally rises with an increase in the CSF total protein (Fishman *et al.*, 1957). This is considered to illustrate the role of molecular weight (or molecular sifting based on molecular volume) in determining the distribution of proteins within the CSF (Felgenhauer, 1974). This will be discussed further.

Alpha Globulins

Several proteins make up the alpha$_1$ globulin peak, including two discrete alpha$_1$ lipoproteins and alpha$_1$ glycoproteins. Haptoglobins, ceruloplasmin, alpha$_2$ lipoprotein, and several other discrete proteins are included with the alpha$_2$ globulins (see Table 6–8A). There are no specific correlations between changes in the concentration of the alpha$_1$ and alpha$_2$ globulins and neurological disease; in clinical practice their measurement is not of diagnostic use.

Beta Globulins

Transferrin, the iron-binding beta$_1$ globulin, is one of several proteins included under the beta globulin peak, as summarized in Table 6–8A. There are two transferrins in the CSF: beta$_1$ transferrin, which is identical to the serum transferrin, and beta$_2$ transferrin. There is some uncertainty about the identity of this latter protein. Some workers have considered it to be a unique protein in the CSF, termed tau-protein, which is absent from serum, whereas other investigators have considered it to be a modified (neuroaminic acid deficient) transferrin which is also present in plasma (Verheecke, 1975). However, no specific correlations of these proteins with neurological disease have been established. The relative concentration of the beta globulins is somewhat higher in normal CSF than in serum, and they, like prealbumin, have a somewhat greater concentration in ventricular fluid than in lumbar fluid. The mechanism and significance of the relative increased concentration in the ventricular fluid are not known.

Gamma Globulins

The voluminous literature regarding the globulins of the CSF (well-summarized by Schultze and Heremans, 1966; Schmidt, 1968; Tourtellotte, 1970; Lumsden, 1972; and Laterre, 1975) has been of special interest to clinicians because of the changes associated with multiple sclerosis and many other inflammatory diseases of the central nervous system (Johnson and Nelson, 1977). The terms *gamma globulins, immunoglobulins,* and *IgG* are derived from the methods used for their assay. Electrophoretic techniques define the *gamma globulins* as a heterogeneous group of proteins with migration at similar rates in an electrical field, whereas the major *immunoglobulins* IgG, IgA, and IgM are measured by radioimmunoassay or immunochemical assay. These three immunoglobulins, normally present in the serum, have also been detected in normal CSF. In addition, minute amounts of IgD and IgE have also been found in normal fluid (Nerenberg *et al.,* 1978).

The concentration of IgG is normally 4.6 ± 1.9 mg/dl; that of IgA is $0.08 \pm .05$ mg/dl; and that of IgM is 0.017 ± 0.005 mg/dl. Thus, the major immunoglobulin in normal CSF is IgG, and most studies have dealt with it. It has a molecular weight of 150,000; many antibodies to both bacteria and viruses are of the IgG class. Extensive data indicate that the increased CSF gamma globulin observed in multiple sclerosis is derived from the inflammatory cells associated with demyelinative lesions and diffusion of the immunoglobulins into the CSF, an example of the sink action of the CSF (Tourtellotte, 1975).

Study of the kinetics of gamma globulin exchange between plasma and CSF, using radioiodinated gamma globulin, has established that the CSF gamma globulin normally originates in the plasma (Cutler *et al.,* 1970). Normally, the concentration of gamma globulin relative to the total protein in lumbar fluid is about two-thirds the ratio found in the serum; there is relatively less gamma globulin in CSF than in plasma. An increased concentration of gamma globulin in CSF has been reported in many inflammatory pathological states. This was first recognized when an abnormal colloidal gold curve (Lange, 1913) was noted in the CSF in neurosyphilis and in a variety of inflammatory disorders, before definition of the gamma globulins. (This empirically devised test will be described later.) The most striking correlations occur with multiple sclerosis, neurosyphilis, subacute sclerosing panencephalitis, progressive rubella encephalitis, many viral meningoencephalitides, and other inflammatory disorders including meningeal sarcoidosis and cysticercosis.

Of special diagnostic interest is the occurrence of an increased gamma globulin in 34 per cent of 104 patients with various brain tumors, reported by Castaigne *et al.* (1972). The data were not corrected for the entry of serum proteins into the CSF. Assuming that the gamma globulin was not derived only from the serum, the finding indicates the presence of inflammatory cells in association with some brain tumors.

In the pathological conditions just listed, the major change has been an increase in the IgG level, with less change in the IgA level. Only recently have techniques become available for measuring IgM in unconcentrated CSF; preliminary data suggest that it is increased in multiple sclerosis and other inflammatory disorders as well (Williams *et al.*, 1978). It has been generally assumed that IgM in CSF is derived from the serum. A single report describes a patient with an immunodeficiency syndrome and a chronic progressive encephalopathy, in whom IgM was present in high concentration in the CSF but undetected in the serum (Lord *et al.*, 1973). This suggests that IgM may be formed in the brain and that it is not necessarily derived from the serum. Radioimmunoassay of IgM, normally present in minute concentration, shows a slight increase in about 50 per cent of patients with multiple sclerosis (Nerenberg *et al.*, 1978). It is increased also with major increases in permeability of the blood-brain barrier, for instance, in purulent meningitis and other conditions with a highly elevated CSF protein. The increase in IgM has been considered to represent a thymus-independent antigenic response (Nerenberg *et al.*, 1978). The clinical usefulness of measuring IgM remains to be determined.

Quantitative Measurement of Gamma Globulin

The normal serum IgG is 15 to 18 per cent of the total serum protein, whereas the normal CSF IgG is only 5 to 12 per cent of the total CSF protein. This difference makes it necessary to relate the CSF IgG level to the other proteins present in the CSF in order to determine whether the CSF IgG is simply serum IgG entering the CSF across a damaged blood-brain barrier, or whether the CSF IgG is partially synthesized within the central nervous system. There is a difference of opinion about the best way of expressing the data. Most laboratories express the CSF gamma globulin as a per cent of the total CSF protein (Lumsden, 1972), whereas some investigators have recommended the use of the CSF albumin (Tourtellotte, 1970), transferrin, or $alpha_2$ macroglobulin (Schliep and Felgenhauer, 1974) as a better denominator than the CSF total protein. The CSF albumin and $alpha_2$ macroglobulin have the advantage of being synthesized entirely outside of the central nervous system, whereas the total protein includes a variable though small percentage of protein presumably synthesized within the central nervous system in pathological conditions.

In many laboratories, the method for measuring total protein has the greatest accuracy, and therefore total protein usually serves as the most useful reference in the interpretation of the CSF gamma globulin in clinical practice. However, with the availability of new techniques for the accurate measurement in CSF of albumin, transferrin, and $alpha_2$ macroglobulin, some laboratories have used the IgG ratio to these proteins in order to interpret an increase in the IgG level. The key issue in choosing the denominator seems to be the accuracy, sensitivity, and reproducibility of the methods used for determining the CSF total protein, albumin, transferrin, or alpha$_2$ macroglobulin. The decision as to which protein is best will depend on the individual laboratory's performance.

Recently, the calculation of the IgG-albumin index has been used to correct the CSF IgG level for the contribution of IgG derived from the blood and for its increased entry across a damaged barrier.

$$\text{IgG-albumin index} = \frac{\text{IgG (CSF)} \times \text{albumin (serum)}}{\text{IgG (serum)} \times \text{albumin (CSF)}}$$

According to Delpech and Lichtblau (1972), 0.85 is the upper normal limit of the index; Olsson and Petterson (1976) used 0.66 and Tibbling *et al.* (1977) used 0.34 to 0.58 as the normal range. Each laboratory must carefully define its normal values if the index is to be used. The index is dependent upon four individual laboratory determinations; methodological errors would subject the index to much variation.

Tourtellotte (1975, 1978) devised a formula to estimate the amount of IgG synthesized each day in the nervous system that contributes to its concentration in CSF. It corrects for the amount of gamma globulin entering CSF from the serum. It requires accurate measurement of the albumin and IgG content of CSF and serum. Several constants were used in the calculation that were derived from the findings in normal subjects. The average synthetic rate in normal subjects was reported as minus 3.3 mg per day, with confidence limits of minus 9.9 to plus 3.3. The formula should prove useful in clinical research, particularly when serial determinations are carried out in the same patient.

Kappa/Lambda Ratios of IgG Light Chains

The IgG molecule can be dissociated to demonstrate that it contains two kinds of polypeptide chains, including two heavy and two light chains. Each heavy chain has a molecular weight of 55,000 and contains about 450 amino acids. Each light chain has a molecular weight of about 22,500 and contains about 210 amino acids. Two types of light chains have been identified: kappa and lambda. Bence Jones proteins, present in CSF and urine in cases of multiple myeloma, are composed of such light chains. In Waldenström's macroglobulinemia, myeloma, and the various forms of monoclonal gammopathy, specific changes in the distributions of kappa and lambda light chains in serum have been identified (Kyle and Greipp, 1978).

There has been recent interest in determining the *light chain* characteristics of the immunoglobulins in CSF (Link and Zettervall, 1970; Vandvik, 1977). In normal subjects, the kappa and lambda chains were about equal in concentration; the kappa/lambda ratio in CSF was about 1.0, similar to the ratio in serum. The ratio was elevated to 2.6 ± 1.3 in multiple sclerosis, with lesser increases in other inflammatory disorders. Eickhoff and Heipertz (1978) studied patients with a variety of neurological diseases and concluded that an increase in the kappa/lambda ratio was common in many inflammatory diseases of the nervous system, including multiple sclerosis. These studies are of special interest regarding the pathophysiology of such diseases, but their role in clinical diagnosis has not been shown.

Myelin Basic Protein

There is special interest in the measurement of myelin basic protein (encephalitogenic protein) in CSF as a potential guide to demyelination in patients with multiple sclerosis (Cohen *et al.*, 1976; Whitaker, 1977; Panitch *et al.*, 1980). Myelin is composed of 70 per cent lipid and 30 per cent protein. The major protein components are proteolipid, myelin basic (encephalitogenic) protein, and an acidic protein or proteins termed the Wolfgram protein. Basic protein has been of special interest because it produces experimental allergic encephalomyelitis in various laboratory animals. It constitutes about 30 per cent of the myelin proteins and has a molecular weight of 18,000, and the number (169) and sequence of its amino acid residues are known.

Whitaker (1977) developed a radioimmunoassay performed on unconcentrated CSF which identified a specific fragment (P-1) of basic protein in the CSF. The P-1 fragment was present in the CSF of patients in the acute phase of an exacerbation of multiple sclerosis, and it was absent in patients who were stable or had a gradually progressive course. The P-1 fragment was also found in the CSF of a patient with acute cerebral infarction. The correlation between changes in the concentration of the P-1 fragment and the activity of the disease awaits further study.

McKhann (1978) also studied myelin basic protein using a radioimmunoassay and found none in normal CSF and elevations only in patients with an acute exacerbation of multiple sclerosis or with acute cerebral infarction. The presence of basic protein was considered as an index of active demyelination, which might be useful as a diagnostic test for the disease. However, its nonspecificity and transient appearance may limit its applicability. Panitch *et al.* (1980) measured CSF antibodies to myelin basic protein. Antibodies were found more frequently in patients with active disease than in patients in remission. Specific correlations have not yet been established between the CSF IgG level, the presence of oligoclonal bands seen with electrophoresis, the concentration of myelin basic protein, and the antibody level to myelin basic protein.

Trace Proteins

There have been many attempts to demonstrate the presence in CSF of proteins that are unique to the CSF and absent from the plasma (Link and Olsson, 1972). In these studies, antisera have been prepared against CSF and then thoroughly absorbed with normal plasma. Proteins not absorbed were considered unique to the CSF. Two such proteins, beta-trace and gamma-trace, have been studied in some detail (Hochwald and Thorbecke, 1962).

Beta-trace protein, a single polypeptide chain with a molecular weight of about 31,000, has been found in normal CSF with immunoelectrophoresis using an antiserum against human CSF, but it is almost absent from the serum. The normal CSF content of beta-trace protein is about 7 per cent of the total CSF protein (about 1.5 to 3.5 mg/dl) but the normal serum level is less than 0.5 mg/dl.

It has been demonstrated in the urine and in extracts of brain tissue but not in renal tissue. Link and Olsson (1972) concluded that its greater concentration in normal CSF indicated synthesis within the central nervous system. They also suggested that an increase in CSF level might reflect severe myelin degradation in disease. Significant increases in the CSF beta-trace level have been reported with aging, cerebrovascular disease, some brain tumors, and multiple sclerosis (Lumsden, 1972). There is some correlation between the CSF level and the CSF total protein level. However, elevation of the beta-trace protein has not been shown to be useful in clinical diagnosis because of its nonspecificity.

Gamma-trace proteins, present in CSF, are probably also present in serum in very low concentrations. Both beta-trace and gamma-trace proteins have also been found in ascitic and pleural fluids, but their functional significance is not known.

Fibronectin

Fibronectin is a high molecular weight glycoprotein (MW about 200,000) found in blood and various tissues and in cultures of fibroblasts and astroglial cells. Its concentration in normal plasma is about 300 μg/ml, using a radioimmunoassay. It has been demonstrated also in normal CSF, where the concentration is 3.0 ± 1.6 μg ml ($\pm$SD). The CSF/plasma ratio of about 0.01 (compared to 0.02 for albumin) suggests that the CSF fibronectin may be derived from the brain as well as from the plasma. This possibility is supported by the findings that astroglial cells release large amounts of fibronectin into the culture medium. Very high CSF levels have been observed with astrocytoma and metastatic carcinoma. However, in multiple sclerosis, the CSF level of 1.6 ± 0.8 μg/ml was about half that observed in the control fluids (Kuusela et al., 1978). The reproducibility and significance of this finding has not been established.

Interferon

Interferon, a protein that inhibits the replication of viruses, is produced by various cells in response to exogenous stimuli. It may be an important factor in the host's defense against viral infections. While major attention has focused on various viruses, other infectious agents, including bacteria, Rickettsia, and Toxoplasma, also stimulate interferon production or release, in vivo and in vitro, with the use of cell cultures. Degne et al. (1976) found interferon in the CSF and serum from about half of a group of patients with acute encephalitis, presumed to be viral, and from about half of a group of patients with multiple sclerosis. The CSF titers appeared to be derived from the serum, where the titers were substantially higher. Significant titers of interferon were not observed in the CSF in noninflammatory disorders of the central nervous system.

Alpha Albumin (Glial Fibrillary Acidic Protein)

Alpha albumin, also termed glial fibrillary acidic protein, is present in brain and has been considered to be localized in astrocytic glial cells. Lowenthal et al. (1978) reported its presence in CSF in about 10 per cent of 244 patients studied.

The positive samples were obtained in heterogeneous neurological disorders, including acute multiple sclerosis, and after severe epileptic seizures. These workers suggested that the protein might appear in the CSF as a result of damage to glial cells. Further study is needed to determine the clinical correlations with the appearance of alpha albumin as well as its significance.

Protein Size and CSF Composition

The relatively low protein content of normal CSF has been considered to depend upon the relative exclusion of macromolecules by the blood-brain barrier determined by the capillary endothelial cells. The importance of molecular size in determining the distribution of the various CSF proteins derived from the serum was first emphasized by Kabat *et al.* (1942), who measured gamma globulin using an immunochemical technique and reported relatively less in CSF than the total protein or albumin concentrations. An extensive literature supports the generalization, but there are also several exceptions to the rule that the CSF protein composition is simply related inversely to molecular weight. Such exceptions include the following: (1) the concentration of transferrin and prealbumin in CSF is relatively greater than can be explained by their molecular weights; and (2) the concentrations of gamma-trace and beta-trace proteins are considerably higher than would be expected on the basis of their molecular weight and serum concentrations (Link *et al.*, 1972).

More recently, Felgenhauer (1974) studied the hydrodynamic radii of various serum proteins and reported discrepancies between molecular weight and hydrodynamic volume (the Einstein-Stokes radius). (See Table 6–8B.) He concluded that the CSF/serum distribution ratios of the various proteins are better correlated with their hydrodynamic radii than with their molecular weight, and that this feature also explains, in part, the electrophoretic characteristics of the various proteins in CSF which originate in the serum. If pinocytosis is the major route whereby proteins cross the endothelial and arachnoid villus cells, macromolecules of various sizes would be expected to cross the barrier at a similar rate. This would favor the relative similarity of the CSF/serum distribution ratios of the various proteins. Further information is needed to clarify the mechanisms involved.

Pathological Patterns in the CSF Proteins

Various classifications have been proposed (Laterre, 1965; Schultze and Heremans, 1966; Schmidt, 1968) for the changes in the distribution of the CSF proteins in pathological conditions. Delineation of the following patterns has proved useful: (1) patterns of increased entry of plasma proteins; (2) patterns secondary to changes in the plasma proteins; (3) patterns of local immunoglobulin production, including oligoclonal bands; and (4) degenerative patterns. Each of these patterns and its diagnostic significance is now discussed.

PATTERNS OF INCREASED ENTRY OF PLASMA PROTEINS. The greater entry of plasma into the CSF results in an increase in total CSF protein; therefore, the immunoelectrophoretic pattern of the CSF more closely resembles that of the plasma. This occurs in two circumstances: (1) increased endothelial cell permeability characteristic of disruption of the blood-brain barrier, and (2) defective reabsorption of CSF proteins by the arachnoid villi or with obstruction in the subarachnoid spaces. The CSF total protein is variably increased in both conditions. As the total protein reaches progressively higher levels, the prealbumin and tau fractions become less prominent because of their dilution by the influx of serum proteins. The macromolecular plasma proteins (including IgM immunoglobulin, beta$_1$ and alpha$_2$ lipoprotein, and fibrinogen), normally largely excluded, become increasingly apparent with progressive CSF protein elevation.

PATTERNS REFLECTING ALTERATIONS IN PLASMA PROTEINS. The changes in the serum noted in the various dysproteinemias are often reflected in the CSF (Schultze and Heremans, 1966). Thus, the usual monoclonal gammopathy seen in the serum with multiple myeloma is also detected in the CSF. Bence Jones proteins are readily seen in the CSF, whereas high molecular weight paraproteins are excluded. The fact that changes in the serum gamma globulins are readily reflected in the CSF makes it necessary to compare the CSF and serum protein electrophoreses in order to interpret an abnormal CSF pattern. *The serum protein electrophoreses should be obtained in all patients with increased CSF gamma globulins to clarify whether the latter have originated in the plasma or whether they represent de novo synthesis within the central nervous system.*.

PATTERNS OF LOCAL IMMUNOGLOBULIN PRODUCTION. In a variety of disorders, the CSF is often characterized by an increase in the gamma globulin fraction with normal plasma immunoglobulin levels. In these cases, there is substantial evidence that the immunoglobulins are synthesized within the central nervous system (Tourtellotte, 1970, Lumsden, 1972). This interpretation has been supported by kinetic studies using radioiodinated gamma globulin in patients with increased CSF gamma globulin levels associated with multiple sclerosis and SSPE (Cutler *et al.*, 1970). Increased CSF levels have been reported in the gamut of chronic and subacute inflammatory diseases of the nervous system, including neurosyphilis, tuberculous meningitis, brain abscess, viral meningoencephalitis, paraneoplastic syndromes, cysticercosis, subacute sclerosing panencephalitis, postvaricella meningoencephalitis, Vogt-Koyanagi-Harada's disease, and sarcoidosis. Minor increases in gamma globulin content are seen often also in the Guillain-Barré syndrome and tuberculoma and in some patients with brain tumor.

The occurrence of an elevated gamma globulin in about 70 per cent of cases of multiple sclerosis is of major diagnostic import. Representative values obtained with a variety of methods are summarized in Table 7–10 (page 310). The normal range for CSF gamma globulin in most laboratories is between 5 and 12 per cent of total protein. The choice of optimal method for the quantitative separation of the CSF proteins is moot. Electrophoretic analysis of concentrated CSF using cellulose acetate is probably in widest use at present.

In pathological conditions, when the total CSF protein becomes elevated because of increased permeability of the blood-brain barrier, the CSF gamma globulin is further increased by the addition of serum protein, which normally contains 15 to 18 per cent gamma globulin. Thus, it is difficult to ascertain the upper normal limit for the CSF gamma globulin as a per cent of the total protein when the CSF total protein is greatly elevated. The CSF gamma globulin may be increased to levels as high as 36 per cent of the total protein and perhaps higher in subacute sclerosing panencephalitis and chronic rubella panencephalitis (Wolinsky *et al.*, 1976), but elevations to levels higher than 30 per cent of the total protein are very unusual in most other neurological disorders.

Tourtellotte's (1975, 1978) formula for estimating the amount of gamma globulin produced each day in the nervous system has been discussed earlier. The calculation depends upon the generalization that in normal subjects all the CSF gamma globulin is derived from the serum. In 127 patients with multiple sclerosis, increased IgG formation within the central nervous system was noted in 86 per cent of those tested. Tourtellotte (1975) found that the figure was higher in the more acute forms of the disease. It tended to increase with age, duration of disease, number of relapses, and elevated CSF leukocytes. However, a number of earlier reports have been unable to relate the elevated CSF gamma globulin to the activity of the disease (Yahr *et al.*, 1954; Laterre, 1965). The Tourtellotte formula appears to be a more sensitive index of changes in IgG turnover than does the measurement of gamma globulin *per se*.

OLIGOCLONAL BANDS.   In addition to the absolute increase noted in gamma globulin content in inflammatory diseases of the nervous system, qualitative changes in the CSF gamma globulins have also been demonstrated in concentrated CSF with agarose gel electrophoresis and with other gels (Johnson and Nelson, 1977; Thompson, 1977). This technique demonstrates discrete bands in the gamma globulin pattern which have been termed *oligoclonal bands*. The term describes a population of proteins, having identical electrophoretic characteristics, that are derived from the same population of immunocompetent cells. A single antigen is presumed to give rise to a single band.

Oligoclonal IgG bands can usually be seen after concentration of CSF about 50 times (using one of several methods such as negative pressure dialysis). The concentrated CSF is applied to agarose gel for electrophoresis, then fixed and stained with amido-black or Coomassie Blue protein stains. Bands have been reported in about 90 per cent of patients with multiple sclerosis (Johnson and Nelson, 1977). This figure is somewhat higher than the 79 per cent reported earlier by Laterre *et al.* (1970). Oligoclonal bands are frequently observed whenever the CSF gamma globulin is increased with the gamut of inflammatory disorders of the nervous system listed earlier (Thompson, 1977). Oligoclonal bands occur more often in these conditions than does an increase in the gamma globulin concentration. The appearance of such bands in the CSF, in the absence of serum banding, is an indication of an inflammatory process in the nervous system even when the gamma globulin level is normal. Examples of oligoclonal banding in a case of multiple sclerosis and subacute sclerosing panencephalitis are shown in Figure 6–4 (page 180). Between 2 and 5 bands have been observed in many inflammatory diseases; rarely, as many as 10 bands have been reported. In patients with multiple sclerosis the band pattern seems to be unique for each patient, and it remains remarkably stable over time. Bands occur rarely in patients with neoplasms, vascular disease, motor neuron disease, and other neurological diseases that are not generally viewed as immunological disorders.

While the usefulness of oligoclonal bands in the diagnosis of multiple sclerosis and the various inflammatory diseases has been emphasized, the functional significance of these restricted populations of IgG is not known.

Oligoclonal bands are very striking in subacute sclerosing panencephalitis, and Norrby and Vandvik (1975) have reported that the activity of some bands could be absorbed by concentrated measles antigens, which indicates that the band material represents antibodies to measles virus. However, some bands are not composed of antimeasles antibody, and Booe *et al.* (1972) have suggested that these may represent antibodies directed against brain antigens. The origin of the multiple oligoclonal bands observed in multiple sclerosis and optic neuritis is less clear. In some patients, bands have been attributed to the measles antigen, but the significance of this finding is not known. Norrby (1978) reviewed the evidence regarding the increase in antibodies to numerous viral antigens in the CSF of multiple sclerosis patients, including measles, rubella, and vaccinia. Their relationship to the pathogenesis of the disease and to the presence of oligoclonal bands is under active investigation (Forghani *et al.*, 1978). At present it seems that multiple sclerosis patients are immunologically different in their responses to various viral antigens, but no specific viral agent has been implicated in the etiology of the disease.

In summary, the multiple oligoclonal bands sometimes observed represent immunoglobulin responses in the nervous system. The specific antigens involved and their relationship to the disease in which they are found is currently under active investigation.

DEGENERATIVE PATTERNS.   There is an extensive literature, largely European (Lowenthal, 1964; Laterre, 1965; Schultze and Heremans, 1966; Schmidt, 1968), directed toward finding unique electrophoretic patterns which might prove highly specific for some neurological diseases. A number of changes have been suggested to serve as an index of degenerative disease of the nervous system. Thus, in a heterogeneous group of neurological disorders (including epilepsy, cerebrovascular disease, and degenerative diseases), reciprocal changes in the concentrations of beta$_1$ globulin and tau fractions have been observed, i.e., a decrease in the beta$_1$ globulin and an increase in tau fraction. Such changes represent greater degradation of transferrin to yield an increase in tau fraction (Schultze and Heremans, 1966). However, it is difficult to assess the significance of these observations. It is my view that *no* specific changes or degenerative patterns of diagnostic importance have been established, apart from the changes in the immunoglobulins described above. In clinical practice at present, the total protein, the per cent gamma globulin (related to total protein, albumin, or transferrin), and the presence of oligoclonal bands are major diagnostic aids. The measurement of the other proteins observed with electrophoresis or immunoelectrophoresis lacks sufficient diagnostic specificity, although it remains of potential interest for clinical investigation.

Colloidal Gold Reactions

In the early years of this century, various colloidal reactions were developed empirically for the analysis of spinal fluid proteins (Lange, 1913; Levinson, 1929; Lups and Haan, 1954). These have largely been replaced by various methods of electrophoretic analysis. The colloidal gold test, now rarely used, is based on the precipitation of a colloidal suspension of gold with 10 serial dilutions of spinal fluid, ranging from 1:0 to 1:5120. Colloidal gold solution, rust in color, is then added to each tube. The change in color in each tube is recorded as follows: 0-no change in color; 1-very slight change to a deeper red; 2-lilac;

3-blue; 4-blue with some precipitation of the colloidal gold; 5-clear supernatant fluid with complete precipitation of the gold. This variable degree of precipitation is influenced by the total protein concentration, the albumin and globulin content, and the amounts and types of globulin subfractions present (Press, 1956). Albumin, alpha globulin, and beta globulin tend to maintain the colloidal suspension, while gamma globulin favors precipitation of the gold.

Three major types of abnormal gold curves are described. With normal fluids, the color is unchanged and the curve is described as flat or 0000000000. The most significant abnormal curve is the first zone curve, 5555443210, which describes maximal precipitation in the first tubes. The second zone curve, 0123454320, describes maximal precipitation in the middle dilutions. The third zone or end zone curve, 0000112345, describes maximal precipitation in the tubes with the most dilute concentration of protein. At one time, the first two curves were considered diagnostic of neurosyphilis and they were referred to as *paretic* and *tabetic* curves, respectively, and the third was called the *meningitic curve*. As the curves were later shown to indicate nonspecific changes in protein content, these pathological terms were dropped. Normal colloidal gold curves may occur in many pathological conditions, despite an increased protein content or pleocytosis. Abnormal gold curves have also been noted with a normal total protein. Correlation of the various colloidal reactions with electrophoretic analysis of the proteins present leads to these conclusions. The first zone curve is a fair index of a substantial increase in gamma globulin in the spinal fluid. The first zone curve is commonly seen with neurosyphilis, multiple sclerosis, and subacute sclerosing panencephalitis, and less often seen with other inflammatory diseases of the central nervous system. The mid zone curve has a similar meaning but usually reflects a lesser elevation of gamma globulin content. The third zone or meningitic curve is most commonly found in fluids with a high protein content and a relative excess of albumin to globulin. These changes account for the facilitation of colloidal precipitation in the very dilute solutions of protein in the end zone tubes. It has been frequently noted in acute purulent meningitis, spinal subarachnoid block, and subarachnoid hemorrhage.

Thompson (1977) reported that only 50 per cent of multiple sclerosis patients had either a first zone (17 per cent) or second zone (32 per cent) curve. This relatively low diagnostic yield illustrates the advantages of the direct measurement of the immunoglobulin level with a more sensitive electrophoretic technique. A number of other nonspecific colloidal tests were used in the past, including the mastic solution, benzoin solution, and paraffin tests (Schmidt, 1968). There seems to be no justification for their continued use in light of the more specific methods available for the study of proteins in biological fluids.

Qualitative Tests of CSF Proteins

Prior to the introduction of electrophoresis for the quantitative measurement of gamma globulin, several qualitative tests were widely used to indicate an increase in the total globulins present. These tests have been antiquated by the quantitative tests just described. They are summarized briefly here only as a guide to the older literature, which commonly describes their use.

Pándy test. The test utilizes a saturated solution of phenol to precipitate the globulins. One drop of CSF is added to 1 to 2 ml of Pándy's solution (a filtered, saturated solution of phenol) in a small test tube. An excess of globulin is indicated by immediate clouding of the solution. The increase may be graded as 1, 2, 3, or 4. In normal CSF there is no change or only a very faint turbidity. The test loses specificity when the total protein is elevated above approximately 100 mg per dl; all high protein fluids will cloud the solution.

Ross-Jones test. This test is based on the precipitation of globulins by concentrated solutions of ammonium sulfate. One ml of CSF is layered over an equal volume of a saturated solution of ammonium sulfate. A white precipitate forming a ring at the junction of the two fluids indicates an excessive concentration of globulins.

The *Nonne-Apelt test* is similar except that the two solutions are mixed rather than layered. A white precipitate indicates excessive globulins in the CSF. Both tests using saturated ammonium sulfate also lose specificity when the total protein is elevated above approximately 100 mg per dl; all concentrated protein solutions precipitate in concentrated ammonium chloride solution.

Concentration Gradient of Proteins Along the Neuraxis

In normal children and adults there is a concentration gradient of protein from a low level in the ventricles, 6 to 15 mg per dl, to an intermediate level in the cisterna magna, 15 to 25 mg per dl, to the highest level in the lumbar sac, 20 to 50 mg per dl (Merritt and Fremont-Smith, 1938). Several mechanisms have been put forth to explain the protein gradient along the neuraxis. So-called stagnation in the lumbar region was suggested by Merritt and Fremont-Smith (1938) as a possible explanation for the relatively increased protein content in the lumbar sac. The subsequent demonstration of an arterial pulse pressure of about 30 mm water in the lumbar region in normal subjects makes the concept of stagnation, or poor mixing, unlikely in the absence of a spinal subarachoid block.

We studied the entry of radioiodinated albumin (RISA) into the CSF following intravenous administration in 5 children with hydrocephalus or brain tumor (Fishman *et al.*, 1958). RISA entered lumbar fluid most rapidly, the cisternal region less rapidly, and the ventricles most slowly. Electrophoretic analysis of ventricular and lumbar fluids also showed that the concentration of albumin in lumbar fluid substantially exceeded that in the ventricular fluid. We concluded that the lumbar subarachnoid space was more permeable than the ventricular system to albumin. Our observations were confirmed by Weisner and Bernhardt (1978), who compared the protein composition of ventricular, cisternal, and lumbar fluid, using both electrophoretic and immunoelectrophoretic techniques. They also found the expected relative decline in prealbumin concentration along the neuraxis as well as a progressive increase in albumin (both absolute and relative to total protein) from ventricular to lumbar fluid.

The data summarized in Table 6–9 support the view that the protein gradient reflects a differential increase in permeability to proteins. (If defective absorption of CSF proteins took place in the lumbar region, one might expect a relative increase in the globulins, which have a greater molecular weight and greater dynamic volume (Einstein-Stokes radius). On the other hand, vesicular

TABLE 6–9   Protein Concentration Gradients in CSF

PROTEIN	VENTRICULAR (27)*	CISTERNAL (33)	LUMBAR (127)
Total protein	25.6 ± 5.9 mg/dl†	31.6 ± 5.8 mg/dl	42.0 ± 5.5 mg/dl
Albumin	8.3 ± 2.5 mg/dl	12.7 ± 4.1 mg/dl	18.6 ± 6.6 mg/dl
% albumin	32.4%	40.2%	44.3%
IgG	0.9 ± 0.4 mg/dl	1.4 ± 0.5 mg/dl	2.3 ± 1.0 mg/dl
% IgG	3.5%	4.4%	5.5%

The data demonstrate that the increasing concentration of protein from the ventricular to lumbar fluids is associated with progressively greater amounts of albumin, both in concentration and as a percentage of the total protein.

Total protein and protein fractions measured by radioimmunodiffusion in ventricular, cisternal, and lumbar cerebrospinal fluid (derived from the data of Weisner and Bernhardt, 1978).

*( ) = number of subjects.

† ± SD.

transport might remove various macromolecules at the same rate.) In summary, the protein concentration gradient in CSF in humans is best explained by the relatively increased permeability of the blood-CSF barrier to proteins in the spinal subarachnoid space. Although this was not demonstrated in cats (Hochwald *et al.*, 1969), there appears to be no better explanation for the findings in patients.

Enzymes

The technical advances that made possible the ready assay of a wide variety of enzymes in the serum have also been extended to the study of the CSF (Lowenthal, 1968). A huge literature has been assembled in the last 30 years, but it is largely disappointing to the clinician because enzyme assays in CSF have provided few data with sufficient diagnostic specificity to warrant their introduction into clinical practice.

Enzymes in the CSF have three possible sources: (1) brain tissue or brain tumors, (2) blood, and (3) cellular elements within the CSF. In probably every instance, the blood enzyme level is higher than the CSF level in normal subjects. Unfortunately, many reports of the CSF enzyme levels in disease have failed to report the concurrent blood enzyme level, the total and differential CSF cellular count, and the CSF protein content. Thus, in evaluating the literature, it is difficult to assess the source of the enzyme level of CSF and the specificity of changes in the enzyme level. (The interpretation of changes in the CSF gamma globulin poses an analogous problem; it is difficult to assess an elevated CSF level without knowledge of the serum level.) It is not surprising that most "abnormal" CSF enzyme levels have been associated with purulent meningitis, brain tumor, or other conditions with evidence of vasogenic edema and increased barrier permeability. Many authors have suggested that increases in CSF enzyme level would prove valuable in clinical diagnosis. However, none of the enzyme assays has been shown to be sufficiently sensitive or specific to warrant its use in clinical practice.

TABLE 6–10   Enzymes Present in CSF

Adenylate kinase (Ronquist *et al.*, 1977)
Aldolase (Schapira, 1962)
Arginine esterase (Briseid *et al.*, 1976)
Aspartate aminotransferase (Savory and Brody, 1979)
Choline acetyltransferase (Aquilonius and Eckern, 1976)
Cholinesterases (Plum and Fog, 1960)
Creatine phosphokinase (Sherwin *et al.*, 1969)
      Isoenzymes (Beatty and Oppenheimer, 1968)
Dehydrogenases
      Isocitric (van Rymenant *et al.*, 1966)
      Lactic (Sherwin *et al.*, 1968)
      Malic (Lowenthal, 1968)
Dopamine beta-hydroxylase (Goldstein and Cubeddu, 1976)
Glucuronidase (Lehrer, 1963)
Leucine aminopeptidase (Green and Perry, 1963)
Lipases (Spiegel-Adolf *et al.*, 1957)
Lysozyme (Klockars *et al.*, 1978)
Phosphatases, acid and alkaline (Colling and Rossiter, 1950)
Phosphohexose isomerase (Thompson *et al.*, 1959)
Proteolytic enzymes (Chapman and Wolff, 1959)
Ribonuclease (Rabin *et al.*, 1977)
Transamines
      Glutamic-oxaloacetic transaminase (Katzman *et al.*, 1957)
      Glutamic-pyruvic transaminase (Lowenthal, 1968)

A lengthy (although incomplete) list of the various enzymes that have been measured is given in Table 6–10. Only a few of these will be discussed in detail. The interested reader should consult the references for further details. There has been special interest in lactic dehydrogenase and its isoenzymes, lysozyme, and creatine phosphokinase. These will be discussed below.

Lactic Dehydrogenase and Its Isoenzymes

The concentration in CSF of lactic dehydrogenase (LDH) and its five isoenzymes has been studied in bacterial and viral meningitis (Beatty and Oppenheimer, 1968; Neches and Platt, 1968). Both conditions were associated with increased LDH levels. The highest levels were found in pneumococcal meningitis, with lesser increases in most cases of influenzal and meningococcal meningitis. There was only a modest elevation in LDH activity in viral infections. However, there was sufficient overlap between the bacterial and viral cases to limit the usefulness of the enzyme assay in differential diagnosis. Isoenzymes 4 and 5 were preponderant in terms of their percentage distribution in bacterial infection. This suggests that these isoenzymes were derived chiefly from granulocytes, because normal CSF, serum, and brain tissue have an isoenzyme pattern characterized by a preponderance of isoenzymes 1 and 2. In mild viral infections, a mild elevation in fractions 1 and 2 was observed. Patients who died from either bacterial or viral meningoencephalitis had marked elevation in fractions 1 and 2; this suggested that extensive brain damage resulted in their release from the tissue into the CSF. There have been no more recent reports extending these observations.

Lysozyme

Lysozyme, an anionic protein whose molecular weight is 14,300, is a constituent of tears (lacrimal fluid), blood, kidney, cartilage, and other tissues. Most of the serum lysozyme is derived from the lysosomes of polymorphonuclear leukocytes and macrophages. The protein is enzymatically active, and it serves to depolymerize the bacterial walls of some bacteria. In normal subjects, the concentration of lysozyme in CSF is less than 1.5 μg per ml. The CSF level is not altered, despite marked increases in the serum level. (One would predict that the CSF level of a protein with a molecular weight of 14,000 would be normally about 1 per cent of the serum level.) Newman *et al.* (1974) have reported the CSF lysozyme levels in 30 patients with various medical and neurological diseases. Increased concentrations were found in 4 patients with bacterial meningitis and in 12 patients with various malignancies affecting the central nervous system, almost all of whom had malignant cells in the CSF demonstrated by cytological study. The highest levels were found in a patient with histiocytic lymphoma, a tumor presumably very high in lysozyme. Lysozyme levels fell with a favorable response to chemotherapy and radiotherapy, along with a fall in the number of malignant cells in the fluid. The authors suggested that lysozyme assay might serve as a useful diagnostic indication of inflammatory or neoplastic disease of the central nervous system and meninges.

Klockars *et al.* (1978) studied lysozyme levels in patients with bacterial or viral meningitis. Nine of 11 patients with bacterial meningitis had increased levels, whereas only 10 of 18 patients with viral meningitis had increased levels. While greater increases were seen in bacterial meningitis, there was considerable overlap between the two groups. The changes in lysozyme concentration paralleled changes in lactic dehydrogenase.

Creatine Phosphokinase (CPK)

CPK catalyzes the reversible reaction between creatine phosphate and ADP to yield creatine and ATP. It is present in highest concentration in skeletal and cardiac muscle, but considerable amounts are also present in brain. There are "brain type" and "muscle type" isoenzymes of CPK which have been found in the serum. The isoenzyme found in CSF is of the brain type, and its concentration is largely independent of the serum enzyme level and CSF protein concentration. Very low levels of CPK were detected in the CSF of control subjects. Increased levels were found in a wide variety of neurological disorders, including seizures, tumors, stroke, and multiple sclerosis (Sherwin *et al.*, 1969).

In summary, none of the available enzyme assays have sufficient specificity to warrant their use as routine diagnostic tests.

Glucose

The CSF glucose is derived solely from the plasma, and its concentration is dependent upon the blood level. The normal range in CSF is between 45 and 80 mg/dl in patients with a blood glucose between 70 and 120 mg/dl; i.e., it is normally 60 to 80 per cent of the blood glucose. Values between 40 and 45 mg/dl are almost always abnormal, and values below 40 mg/dl are invariably abnormal. Hyperglycemia elevates the CSF glucose, and its presence may mask a depressed CSF level; thus, a CSF glucose of 60 mg/dl may represent a pathologically low level in the presence of a sustained blood glucose level of 200 mg/dl. The CSF/blood glucose ratio falls below 0.6 with progressive increases in the blood glucose level. The mechanism of this fall in ratio depends upon the kinetics of glucose transfer between blood and CSF.

Membrane Transport of Glucose

It is well established that the transfer of glucose into the CSF and brain from the blood depends upon facilitated diffusion (Fishman, 1964; Crone, 1965; Siesjo, 1978). Carrier-facilitated diffusion assumes that a lipid insoluble compound such as glucose crosses cellular membranes by combining with a mobile component of the membrane, a membrane carrier which shuttles glucose across the membrane. This mechanism, with its characteristic features (saturation kinetics, stereospecificity, bidirectionality, competitive inhibition, and counterflow), is an equilibrating system and is not dependent on active transport.

Active transport is characterized by energy dependence and usually by movement of the solute against a concentration difference, which has not been demonstrated to occur in blood-CSF transfers of hexoses. There is substantial evidence that transfer of glucose across the capillary endothelium, the choroid plexus, and the cell membranes of neurons and glia is dependent upon specific membrane carrier transport systems (Betz *et al.*, 1979). Siesjo (1978) has provided a thoughtful analysis of the abundant literature that supports this generalization.

The CSF/Blood Glucose Ratio

Several mechanisms are responsible for the maintenance of the normal CSF/blood glucose ratio of about 0.6. A steady-state ratio of less than 1.0 indicates that the net rate of entry of glucose into CSF is less than the net rate of removal of glucose from CSF. There are two mechanisms for the entry of glucose into CSF from plasma across the multiple membranes of the barrier: (1) carrier-facilitated diffusion and (2) simple diffusion. The former is quantitatively much more important; the rate of facilitated diffusion is many times faster than that of simple diffusion at normal blood levels.

There are two major mechanisms for the removal of glucose from CSF: (1) bulk flow of CSF into the venous system, which is a minor factor in maintenance of a CSF/plasma glucose ratio of less than 1.0 and (2) glucose utilization by arachnoidal, ependymal, neuronal, and glial elements close to the CSF. The quantitative role of glucose utilization by each of these cellular elements in maintaining the CSF/blood ratio is not known, but together they determine the normal distribution ratio of 0.6. The concentration of glucose in brain is about 20 mg/dl (Seisjo, 1978); thus, normally the brain serves as a sink for the blood glucose of 100 mg/dl and the CSF glucose of 60 mg/dl.

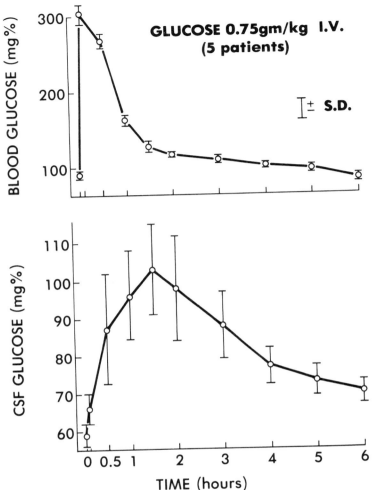

Figure 6-5   The response of the CSF glucose to acute hyperglycemia in five patients. Five minutes after the intravenous injection of 50 per cent glucose, 0.75 gm/kg, the average venous glucose was 300 mg/dl; it approached the average control level 2 to 3 hours thereafter. The lumbar CSF glucose rose slowly, a minor increase was detected 5 minutes after the injection, and peak levels were observed after 90 to 120 minutes. Control levels were not approached for 4 to 6 hours after the injection. (Data previously published in part, Fishman, 1963.)

Dependency upon the Blood Glucose

Changes in the blood glucose level are reflected in parallel changes in the CSF glucose level. A variable time is required before the CSF glucose reaches a steady-state equilibrium with the blood glucose. Thus, the CSF glucose level will not reach a maximum for about two hours after rapid intravenous injections of 50 ml of 50 per cent glucose, and it does not reach equilibrium for about four hours. Figure 6–5 illustrates this response in 5 adult subjects (Fishman, 1963). There is probably a similar delay in the lowering of the spinal fluid glucose level in response to insulin-induced hypoglycemia, although such data on humans are lacking. With a sudden drop in the blood glucose level following intravenous administration of insulin, the CSF glucose level may exceed the blood level for a brief time. Thus, the CSF glucose level at any moment is a complex function of the blood glucose level during the previous four hours. *Therefore, when the CSF glucose is of great diagnostic importance, CSF and blood glucose levels should be obtained simultaneously, with the patient in a fasting state of at least four hours.*

Glucose Concentrations at Different Levels

The glucose content of the ventricular fluid is usually higher than that of the cisternal fluid, and the latter is slightly higher than that of the lumbar fluid. Merritt and Fremont-Smith (1938) described the ventricular and lumbar fluid glucose levels drawn simultaneously from 16 patients without meningitis. The ventricular fluid concentration was between 6 and 18 mg greater than the lumbar level in 13 patients, but it is not clear whether these patients were in a steady-state. (The changes induced by meningitis in the glucose levels of fluid from different levels of the spine will be discussed in Chapter 7.) p260

Glucose enters the CSF via the choroid plexus as well as by transcapillary movement into the extracellular fluid space of the brain and cord, which is contiguous with the CSF. It does not enter the CSF solely in the ventricles, as evidenced by the rapid rise in the glucose level above and below a ligature placed about the thoracic cord following intravenous injections of glucose. Riser and Mériel (1927) experimentally demonstrated similar increases in the cisternal and lumbar fluid levels in dogs as well as in patients with a complete thoracic block due to cord tumor. However, Merritt and Fremont-Smith (1938) reported that the glucose in cisternal fluid was increased to a much higher level than that of the lumbar fluid after an oral glucose load administered to patients without spinal subarachnoid block. (The time course of these changes was not described.) Despite these somewhat divergent reports, it is reasonable to conclude that glucose enters the extracellular fluid of the brain and spinal cord by carrier-mediated transport, and thus it freely equilibrates with the CSF along the neuraxis.

Increased CSF Glucose Levels

An increase in CSF glucose is of no diagnostic significance apart from reflecting the presence of hyperglycemia within the four hours before lumbar puncture. The CSF glucose is relatively increased in both premature infants and the newborn, in whom the CSF/plasma ratio of glucose is 0.8 or greater (Sarff *et al.*, 1976). The explanation for the ratio approaching unity in the neonatal period is not clear; it may reflect the normally greater permeability of the blood-brain barrier at this age to macromolecules. Another factor is the much greater rate of cerebral blood flow in infancy, when it is about 100 ml per 100 gm per minute (Kennedy and Sokoloff, 1957).

With increasing blood glucose levels, the CSF glucose level is secondarily elevated, but to a lesser degree than the blood glucose level. This decrease in the CSF/blood ratio is a reflection of the saturation kinetics that characterizes carrier-facilitated transport at high substrate concentrations. Thus, the CSF/blood ratio falls to about 0.5 with a blood glucose of 500 mg/dl and to about 0.4 with a blood glucose level of 700 mg/dl. There are insufficient data to be more specific, but the ratios given reflect my clinical experience and isolated case reports in the literature. The observation is clinically relevant because hyperglycemia may mask meningitis. For instance, a CSF level of 70 mg/dl would be considered abnormally low in the presence of a blood glucose of 250 mg/dl if the blood level had been elevated to such concentrations for two hours.

Decreased CSF Glucose Levels

The CSF glucose level may be abnormally low (hypoglycorrhachia) in several diseases of the nervous system as well as with hypoglycemia, as indicated in Table 6–11. Thus, the CSF glucose level is characteristically decreased in acute purulent meningitis; levels below 5 mg/dl (approaching the detection limits of the analytic method) are not uncommon. Low levels, generally ranging between 20 and 40 mg/dl, are also seen in tuberculous meningitis and in the various fungal meningitides such as torulosis and coccidioidomycosis (see Chapter 7). A similarly low spinal fluid glucose level is also characteristic of diffuse meningeal neoplasia (carcinomatous meningitis), in which sheets of neoplastic cells infiltrate the meninges. The tumor cells may be visible only microscopically at postmortem examination. Tumors repsonsible for this syndrome include the various gliomas, sarcoma, lymphoma, meningeal leukemia, melanoma, and metastatic carcinoma from the lung, breast, gut, and elsewhere (Olson *et al.*, 1974). Most frequently the protein level is elevated, and there is a mild pleocytosis, suggesting an inflammatory process, as well as malignant cells. Rarely, the CSF may have a normal protein level and total cell count despite the presence of malignant cells and a low glucose level. A reduced CSF glucose level is commonly noted in sarcoidosis involving the meninges and in other diffuse granulomatous infiltrations of the meninges, including cysticercosis. Similarly, a

TABLE 6–11   Low CSF Glucose Syndromes

Acute purulent meningitis
Tuberculous meningitis
Fungal meningitis
Meningeal sarcoidosis
Carcinomatous meningitis (diffuse meningeal neoplasia)
Primary amebic meningitis (*Naegleria*)
Meningeal cysticercosis
Meningeal trichinosis
Acute syphilitic meningitis
Chemical meningitis (following intrathecal therapy)
Subarachnoid hemorrhage
Viral meningitis—glucose is usually normal.
    Exceptions: mumps meningitis (25% cases), herpes simplex and herpes zoster
    (occasionally reduced)
Hypoglycemia
Rheumatoid meningitis
Lupus myelopathy

low CSF glucose level may rarely occur in neurosyphilis, specifically in acute syphilitic meningitis and in general paresis (Merritt *et al.*, 1946).

Although the CSF glucose level is usually normal in most cases of viral meningitis, a low level occurs in 25 per cent of patients with acute mumps meningoencephalitis (Wilfert, 1969) and in some patients with herpes simplex encephalitis (Sarubbi *et al.*, 1973). The CSF glucose level may remain depressed for one to two weeks following adequate treatment of bacterial meningitis, at a time when the pleocytosis and protein have returned to essentially normal levels (Swartz and Dodge, 1965).

A low CSF glucose level may also be noted in bloody spinal fluid due to subarachnoid hemorrhage, however caused. The precise incidence of this finding is not established, because often the CSF glucose has not been systematically analyzed in patients with obvious subarachnoid hemorrhage. Merritt and Fremont-Smith (1938) reported that 7 of 199 patients with cerebral hemorrhage had a CSF glucose level below 30 mg/dl and that 15 per cent of these cases had a glucose level below 50 mg/dl. In a small group of patients, Troost *et al.* (1968) observed that the low CSF glucose levels occurred most frequently four to eight days after the hemorrhage. Sambrook *et al.* (1973) studied the CSF glucose during the first ten days after subarachnoid hemorrhage or stroke, reporting a glucose level below 40 mg/dl in 4 of 24 patients with subarachnoid hemorrhage. The maximum fall occurred between the first and the sixth day, and it appeared to depend upon the extent of rebleeding. No other specific changes were noted in the CSF glucose level in subarachnoid hemorrhage or stroke.

A low CSF glucose level has also been noted with transient meningeal reactions to the intraspinal injection of radioiodinated serum albumin (Barnes and Fish, 1972) and with the chemical meningitis induced by Pantopaque myelography (Wishler, 1978). In these cases of transient chemical meningitis, cultures for bacterial contamination have been negative.

The Mechanism of Decreased Glucose Levels

Several factors play a role in the pathogenesis of decreased CSF glucose levels, including the rate of glucose utilization and the rate of glucose entry. The reduction of CSF glucose concentration in purulent meningitis reflects, in part, increased glycolysis by polymorphonuclear leukocytes, particularly when these cells are in a state of active phagocytosis (Petersdorf and Harter, 1961). In these cases, the low glucose level is associated with an increased CSF lactate level. However, the increase in granulocytes is often small; the cells often are insufficient to account for the depression in light of the constant supply of glucose from the circulation. Bacteria also utilize glucose; however, quantitative studies of the glycolytic rates of bacteria *in vitro* and *in vivo* strongly suggest that there are insufficient bacteria in meningitis to be a major factor (Goldring and Harford, 1950; Baltch and Osborne, 1957). *In vitro* studies of glucose utilization by bacteria and leukocytes are very limited analogs of *in vivo* circumstances, because they do not allow for the rapid entry of glucose into the CSF made possible by the cerebral circulation. An increased CSF lactate concentration probably always occurs with a low CSF glucose level from any cause except hypoglycemia, reflecting increased anaerobic glycolysis by cellular elements close to the CSF.

Evidence in support of the induction of a low CSF glucose level by granulocytes was obtained by Petersdorf and Harter (1961). They showed that irradiated leukopenic dogs did not respond to pneumococcal meningitis with a pleocytosis, nor did depression of the glucose level occur. This does not necessarily mean that granulocytes utilize the glucose sufficiently to depress its concentration. Rather, a key factor might be the effects of granulocytic membranes *per se* on brain metabolism; pus has been shown to increase glycolysis by the cerebral cortex, studied *in vitro* (Fishman *et al.*, 1977). The failure to depress the CSF glucose level in leukopenic dogs may have been due to the absence of pus.

The early work of Sifontes *et al.* (1953) showed inhibition of the entry of glucose into the CSF of children with tuberculous meningitis, following intravenous loads. A similar study in patients with diffuse meningeal carcinomatosis also suggested that the low CSF glucose levels in this disease were also related to impaired membrane transfer of glucose (Fishman, 1964). Studies of experimental pneumococcal meningitis in dogs showed that the facilitated membrane transport of glucose (measured with a nonmetabolized glucose analog, 3-O-methyl glucose) was inhibited bidirectionally (Prockop and Fishman, 1968). However, we concluded that inhibition of carrier transport was not an important factor in the pathogenesis of low CSF glucose levels in our laboratory model of pneumococcal meningitis; meningitis caused a noncarrier-dependent increase in glucose entry via simple diffusion which was greater than the inhibition of carrier transport, resulting in a net increase in glucose entry. It is noteworthy that inhibition of the glucose carrier mechanism was demonstrated; it is possible that such inhibition may operate in other forms of hypoglycorrhachia in which barrier permeability is less affected and polymorphonuclear responses are minimal, such as the various forms of chronic meningitis described earlier.

Carrier inhibition may also be important when a persistent lowering of CSF glucose occurs following treatment of bacterial meningitis. Occasionally, such patients recovering from purulent meningitis have a fluid with a minimal pleocytosis, negative cultures, and a normal lactate concentration which suggests that glycolysis is normal.

In summary, the major factors responsible for a low CSF glucose level in meningeal disorders include (1) increased glucose utilization due to an increase in anaerobic glycolysis, chiefly in adjacent brain and spinal cord, and to a lesser degree by polymorphonuclear leukocytes; and (2) inhibition of the entry of glucose due to alterations in the membrane carrier system responsible for the transfer of glucose from blood to CSF. The importance of increased glucose utilization is supported by the increase in CSF lactate content which is characteristically found with a low glucose level. While inhibition of glucose transport in meningitis might be of importance, this remains a largely hypothetical issue, despite the experimental demonstration of such inhibition (Fishman, 1964; Prockop and Fishman, 1968; Cooper *et al.*, 1968). Lastly, a low CSF glucose level in the absence of hypoglycemia indicates the presence of a *diffuse,* generalized meningeal disorder, but may be present below a spinal block due to neoplasm. It does *not* occur with localized meningitis or cerebritis.

Fructose Levels in CSF

The concentration of fructose in biological fluids is very low. Plasma levels were less than 2.0 mg/dl in 29 of 40 patients, and between 2.2 and 4.6 mg/dl in the others. Curiously, the concentration in lumbar CSF is higher than in plasma; it ranged from 1.8 to 13 mg/dl in 39 of 40 patients (Wray and Winegrad, 1966). The mechanism underlying this concentration difference is not known. Fructose given intravenously has limited entry into the CSF, presumably because it enters only by simple diffusion; fructose apparently has no affinity for the carrier transport system for sugars across the choroid plexus or capillary endothelial cells. It seems likely that fructose is an end product of brain metabolism. Wray and Winegrad (1966) found that there was a close correlation between the glucose and fructose concentrations. They suggested that the increased CSF levels of fructose in diabetes are derived from the brain (see Polyols, page 250).

Sodium

The sodium ion is the major cation present in the plasma and CSF. While the normal range of concentrations in both fluids is about the same, varying between 133 and 145 meq per l, the absolute concentration is slightly greater in plasma than in CSF when the difference in water content of the two fluids is taken into account, that is, when the data are expressed in milliequivalents per kilogram of plasma water and CSF water. Plasma is about 92 per cent water and CSF is 99 per cent water; hence a sodium level of 140 meq per l in each body fluid actually represents a concentration in plasma of 152 meq per l plasma water and in CSF of 141 meq per l CSF water; thus, the CSF/plasma concentration ratio is about 0.93.

There is an extensive literature, reviewed by Davson (1966) and Katzman and Pappius (1973), regarding the effect of the Donnan equilibrium upon the distribution of sodium between both fluids. The Donnan equilibrium describes the effect of proteins, which are negatively charged, upon the distribution of ions across a semipermeable membrane. These authors also reviewed the theoretical effects of the small steady-state difference in the electrical potential between the CSF and blood (the CSF is about 5 mv positive to the blood), upon the distribution of sodium. Thus, according to Katzman and Pappius (1973), theoretically the plasma sodium concentration should exceed the CSF sodium concentration between 6 and 17 per cent because of the Donnan effect and the difference in electrical potential. The fact that such differences in sodium concentration between the two compartments are *not* found indicates that active secretory processes help maintain the concentration of sodium in CSF. The latter is modified also by osmotic forces that are responsible for the maintenance of equal osmolalities in both fluids and by the ready transfer of water between the two fluids.

Current concepts of the mechanism of CSF formation, reviewed in Chapter 3, indicate that the rate of CSF formation is determined by the rate of sodium transfer across the choroid plexus and by the addition of sodium and water by transcapillary exchange within the brain's extracellular fluid space (extrachoroidal CSF formation). Both the rate of CSF formation and the rate of radioactive sodium entry are relatively constant in the face of many physiological and pharmacological manipulations. However, the concentration of sodium in CSF does change, paralleling alterations in the plasma level. In dogs, the half-time for radiosodium to reach equilibrium in the CSF was about 2 hours (Fishman, 1959). In cats, there was a time lag of only about 60 minutes for the CSF sodium level to reach a maximum after an acute elevation of the plasma sodium level (Pape and Katzman, 1970). The rapid equilibration of sodium between the two compartments seen experimentally is also observed in humans. Parallel changes in CSF sodium concentration are also the rule in hyponatremia and hypernatremia, although the precise time course is not known.

CSF Sodium in Disease

In hyponatremia and hypernatremia, the CSF sodium level changes in the same direction as the plasma level, but the CSF changes are often lesser in degree. The mechanism of this modulation is not entirely clear. In most reports, the plasma and CSF osmolalities have not been given, nor has it been clear whether a patient may have been in a new steady-state such as that observed in chronic states of asymptomatic hyponatremia or hypernatremia. Presumably, in the adapted (asymptomatic) state the concentration difference between plasma and CSF is minimal. Representative changes reported in the literature are given in Table 6–12. Little information is to be gained from the measurement of the CSF sodium in clinical practice. In the face of marked hyponatremia or hypernatremia, the physician may assume that the CSF sodium level will follow the plasma level, unless the plasma level is changing so rapidly that there might be a lag of some hours before a new equilibrium is reached.

Potassium

The concentration of potassium in CSF is very stable. The normal mean value is 2.88 ± 0.15 meq/l in the presence of a normal serum potassium of 4.5

TABLE 6–12   Sodium Levels in CSF and Plasma

	N*	CSF	PLASMA	REFERENCE
		$mEq/l \pm SD$†		
Controls	23	147 ± 3	138 ± 3	Bradbury et al., 1963
	20	141 ± 6	141 ± 7	Cooper et al., 1955
	13	145 ± 3	140 ± 4	Salminen et al., 1962
	40	142 ± 3	138 ± 3	Sambrook et al., 1973
Hypernatremia	3	158–179	164–185	Cooper et al., 1955
Hyponatremia	1	119	116	Cooper et al., 1955
Tuberculous meningitis	5	165 ± 3	132 ± 5	Cooper et al., 1955
	5	140 ± 4	135 ± 4	Bradbury et al., 1963
Uremia	5	138 ± 5	146 ± 5	Salminen et al., 1962
Cirrhosis	5	136 ± 5	145 ± 5	Salminen et al., 1962
Acute cerebral infarction	10	143 ± 8	146 ± 9	Cooper et al., 1955
Subarachnoid hemorrhage	24	142 ± 6	138 ± 4	Sambrook et al., 1973

*N: number of subjects.
†The values have been expressed to the nearest whole number.

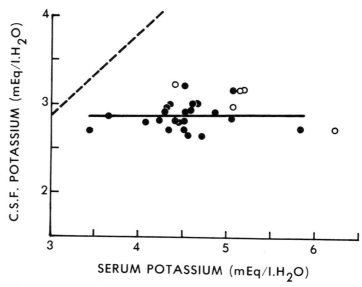

Figure 6-6 Stability of the CSF potassium. The relation of lumbar CSF potassium to serum potassium for subjects with normal "barriers" (solid circle) and subjects with acute tuberculous meningitis (hollow circle). The solid line is the regression line for those with normal barriers; the interrupted line indicates the theoretical ratio between the two compartments if the CSF was a plasma dialysate (from Bradbury *et al.*, 1963).

meq/l. The CSF potassium is little affected by changes in the plasma level. The CSF has a normal range of 2.7 to 3.9 meq/l, despite plasma levels that vary between 3.4 and 5.8 meq/l (Bradbury *et al.*, 1963). These data are illustrated in Figure 6–6. Such degrees of hypokalemia and hyperkalemia would be sufficient to cause characteristic changes in the electrocardiogram. The CSF potassium has been studied in various neurological disorders, including tuberculous meningitis, brain tumor, uremia, and cirrhosis; no significant changes have been reported (Salminen *et al.*, 1962; Katzman and Pappius, 1973).

It is noteworthy that subarachnoid hemorrhage, which results in hemolysis of red cells with the release of potassium into the CSF, does not result in an increase in CSF potassium level. This finding illustrates the presence of a highly efficient system for removing potassium from the CSF. In fact, Sambrook *et al.* (1973) showed that subarachnoid hemorrhage actually resulted in a slight but significant *decrease* in CSF potassium over the first five to ten days to levels as low as 2.1 meq/l. This decrease appeared to correlate with the occurrence of drowsiness and mental confusion. This unexpected observation suggests that the chemical meningitis initiated by blood in the subarachnoid space activates cellular mechanisms that facilitate the removal of potassium, presumably by glial and endothelial cells (Goldstein *et al.*, 1979).

Most of these patients also had low CSF glucose levels, which suggests that increased glycolysis by cellular elements in close proximity to the CSF might play a role in an intracellular shift of potassium. These workers also described elevation of the CSF potassium to levels as high as 4.5 meq/l in a few patients with cerebral infarction. Presumably, in these patients, sufficient potassium was released into the CSF from infarcted tissue to exceed the cellular transport systems which remove potassium from the CSF.

The CSF has a low potassium content compared with that of the plasma and particularly compared with the intracellular concentration of potassium in brain, which is about 100 meq/l. It is of special interest that the CSF potassium rises rapidly after death (Fraschini *et al.*, 1963; Paulson and Stickney, 1971). Naumann (1958) studied the postmortem changes in cisternal fluid potassium in 157 subjects. The CSF level ranged between 5.6 and 40 meq/l, and the degree of elevation correlated roughly with the time interval after death. The mean level was 21 meq/l when autopsy was performed an average of 10.5 hours after death. The striking elevation in CSF potassium after death is considered to be a consequence of the depletion of tissue ATP and failure of the ion pump, sodium-potassium activated ATPase.

Potassium ions alter brain excitability by their depolarizing effects on cellular membranes. Bourke *et al.* (1972, 1979) also demonstrated that high extracellular potassium causes astroglial swelling. Teleologically, there is a clear need to protect the CSF and the extracellular fluid from changes in concentration of this cation. The mechanism underlying the fine control of the CSF potassium has been extensively studied in laboratory animals. Experimentally, when the serum potassium is acutely lowered by the administration of glucose and insulin, there is a slight reduction in the CSF potassium (Bekaert and Demeester, 1954). It is noteworthy that Ames *et al.* (1965) showed a slight gradient in the potassium concentration at different loci in the CSF of cats. Thus, it was slightly higher in choroid plexus fluid than in the cortical subarachnoid space. This indicates that although newly formed CSF has a low potassium level, there are mechanisms for the removal of additional potassium as it moves through the CSF pathways. The experimental elevation of the plasma potassium to levels as high as 10 meq/l was sufficient to cause fatal cardiac arrest without changing the cisternal fluid level (Bekaert and Demeester, 1954).

The work of Ames *et al.* (1965) showed that the active transport systems of the choroid plexus play an important role in limiting the concentration of potassium in newly formed CSF. The enzyme sodium-potassium activated ATPase, which is inhibited by cardiac glycosides, is considered to be of key importance in this process. However, as noted earlier, there are cellular mechanisms in brain other than those in the choroid plexus that maintain very low levels of potassium in the brain's extracellular fluid. Electrophysiological studies of the cortex with potassium-sensitive electrodes suggest that glial cells serve as a sink for the potassium released into the extracellular fluid (Katzman, 1976). It also seems certain that there is a transport system, apart from the choroid plexus, capable of moving potassium from the CSF and extracellular fluid into the blood. *In vitro* data indicate that the capillary endothelial cells of the brain have this key function (Goldstein, 1979).

Calcium

The normal values obtained in several published series for the calcium levels in CSF and plasma are given in Table 6–13. The CSF calcium levels have varied between 2 and 3 meq per 1 and the total serum levels between 4 and 5 meq per 1.

TABLE 6–13   Normal CSF and Serum Calcium Levels

N*	CSF mEq/l (±SD)	SERUM mEq/l (±SD)	REFERENCE
45	3.01 ± 0.08	5.38 ± 0.95	McCance and Watchhorn (1931)
49	2.48 ± 0.01	4.99 ± 0.02	Merritt and Bauer (1931)
51	2.65 ± 0.07	4.72 ± 0.03	Herbert (1934)
68	2.22 ± 0.19	–	Decker et al. (1964)
16	2.11 ± 0.07	4.77 ± 0.07	Woodbury et al. (1968)

*N: number of subjects.

The more recent reports of Decker *et al.* (1964) and Woodbury *et al.* (1968) provide somewhat lower normal values than does the earlier literature. This probably reflects methodological differences, such as the recent use of atomic absorption spectroscopy.

Calcium is present in serum in at least two forms. About one-third to one-half is bound to albumin, and the balance is the ionized, diffusible fraction. While the concentration of calcium in CSF roughly approximates the diffusible fraction in serum, published experiments indicate that the ionized fraction in serum is somewhat greater than the CSF level. In addition, Merritt and Bauer (1931) showed that the CSF calcium level was independent of the serum protein level. These observations, plus the evidence that the CSF calcium is little or not at all affected by hypoparathyroidectomy, infusion of calcium salts, or parathormone, or by changing the ionizable serum calcium with EDTA, support the conclusion that the CSF calcium level is determined by a secretory process. It does *not* simply represent the diffusible or ionized calcium present in the serum (Katzman and Pappius, 1973, Goldstein *et al.*, 1979).

Studies of the kinetics of radiocalcium exchange between blood and CSF using ventriculo-cisternal perfusion have also indicated that calcium entry into CSF is dependent largely upon an active or carrier-mediated transport process and somewhat upon passive diffusion (Oppelt *et al.*, 1963; Graziani *et al.*, 1965, 1967). While the addition of ouabain to the ventricular fluid inhibits both CSF formation and calcium influx at the choroid plexus, it is also likely that calcium entry into the CSF and extracellular fluid depends upon carrier-mediated transport systems in capillary endothelial cells of the brain and spinal cord. The concentration of calcium is uniform in the ventricles and lumbar sac in humans, although in dogs and monkeys the lumbar levels are slightly higher.

The effects of parathormone on the CSF calcium are complex (Katzman and Pappius, 1973). Experimentally, parathormone appears not to be essential for the maintenance of the normal CSF calcium level when the serum calcium level is normal, but it does have an effect at very low serum calcium levels. It is noteworthy that hyperparathyroidism is a cause of the syndrome of benign intracranial hypertension, whose pathophysiology is not known. An animal model of this syndrome, which might help to clarify the mechanisms involved, has not been reported.

The CSF calcium is not affected by diseases of the nervous system, although it must be added that there are limited published data about this point. Thus, no changes have been reported in epilepsy, parkinsonism, or cerebrovascular disease, or in purulent meningitis despite a major increase in the CSF protein. There are isolated reports of a slight decrease in CSF calcium levels secondary to severe hypocalcemia (McQuarrie *et al.*, 1941). The calcium level is even maintained in CSF post mortem, unlike the potassium and magnesium concentrations, which increase rapidly after death (Naumann, 1958). This reflects the relatively low calcium content of brain cells and the fact that this cation is tightly bound to intracellular structural elements. Thus, there appears to be little basis for measuring the CSF calcium level in clinical practice. The recent report of Jimerson *et al.* (1979) that the CSF calcium level falls very slightly during mania is open to question regarding its specificity or significance.

Phosphorus

An extensive early literature regarding the inorganic phosphorus (largely phosphate) present in CSF in various neurological diseases was summarized by Friedman and Levinson (1955). The concentration of inorganic phosphorus in normal CSF averaged about 60 per cent of the serum level. The normal range in the CSF varied between 1.2 and 2.0 mg/dl with an average of 1.6 mg/dl, compared to an average serum level of about 4.0 mg/dl. The phosphorus content of the CSF was unaffected by large increases in the serum level. Even with a serum phosphorus level as high as 7.0 mg/dl, a normal CSF phosphorus level was observed. There were no specific relationships between the CSF level and neurological disease. However, there was a definite relationship between the inorganic phosphorus level and the CSF protein concentration. Thus, as the CSF protein became progressively higher, the CSF phosphorus level was increased in meningitis, polyneuritis, and brain tumor, reflecting the increased permeability of the barrier to serum proteins in these conditions. The highest CSF phosphorus level observed was 4.4 mg/dl in a patient with tuberculous meningitis. Recent studies by Goldstein *et al.* (1979) confirmed the stability of the CSF phosphorus level in the face of changing serum levels.

An old literature dealt with the effects of CSF phosphate in the genesis of uremic twitches (Harrison *et al.*, 1936; Harrison and Mason, 1937). Thus, the intracisternal injection of phosphate induced twitches in dogs. Although Freeman *et al.* (1962) observed in 17 patients with uremia that the CSF to serum phosphate ratio was not altered, 5 patients with twitching had CSF phosphate levels greater than 3.8 mg/dl. However, some patients with uremic twitches had normal serum and CSF phosphate levels (Harrison *et al.*, 1936). The role of the CSF phosphate and its relationship to calcium metabolism in the genesis of the uremic syndrome need further study (Arieff and Massry, 1974).

Magnesium

There has been considerable interest in the magnesium level, because it is the sole cation whose concentration in CSF is substantially greater than that in serum (Cohen, 1927). The values obtained in several different series, using a variety of methods, demonstrate that the CSF level is about 30 per cent greater than the serum level (see Table 6–14). The CSF level usually lies between 2.0 and 2.5 meq/l and the serum level between 1.5 and 2.0 meq/l. Moreover, about

TABLE 6–14   Normal CSF and Serum Magnesium Levels

N*	CSF mEq/l (±SD)	SERUM mEq/l (±SD)	REFERENCE
10	2.43 ± 0.05	1.95 ± 0.15	Stutzman and Amatuzio (1952)
10	2.57 ± 0.11	1.98 ± 0.05	Harris and Sonnenblick (1955)
20	2.35 ± 0.20	1.49 ± 0.09	Friedman and Rubin (1955)
38	2.24 ± 0.01	1.62 ± 0.07	Hunter and Smith (1960)
67	1.93 ± 0.03	1.52 ± 0.04	Pallis *et al.* (1965)
11	2.24 ± 0.10	1.67 ± 0.14	Woodbury *et al.* (1968)
122	2.29 ± 0.10	1.75 ± 0.20	Heipertz *et al.* (1979)

*N: number of subjects

one third of the serum level is bound to the serum protein, and thus the concentration difference of the diffusible or ionized fraction between both compartments is even greater. The small electrical potential difference between the CSF and blood (CSF is 5 mv positive) would favor a lower concentration of magnesium in CSF. Thus, despite the electrochemical potential and the effect of binding magnesium to serum proteins, the CSF magnesium is maintained at a higher level. This illustrates the importance of active transport mechanisms in maintaining the concentration difference (Katzman and Pappius, 1973). Newly formed choroidal CSF has a somewhat higher magnesium level than lumbar CSF, and while it is likely than an ATP-dependent active transport is involved, only limited pertinent data are available.

The relative constancy of the CSF magnesium level despite major changes in the plasma level has been observed by many investigators. Thus, an acute elevation of the serum content by intravenous infusion of magnesium sulfate to serum levels as high as 700 per cent of the control level, given over several hours, increased the CSF level by only 20 per cent (Kemeny *et al.*, 1972). Similarly, a reduction in the serum level to very low levels, obtained with a magnesium-free diet, failed to reduce the CSF level or induced only a minor drop (Chutkow and Meyers, 1968). Thus, there are potent homeostatic mechanisms for maintaining the CSF level within narrow limits. Although there is an active transport system for magnesium in the choroid plexus, it seems likely that the control mechanism involves cellular elements throughout the central nervous system, presumably including capillary endothelial cells as well as glial cells. It is noteworthy that the CSF magnesium level, like that of potassium, increases rapidly after death as energy-dependent transport systems fail to maintain magnesium within brain cells (Naumann, 1958).

Both hypermagnesemia and hypomagnesemia, when severe, have profound neurological effects, such as hypermagnesemic paralysis and hypomagnesemic seizures (Fishman, 1965). The striking modulating effects of the magnesium ion on brain excitability indicate the need for maintenance and control of the magnesium level in CSF and in the brain's extracellular fluid. The cellular mechanisms involved are not understood, and they require further elucidation.

The CSF magnesium level is unchanged in a wide variety of neurological disorders. One exception is severe purulent meningitis, in which the CSF level is decreased nearly to the serum level (Cohen, 1927). There are a few reports of severe hypomagnesemia wherein the CSF level was slightly decreased, in patients with cirrhosis, alcoholism, and various forms of meningitis (Woodbury *et al.*, 1968). However, no consistent relationship was observed between the serum and CSF levels, nor was any diagnostic specificity established.

Chloride

An early interest in the CSF chloride was initiated by the observations that it served as the major anion of CSF and that its concentration exceeded the plasma level (Mestrezat, 1912). Another reason was that convenient laboratory methods for measuring chloride were available long before the introduction of the routine measurement of sodium or potassium levels in body fluids. (Until the introduction of the flame photometer in the late 1940's for the determination of sodium and potassium in clinical practice, their measurement was a laborious research procedure in limited use.)

The early method for measuring chloride usually expressed the chloride concentration in terms of mg sodium chloride per 100 ml. When this value is divided by the molecular weight of sodium chloride (58.5), the data are expressed as meq per l, and this conversion is used here in referring to the older literature. Merritt and Fremont-Smith (1938) reported that the CSF level ranged between 120 and 129 meq per l and the serum level between 97 and 113 meq per l. More recently, Sambrook *et al.* (1973) reported the normal CSF range in 40 subjects as 119.1 ± 3.3 meq per l, and the plasma range as 102.1 ± 3.4 meq per l. Thus, the concentration of the CSF chloride is normally 15 to 20 meq greater in CSF than in serum.

There has been some uncertainty as to whether this concentration difference is a result chiefly of the Donnan effect and the electrical potential difference between blood and CSF, or whether active transport of chloride must be invoked to explain the gradient (Davson, 1967; Wright, 1978; Bourke, 1979). The electrical potential between blood and CSF favors a greater concentration of chloride in CSF; the anion would move passively into the CSF because of the electrochemical gradient, although this potential difference alone appears insufficient to account for the total concentration difference. The fact that the CSF chloride level tends to fall whenever the CSF protein is substantially increased reflects a passive mechanism attributable to the Donnan effect. Thus, in patients with a CSF protein level greater than 1000 mg/dl, the usual difference between the CSF and serum chloride of 15 to 20 meq per l falls to about 10 meq per l.

The dependence of the CSF chloride level upon the plasma chloride indicates the passive distribution of chloride between the two fluid compartments. The CSF chloride follows changes in the plasma chloride with hypochloremia and hyperchloremia (Merritt and Fremont-Smith, 1938). This has also been studied experimentally. While the CSF chloride level follows changes in the serum level, the adjustment is not complete, so that the CSF/plasma ratio decreases with a rise in plasma concentration and increases with a fall in the serum chloride level (Bradbury *et al.*, 1963, 1969).

Additional data indicate that the maintenance of the CSF chloride level is not entirely passive. The movement of chloride, studied radioisotopically, appears to be closely coupled to the movement of the sodium ion, which is dependent upon both carbonic anhydrase and sodium-potassium activated ATPase. It has been pointed out by Davson (1967) and by Katzman and Pappius (1973) that secretory activity involving one ion affects the migration of other ions. It may be difficult to determine whether an ion is specifically transported or whether it is passively distributed secondary to secretory activity involving another ion in the system. The rate of entry of radiochloride with the CSF is inhibited by acetazolamide to the same degree as CSF production and the entry of radiosodium. This has been interpreted to reflect the dependence of both sodium and chloride transport upon carbonic anhydrase, although the drug appears not to directly alter choroid plexus secretion of chloride.

The ability of furosemide to inhibit CSF formation (see Chapter 3) is of interest because the drug is considered to act primarily on active chloride transport in the renal tubule. Its effects on sodium transport are probably secondary, although coupled to chloride transport. A similar mechanism in the choroid plexus would help explain the differential effects of the two drugs on choroid plexus. Wright's (1978) extensive studies of anion transport in frog choroid plexus indicate some of the complexities of the regulation of the CSF anion content that are probably analogous to the mechanism in the human. In addition, extrachoroidal mechanisms in brain probably play a role in the regulation of the CSF chloride (Bourke et al., 1979). In summary, it seems likely that the maintenance of a CSF/plasma chloride ratio of about 1.2 depends upon an ion-specific membrane transport system, despite the apparent passive dependency of the CSF chloride level upon the plasma chloride concentration and the CSF protein concentration.

Early workers emphasized that a low CSF chloride was characteristic of tuberculous meningitis (Mestrezat, 1912). Subsequently, it became clear that a low CSF chloride had no diagnostic significance apart from serving to indicate the common occurrence of hypochloremia in such patients (Merritt and Fremont-Smith, 1938). In tuberculous meningitis, hypochloremia was often a reflection of salt depletion due to vomiting, but it also was due in some patients to the then unrecognized syndrome of inappropriate secretion of antidiuretic hormone (ADH). The latter was not defined by Bartter and Schwartz (1967) until many years after Mestrezat's monograph.

To recapitulate, the CSF chloride level is normally 15 to 20 meq higher than the serum level. The CSF chloride level is slightly reduced in the presence of a very elevated CSF protein level. The CSF chloride level follows the serum level in both hyperchloremia and hypochloremia, although the absolute changes in the CSF are usually less than the change in plasma level. The data indicate that there are no indications for the measurement of the CSF chloride in clinical practice.

Acid-Base Balance

There have been extensive studies of CSF acid-base balance in normal subjects and in patients with various systemic disorders. They have been concerned with the control of respiration, the occurrence of metabolic encephalopathy, and the changes associated with head injury, stroke, and meningitis. Laboratory studies involving various species have established the presence of homeostatic mechanisms that favor the maintenance of a relatively constant pH in the CSF and the contiguous extracellular fluid of the brain despite changes in systemic arterial pH. The changes in CSF pH that occur in response to arterial pH changes depend upon the blood-brain barrier (see Chapter 3), which is relatively impermeable to hydrogen and bicarbonate ions, in contrast to the ready transfer of carbon dioxide across its membranes. Another factor that plays an important role in acid-base balance is the hydrogen ion sensitive chemoreceptors of the brain stem respiratory center, which regulate pulmonary ventilation and thus stabilize the pH in response to changes in the CO_2 level. The carbon dioxide-bicarbonate system is the major buffer of the acidity in the CSF, because the proteins present are much too dilute to play a significant role (Siesjo, 1972). There is also evidence for the active transport of bicarbonate from the CSF by glial cells. The cerebral circulation is also very pH-dependent; this serves to regulate the clearance of CO_2 and hydrogen ions from the brain and CSF.

In summary, four factors contribute to the maintenance of a stable CSF pH when there are major alterations in the pH of the arterial blood. These include (a) alterations in respiratory rate; (b) alterations in cerebral blood flow; (c) regulation of CSF bicarbonate concentrations; and (d) possibly, the buffering capability of brain tissue (Brooks et al., 1965; Siesjo, 1972).

In clinical practice, the acid-base parameters of CSF and serum are measured using specific electrodes for pH and pCO_2, and the bicarbonate level is calculated using the Henderson-Hasselbalch equation. The Astrup equilibration technique used to directly measure the CSF pCO_2 must be employed with special care to minimize the number of transfers of the CSF in order to avoid diffusional loss of CO_2 and overestimation of the pH. Such technical factors probably are responsible for some of the variation in reported values.

Normal Subjects

In normal subjects, the pH of CSF is slightly lower than the arterial blood pH, the pCO_2 is higher, and the bicarbonate level is about equal. Cisternal and lumbar fluids obtained at the same time in normal subjects in a steady-state have very similar pH, pCO_2, and bicarbonate levels. However, during rapidly changing conditions, particularly respiratory alkalosis and acidosis, the lumbar CSF is slow to respond whereas the cisternal fluid will more rapidly reflect changes in systemic acid-base parameters (Siesjo, 1972). It is noteworthy that a close similarity in the acid-base characteristics of jugular venous blood and lumbar CSF allows the estimation of CSF pCO_2 from the arterial pCO_2 and the jugular venous pCO_2 tensions. Table 6–15 summarizes the data obtained in various reports of the pH, pCO_2, and bicarbonate values in arterial blood and CSF of normal subjects.

The usual CSF pH of about 7.32 is about 0.08 pH unit lower than the arterial blood level of 7.40; the CSF pCO_2 of about 48 mm Hg is about 8 mm Hg higher than the blood level of 40 mm Hg; the bicarbonate level of about 23 meq per l is about the same in both fluids. The interested reader is referred to the extensive literature on the role of spinal fluid pH in the regulation of respiration (Leusen, 1972; Dempsey et al., 1974).

**TABLE 6–15   Acid-Base Balance in CSF and Arterial Blood
in Normal Subjects**

		pH		CARBON DIOXIDE TENSION (pCO₂ mm Hg)		BICARBONATE (mEq/l)	
REFERENCE	N†	CSF*	Art‡	CSF*	Art‡	CSF*	Art‡
Bradley and							
Semple (1962)	23	7.307	7.397	50.5	41.1	23.3	25.3
	4	7.276 (C)		49.9 (C)		23.7 (C)	
	4	7.279 (L)		49.6 (L)		23.7 (L)	
Manfredi (1962)	15	7.34	7.40	49	42		
Pauli et al. (1962)	10	7.339	7.422	45	35.4	22.5	22.6
Schwab (1962)	15	7.349	7.424	45.2	37.5	23.6	24.9
Buhlman et al. (1963)	12	7.31	7.40	46.5	38.0	22.0	22.8
Fisher and Christianson	6	7.370 (C)	7.435	42.8 (C)	38.9	23.38 (C)	25.34
(1963)		7.370 (L)		42.1 (L)		23.29 (L)	
Severinghaus et al.	4	7.328	7.424	49.4	40.1	24.7	25.9
(1963)							
Mitchell et al. (1965)	12	7.326	7.409	50.2	39.5	21.5	24.8
Posner et al. (1965)	35	7.311	7.414	47.9	38.3	22.9	23.4
Sambrook et al. (1973)	40	7.335	7.410	46.8	40.7	25.8	22.2
Plum and Price (1973)	6	7.328 (C)	7.428	42.9 (C)	38.1	22.1 (C)	24.7
		7.307 (L)		43.8 (L)		21.5 (L)	

*Lumbar CSF except when cisternal (C) and lumbar (L) samples directly compared
†N: number of subjects
‡Art: arterial blood

Acid-Base Balance of Lumbar and Cisternal Fluid

The acid-base balance of lumbar and cisternal fluid is subject to considerable variation. These differences have been noted in normal subjects (see Table 6–15), and they may be magnified during illness or a rapidly changing metabolic or respiratory state. Plum and Price (1973) have studied simultaneously the pH, carbon dioxide tension (pCO₂), and the bicarbonate concentration in CSF from both locations and in arterial and jugular venous blood. A small but consistent difference between the two CSF compartments was noted in normal subjects, with the pH lower (mean difference 0.039 unit) and the pCO₂ higher (mean difference 3.8 mm Hg) in lumbar than in cisternal fluid; the bicarbonate concentrations were equal statistically. The pCO₂ of the cisternal fluid was about 1 mm Hg higher than the mean of the arterial and jugular venous values. The differences in CSF from the two sites were considered to reflect differences in the ratio of local metabolism (hydrogen ion production) to the blood flow removal of metabolites in the two regions. The authors concluded that sampling of lumbar CSF in acutely ill patients may provide *unreliable* information about cerebral acid-base status.

Paradoxical pH Reactions

The blood-brain barrier to carbon dioxide and bicarbonate greatly influences the pH changes in the CSF that occur in response to changes in the pH of the blood. The CSF compartment is rapidly permeable to carbon dioxide and only slowly permeable to changes in the blood bicarbonate levels. This is reflected in the fact that changes in the arterial CO₂ tension (respiratory acidosis and alkalosis) are followed rapidly by a CSF pH that *parallels* the blood pH.

However, the acute responses to changes in the blood bicarbonate concentration (obtained with metabolic acidosis and alkalosis) are more complex and have been termed *paradoxical pH reactions* (Leusen, 1972; Siesjo, 1972). Experimentally, when animals are given intravenous hydrochloric acid, there is actually a transient *increase in* CSF pH before it begins to fall to parallel the decrease in blood pH. This occurs because the intravenous acid causes hyperventilation with loss of CO_2 from both the blood and CSF compartments. The relative preservation of the CSF bicarbonate level thus results in transient CSF alkalosis, despite systemic acidosis. Similarly, the rapid intravenous infusion of sodium hydroxide results in a transient *decrease* in CSF pH before it begins to rise to parallel the increase in blood pH. The intravenous alkali causes hypoventilation and CO_2 retention within the blood and CSF compartments, thereby causing a transient CSF acidosis, despite systemic alkalosis. The paradoxical reactions are transient, lasting no more than a few hours. They are largely laboratory curiosities, with occasional exceptions reported, because in the clinical setting the CSF pH is usually maintained close to normal, despite systemic changes in blood pH due to metabolic or respiratory acidosis or alkalosis.

With sustained derangement of the blood pH, whatever the cause, the CSF pH will be altered in the same direction as that of the blood. The evidence obtained experimentally and in patients shows that homeostatic mechanisms favor stabilization of the pH of the CSF and extracellular fluid. The findings reported in patients with systemic acidosis and alkalosis are summarized in the following sections.

Metabolic Acidosis

The severe systemic acidosis observed in uremia, diabetic ketoacidosis, and methyl alcohol intoxication reportedly depresses the blood pH to levels as low as 7.10 and lower (Posner and Plum, 1967; Fencl *et al.*, 1969; Siesjo, 1972; Plum and Price, 1973). However, the CSF is usually maintained at a level close to its normal pH of 7.32, or is only slightly decreased. There have been occasional reports of a minor pH shift in the alkaline direction, the paradoxical reaction just described.

The published data from several laboratories are summarized in Table 6–16. The stabilization of the CSF pH in the face of systemic acidosis appears to depend, in part, upon a greater decrease in pCO_2 in the CSF than in the blood, which is probably due to the considerable increase in cerebral blood flow induced by acidosis. There is also a smaller decrease in the bicarbonate concentration of the CSF than in the blood; the CSF level is clearly greater than the blood level in each of the series of patients recorded in Table 6–16. The mechanisms underlying the preservation of the CSF bicarbonate are not entirely clear; its occurrence suggests that the active transport of bicarbonate is of key importance in protecting the pH of the CSF. This probably takes place in glial cells and endothelial cells and in the choroid plexus (Maren, 1972; Siesjo, 1978).

Metabolic Alkalosis

The systemic metabolic alkalosis associated with chronic loss of gastric fluid, liver disease, or the chronic ingestion of alkali results in an increase in arterial

TABLE 6–16   Effect of Metabolic Acidosis on Acid-Base Characteristics of Arterial Blood and CSF

Reference	Condition	N*	pH		Carbon Dioxide Tension (pCO₂ mm Hg)		Bicarbonate (mEq/l)	
			CSF	Art†	CSF	Art†	CSF	Art†
Bradley and Semple (1962)	Normal	23	7.307	7.397	50.5	41.1	23.3	25.3
	Metabolic acidosis	5	7.322	7.300	39.8	33.8	19.1	17.0
Pauli et al. (1962)	Normal	10	7.339	7.422	45.0	35.4	22.5	22.6
	Metabolic acidosis	11	7.353	7.298	29.2	22.7	15.1	11.6
Schwab (1962)	Normal	15	7.349	7.424	45.2	37.5	23.6	24.9
	Metabolic acidosis	12	7.372	7.305	34.1	26.9	18.9	13.5
Mitchell and Singer (1965)	Normal	12	7.326	7.409	50.2	39.5	25.1	24.8
	Metabolic acidosis	5	7.319	7.334	38.2	31.1	18.6	16.5
Posner et al. (1965)	Normal	35	7.311	7.414	47.9	38.3	22.9	23.4
	Metabolic acidosis	17	7.276	7.200	25.4	20.3	11.6	8.6
Fencl et al. (1969)	Normal	4	7.279	7.357		46.0	24.0	
	NH₄Cl chronic	3	7.275	7.248		36.8	20.0	
Plum and Price (1973)	Normal	6	7.307	7.428	43.8	38.1	21.5	24.7
	Metabolic acidosis	10	7.264	7.264	31.5	22.0	13.9	10.1

*N: number of subjects
†Art: arterial blood

blood pH from about 7.41 to levels of about 7.52 and higher. However, the CSF pH is little affected, usually rising from its normal level of about 7.32 to about 7.37. The data from several published series are summarized in Table 6–17. Occasionally, the paradoxical pH reaction has been observed, with an actual fall in CSF pH from 7.31 to 7.29 despite an increase in arterial blood pH from 7.40 to 7.44, following the intravenous administration of sodium bicarbonate (Bradley and Semple, 1962). The major factor responsible for the preservation of the CSF pH in the face of systemic metabolic acidosis is the relatively smaller increase of bicarbonate in CSF than in the arterial blood (Siesjo, 1972; Plum and Price, 1973). The cellular basis for this homeostatic mechanism, which probably involves active transport of bicarbonate by glia and endothelial cells, requires further study.

Respiratory Acidosis

Chronic respiratory acidosis occurs in association with chronic obstructive pulmonary disease or paralytic pulmonary insufficiency. The changes in CSF acid-base balance have been studied experimentally and in patients (Bleich et al., 1964; Bulgar et al., 1966; Huang and Lyons, 1966; Fencl et al., 1969; Plum and Price, 1973). The arterial blood pH falls from a normal value of 7.41 to levels of about 7.37, and with severe hypercarbia to levels as low as 7.29, reflecting the greatly increased arterial pCO₂ level. The pH of the CSF falls in parallel fashion, maintaining a pH of about 0.10 unit lower than the arterial pH, similar to the difference seen in normal subjects. The values obtained in several published

TABLE 6–17　Effect of Metabolic Alkalosis on Acid-Base
Characteristics of Blood and CSF

REFERENCE	CONDITION	N*	pH CSF	pH Art†	CARBON DIOXIDE TENSION (pCO₂ mm Hg) CSF	Art†	BICARBONATE (mEq/l) CSF	Art†
Schwab *et al.* (1962)	Normal	15	7.349	7.424	45.2	37.5	23.6	25.2
	Metabolic alkalosis	5	7.380	7.492	44.4	37.1	25.1	29.1
Bradley and Semple (1962)	Normal	11	7.311	7.406	49.4	40.1	22.9	25.2
	NaHCO₃ adm. acute	5	7.299	7.445	49.3	39.5	22.5	27.3
	adm. chronic	6	7.302	7.434	54.8	44.7	25.2	30.2
Mitchell and Singer (1965)	Normal	12	7.326	7.409	50.2	39.5	25.1	24.8
	Metabolic alkalosis	3	7.337	7.523	60.6	48.2	30.6	38.4
Posner *et al.* (1965)	Normal	35	7.311	7.414	47.9	38.3	22.9	23.4
	Metabolic alkalosis	4	7.390	7.542	54.4	42.1	30.5	36.0
Mitchell and Singer (1965)	Normal	1	7.318	7.417	48.7	39.8	24.0	25.3
	NaHCO₃ adm. chronic	1	7.320	7.460	50.4	43.2	24.6	30.3
Plum and Price (1973)	Normal	6	7.307	7.428	43.8	38.1	21.5	24.7
	Metabolic alkalosis	5	7.281	7.497	50.0	40.4	23.0	30.9

*N: number of subjects
†Art: arterial blood

series are listed in Table 6–18. The data illustrate that the changes in pH, pCO_2, and bicarbonate are closely parallel in both compartments. A drop in arterial blood pH to a level of about 7.3 is needed before the CSF pH begins to fall, and similarly the CSF pH is not altered until the arterial pCO_2 is greater than 55 mm Hg (Plum and Price, 1973). Many patients have a variable degree of cerebral hypoxia associated with severe respiratory acidosis. This may aggravate the severity of the acidosis in CSF because of increased concentrations of lactic acid produced secondary to the increased rate of glycolysis induced by hypoxia (Siesjo, 1978).

Respiratory Alkalosis

Respiratory alkalosis may occur as a result of hyperventilation associated with head injury, pregnancy, salicylate poisoning, or liver disease, as well as in normal humans adapting to higher altitudes (Pauli *et al.*, 1962; Severinghaus *et al.*, 1963; Mitchell *et al.*, 1965; Plum and Price, 1973). The arterial blood pH is elevated, often from the normal pH level of 7.41 to levels as high as 7.61. The CSF pH may be unchanged or rise slightly. The findings in several published studies of patients are summarized in Table 6–19. The data include the findings of Severinghaus *et al.* (1963) regarding acclimatization at high altitudes; the CSF pH was little affected, but the CSF bicarbonate and pCO_2 levels fell parallel to the decreases observed in arterial blood pH. Again, these observations indicate that the regulation of CSF pH involves the control of CSF bicarbonate levels, which is dependent upon the active transport of bicarbonate.

TABLE 6–18   Acid-Base Characteristics of Arterial Blood and Lumbar CSF in Respiratory Acidosis

REFERENCE	CONDITION	N*	pH		CARBON DIOXIDE TENSION (pCO$_2$ mm Hg)		BICARBONATE (mEq/l)	
			CSF	Art†	CSF	Art†	CSF	Art†
Schwab (1962)	Normal	15	7.349	7.424	45.2	37.5	23.6	24.9
	Mild respiratory acidosis	7	7.310	7.387	60.0	52.3	28.5	29.3
	Severe respiratory acidosis	9	7.299	7.389	60.8	51.7	28.1	29.0
Buhlman et al. (1963)	Normal	12	7.31	7.40	46.5	38.0	22.0	22.8
	Respiratory acidosis	6	7.22	7.34	70.0	56.0	26.7	29.8
Fisher and Christianson (1963)	Normal	8	7.34	7.41	45.3	38.3	23.2	23.7
	Respiratory acidosis	11	7.28	7.38	68.3	61.7	30.5	34.8
Mitchell et al. (1965)	Normal	12	7.326	7.409	50.2	39.5	25.1	24.8
	Respiratory acidosis	3	7.314	7.382	66.5	49.2	32.0	31.4
Posner et al. (1965)	Normal	35	7.311	7.414	47.9	38.3	22.9	23.4
	Respiratory acidosis	11	7.273	7.374	71.1	67.3	30.9	37.9
Huang and Lyons (1966)	Normocarbia	23	7.343	7.423	47.0	39.5	24.25	24.67
	Hypercarbia	10	7.322	7.377	54.2	47.2	26.65	26.53
	Severe hypercarbia	4	7.214	7.297	84.4	76.2	32.35	35.55
Plum and Price (1973)	Normal	6	7.307	7.428	43.8	38.1	21.5	24.7
	Respiratory acidosis	10	7.241	7.337	78.3	66.3	33.4	34.7

*N: number of subjects
†Art: arterial blood

TABLE 6–19   Acid-Base Characteristics of Arterial Blood and Lumbar CSF in Respiratory Alkalosis

REFERENCE	CONDITION	N*	pH		CARBON DIOXIDE TENSION (pCO$_2$ mm Hg)		BICARBONATE (mEq/l)	
			CSF	Art†	CSF	Art†	CSF	Art†
Schwab (1962)	Normal	15	7.349	7.424	45.2	37.5	23.6	24.9
	Respiratory alkalosis	13	7.338	7.456	45.2	34.3	23.0	24.4
Pauli et al. (1962)	Sea level	10	7.339	7.422	45.0	35.4	22.5	22.6
	3261 m; 1–14 days	4	7.350	7.452	40.4	28.4	20.7	19.6
Severinghaus et al. (1963)	Sea level	4	7.328	7.424	49.4	40.1	24.7	25.9
	3800 m; 2 days	4	7.338	7.485	39.6	31.7	20.4	24.1
	3800 m; 8 days	4	7.336	7.484	39.2	29.2	20.1	22.2
Fisher and Christianson (1963)	Normal	3	7.33	7.44	52.1	42.0	26.3	28.0
	Hyperventilation	3	7.36	7.61	48.8	32.2	25.9	28.1
Mitchell et al. (1965)	Normal	12	7.326	7.409	50.2	39.5	21.5	24.8
	Pregnancy	7	7.336	7.444	41.4	31.1	20.9	21.2
Posner et al. (1965)	Normal	35	7.311	7.414	47.9	38.3	22.9	23.4
	Respiratory alkalosis	16	7.335	7.481	33.3	24.0	16.8	17.6
Huang and Lyons (1966)	Normocarbia	23	7.343	7.423	47.0	39.5	25.74	25.87
	Hypocarbia	17	7.358	7.474	43.0	33.6	24.33	24.60
Plum and Price (1973)	Normal	6	7.307	7.428	43.8	38.1	21.5	24.7
	Respiratory alkalosis	16	7.305	7.528	41.0	27.6	19.7	22.6

*N: number of subjects
†Art: arterial blood

Primary Acidosis of the CSF

Acidosis of the CSF in the presence of normal arterial blood pH has been observed in patients with primary subarachnoid hemorrhage, head injury, cerebral infarction, and purulent meningitis (Sambrook *et al.*, 1973; Bland *et al.*, 1978; Brook *et al.*, 1978). These are examples of *primary* acidosis of the CSF. The acidosis is secondary to metabolic changes involving the cerebrum; such events are reflected in the subarachnoid space, and they occur independently of a change in systemic acid-base balance. Froman and Crampton-Smith (1967) reported a reduction in CSF pH and an increase in the CSF lactate level in patients with subarachnoid hemorrhage. They suggested that hyperventilation in some patients might be due to the CSF acidosis. These workers also suggested that a low CSF glucose level in subarachnoid hemorrhage was indicative of increased rates of glycolysis and lactate production. They concluded that these changes were attributable to the presence of hemolyzed red cells *per se* in the subarachnoid space.

Sambrook *et al.* (1973) also reported primary CSF acidosis in patients with subarachnoid hemorrhage, in whom a pH as low as 7.12 was reported. The acidosis was usually maximal four to six days after the onset, and lactate levels were elevated three to four times above the normal level of 1.55 ± 0.42 mmole per l. While all the patients with CSF acidosis had increased lactate levels, some patients had elevated lactate levels with a normal pH, illustrating the presence of homeostatic mechanisms that maintain a constant CSF pH.

In some patients, even though the red blood cells disappeared from the CSF after three or four days, the CSF lactic acid levels did not return to normal until six to ten days after the subarachnoid hemorrhage. This observation indicates that subarachnoid hemorrhage may have a protracted effect on the metabolism of adjacent cerebral tissue. The chemical meningitis induced by hemolyzed red cells (see discussion of subarachnoid hemorrhage) is associated with inflammatory cells in the leptomeninges that probably also contribute to the increased lactate production. Analogous data have been obtained from purulent CSF; a primary CSF acidosis in association with increased glycolysis and lactic acid production has been documented. The observation that membrane preparations of granulocytes induce increased glycolysis and lactic acid production by brain cortical slices *in vitro* (Fishman *et al.*, 1977) supports the hypothesis that increased glycolysis by the cerebral cortex in patients with meningitis contributes to the persistent lactic acidosis observed in the CSF. There are reports of primary CSF acidosis in patients following convulsive seizures (Brooks and Adams, 1975). This finding also reflects increased cerebral glycolysis.

In summary, studies of acid-base balance in the CSF have elucidated the consequences of systemic acid-base changes and those associated with primary diseases of the nervous system. However, the application of such analyses to clinical practice has proved to be quite limited. First, lumbar CSF analyses do not necessarily accurately reflect the changes that take place in brain (Plum and Price, 1973). Second, and more important, the CSF data, while of interest, do not enter into the decisions of the clinician regarding management as does the direct measurement of arterial blood gases.

Oxygen

There are several reports of oxygen levels in cisternal fluid and lumbar CSF in both normal and pathological conditions. The data indicate that the CSF levels reflect the cerebral tissue oxygen tension *per se* rather than the cerebral arterial oxygen tension, because it is much lower and particularly because inhalation of 5 per cent carbon dioxide in atmospheric air raises cisternal fluid oxygen tension despite the fact that this has no effect on arterial oxygen tension. The increase in cisternal oxygen occurs as a result of increased cerebral blood flow, which is responsible for an increase in brain tissue oxygen. Thus, Jarnum *et al.* (1964) suggested that the cisternal oxygen tension is an expression of the "available oxygen to the brain" and that changes in oxygen tension could reflect changes in cerebral blood flow as well as cerebral metabolism. Rossanda and Gordon (1970) found that the oxygen tension in lumbar CSF in patients without brain lesions was 43.0 ± 10.8 mm Hg. With a normal arterial oxygen tension of 104 mm Hg, the jugular venous blood oxygen tension was usually greater than the lumbar CSF oxygen tension. They noted no significant difference between lumbar and cisternal fluid oxygen tensions, although Ganshirt (1966) reported cisternal fluid oxygen tension to be 6 mm Hg greater than the lumbar fluid tension in normal subjects. There is a paucity of available data regarding CSF oxygen in pathological states, and these findings should be considered only tentative.

Lactic and Pyruvic Acids

There was early interest in the lactic acid content of CSF because its elevation was observed in purulent meningitis (Levinson, 1929). In recent years, there has been a renewed interest in the diagnostic value of an increased CSF lactate level in the identification of purulent meningitis and partially treated bacterial meningitis, in contrast to the usually normal lactate level in viral meningitis (Brook *et al.*, 1978; D'Souza *et al.*, 1978; Kormorowski *et al.*, 1978). An increased CSF lactate level has also been recognized as a characteristic finding in acute cerebral infarction, reflecting the occurrence of tissue acidosis and increased anaerobic glycolysis (Zupping *et al.*, 1971).

The concentration of lactic acid relative to that of pyruvic acid in normal biological fluids is approximately 20 to 1; this ratio depends in part upon the activity of the enzyme lactic dehydrogenase. The lactate/pyruvate ratio reflects the redox state in the brain; there is substantial evidence, well summarized by Siesjo (1978), that whenever cerebral glycolysis is increased (whether from hypoxia, ischemia, seizures or meningitis), the lactate and pyruvate concentrations of brain and CSF, and the lactate/pyruvate ratio, are characteristically increased.

The concentration of lactic acid in brain is dependent directly upon the rate of lactate production in brain. There is substantial evidence in patients and in experimental animals that the blood and CSF lactate concentrations are largely independent of each other (Posner and Plum, 1967). Thus, in dogs, the intravenous infusion of sufficient lactic acid to raise the blood level sixfold failed to increase the CSF concentration. Similarly, an increased CSF lactate level is commonly associated with a normal blood lactate level, which led Posner and Plum (1967) to conclude that the CSF lactate level reflects chiefly the concentration of lactate in brain. There is some variation in the literature regarding normal lactate and pyruvate levels in plasma; this may reflect the failure to rapidly deproteinize blood in order to halt continued lactate production by blood cells. Plasma levels fluctuate with exercise and the postprandial state. There is a slightly greater lactic acid content in normal jugular venous blood than in arterial blood, representing the lactate production of the brain. The lactic acid content of normal lumbar CSF is slightly higher than the arterial and jugular venous blood levels. The normal range of lumbar CSF values in most reports ranges between 10 and 20 mg/dl (1.1 to 2.2 meq or mmole/l), and most patients with purulent meningitis have levels above 35 mg/dl ranging to values above 100 mg/dl (11 mmole/l) (Brook *et al.*, 1978; D'Souza *et al.*, 1978; Kormorowski *et al.*, 1978). Posner and Plum (1967) reported lumbar CSF lactate levels in normal subjects to be 1.58 ± 0.03 meq/l, higher than the arterial blood levels of 0.97 ± 0.13 meq/l.

Zupping *et al.* (1971) studied the CSF and blood lactate and pyruvate levels in control subjects and in patients with cerebral infarction. They reported the normal CSF lactate to be 2.03 ± 0.12 meq/l, higher than the arterial and jugular venous blood lactate levels, which were both 1.81 ± 0.14 meq/l. The CSF pyruvate was 0.079 ± 0.004 meq/l; the jugular venous blood pyruvate was 0.107 ± 0.004 meq/l, the arterial blood pyruvate was 0.109 ± 0.006 meq/l. Thus, in control subjects, the lactate/pyruvate (L/P) ratio was 26 in lumbar CSF, and 17.6 in both arterial and jugular venous blood. These authors found that the CSF lactate and pyruvate were both elevated in brain infarction, with a minor increase in the L/P ratio reflecting brain tissue lactic acidosis.

The CSF lactate levels and L/P ratios in ventricular fluid have been studied by Raisis *et al.* (1975) in patients with communicating and noncommunicating hydrocephalus, before and after a surgical shunt. A drop in the ventricular fluid lactate level and the L/P ratio was observed in postoperative patients who preoperatively had increased intracranial pressure. These investigators concluded that hydrocephalus, when responsible for intracranial hypertension and diminished cerebral perfusion, causes sufficient cerebral ischemia to increase lactate production and to elevate the L/P ratio.

The recent renewed interest in the CSF lactate levels in the diagnosis of meningitis has been fostered by the ready availability of the enzymatic method for its accurate determination in biological fluids. Multiple reports (Brook *et al.*, 1978; Kormorowski *et al.*, 1978; Controni *et al.*, 1977) conclude that the CSF lactate level is almost always elevated in untreated bacterial or fungal meningitis and that it is generally normal in viral meningitis. In partially treated meningitis, intermediate lactate levels have been reported, and a decreasing lactate level has been considered evidence of effective medication and resolution of the infection. However, D'Souza *et al.* (1978) emphasized the considerable overlap in CSF lactate levels among three crucial groups of patients: those with viral meningitis, those with partially treated bacterial meningitis, and those with tuberculous meningitis. Such overlap limits the value of measuring the CSF lactate in the differential diagnosis of these disorders.

Other conditions in which the CSF lactate is generally elevated include all the meningeal disorders associated with depressed CSF glucose levels, discussed earlier. While a mild or moderate elevation in lactate level is often observed with a normal CSF glucose level, a very low CSF glucose level has been invariably associated with a substantial increase in lactate level. This indicates increased anaerobic glycolysis by the adjacent cerebral tissue or by cellular infiltrates in the leptomeninges, in the pathogenesis of the reduction in glucose content and the increases in lactate and the L/P ratio.

In summary, the measurement of CSF lactate levels and the lactate/pyruvate ratio have been considered by several investigators to be clinically useful in the differential diagnosis of disorders associated with a low CSF glucose level and as a guide to the response to therapy. However, the overlapping concentrations seen in viral, bacterial, and tuberculous meningitis pose limitations to their diagnostic value in clinical practice.

Amino Acids

Study of the amino acid content of biological fluids has been facilitated by the availability of automated amino acid analyzers for the separation and quantitation of the free amino acids in protein-free filtrates. In many reports, the CSF and plasma values were not obtained simultaneously, nor is the reader informed whether the patients were fasting. Humoller et al. (1966) studied the CSF and plasma obtained from 5 normal fasting subjects at the time of spinal anesthesia. The total free amino acid content of plasma, 228 μmole/dl, was about three times the CSF level, 80 μmole/dl. Glutamine was the major amino acid, about 58 μmole/dl, in both compartments; it composed about 73 per cent of the total amino acids in CSF but only 24 per cent of the plasma pool. The distribution of the other free amino acids in both fluids was quite different.

The distribution of the free amino acids in the lumbar CSF and plasma of 37 fasting normal subjects has been summarized in Table 6–20. These findings differ slightly from earlier reports of adults (Perry et al., 1961; Dickinson et al., 1966; Van Sande et al., 1970; Gjessing et al., 1972). McGale et al. (1977) identified and quantified 23 amino acids; trace quantities of 8 other amino acids were also detected. Preliminary data showed no differences in the amino acid composition of ventricular and lumbar fluid, with the exception of glycine, serine, and glutamine. The glycine and serine concentrations were significantly higher in ventricular fluid, whereas the glutamine concentration was significantly lower in ventricular fluid.

The findings in newborn infants have been reported by Heiblim et al. (1978). The children ranged in age from 1 to 30 days, with a median age of 18 days; meningitis was excluded, but the infants were receiving intravenous glucose and electrolyte solutions. The CSF protein ranged between 16 and 70 mg/dl. The CSF amino acids in the newborn infants were increased compared to the findings in normal adults. The increases were even greater in infants with febrile convulsions and bacterial meningitis. There was a generalized increase in all the amino acids in both conditions, but the increases were greater in meningitis than in febrile convulsions. Proline, not usually seen in normal CSF, was greatly increased in both conditions but more so in meningitis. These workers

TABLE 6–20 Amino Acids in CSF and Plasma: 37 Normal Men and Women

Amino Acid	Mean CSF Concentration ($\mu mol/l$)	Mean Plasma Concentration ($\mu mol/l$)	CSF : Plasma Concentration Ratio
Alanine and citrulline	34.3	488.5	0.08
2-Aminobutyric acid	3.5	29.8	0.14
Arginine	22.4	80.9	0.31
Asparagine	13.5	111.7	0.12
Glutamic acid	26.1	61.3	0.40
Glutamine	552.0	641.0	0.86
Glycine	5.9	282.7	0.02
Histidine	12.3	79.8	0.16
Isoleucine	6.2	76.7	0.09
Leucine	14.8	155.3	0.10
Lysine	20.8	170.7	0.12
Methionine	2.5	27.7	0.10
Ornithine	3.8	73.5	0.06
Phenylalanine	9.9	64.0	0.17
Phosphoethanolamine	5.4	5.1	1.05
Phosphoserine	4.2	8.3	0.58
Serine	29.5	139.7	0.23
Taurine	7.6	77.2	0.11
Threonine	35.5	165.5	0.25
Tyrosine	9.5	73.0	0.14
Valine	19.9	308.6	0.07

(From McGale *et al.*, 1977)

could not confirm a previous report of Buryakova and Sytinsky (1975) that gamma aminobutyric acid, although not detected in normal CSF, was present during acute meningitis.

The mechanism for the elevations in CSF amino acids found in purulent meningitis and febrile convulsions is not clear. Several factors have to be considered, including increased permeability of the blood-brain barrier, inhibition of choroid plexus transport of amino acids from CSF to blood, and alterations in brain metabolism. There are specific membrane transport systems in the blood-brain barrier for acidic, basic, and neutral amino acids; these systems are located in the capillary endothelial cells of the brain. Specific transport systems also have been identified in the choroid plexus as well as in brain cell membranes studied *in vitro* utilizing brain slices. Thus, there are many factors affecting the concentration of each free amino acid that are exceedingly complex (Oldendorf, 1973).

There are several reports of changes in the concentration of some of the amino acids in brain in neurological diseases other than purulent meningitis and febrile convulsions. Van Sande *et al.* (1970) reported that the levels of 15 amino acids were significantly increased in parkinsonism, most notably citrulline, lysine, histidine, and arginine. These abnormalities persisted with oral L-dopa therapy, and the levels of leucine, isoleucine, and valine were even higher. However, Gjessing *et al.* (1974) could not confirm these observations. In a study of old age and parkinsonism, the latter investigators concluded that such changes were not specific for parkinsonism but reflected the age of the patients. In older patients whose mean age was 70 years, the concentration of 11 amino acids was higher than that found in younger patients whose mean age was 38 years. These included glutamine, glycine, alanine, citrulline, alpha aminobutyric acid, valine, methionine, isoleucine, leucine, phenylalanine, and lysine. They also reported a decrease in homocarnosine and aspartate in old age. In parkinsonism, only tyrosine, phenylalanine, tryptophan, and arginine were slightly elevated. The changes noted with age and their mechanism and significance have not been explained and require further study.

Gamma Aminobutyric Acid (GABA)

There has been special interest in the amino acid gamma aminobutyric acid (GABA) because of its role as a major inhibitory neurotransmitter in the brain and spinal cord, where it is present in high concentration. Reliable measurement of GABA in CSF has been difficult because of the limited sensitivity of the Ninhydrin detection method used in conventional amino acid analysis (Perry and Hansen, 1976). However, Wood *et al.* (1978) have verified the presence of GABA in normal CSF in low concentrations, about 150 pmole per ml, and this has been confirmed by others (Enna *et al.*, 1977; Manyam *et al.*, 1978). The concentration of GABA is reduced about 50 per cent in patients with Huntington's chorea, and similar low levels *may* be present in patients at risk prior to the onset of symptoms (Manyam *et al.*, 1978). The data now available regarding the specificity of this finding are insufficient to establish the assay of GABA as such a diagnostic test. Thus, Faull *et al.* (1978), using mass spectrometry, a very sensitive method, found overlapping CSF GABA levels in patients with Huntington's chorea, schizophrenia, manic-depressive psychosis, and tardive dyskinesia!

Welch *et al.* (1976) have studied the GABA in CSF obtained from patients with migraine during headache attacks and during headache-free intervals, and from patients with tension headache during headache-free intervals. Their method was too insensitive to detect the presence of GABA in asymptomatic patients, but the CSF GABA level was significantly elevated in 5 of 6 subjects during a migraine headache. These workers have also reported an increase in CSF GABA during cerebral ischemia and infarction. They suggested that the increase in CSF GABA during migraine attacks may reflect the cerebral ischemia that occurs during the vasoconstrictor phase of the headache. Buryakova and Sytinski (1975) also reported the presence of GABA in purulent meningitis, although this was not confirmed by Heiblim *et al.* (1978). Thus, despite theoretical interest in GABA, its assay has not yet been shown to provide reliable diagnostic information.

Ammonia and Glutamine

At physiologic pH, 90 per cent or more of ammonia is in the ionized form, and only 10 per cent of the blood ammonia is un-ionized and therefore freely diffusible across membranes. Ammonia, which is toxic to the nervous system, combines with alpha ketoglutarate in the brain to yield glutamine. Glutamine formation in brain serves as a means of protecting the nervous system from the toxic effect of ammonia. The concentration of ammonia in normal CSF is about one third to one half of the arterial blood ammonia level. Muting *et al.* (1968) reported that CSF levels in 20 normal subjects ranged between 11 μg/dl and 37 μg/dl; blood ammonia levels were between 29 and 136 μg/dl in 200 normal subjects. Moore *et al.* (1963) reported CSF values in 12 normal subjects of 34 ± 12 (SD) μg/dl. In hepatic failure, both arterial and CSF levels were elevated, and the CSF/blood ratio rose to 0.6. This relatively greater rise of CSF ammonia was not explained by changes in pH of the two fluids (Moore *et al.*, 1963). It may be related to the conversion of ammonia in brain to glutamine, which is rate-limited.

There is a good but inconstant correlation between the increase in CSF ammonia concentration and the degree of hepatic encephalopathy. An increase in CSF glutamine is an indirect measure of increased brain ammonia that correlates well with hepatic encephalopathy. There are technical difficulties in sampling and measuring ammonia in CSF because of its rapid volatilization. The glutamine assay is a more clinically useful index of hepatic (porto-systemic) encephalopathy than is the direct measurement of the CSF ammonia.

Walshe (1951) first reported elevated CSF glutamine levels in hepatic encephalopathy, a finding that has been subsequently confirmed by many laboratories (Gilon *et al.*, 1953; Brandstetter and Barzilai, 1960; Caesar, 1962; Plum, 1971). The normal level has ranged between 5 and 23 mg/dl. The data are summarized in Figure 7–1 (page 305). Most patients with hepatic coma have concentrations which range between 25 and 95 mg/dl. Values over 35 mg/dl are almost always associated with encephalopathy.

Hourani *et al.* (1971) measured the CSF glutamine in 86 patients. In 51 patients without liver disease, the mean CSF glutamine was 12.6 ± 5.1 mg/dl. In 9 patients with liver disease but without encephalopathy, the mean value was 21.6 ± 6.2 mg/dl, and in 26 patients with varying degrees of pre-coma and coma, it was about 40.3 ± 14 mg/dl. The highest level observed in this series was 75 mg/dl. The measurement of the CSF glutamine appears well established as a valuable diagnostic test in the evaluation of patients with suspected hepatic encephalopathy.

Alpha Ketoglutaramate

Alpha ketoglutaramate (α-KGM) is a metabolite of glutamine that was identified in the CSF of patients with hepatic encephalopathy (Duffy *et al.*, 1974; Vergara *et al.*, 1974). The level of α-KGM was less than 11 μmole/l in control subjects, the mean was 6.1 ± 1.8 (SE) μmole/l. In hepatic encephalopathy, there was an increase in the α-KGM level in CSF that roughly paralleled the severity of the encephalopathy. In hepatic coma, the CSF level was 76.7 ± 11.5 (SE) μmole/l. It appears that an increased α-KGM has no more diagnostic specificity than an elevation in its precursor, glutamine. In view of the greater ease with which glutamine can be measured, it is preferred for diagnostic testing.

Urea and Creatinine

The concentration of urea in CSF is slightly less than that of the serum in the steady-state, and changes in the serum level are followed by parallel changes in the CSF level. The time necessary for urea to reach equilibrium in CSF accounts for the transient osmotic effects of intravenous loads of hypertonic urea. In normal subjects in the steady-state, the urea content is about 4.7 mmole/l in CSF and 5.4 mmole/l in plasma (Bradbury *et al.*, 1963).

The normal concentration of creatinine in CSF varies between 0.5 and 1.9 mg/dl, averaging about two-thirds of the plasma creatinine level. The data were not corrected for the binding of creatinine to plasma proteins. Increased plasma creatinine levels in patients with renal insufficiency are accompanied by elevated CSF levels (Cockrill, 1931).

Cyclic Nucleotides

There has been interest in measuring the concentration in CSF of cyclic adenosine monophosphate (cAMP) and cyclic guanosine monophosphate (cGMP), because the brain and spinal cord contain large amounts of both nucleotides as well as the enzymes for their synthesis and degradation. Brooks *et al.* (1977) showed that both the lumbar fluid cAMP and cGMP levels remained constant despite a 40-fold increase in the plasma levels of cAMP or following a minor increase in the plasma cGMP level obtained with intravenous glucagon infusion. These observations indicate that in patients with an intact blood-brain barrier, measurement of the cAMP and cGMP levels in CSF can be considered to reflect cerebral metabolism rather than the blood level.

The normal lumbar CSF contains 5 to 30 nmole/l of cAMP. Elevations of the cAMP level have been reported in ischemia, migraine, seizures, and head injury (Cramer *et al.*, 1973; Rudman *et al.*, 1976; Welch *et al.*, 1976). However, with severe head injury causing coma, the ventricular fluid cAMP was strikingly depressed to levels as low as 1 nmole/l (Fleisher *et al.*, 1977). The authors have suggested that this depletion did not represent a nonspecific consequence of brain damage. They proposed a specific effect of trauma upon the adenyl cyclase system which generates cAMP; perhaps the depressed levels were a consequence of the depletion of the brain's ATP that follows tissue hypoxia.

Kassan and Kagen (1978) reported a threefold increase in CSF cGMP in patients with systemic lupus and neurological involvement but without any change in cAMP level. However, the elevated cGMP levels were correlated with the total white count in the CSF, which suggests that the inflammatory cells might explain the elevation. In control patients, cGMP was 0.68 nmole/l ± 0.14; in patients with systemic lupus, it was 2.4 nmole/l ± 0.44. They suggested that the increase in cGMP reflected changes in brain metabolism which might have diagnostic value.

Hypoxanthine

Interest in the hypoxanthine content of CSF was initiated by observations that concentrations of the metabolites of adenine nucleotides—adenosine, inosine, and hypoxanthine—are increased in tissue hypoxia. Meberg and Sangastad (1978) studied infants with hypoxia due to the idiopathic respiratory distress syndrome as well as older children with meningitis, seizures, and leukemia. The hypoxanthine levels in blood-free CSF ranged between 0 and 3 μmole/l in miscellaneous diseases without hypoxia. In hypoxic children, the CSF levels were increased to as high as 28 μmole/l. Hypoxanthine was also increased in purulent meningitis and meningeal leukemia. There was no correlation between the total hypoxanthine level and the CSF protein concentration. The relation between the CSF and blood hypoxanthine level has not been defined, nor have its turnover or possible toxic effects been studied.

Uric Acid

The uric acid content of CSF varies with changes in the serum level. Carlsson and Dencker (1973) studied uric acid levels in normal subjects and in alcoholic and schizophrenic patients. In normal patients, the CSF concentration was 0.25 ± 0.02 mg/dl (SEM) and the serum level was 5.50 ± 0.53 mg/dl (SEM); the CSF/serum ratio was about 0.05. Similar data were obtained by Wolfson *et al.* (1947). The CSF uric acid was increased about twofold in alcoholic withdrawal states to 0.44 ± 0.02 mg/dl (SEM) without any change observed in the serum level. Most of the uric acid in serum is bound to serum albumin. Thus, it is likely that the elevated CSF uric acid levels noted in alcoholism are a nonspecific consequence of an increased CSF protein concentration. An analogous increase has been observed in patients with purulent meningitis.

Carlsson and Dencker (1973) suggested that an increase in CSF uric acid might reflect alterations in nucleic acid catabolism in alcoholic withdrawal states. Increased CSF uric levels were also observed in patients with cerebral atrophy. However, the data regarding changes in the CSF uric acid content were not corrected for binding to albumin, and the specificity of the reported changes is questionable. No data are available regarding the mechanism for the removal of uric acid from the CSF. The existence of active transport of various organic acids by the choroid plexus from the CSF to the blood (discussed in Chapter 3) suggests that such a mechanism might also serve to clear uric acid from the CSF as well.

Biogenic Amines

The identification of a decreased concentration of dopamine in the brain of patients with parkinsonism initiated study of various monoamine metabolites in CSF in the gamut of extrapyramidal diseases, including dystonia, tardive dyskinesia, and Huntington's chorea, as well as in the various organic dementias (Gottfries *et al.*, 1969; Moir *et al.*, 1970; Chase *et al.*, 1973; Manyam *et al.*, 1978). A parallel interest has been expressed, largely in the psychiatric literature, regarding the various biogenic amines in affective illness, manic-depressive psychosis, autism, and schizophrenia (Post *et al.*, 1975; Asberg *et al.*, 1976; Vestergaard *et al.*, 1978). This often very speculative, at times contradictory, and rapidly expanding literature will be only briefly summarized.

The CSF has been studied with regard to its content of dopamine, serotonin, and norepinephrine and their major metabolites, respectively homo-vanillic acid (HVA), 5-hydroxyindoleacetic acid (5-HIAA), and 3-methoxy-4-

hydroxy-phenylethyleneglycol (MHPG). The use of the *probenecid test* was introduced in the study of these compounds because probenecid inhibits the active transport of a wide variety of organic acids and biogenic amines from CSF to blood by the choroid plexus. Probenecid also serves as a competitive inhibitor of binding of some organic acids in serum and brain (Fishman, 1966; Korf *et al.,* 1971; Perel *et al.,* 1974). Its effect on the transport of organic acids by the choroid plexus is quite analogous to its effect on renal tubular transport, although its direct effects on the brain are less well understood. (See discussion of blood-brain barrier to penicillin in Chapter 3.) Probenecid has been administered to patients with several pathological conditions to obtain an increase in monoamine concentration in the CSF. The use of the drug amplifies differences in the concentrations of some metabolites that were not otherwise apparent. The findings in normal subjects and in disease will be summarized.

Dopamine and Homovanillic Acid (HVA)

The decrease in dopamine content of the brain, first reported in parkinsonism, was shown to occur also in presenile dementia (Alzheimer's disease) and senile dementia. These observations prompted studies of the dopamine content in CSF as well as of its major metabolite, homovanillic acid (HVA), in various diseases of the basal ganglia as well as in psychiatric disorders. Lower levels of HVA in lumbar CSF were reported in parkinsonism, senile and presenile dementia, and depressive psychosis (Gottfries *et al.,* 1969; Moir *et al.,* 1970; Gottfries *et al.,* 1971), although there was considerable overlap in the values, and the control patients were not age matched. The latter is of considerable importance because the concentration of HVA in the lumbar CSF of normal humans has a rather wide range. Gottfries *et al.* (1971) reported HVA levels of 30 ± 12 μg per ml (SD) in old persons (aged 71 to 81 years); in younger persons (aged 18 to 54 years) the level was 60 ± 32 μg per ml (SD). No significant changes in HVA levels were noted in schizophrenia.

There are substantial data, largely derived from animal experiments, indicating that changes in the CSF levels of monoamine metabolites reflect changes in the corresponding amines in the brain, but the CSF level is dependent also upon the normal function of the removal mechanism for the metabolites from the brain and CSF. These dual factors make it difficult to assess the significance of a change in CSF level. Does a given change represent a change in cerebral metabolism or an altered rate of removal? Thus, high values of HVA (as well as of 5-HIAA) have been demonstrated in hydrocephalic adults and children and in patients with purulent meningitis (Ashcroft and Sharman, 1960; Andersson and Ross, 1969; Bakke *et al.,* 1974). These increases have been attributed to impaired choroid plexus function in hydrocephalus and in purulent meningitis. However, it is difficult to exclude a change in cerebral metabolism involving dopamine or HVA metabolism in such cases. To date, the changes in dopamine and HVA levels in CSF have not proved sufficiently specific to warrant their measurement as an aid to diagnosis.

There has been considerable interest in the dopamine hypothesis of schizophrenia, which states that schizophrenia may be related to a relative excess of dopamine-dependent neuronal activity. There are conflicting reports regarding the dopamine and HVA levels in CSF in schizophrenia, and to date no consistent changes have been established in any psychiatric illness (Meltzer *et al.*, 1976).

Serotonin and 5-HIAA

Serotonin (5-hydroxytryptamine) and its metabolite 5-hydroxyindoleacetic acid (5-HIAA) were studied in the CSF in various neurological and psychiatric disorders (Bowers *et al.*, 1969). The normal 5-HIAA level was 0.04 ± 0.01 μg per ml, with levels of 0.02 ± 0.01 μg per ml (SD) reported in presenile dementia, and lower levels in parkinsonism (Gottfries *et al.*, 1969). Low levels have also been reported in depression, and Asberg *et al.* (1976) have suggested that low levels may have predictive value in indicating the suicide-prone patient! The possibility of validating this hypothesis seems remote.

Ventricular fluid concentrations of HVA and 5-HIAA, the respective metabolites of dopamine and serotonin, were measured by Tabbador *et al.* (1978a) in 57 patients undergoing thalamotomy for the relief of movement disorders. The diseases included were Parkinson's disease, dystonia, cerebral palsy, multiple sclerosis, and post-traumatic or posthypoxic encephalopathy. The lowest mean HVA level (119 ng per ml) occurred in parkinsonism. There were diminished concentrations in patients with diffuse brain dysfunction, including postanoxic and post-traumatic encephalopathy, and with diffuse cerebral multiple sclerosis. There was considerable variation in the other disease categories. There were no significant changes in 5-HIAA levels in any of the patient groups. Tabbador *et al.* (1978b) also found that the ventricular fluid levels of HVA were significantly lower in patients with adult onset dystonia than in childhood onset torsion dystonia. The decrease in CSF concentration may be a reflection of decreased HVA levels in brain adjacent to the cerebral ventricles.

Norepinephrine and MHPG

The measurement of norepinephrine (NE) in CSF has been difficult, because its usual concentration is at the lower limits of detection with the fluorescent methods available (Ziegler *et al.*, 1976). Most investigators have reported CSF levels of about 100 to 300 pg per ml, approximately 60 per cent of the mean plasma NE level. Dietary intake of large amounts of foods containing a source of monoamines (bananas, cocoa, etc.) may be a source of increased levels in blood and CSF, and dietary controls are needed to avoid such errors. There is also a gradient in the concentration of NE in CSF obtained from various levels. Ziegler *et al.* (1976) showed that NE levels differ in the first 20 ml of CSF removed by lumbar puncture; the CSF concentration in the first 4 ml removed was about 25 per cent less than the concentration of the 16th to the 20th ml of CSF removed. (It is possible that the concentration of NE in lumbar CSF chiefly reflects NE derived from the spinal cord; CSF adjacent to the cauda equina has less NE than the thoracic spinal cord.) *It is clearly necessary for investigators to remove standard volumes of CSF to avoid errors due to such concentration gradients.* MHPG (3-methyoxy-4-hydroxyphenylethyleneglycol) is the major metabolite of NE in brain, and its CSF levels are about 40 times those of NE. MHPG appears to be evenly distributed throughout the CSF; there are similar concentrations of the metabolite in lumbar and ventricular fluid (Chase *et al.*, 1973; Sjostrand *et al.*, 1975). The norepinephrine in CSF appears to be derived from the central nervous system rather than from peripheral sources of norepinephrine; i.e., there is a blood-brain barrier for norepinephrine. (A patient with a pheochromocytoma had markedly elevated blood levels, 9680 pg per ml, but a normal CSF level of 200 pg per ml.)

Chase *et al.* (1973) have suggested that the MHPG level in CSF is an index of norepinephrine metabolism in the central nervous system. These workers reported that the MHPG level was about the same in ventricular and lumbar fluid, whereas the ventricular HVA was 10 times the lumbar fluid level and the ventricular 5-HIAA was 4 times the lumbar level. Thus, there was a variable correlation between CSF norepinephrine levels and its metabolites MHPG and VMA. This may reflect differences in the half-life of the three compounds, in part related to their kinetics for transport by the choroid plexus and capillary endothelial cells. Chase *et al.* (1973) found that the MHPG levels in lumbar CSF were the same in normal subjects and in patients with parkinsonism, dystonia, Huntington's chorea, and Down's syndrome; the level was about 15.0 ± 2.3 mg/ml (SD) in all patients studied. Studies of the CSF catecholamine levels in cerebral infarction and hemorrhage by Meyer *et al.* (1973) revealed greatly increased norepinephrine levels in hypertensive cerebral hemorrhage. These workers raised the question that the increased CSF concentration might play a part in the pathogenesis of diaschisis. However, there are no further data available regarding this hypothesis.

There has been much interest in the NE level in CSF of patients with affective disorders, including manic-depressive illness (Chase *et al.*, 1973; Ziegler *et al.*, 1976; Post *et al.*, 1978). It has been suggested that alterations in mood or motor activity may be associated with changes in central norepinephrine metabolism. Study of the metabolites of norepinephrine in psychiatric disorders, notably affective illness, has raised some interesting questions. Recently, Post *et al.* (1978) applied a sensitive radioenzymatic assay in patients with manic and depressive illness. They showed that probenecid produced an elevation in CSF norepinephrine. Although no differences were found between control subjects and depressed patients, the CSF norepinephrine levels were increased in the manic phases of illness. Thus, study of lumbar fluid levels of norepinephrine and its metabolite MHPG has shown some correlations with neurological and psychiatric illness, the significance of which requires further study.

To recapitulate, despite the intense interest in the study of the biogenic amines in the CSF in various neurological and psychiatric disorders, changes in their concentrations have not yet proved sufficiently specific to establish a basis for their measurement in clinical diagnosis.

Histamine

The older literature regarding the presence of histamine in CSF was summarized by Schain (1960). The bioassay in use failed to exclude inflammatory cells in the CSF as a source. There are no known correlations relating histamine levels to neurological disease. In view of recent interest in the properties of histamine as a neurotransmitter, this subject appears worthy of further investigation.

Acetylcholine

The importance of acetylcholine (ACh) as a central neurotransmitter prompted a variety of studies to measure its concentration in CSF. Experimentally, electrical or chemical stimulation of the brain in animals given eserine caused ACh to appear in the CSF. Major limiting factors have been the insensitivity of the various bioassay methods available for its quantitation and the great lability of acetylcholine in CSF. The addition of the anticholinesterase neostigmine as a preservative, by Tower and McEachern (1949), or physostigmine, introduced by Duvoisin and Dettbarn (1967), made it possible to show the presence of acetylcholine in CSF. In the past, the bioassay procedures used the dorsal muscle of the leech, the mollusc heart, frog lung, and more recently, the physostigmine-sensitized frog rectus abdominis muscle (Duvoisin and Dettbarn, 1967).

Early investigators found variable amounts of ACh present in the CSF in a wide variety of disease states, including psychoses, general paresis, alcoholic polyneuritis, and convulsive seizures (Schain, 1960). Tower and McEachern (1948) found increased ACh levels following head injury. Kunkle (1959) reported acetylcholine in the CSF of 5 of 9 patients with migraine headaches, but none was found in 35 of 37 patients without migraine; the 2 remaining patients of the latter group were subject to grand mal seizures. The presence of ACh in the CSF following head injury prompted Ward's (1950) study of atropine in the treatment of head injury. Sahar (1966) reported elevated ACh levels following brain surgery, but he found no relationship between the ACh level in CSF and the state of consciousness. The more sensitive assay technique of Duvoisin and Dettbarn (1967) identified ACh activity in normal CSF; the normal level was 1.79 ± 0.51 mg/dl. The level was increased in a few patients with epilepsy but was not changed in patients with parkinsonism. Lumbar CSF may not be representative of ventricular fluid or fluid obtained from the cortical subarachnoid space. In view of the rapid degradation of acetylcholine by the enzyme acetycholinesterase present in the CSF and in brain, it is possible that changes in ACh concentration in the CSF adjacent to the cerebrum may not be discernible in lumbar fluid.

Choline

There has been some interest in the measurement of choline in CSF, because it is a precursor for the formation of acetylcholine as well as an end product of its metabolism. As noted, acetylcholine is difficult to measure in CSF. In contrast, choline is a rather stable compound, and its concentration has been measured in normal subjects and in patients with extrapyramidal disorders. Aquilonius et al. (1972), using an enzymatic assay, reported that the lumbar CSF concentration is quite constant, ranging between 1.5 and 3.5 nmole/ml. The presence of red blood cells, up to 500 per mm^3, did not affect the CSF choline level. The choline concentration was about 25 times the concentration of acetylcholine reported by Duvoisin and Dettbarn (1967). In a small group of patients, the ventricular fluid choline levels were somewhat higher than in lumbar fluid, although there is evidence obtained with ventriculo-cisternal perfusion that choline is actively removed from the CSF (Cserr, 1971). Aquilonius *et al.* (1972) reported that the choline level in lumbar CSF was not altered in parkinsonism, nor was it influenced by anticholinergic therapy or by L-dopa. The choline concentration was significantly reduced in Huntington's chorea, both without therapy and with the administration of phenothiazines. The concentration appeared to be increased in the ventricular fluid from patients with intention tremor.

It is difficult to interpret these observatons. Choline in CSF can be derived from the plasma choline as well as from the brain as a product of acetylcholine or phospholipid metabolism. The source of the changes in choline concentration is not clear; their explanation will require further study.

Prostaglandins

Growing interest in the physiological role of various prostaglandins in animal tissues and their role in inflammation has been extended to the nervous system and to the study of the CSF in patients (Wolfe, 1975). The prostaglandin PGF_2 alpha, whose precursor is the polyunsaturated fatty acid arachidonic acid (C20:4), is the predominant prostaglandin in brain, although other prostaglandins have also been identified. There are technical difficulties in the measurement of the prostaglandins in CSF because of their great dilution. Gas chromatography with mass spectrometry is apparently sufficiently sensitive for their assay in small volumes of CSF.

Cory *et al.* (1976) studied PGF_2 alpha in CSF and found that the majority of patients had levels below 2 ng per ml, although levels in excess of 10 ng per ml were also reported. Their preliminary data showed that ventricular fluid levels were lower than lumbar levels and that the presence of red or white blood cells did not cause an elevation of the PGF_2 alpha content. However, the data suggested that elevations occurred with acute demyelinative lesions.

Wolfe (1975) reported "normal" PGF_2 alpha levels to be 92 pg per ml in fluids obtained at pneumoencephalography, with fivefold elevations in patients with epilepsy and tenfold increases in patients with meningitis or encephalitis. Similar increases were reported in subarachnoid hemorrhage, but the level apparently failed to show any correlation with the occurrence of vasospasm. A preliminary study of lumbar CSF during a migraine attack did not reveal an elevation in the prostaglandin level. Thus, further study is needed to establish the origin and significance of changes in prostaglandin concentration.

Polyamines

The availability of analytical methods for the detection of several polyamines in the CSF has prompted special interest in polyamine measurement as a diagnostic tool for malignancy and as an index of response to cancer chemotherapy. The polyamines spermidine, spermine, and their precursor putrescine are widespread in various tissues. The relative and absolute amounts of these compounds vary with cell type and the physiological state of the cells. Although their precise function has not been determined, *in vitro* and *in vivo* studies have linked the polyamines to the metabolism and function of the nucleic acids and thus to cellular proliferation and division (Marton, 1976).

Polyamines are polycationic in nature, and they form complexes with polyanionic compounds (RNA, DNA) and with nucleic acid-containing structures and membranes. They are usually increased in rapidly growing tissues and in malignancies. The major polyamines found in blood and CSF are present in the micromole per liter range. Several methods have been developed for their assay, including specific enzymatic assays, radioimmunoassay, gas-liquid chromatography, mass spectrometry, and ion-exchange column chromatography (Seiler, 1977). The polyamines in biological fluids are present both in the free form and as conjugates.

Marton *et al.* (1976) reported that spermine was not found in normal CSF, but low concentrations of putrescine and spermidine were found in the fluids of patients with apparently normal CSF. In these patients, the mean putrescine concentration was 184 ± 54 pmole/ml (SD), and the spermidine concentration was 150 ± 48 pmole/ml (SD). These two polyamines were increased in the CSF in a variety of brain tumors to levels as high as 2000 pmole/ml. The highest levels were seen in patients with medulloblastoma and meningeal seeding. Marton (1976) suggested that the concentrations of putrescine and spermidine may prove useful in following the course of patients with medulloblastoma and their response to therapy.

The relationship between the polyamine level and the CSF protein or cell count has not been established, nor has it been made clear whether there are concentration differences in ventricular, cisternal, and lumbar fluid. Data regarding the changes associated with purulent meningitis or cerebral infarction are not available. The mechanism and time course of the clearance of polyamines from the CSF have not yet been defined.

Lipids

The concentration of the total lipids in normal CSF is very low, only about 1.0 to 2.0 mg/dl, which is less than 0.2 per cent of the serum level. The literature regarding the normal lipid composition of the CSF is sparse, reflecting the technical difficulties in quantitative measurement of such minute amounts. However, the various phospholipids, including lysolecithin, sphingomyelin, lecithin, free and esterified cholesterol, and phosphatidyl inositol and phosphatidyl ethanolamine (composing cephalin) have been measured. Representative values from three laboratories are summarized in Table 6–21.

Phospholipids

The phospholipids in normal CSF are only about 1.5 per cent of the total in normal serum. McArdle and Zilkha (1962) studied the CSF phospholipids in various neurological disorders. Their values in control subjects were similar to those of Illingworth and Glover (1971) and others (see Table 6–21). They

TABLE 6–21   Lipid Content of Normal CSF: Representative Values

	Tourtelotte and Haerfr (1969)	Tichy et al. (1970)	Illingworth and Glover (1971)
Total lipids	1.25 mg/dl	1.03 mg/dl	—
Total phospholipids	0.37 mg/dl	0.49 mg/dl	0.60 mg/dl
Lysolecithin			6.7 per cent
Sphingomyelin			20.3 per cent
Lecithin			54.0 per cent
Phosphatidyl inositol ⎫			4.5 per cent
Phosphatidyl ethanolamine ⎬ cephalin			13.1 per cent
Phosphatidic acid ⎭			3.1 per cent
Choline phosphoglycerides		0.22 mg/dl	
Total cholesterol	0.40 mg/dl	0.31 mg/dl	0.54 mg/dl
Free	28 per cent	42 per cent	35 per cent
Esterified	72 per cent	58 per cent	65 per cent

separated the phospholipids into four major constituents: (a) lysolethicin and inositol phosphatide; (b) sphingomyelin; (c) lecithin; (d) phosphatidyl serine and phosphatidyl ethanolamine. They confirmed the similarity in percentage distribution of the phospholipid composition of normal CSF to that of plasma. Inflammatory lesions, stroke, and brain tumor were associated with an elevation in the total phospholipid present in CSF, and the percentage composition reflected that of plasma with a relatively low cephalin content (phosphatidyl ethanolamine). With disorders of the myelin, including multiple sclerosis, amyotrophic lateral sclerosis, and radicular polyneuritis, they observed an elevated total phospholipid content in CSF, but the cephalin fraction was often particularly raised as was the sphingomyelin fraction, changes which simulated the phospholipid concentration of white matter (McArdle and Zilkha, 1962).

More recently, Pedersen (1974) reported contrary findings, namely a decrease in CSF phospholipids in multiple sclerosis. These data require further substantiation.

Fatty Acid Composition of the Major Lipids

Illingworth and Glover (1971) studied the composition of the fatty acids in the following major lipids of the CSF: the cholesterol esters, phospholipids, and the triglyceride plus nonesterified fatty acid (NEFA) fractions (see Table 6–21). They analyzed large volumes (200 ml) of pooled CSF from children and adults. The individual fatty acids present in the cholesterol esters included oleate and linoleate. The phospholipids had high proportions of palmitate, stearate, and arachidonate. There was a greater resemblance between the fatty acid compositions of CSF and brain (with particular regard to the phospholipids) than between those of CSF and plasma. This was seen with the comparatively high concentration of phosphatidyl serine and phosphatidyl ethanolamine (cephalins) in CSF. These probably originate in brain, where they constitute an important lipid constituent, composing about 50 per cent of the total phospholipids in both white and gray matter.

Berry *et al.* (1965) also studied the fatty acids after chemical extraction, using gas-liquid chromatography. Although the total amount present was very small, over 30 individual fatty acids were identified, ranging from decanoic acid (C10:0) to nervonic acid (24:1). About 60 per cent of the fatty acids were saturated; 30 per cent had a single double bond; the remaining 10 per cent were polyunsaturated fatty acids. Palmitic acid (C16:0) was shown as the major fatty acid present, composing about 30 per cent of the total fatty acids in CSF. Arachidonic acid (C20:4) was the major polyunsaturated fatty acid present. No significant differences were observed between the findings in normal subjects and those in patients with multiple sclerosis or metachromatic leukodystrophy. The recent demonstration of the edema-producing effects of polyunsaturated fatty acids, such as arachidonic acid, suggests that further study of the polyunsaturated fatty acids in CSF may prove rewarding (Chan and Fishman, 1978).

Cholesterol

Cholesterol is present in both the free and esterified forms, the former composing about one. third and the latter two thirds of the fluids of the total cholesterol in CSF (see Table 6–21). In light of the high cholesterol content of serum, the CSF cholesterol is nonspecifically increased in pathological conditions associated with an increased CSF protein.

There is an extensive literature regarding CSF changes in free and esterified cholesterol in multiple sclerosis, summarized by Pedersen (1974). Technical difficulties have resulted in conflicting data. No consistent changes in total or esterified cholesterol have been established in multiple sclerosis or other diseases of the nervous system.

Desmosterol

A biochemical test for the diagnosis of brain tumor was introduced, based on the observation that desmosterol (2,4-dehydrocholesterol) appeared in the CSF after the administration of triparanol, a drug that blocks the conversion of desmosterol to cholesterol (Fumagalli and Paoletti, 1971). Weiss *et al.* (1972) confirmed this observation as well as the presence of an increased cholesterol level in the CSF of patients with brain tumor. However, a definite increase in CSF desmosterol (greater than 0.1 μg per ml) was observed in only 60 per cent of patients with gliomas. Thus, these observations are of theoretical interest, but the test does not have sufficient specificity to appear useful in clinical practice.

Lipoproteins

The very small concentration of total lipids in CSF, about 1.0 to 2.0 mg/dl, includes also small amounts of lipoproteins. The electrophoretic pattern of the CSF lipoproteins differs from that of serum. The lipoproteins in normal serum occur in two major electrophoretic fractions corresponding to the alpha$_1$ globulin and beta globulin bands, and they represent about 25 to 30 per cent and 50 to 60 per cent, respectively, of the protein-bound lipids. A small fraction, about 3 per cent, of the lipoproteins appears as alpha$_2$ lipoproteins, and the remaining 10 to 20 per cent consists of chylomicrons; these lipoproteins are absorbed to the filter paper at the application site of the CSF sample prior to electrophoresis (Dencker and Swahn, 1961; Schultze and Heremans, 1966). The electrophoretic analysis of CSF lipoproteins requires concentration prior to electrophoresis as well as prompt study shortly after spinal puncture. This is necessary because the lipids in the lipoproteins are easily dissociated from the proteins following refrigeration, which alters their electrophoretic pattern.

Dencker and Swahn (1961) found that normal CSF contained only one discrete band, alpha$_1$ lipoprotein, and that beta lipoprotein was not observed in normal fluids, multiple sclerosis, or neurological disorders with a normal CSF protein. However, in patients with brain tumor or meningitis, a definite beta lipoprotein band was readily identified. This appeared to be derived from the serum along with the other serum proteins which more readily enter the CSF when there is a defective blood-brain barrier. No more specific changes in the CSF lipoproteins have been reported and there has been little interest in their measurement in clinical diagnosis. Thus, while these observations are of theoretical interest, the test does not have sufficient specificity to appear useful in clinical practice.

Hormones

Pituitary Hormones

The major pituitary hormones, including corticotropin (ACTH), growth hormone, thyrotropin, prolactin, luteinizing hormone (LH) and follicle stimulating hormone (FSH), have been measured in the serum and CSF with radioimmunoassay methods (Schaub *et al.*, 1977). These studies have dealt chiefly with patients harboring a variety of pituitary tumors. The CSF often has been obtained at the time of pneumoencephalography.

Jordan *et al.* (1976) reported very low concentrations of these hormones in control subjects and in patients with heterogeneous neurological diseases, including brain tumor, seizures, hydrocephalus, multiple sclerosis, and Alzheimer's disease. The CSF hormone levels were not affected in patients with pituitary tumors which were totally intrasellar in location. Even in patients with markedly elevated plasma hormone levels, such as those observed in Nelson's syndrome, acromegaly, and hyperprolactinemia, the CSF hormone levels were unchanged. In marked contrast, patients with suprasellar extension of a pituitary tumor almost always had an elevated CSF concentration of one or more of the adenohypophyseal hormones; this was found in 21 of 22 such patients. The CSF concentrations of prolactin, LH, and FSH were elevated more commonly than were the other pituitary hormones. The hormone levels also fell toward normal with radiation therapy. Jordan *et al.* (1976) concluded that the increased CSF hormone levels could serve as a useful and sensitive screening procedure to establish the presence of suprasellar extension of a hormone secreting tumor. These authors also reported that one patient with pseudotumor cerebri had an elevation of CSF prolactin and luteinizing hormone that was not explained.

Prolactin in CSF has been assayed in various conditions, including pregnancy and pituitary adenoma, by Assies *et al.* (1978). They found the CSF level to depend upon the plasma level. The CSF level was not *per se* indicative of the presence of a pituitary tumor, with or without suprasellar extension, or of its absence. Low CSF/plasma prolactin ratios were found in some patients with suprasellar extension. Jordan *et al.* (1979) considered a CSF to plasma prolactin ratio of 0.2 or greater in a nonpregnant patient, or an increase in the CSF prolactin level during stimulatory testing, to be strongly suggestive of suprasellar extension of a pituitary tumor.

Cortisol

Cortisol in plasma is present as free cortisol, protein-bound cortisol, and conjugated cortisol, a water soluble metabolite. Free cortisol, the active form of the hormone, is lipid soluble and readily equilibrates between plasma and CSF, whereas the other forms of cortisol are excluded from the CSF (Christy and Fishman, 1961; Rodrigues, 1976).

Insulin

With the use of a radioimmunoassay, Rafaelson *et al.* (1966) reported the mean insulin level in the CSF of 18 fasting subjects to be 3.7 mμ per ml; simultaneous blood serum levels had a mean of 36 mμ per ml. No data are available regarding concentration differences at various loci in the CSF, nor has the time course for insulin exchange between serum and CSF been defined.

Thyroid Hormone

The total and dialyzable thyroxine in CSF and in serum was measured in 33 euthyroid patients with various neurological disorders and in 2 hypo- and 2 hyperthyroid patients by Hansen and Siersbaek-Nielson (1969). Total and dialyzable thyroxine in CSF were influenced by the protein concentration in CSF and by the thyroxine levels in serum. The mean values for free thyroxine were almost identical in serum and CSF, suggesting a free passage of free thyroxine across the blood-brain barrier. The total binding capacity of thyroxine was found to be higher in CSF than in serum samples diluted to the same protein concentration as in CSF. This occurrence was probably due to the higher concentration of prealbumin in CSF, which has a specific thyroxine-binding affinity. The T_3, T_4, and thyroxine-binding albumin and globulin of CSF were studied by Hagen and Elliott (1973), who concluded that thyroid hormone transport in CSF qualitatively resembled that in serum.

Chorionic Gonadotropin

Delfs (1957) reported chorionic gonadotropin in the CSF of women during normal pregnancy as well as with choriocarcinoma. CSF levels averaged 0.5 per cent of the serum concentrations in normal pregnancy, and in choriocarcinoma with cerebral metastases the percentages were elevated to 2 per cent. The relationship of the CSF level to increasing serum levels was not well defined. No more recent data are available to indicate whether the CSF hormone level might have diagnostic value in establishing the presence of metastatic disease in the central nervous system.

Gastrin and Cholecystokinin

These two peptide hormones, first isolated from the antrum and jejunum, have also been identified in brain tissue by use of a sensitive radioimmunoassay. Rehfield and Kruse-Larsen (1978) also demonstrated their presence in normal CSF, with a mean gastrin concentration of 3.4 pmole/l and a mean cholecystokinin of 14 pmole/l. The molecular configuration of the peptides in CSF was considered similar to that in brain. The physiological role of these hormones in the central nervous system is currently under active study.

Somatostatin

Somatostatin, a polypeptide hormone that inhibits the release of growth hormone and thyrotropin, was found in high concentration in the hypothalamus by Patel et al. (1977). Only small amounts were detected in other parts of the brain and spinal cord. The CSF in 7 patients without neurological disease contained somatostatin ranging in concentration from 15 to 55 pg per ml. In 20 of 24 patients with various neurological diseases of the brain and spinal cord, the somatostatin levels were increased, suggesting nonspecific leakage from brain tissue. These included patients with traumatic myelopathy, disc disease, multiple sclerosis, tumor, and bacterial and fungal meningitis. The highest somatostatin values were found in patients with medulloblastoma and cryptococcal meningitis. Although this finding correlated with an increase in CSF protein, the hormonal concentration in 5 patients was increased although the CSF protein was normal. In such patients, the authors considered that the CSF somatostatin level may prove to be a useful indication of disease in the central nervous system.

Endorphin

Beta endorphin is a brain peptide with potent morphine-like activity (perhaps the body's endogenous opiate), that is structurally related to the anterior pituitary hormone beta lipotropin. Jeffcoate et al. (1978) developed a radioimmunoassay for beta endorphin in plasma and CSF and found its concentration in lumbar CSF to be consistently greater than the plasma concentration in patients with nonendocrine diseases. CSF levels as high as 145 pmole per l were recorded with a plasma level of less than 10 pmole per l. The CSF beta endorphin concentration exceeded that of beta lipotropin, suggesting that the latter did not account for the endorphin measured. The authors concluded that endorphin was secreted in the brain with subsequent entry into the CSF.

Other Peptides

The presence of biologically active peptides in CSF was suggested by Chapman and Wolff's (1959) observation that the polypeptide bradykinin could be identified using a bioassay dependent upon rat uterus or guinea pig ileum. They suggested that it was present in a variety of inflammatory or degenerative disorders of the nervous system. It seems likely that recent methodological advances in the measurement of peptides in biological fluids will expand our knowledge of various peptides in the CSF in the future.

Vitamins

Limited data are available regarding the concentration in CSF of the various vitamins. The fat soluble vitamins A and D are essentially absent from the CSF despite their high concentration in brain, which reflects their insolubility in aqueous media. In rabbits, the water soluble vitamins, ascorbic acid, folate, and pyridoxine (free-form), are present in the CSF in higher concentrations than in the plasma. The concentration of thiamine (the free, nonphosphorylated form) differs in being slightly lower in CSF than in plasma. Spector (1977, 1978) summarized the evidence that active transport systems in the choroid are responsible for maintaining the higher concentrations found in the CSF. The data in humans regarding the distribution of ascorbic acid, inositol, and folates reveal it to be similar to that in laboratory animals. The CSF concentrations of these three vitamins were 2.5 to 5.0 times greater than the plasma level, uncorrected for binding to albumin, which may mask an even greater difference in concentration of the free vitamin.

With the use of a sensitive bioassay system for the measurement of thiamine, Baker *et al.* (1964) reported a mean CSF value of 4 mμg per ml with a mean serum level of 21 mμg per ml. The method did not differentiate between free thiamine or the three phosphate derivatives of thiamine, i.e., thiamine monophosphate, diphosphate, and triphosphate.

Vitamin B_{12} differs from the other water soluble vitamins in that the serum level greatly exceeds the CSF level, uncorrected for the binding of B_{12} to serum proteins. The serum levels were about 300 pg per ml in the serum and 15 pg per ml in the CSF (Schrumpf and Bjelke, 1970). Specific changes in the CSF concentration of the various vitamins in neurological disease have not been established.

Polyols

Polyols are polyhydric alcohols derived from aldoses or ketoses which have been separated and quantitatively measured in biological fluids using gas-liquid chromatography or mass spectrometry. Servo *et al.* (1977) identified five polyols in CSF, including arabinitol, anhydroglucitol, mannitol, sorbitol, and myoinositol, which together represent 90 to 95 per cent of the total polyol concentration present. The total polyol concentration in CSF was 340 ± 105 μmole per l, approximately twice the plasma concentration, 148 ± 30 μmole per l. There were no apparent correlations between the CSF level and age, sex, or the plasma concentration. The authors concluded that the polyols of the CSF most likely originate from the brain or spinal cord, since entry from the plasma against a concentration gradient seemed unlikely.

Myoinositol is a component of the myoinositol-containing phospholipids, the phosphoinositides, which serve as an important constituent of the cellular membranes of the brain and other organs. Its concentration in normal plasma was 1.09 ± 0.21 mg/dl (SD) and in normal CSF 2.55 ± 0.59 mg/dl (SD) (Garcia-Bunuel and Garcia-Bunuel, 1964). It is intriguing that its concentration in CSF is more than twice the concentration in plasma, similar to the distribution of fructose. These compounds probably are derived from the central nervous system. Specific changes have not been reported with neurological disease.

Other Solutes

Iron

Early investigations established the presence of iron in normal CSF, and several reports indicated abnormal increases of iron content in neurosyphilis, parkinsonism, Sydenham's chorea, and schizophrenia. Rather high levels were reported in the CSF (between 30 and 200 μg per dl), which proved to be incorrect. Kjellin (1966) restudied the problem with a spectrophotometric method, paying special attention to avoid contamination of glassware with iron and contamination of the sample with cellular elements. Normal CSF was found to have very much lower iron levels than previously reported; the normal was 0.01 to 0.02 μg per ml (1 to 2 μg per dl). Kjellin (1966) found that the level was increased in the presence of an increased CSF protein content. It is likely that most of the CSF iron is bound to transferrin. The iron content of serum is about 10,000 times the CSF level, and any contamination of the CSF with serum at the time of sampling would be expected to increase the CSF levels. No specific correlations between the CSF and serum iron have been established with regard to age, sex, or disease state.

Lithium

The introduction of lithium salts in the treatment of psychiatric disorders has prompted study of its distribution in the CSF and brain tissue. Terhaag *et al.* (1978) found that lithium reached a maximum in CSF about four hours after oral administration. The steady-state concentration ratio between CSF and plasma was about 0.44, and the authors concluded that the lithium concentration in CSF approximates the concentration in brain.

Bromide

An early interest in the steady-state distribution of bromide between serum and CSF revealed a plasma/CSF ratio of 2.5 to 3.0. This relative exclusion of bromide from the CSF was considered to be a result of the blood-brain barrier. The choroid plexus was later shown to actively transport bromide from the CSF. Walter's bromide test determined the plasma/CSF bromide ratio after an oral dose of sodium bromide. Its application to various clinical disorders was summarized in detail by Katzenellenbogen (1935). The ratio fell; i.e., the CSF levels were increased in many conditions associated with an increased CSF protein. A modification of the test using radioactive bromide was later introduced and applied to the study of tuberculous meningitis (Rangan and Virmani, 1976). Its specificity is doubtful. The bromide test is of largely historical interest today.

Aluminum

The CSF aluminum levels fell within 2 to 7 ppm in 180 patients (Delaney, 1979). The normal range has been reported to lie between 2 and 5 ppm. No correlations were observed between the aluminum level and CSF protein or neurological disease, apart from a significantly *low* level of aluminum in 10 patients with Alzheimer's disease. The significance of this observation is uncertain.

Trace Metals

A wide range of trace metals has been detected in minute concentration in CSF, including boron, silicon, chromium, manganese, zinc, rubidium, and others (Gooddy *et al.,* 1974, 1975). Whether the trace metals are present in free form or incorporated in or bound to various proteins is not known. No specific changes in the CSF content of the trace metals in neurological disease have been defined.

CHAPTER 7

CEREBROSPINAL FLUID FINDINGS IN DISEASES OF THE NERVOUS SYSTEM

This chapter summarizes the changes observed in the CSF in various diseases. It emphasizes the laboratory data that are useful in differential diagnosis.

Cerebrospinal Fluid in Infancy

The CSF composition is different in prematurity and normal infancy than in older infants, children, and adults. The differences involve the appearance, cell count, and protein and glucose levels. The color of the CSF in the neonate is usually xanthochromic; it varied from light to golden yellow in appearance in most of the 135 normal newborn infants studied during the first 24 hours of life by Naidoo (1968). None of these infants had evidence of subarachnoid bleeding. Earlier reports that red cells were commonly observed in the CSF of neonates were probably attributable to needle trauma. The high incidence of bilirubin staining of neonatal CSF is explained by increased CSF protein levels and by the relatively high serum levels of bilirubin found in neonates. Nasralla *et al.* (1958) reported the mean CSF bilirubin in 49 premature infants to be 0.61 mg/dl; it was 0.24 mg/dl in 34 full-term infants and 0.10 mg/dl in older control subjects. Both direct (free) and conjugated bilirubin are bound to serum albumin; together they contribute to the yellow color of serum. Conjugated bilirubin is more readily dissociated from the albumin, and it enters the urine and CSF. Both free and conjugated bilirubin are found in the CSF and together compose the total bilirubin that has been measured (see Pigments, Chapter 6).

The increased CSF protein is considered to occur as a consequence of immaturity of the blood-brain barrier in the neonate, i.e., it reflects the relatively increased permeability of the capillary endothelial cells to macromolecules, for which there is extensive experimental evidence (Rapoport, 1976). The presence of alpha-fetoprotein, which is derived from the plasma, in the CSF of neonates is an analogous example of the increased permeability of the barrier in neonates (Seller and Adinolfi, 1975).

253

The differentiation between subarachnoid hemorrhage and a traumatic lumbar puncture is difficult in the neonate (see Chapter 6). Chaplin *et al.* (1976) devised a way to confirm the diagnosis of subarachnoid hemorrhage in infants who have been transfused with adult blood *after* subarachnoid bleeding. This was based on the ratio of fetal to total hemoglobin found in peripheral blood and in the CSF. Hellstrom and Kjellin (1971) reported that spectrophotometry of the CSF is useful in differentiating subarachnoid hemorrhage from bilirubin staining. This determination was based on calculating the contributions of oxyhemoglobin and the red cell count to the pigmentation of the CSF.

The average white cell count in several studies was 6 to 7 cells per mm^3 (Widell, 1958; Naidoo, 1968) with a range extending upward to 32 cells per mm^3. The elevated CSF protein levels found by Naidoo (1968) confirmed earlier reports that CSF protein was elevated in the neonate. The mean level was 73 mg/dl, with a range varying between 40 and 148 mg/dl. Otila (1948) reported that the CSF glucose was close to the plasma level in both neonates and infants.

The more recent study of Sarff *et al.* (1976) has provided the most complete data regarding the CSF in full-term and premature infants. The infants had clinical findings suggestive of infection, which prompted diagnostic lumbar puncture; they constituted a high-risk group because of such problems as maternal illness and unexplained jaundice. However, all infants with evidence of bacterial or viral meningitis were excluded. The findings in 87 full-term and 30 premature high-risk infants are summarized in Table 7–1.

The white blood cell counts were the same in both groups. The data indicate that a WBC count greater than 30 per mm^3 (i.e., greater than 2.5 SD above the

TABLE 7–1   Cerebrospinal Fluid in Full-term and Premature Neonates*

	FULL-TERM	PREMATURE
WBC count (cells per mm^3)		
No. of infants	87	30
Mean	8.2	9.0
Median	5	6
SD	7.1	8.2
Range	0–32	0–29
± 2 SD	0–22.4	0–24.4
Percentage PMN†	61.3%	57.2%
Protein (mg per dl)		
No. of infants	35	17
Mean	90	115
Range	20–170	65–150
Glucose (mg per dl)		
No. of infants	51	23
Mean	52	50
Range	34–119	24–63
CSF/blood glucose ratio		
No. of infants	51	23
Mean	0.81	0.74
Range	0.44–2.48	0.55–1.55

*High-risk infants without meningitis who required lumbar puncture.
†PMN: Polymorphonuclear cells.
(Derived from Sarff *et a l.,* 1976)

mean) would be considered pathological. The polymorphonuclear finding of about 60 per cent appears to reflect the differential WBC count in blood. The red blood cell counts varied greatly, with a range of 0 to 45,000 cells per mm³ attributable to needle trauma. (The investigators did not correct the white cell count or protein level for the added blood.) The occurrence of increased CSF protein levels in full-term and premature infants was confirmed. Otila's (1948) earlier study differed somewhat in that the CSF protein was higher in premature infants than in infants at term.

The relatively elevated CSF protein content of the neonate reaches normal levels during the first few months of life. Krieg (1979) gives the following ranges: age 1 to 30 days, 20 to 150 mg/dl; 30 to 90 days, 20 to 100 mg/dl; 3 to 6 months, 15 to 50 mg/dl; 6 months to 10 years, 15 to 30 mg/dl. The upper normal limit increases slightly with age. Naidoo (1968) reported similar findings in infants.

The observation that the CSF glucose level in neonates more closely approximates the blood glucose level when compared to the findings in older children and adults has been explained as an example of the immaturity of the barrier. However, other factors may be of importance. First, the smaller mass of the immature brain (despite its high rate of glycolysis) utilizes less glucose than in maturity. Second, the glucose in the extracellular fluid is more rapidly replenished by the very high rate of cerebral blood flow that characterizes the immature nervous system (Kennedy and Sokoloff, 1957). No data are available regarding the quantitative importance of these factors. The CSF/blood glucose ratios of 0.81 and 0.74 were substantially higher than the usual ratio in adults of 0.50 to 0.65, in the presence of a normal blood sugar level.

Sarff *et al.* (1976) compared the CSF values from their neonatal patients to those from infants with meningitis. *No single test of the CSF proved absolutely reliable for the differentiation of uninfected from infected infants,* thus, one ten-day-old infant had a normal CSF despite culture-proven *E. coli* meningitis. The CSF findings in neonates may be difficult to distinguish from those observed in cases of congenitally or postnatally acquired viral meningitis, congenital syphilis, or toxoplasmosis.

Cerebrospinal Fluid After Death

Recent interest in methods for the determination of "brain death" prompted Paulson and Stickney's (1971) study of 150 cadavers on whom an autopsy was performed. Cases of known head trauma were excluded. Cisternal punctures were performed, and 20 to 25 ml of CSF were removed for chemical analysis. The authors commented that the CSF pressure was above zero in many cases, but no quantitative measurements were reported although earlier workers had reported that recordable pressures could be obtained for as long as 24 hours after death. (The origin of such postmortem pressures is not clear in view of the dependency of the intracranial pressure upon the systemic arterial and venous pressures.)

The CSF sodium levels averaged 128 mEq/l in 17 cadavers. Similarly, there was little change in the CSF chloride level, which averaged 113 mEq/l, suggesting slight dilution of sodium and chloride. The serum levels were not obtained. There was a striking increase in the CSF potassium, ranging from 2.3 to 57.0

mEq/l, with an average of 31.0 mEq/l in 26 cadavers. Although Fraschini *et al.* (1963) suggested that the rate of elevation of the CSF potassium after death might be useful in forensic medicine to determine the precise time of death, no quantitative data are available to support the suggestion. There was a decrease in the CSF glucose, which was roughly related to the time elapsed after death. The enzymes beta-glucuronidase, acid phosphatase, creatine phosphokinase, and lactic dehydrogenase were also measured. There were variable degrees of elevation in these enzymes, presumably derived from cerebral tissue adjacent to the cisterna magna, but precise correlation with the time of death was not possible. Thus, the major and most striking postmortem change was the increased CSF potassium, presumably derived from the ATP-depleted brain adjacent to the cisterna magna.

Purulent Meningitis

In the diagnosis and treatment of acute purulent meningitis, the CSF findings are essential to establish the diagnosis, the causative organism, and the choice of antibiotic. Repeated lumbar puncture also serves as a guide to the clinical course and management. Merritt and Fremont-Smith (1938) reviewed the CSF findings in 163 cases of purulent meningitis due to the following bacterial agents: meningococcus (64 cases), pneumococcus (41 cases), streptococcus (39 cases), staphylococcus (13 cases), and *Hemophilus influenzae* (6 cases). Their data illustrate well the pattern of the CSF changes in untreated acute purulent meningitis and are summarized here.

The CSF pressure, measured at first puncture, was found to be increased in over 90 per cent of the cases. The pressure was between 200 mm and 500 mm in 75 per cent and between 500 to 1000 mm in 15 per cent. The pressure was more likely to be normal if the puncture was made very early in the course of the disease or if subarachnoid block developed. As the disease progressed, the pressure became progressively higher (these patients were studied prior to the introduction of antibiotic therapy). It returned to normal with recovery from the infection. Fluids examined in the early stages of the disease were "ground glass" in appearance, or only slightly turbid. Turbid fluid often has a greenish tinge (Tugwell *et al.*, 1976). Later they become cloudy or frankly purulent. A fine or coarse coagulum formed in nearly all fluids, and the supernatant was usually slightly yellow, reflecting the increased protein concentration. Occasionally, in granulocytopenic patients, the CSF may contain few leukocytes and yet may appear turbid because of the presence of huge numbers of bacteria.

Cells

At the time of first puncture, the CSF generally showed a marked pleocytosis of between 1000 and 10,000 white cells per ml^3. The range of cell counts found at first puncture in 152 cases studied by Merritt and Fremont-Smith (1938) is given in Table 7–2. Polymorphonuclear leukocytes usually constituted 90 to 95 per cent of the total white cell count. Small and large lymphocytes and macrophages were also present. (The absence or presence of eosinophils was not

TABLE 7–2   Lumbar Fluid: Initial Findings in Purulent Meningitis

	MENINGO-COCCUS	PNEUMO-COCCUS	STREPTO-COCCUS	STAPHYLO-COCCUS	H. influenzae	TOTAL	PER CENT
Cells per mm³							
(152 patients)							
Under 100	1	0	0	1	0	2	1
100 to 1000	5	3	7	2	1	18	12
100 to 10,000	39	31	27	8	4	109	72
10,000 to 20,000	11	2	2	1	0	16	10
over 20,000	6	0	1	1	0	7	5
Protein (mg per dl)							
(157 patients)							
Under 45	1	0	1	1	0	3	2
45 to 100	7	2	7	3	0	19	12
100 to 500	39	29	23	4	5	100	64
500 to 1000	7	6	8	1	0	22	14
1000 to 2000	10	3	0	0	0	13	8
Glucose (mg per dl)							
(154 patients)							
Under 10	13	12	8	0	2	35	23
10 to 40	38	19	19	8	3	87	57
40 to 50	2	3	3	2	0	10	6
50 to 60	5	1	4	0	1	11	7
Over 60	3	2	5	1	0	11	7

(Derived from Merritt and Fremont-Smith, 1938)

stated.) Counts under 100 cells per ml³ were found only twice; 90 and 40 cells, in cases due to meningococcus and staphylococcus respectively. Occasionally, in patients with meningococcal meningitis, especially infants, the fluid was an almost pure suspension of organisms with very few cells; with recovery there was a rapid decrease in total cell count, and the relative percentage of lymphocytes and mononuclear cells increased.

The question of the number of white cells that may persist after the adequate treatment of bacterial meningitis has been studied by Chartrand and Cho (1976). A persistent pleocytosis of more than 30 white cells per mm³ was commonly seen in children adequately treated for bacterial meningitis. It occurred in 13 of 21 (62 per cent) children with *H. influenzae* meningitis and in 2 of 9 (22 per cent) with pneumococcal meningitis. A pleocytosis alone was not considered an indication for prolonging therapy. The significance of the persistent pleocytosis was not defined. It was not associated with duration of illness, prior therapy, complications, or relapse.

Swartz and Dodge (1965), in an extensive review of bacterial meningitis, observed no relation between the height of the pleocytosis and the clinical outcome. The highest cell count that they observed was 87,000 per mm³ in a patient with pneumococcal meningitis. With a cell count of this magnitude, one should consider the possibility of intraventricular rupture of a brain abscess, but in their patient this diagnosis was excluded.

Protein

The protein content of the CSF at the time of the first puncture in 157 cases studied by Merritt and Fremont-Smith (1938) is shown in Table 7–2. Protein levels between 100 and 500 mg/dl occurred in about two thirds of the cases. Normal protein values (under 45 mg/dl) were found in less than 2 per cent of cases. Values between 500 and 1000 mg/dl were not uncommon, occurring in 14 per cent of cases, and a protein content greater than 1000 mg/dl was found in only 8 per cent (13 cases). Protein values greater than 1000 mg/dl were often associated with evidence of spinal subarachnoid block (e.g., rapid fall in CSF pressure to a very low level after removal of only a small volume of fluid, as well as abnormal responses to the Queckenstedt test).

The factors responsible for an increased CSF protein have been discussed earlier (see Chapter 6). It is noteworthy that Weiss *et al.* (1967) have reported increased mortality in patients with meningitis, when CSF proteins are above 280 mg/dl. The CSF protein returns to normal promptly with therapy. In children with pneumococcal meningitis, the protein returned to normal in most cases after 8 to 10 days of treatment (Chartrand and Cho, 1976).

The CSF immunoglobulins are characteristically increased in purulent meningitis. Smith *et al.* (1973) found IgM, IgG, and IgA levels increased in patients with viral, purulent, and tuberculous meningitis (see Table 7–3). The changes were greatest in purulent meningitis. The changes in viral meningitis were greatest late in the course of the illness. IgM and IgA levels were greatest in purulent meningitis. IgG levels were greatest late in viral and tuberculous meningitis. The corresponding serum immunoglobulin levels were not obtained.

Glucose

The glucose content at the time of the first puncture in 154 patients studied by Merritt and Fremont-Smith (1938) is summarized in Table 7–2. It was usually moderately or greatly reduced, often below 40 mg/dl, and below 10 mg/dl in 23 per cent of the cases. (When the CSF glucose level is reported as "zero," it is probably more correct to say "less than 5 mg/dl," which is about the sensitivity of most methods used to assay glucose.) The glucose level was over 50 mg/dl in 14 per cent of cases. This was found in some patients tapped early in the course of the disease as well as in patients with concomitant hyperglycemia. Thus, a CSF

TABLE 7–3   CSF Immunoglobulins in Meningitis

GROUP	NUMBER	Immunoglobulin (mg/dl ± SD)		
		IgM	*IgA*	*IgG*
Normal	20	0	0.4±0.6	3.1± 1.2
Viral meningitis (early)	35	0.5±0.6	1.0±0.4	3.8± 2.2
Viral meningitis (late)	5	1.6±1.3	1.2±0.9	11.7± 6.7
Purulent meningitis	24	4.3±5.9	4.1±5.5	9.9± 8.2
Tuberculous meningitis	6	1.6±1.5	3.8±0.4	23.6±14.2

(After Smith, Bannister, and O'Shea, 1973)

glucose level of 50 and 60 mg/dl would probably be abnormal in patients with a blood glucose level of 200 mg/dl or more just prior to the diagnostic tap (see Chapter 6).

The CSF glucose must be analyzed promptly after the sample is obtained. The glucose level will be factitiously reduced when a purulent fluid stands at room temperature unless glycolysis is stopped with fluoride.

The CSF glucose level is of special diagnostic significance in the evaluation of cellular fluids. A low CSF glucose level in a grossly purulent fluid is presumptive evidence of a bacterial meningitis. A low glucose level is indicative of a *diffuse* leptomeningeal inflammatory process as opposed to focal sepsis. However, a persistently normal CSF glucose in the presence of a granulocytic pleocytosis is more often indicative of a focal collection of pus, such as brain abscess, extradural abscess, or subdural empyema, or of venous sinus thrombophlebitis. Weiss *et al.* (1967) have reported an increased mortality due to purulent meningitis in patients with a glucose level less than 13 mg/dl.

The rate of return of the CSF glucose level to normal often parallels the clinical response, as does the return of the cell count and the protein level to normal. However, occasionally the CSF glucose level may remain depressed for as long as 7 to 10 days after the other CSF changes have returned to normal levels. The mechanism of the prolonged depression of the glucose level is probably related to the persistence of an increased rate of glycolysis in the nervous tissue adjacent to the leptomeninges. This is considered the most important factor in the pathogenesis of most cases of low CSF glucose, independently of the cause (see Chapter 6).

Lactic Acid

The factors influencing the CSF lactate levels have been discussed in Chapter 6. In patients with untreated bacterial or fungal meningitis, the CSF lactate level is almost invariably elevated and inversely related to the CSF glucose levels (Brook *et al.*, 1978; Kormorowski *et al.*, 1978; Controni *et al.*, 1977; D'Souza *et al.*, 1978). The CSF lactate levels are usually 2 to 4 times greater than the normal concentration of about 1.6 mEq/l. The return of the lactate level to normal occurs on a similar time course as that observed with glucose. D'Souza *et al.* (1978) showed that there was sufficient overlap in the CSF lactate levels observed in patients with viral meningitis, tuberculous meningitis, and partially treated bacterial meningitis to limit its value in the differential diagnosis of these disorders. Brook *et al.* (1978) also showed that primary CSF acidosis occurs in patients with purulent meningitis, which reflects increased lactic acid production by the brain and by polymorphonuclear granulocytes.

Other Constituents

The changes in lactic dehydrogenase and its isoenzymes in bacterial meningitis have been summarized in Chapter 6.

The assay of cyclic nucleotides in CSF has been discussed in Chapter 6. Recently, Weitzman *et al.* (1979) reported changes in the cyclic adenosine monophosphate (cAMP) level of CSF in bacterial meningitis. The mean level in purulent CSF was 0.5 nmole/l, *less* than half of control level. They did not consider the decrease to be secondary to bacterial or leukocytic metabolism. They suggested that the depressed levels might reflect decreased cAMP levels in brain related to the encephalopathy associated with the meningitis.

Ventricular and Cisternal Fluids in Purulent Meningitis

Merritt and Fremont-Smith (1938) reported that the cisternal fluid findings in patients with acute purulent meningitis showed changes similar to those observed in lumbar fluid, with some minor differences. The cisternal and lumbar fluids were under the same pressure except in the presence of a spinal subarachnoid block, when the lumbar pressure was lower. The protein level and cell count were usually increased less in cisternal fluid than in lumbar fluid, reflecting the ready admixture of cisternal fluid with the large volume of ventricular fluid.

Merritt and Fremont-Smith (1938) also compared the ventricular and lumbar fluids in 20 patients, obtained at the same time or within a few hours of each other. Only one of the 20 patients had a normal ventricular fluid cell count; in the rest, there was a pleocytosis that was usually considerably less than that found in lumbar fluid. Thus, most of the patients had greater evidence of meningitis than of ventriculitis, although in one patient with meningococcal meningitis there were 3 times as many cells found in the ventricular fluid (15,000) than in the lumbar fluid (5000). The ventricular fluid protein was normal in 4 of the patients; in the rest, it was elevated but less than the corresponding lumbar fluid protein level.

The glucose level was always higher in the ventricular fluid than in the lumbar or cisternal fluid. In 13 of the 20 patients, the ventricular glucose level was normal despite distinct depression of the lumbar glucose level. In the rest, the ventricular glucose level was depressed, but never to the level of the corresponding lumbar fluid glucose. A low ventricular fluid glucose level indicates the presence of ventriculitis; a normal level indicates sparing of the ependymal surfaces and subependymal brain despite marked involvement of the leptomeninges.

CSF Changes with Therapy

The return of the CSF toward normal with therapy is usually prompt and parallel to the overall clinical improvement, namely, improved state of consciousness and reduced fever, headache, and meningeal signs. Twenty-four hours after institution of appropriate antimicrobial therapy, the CSF sediment should reveal no organisms, and cultures should be sterile. Mathies (1978) analyzed the CSF improvements in children being treated for influenzal meningitis. The total cell count was often increased on the first day of therapy; this finding should not necessarily be construed to mean failure of therapy. Significant reduction in white cell count was found by day 3 of therapy, and by day 7 most patients had fewer than 500 white cells. The fall in the proportion of white cells that were polymorphonuclear granulocytes paralleled the reduction in total cell count; the majority of cells did not become mononuclear until after the third day of therapy. The CSF glucose usually returned to normal most rapidly, and by day 3 at least 80 per cent of the patients had spinal fluid glucose levels higher than 40 mg per dl. When the patient was afebrile for 5 days, the CSF cell count was usually less than 30 per mm³, and the CSF glucose and protein levels generally were approaching normal.

However, it is important to note that some patients have persistent depression of the CSF glucose levels for 10 or more days despite clinical improvement and improvement in other CSF changes. It is presumed that this represents a persistent defect of membrane transport of glucose or a persistent increase in glycolysis by the adjacent cerebral tissue for an extended period of time.

Repeat Lumbar Puncture in the Diagnosis of Meningitis

The early diagnosis of purulent meningitis is often very difficult, particularly in infancy when the appearance of meningeal signs may be quite delayed. Moreover, the initial lumbar puncture may prove negative and the development of typical CSF changes be delayed for hours to a few days, when a repeat puncture reveals cells and positive cultures. In such patients, the initial blood cultures often have been positive. Such a delayed onset raises the question of whether a lumbar puncture in the presence of bacteremia induces meningitis. While this has been demonstrated experimentally in dogs (Petersdorf *et al.*, 1962), there is uncertainty about its occurrence in patients. However, in view of this possibility, repeated CSF examination has been recommended in infants when the blood culture is positive at the time of a negative lumbar puncture (Kindley and Harris, 1978).

Bacteriological Tests

Gram's stain and both anaerobic and aerobic cultures in the examination of the CSF in patients suspected of having purulent meningitis are fundamental to the appropriate diagnosis and treatment of such patients. The reader is referred to Henry (1979), an excellent resource for bacterial methods. Tugwell *et al.* (1976) reported that stained smears of CSF sediments were positive for gram-positive diplococci in only 71 per cent of 42 cases of pneumococcal meningitis. Cultures were positive in 81 per cent of the cases. Because of the delay in getting such data, several other laboratory tests of CSF have been devised to make a specific bacterial diagnosis more rapidly. These include tests for specific bacterial antigens and bacterial endotoxin and the nitroblue tetrazolium dye test for actively phagocytosing granulocytes.

SPECIFIC BACTERIAL ANTIGENS (THE CIE TEST). The presence of specific bacterial antigens in CSF can be determined with newly developed techniques that are quite rapid and sensitive (Rytel, 1976; Levin *et al.*, 1978). Countercurrent immunoelectrophoreses (CIE), using commercially available antisera, are available for the five major pathogens of bacterial meningitis including *H. influenzae B; N. meningitides A, B, C, X, Y, Z, W 128; S. pneumoniae 1–30;* group B beta-hemolytic streptococci; and *E. coli K1.* There is also antigenic crossover between several of the latter bacterial antigens; a positive CIE for *H. influenzae B* in a neonate is also compatible with *E. coli* meningitis (McCracken, 1976). An adverse prognosis has been correlated with the height and persistence of the spinal fluid antigen. However, the concentration of bacteria may be a more important determination of prognosis than the concentration of antigen (Feldman, 1977).

The sensitivity of the CIE test is limited because of small concentrations of bacteria in some patients. Therapeutic decisions regarding the choice of antibiotics cannot yet be made on the basis of CIE testing alone because of the insufficient specificity of the antigenic response due to the antigenic crossover between various bacteria (Whittle *et al.*, 1975; Coonrod and Drenan, 1976).

Endotoxin Detection: The Limulus Lysate Test.   Endotoxin, a lipopolysaccharide constituent of the cell wall of gram-negative bacteria, has been measured in the CSF. The Limulus lysate test is a commercially available, specific, sensitive, and rapid assay for the presence of endotoxin. A lysate of the amebocytes of the horseshoe crab (*Limulus polyphemus*) forms a gel in the presence of endotoxin; the test becomes positive in the presence of as little as 0.05 nanogram of endotoxin derived from gram-negative bacteria associated with meningococcal meningitis or *H. influenzae B* meningitis. While the test has proved positive in most cases of gram-negative bacterial meningitis, it also may be positive with *Candida* or *Aspergillus* infections because they too produce endotoxin; the test remains negative with aseptic meningitis (Nachum *et al.*, 1973; Ross *et al.*, 1975; Rytel, 1976).

However, the sensitivity of the Limulus lysate test is limited if the concentrations of bacteria are small (Feldman, 1977). The persistence and amount of endotoxin appear to correlate with increasing morbidity and mortality (McCracken and Sarff, 1973). The test appears to serve only as a diagnostic adjunct, because it does not identify the specific bacterial cause, although it implicates the spectrum of gram-negative organisms.

Nitroblue Tetrazolium Dye Test (NBT).   The reduction of NBT dye to form formazan (changing from a pale yellow to a dark blue color) occurs secondary to the presence of superoxide free radicals. These are generated by activated polymorphonuclear granulocytes during phagocytosis. The NBT test uses the dye to determine the presence of activated granulocytes in CSF as an index of purulent meningitis (Zwibel and Schwartzman, 1974). It has not yet been established whether the test is sufficiently sensitive and specific to be useful in routine clinical diagnosis.

Aseptic Meningeal Reaction due to Extradural Sepsis

In the preantibiotic era, extradural septic foci occurred frequently in patients with mastoiditis or sinusitis. While extradural septic collections have become unusual in clinical practice, they still are seen, and their diagnosis may be difficult. Merritt and Fremont-Smith (1938) summarized the findings in 34 such patients with mastoiditis and petrositis. The intracranial pressure was elevated in 21 of the 34 patients. The elevation was attributed to thrombophlebitis and occlusion of the adjacent lateral venous sinus. A polymorphonuclear pleocytosis was noted in 29 of 31 cases; there were 10 to 50 cells per mm^3 in 45 per cent of the cases, 50 to 1000 cells per mm^3 in 35 per cent of the cases, and 1000 to 7000 cells per mm³ in 13 per cent of the cases. The CSF protein content was increased in 60 per cent of the cases, ranging between 45 and 100 mg/dl. The CSF glucose level was normal, except in those patients who had developed the complication of a generalized leptomeningitis. The CSF findings in cases of extradural septic foci were often indistinguishable from those associated with encapsulated brain abscess and subdural empyema. The findings in spinal epidural abscess are similar to those observed with intracranial extradural sepsis (Baker *et al.*, 1975). Evidence of spinal block develops rapidly: the initial pressure is then reduced, and the CSF may be difficult to obtain ("dry" tap).

Subdural Empyema

Subdural empyema occurs in settings similar to those associated with extradural sepsis, including mastoiditis, sinusitis, and metastatic infection from a remote focus. The CSF findings are similar to those associated with extradural sepsis or brain abscess. The CSF pressure is commonly elevated, and the fluid contains from fewer than 100 to a few thousand leukocytes, predominantly polymorphonuclear cells. The protein is usually greater than 100 mg/dl. The glucose is normal, and the fluid reveals no organisms on smear or culture (Kaufman *et al.*, 1975).

Brain Abscess

Recognition of the hazards of lumbar puncture in patients with brain abscess (see Chapter 5), as well as the recent availability of computed tomography as a diagnostic aid, has resulted in fewer diagnostic lumbar punctures in such patients. There is substantial circumstantial evidence that lumbar puncture may aggravate a pre-existing cerebral herniation because of the cerebral edema associated with brain abscess. Thus, Garfield (1978) described deterioration in the level of consciousness in 41 of 140 patients during the 48 hours after lumbar puncture. Carey *et al.* (1972) attributed the death of 5 patients, an 8 per cent mortality, to lumbar puncture. Despite these hazards, patients showing signs of concurrent meningitis may require a diagnostic lumbar puncture for bacteriological studies.

The CSF findings vary greatly depending upon the stage of the abscess and whether it is acute, chronic, well-encapsulated, or associated with evidence of cerebritis or meningitis. Despite the dramatic evidence of extensive brain edema in the area surrounding abscesses, well visualized with computed tomography, the lumbar pressure is often not much elevated. Thus, Kiser and Kendig (1963) reported pressures above 250 mm in only 25 per cent of patients. Garfield's review (1978) of the series of Bonnae and colleagues indicates that the diagnostic value of the CSF findings in patients with brain abscess is limited. In 208 examinations (in a series of 326 patients), the white cell count was below 11 per mm³ in 63 cases, between 11 and 500 per mm³ in 87 cases, and above 500 per mm³ in 58 cases. The cellular responses varied between a solely lymphocytic response, usually with a low total white count, and a predominantly polymorphonuclear response in the presence of cerebritis, ruptured abscess, or diffuse meningitis. Carey *et al.* (1972) found that approximately one third of patients with established brain abscesses had a normal cell count of less than 5 per mm³.

Table 7–4 summarizes the CSF findings in five large groups of patients with brain abscess, both chronic and acute. The intracranial pressure was normal in 38 per cent of cases. The white cell count was normal in 29 per cent. Cell counts greater than 500 per mm³ occurred in the presence of cerebritis and meningitis. With rupture of a brain abscess, many thousands of white cells were observed. There were corresponding changes in the CSF protein.

The changes in the CSF glucose indicate that 21 per cent of 112 patients had a glucose below 40 mg/dl (curiously, these authors used 40 rather than 45 mg/dl as the lower limit of normal). A reduction in the CSF glucose (in the absence of hypoglycemia as the cause) indicates a *diffuse* leptomeningitis rather than localized inflammatory disease (see Chapter 6); in the presence of brain abscess it is indicative of probable abscess rupture.

CSF cultures are negative with an encapsulated abscess, except in cases of concomitant abscess rupture and meningitis. Merritt and Fremont-Smith (1938) observed that the pleocytosis was generally greatest in the early stages and that it decreased with encapsulation of the abscess. With extension of the abscess toward the ventricles or to the subarachnoid space, the cellular responses were increased further. These workers emphasized the diagnostic significance of a relatively high "poly" count in the fluid as a sign of abscess in the differential diagnosis of intracranial mass lesions, although there are exceptions with some cases of glioblastoma, which may also show a polymorphonuclear pleocytosis (see Brain Tumor).

TABLE 7–4   Summary of Lumbar Fluid Changes Associated With Brain Abscess

			Number of Patients	Per Cent
Pressure	<200 mm		38	38
	200–300 mm		35	35
	>300 mm		26	26
		Total	99	
White cells	*per mm³*			
	<5		61	29
	5–100		81	38
	>100		71	33
		Total	213	
Protein	*mg per dl*			
	<50		26	24
	50–100		38	35
	>100		44	41
		Total	108	
Glucose	*mg per dl*			
	>40		89	79
	<40		23	21
		Total	112	

(Derived from Kiser and Kendig, 1963; Garfield, 1978; Carey *et al.*, 1972; Sampson and Clark, 1978; Rosenblum *et al.*, 1978)

Tuberculous Meningitis

The clinical manifestations of tuberculous meningitis and the changes in the CSF are quite variable, reflecting the stage of the disease. The findings depend upon the severity of vascular involvement, ischemic infarction, and hydrocephalus, and the tuberculous encephalopathy which is in part due to the degree of brain edema (Tandon, 1978). A firm diagnosis depends upon identification in the CSF of tubercle bacilli, by smear, culture, or guinea pig inoculation. However, several changes in the fluid are fairly characteristic of the disease. Typically, the CSF is clear and colorless and may show a pellicle or cobweb clot on standing at room temperature or after refrigeration, reflecting the presence of fibrinogen in the fluid. There is usually a moderate pleocytosis, generally not in excess of 500 per mm^3, composed largely of lymphocytes and mononuclear cells. In the early stages of the disease and sometimes during the course of the illness, a predominantly polymorphonuclear cellular response is noted which may confuse the clinician. The CSF protein level is usually moderately elevated, and the glucose level is characteristically depressed. Thus, the CSF changes may simulate those associated with the gamut of subacute meningitides, including fungal meningitis, sarcoid and other forms of granulomatous meningitis, carcinomatous meningitis, and some viral meningitides, most notably herpes simplex and mumps.

Merritt and Fremont-Smith (1938) reported the findings in 84 cases. About 80 per cent of the patients had increased pressure at the time of first puncture. Ten per cent developed partial or complete spinal block during the course of the illness. While 85 per cent of the patients had a cell count between 50 and 500 per mm^3, 9 per cent of them had 500 to as many as 2021 per mm^3 during the course of the illness (in the preantibiotic era). While lymphocytes and mononuclear cells predominated, polymorphonuclear cells averaged about 20 per cent of the total count. They composed more than 50 per cent of the white cells in 10 per cent of the cases. The proteins were mildly to moderately increased in almost all cases. Values in excess of 500 mg/dl were usually associated with complete or partial spinal (manometric) block.

As the disease progressed, the glucose level was reduced in almost all cases, usually to a lesser degree than in acute purulent meningitis; the average was 28 mg/dl in 264 samples. Kennedy and Falton (1979) reported a recent series of cases with closely similar findings. Table 7–5 gives the CSF findings in another series of 35 patients. The data are similar to those just summarized. There was a somewhat higher mortality rate in patients with a greater pleocytosis, but the glucose and protein levels had no predictive value.

There are substantial variations in the CSF findings commensurate with the variations in the initial presentation and the course and stage of the disease. Thus, the CSF may be normal or almost normal in some cases despite the presence of widespread tubercles in the meninges. Kocen and Parsons (1970) suggested that this occurs because miliary cerebral tuberculomas may give rise to neurological symptoms and signs prior to involvement of the leptomeninges. According to various published series, the incidence of a low CSF glucose at the time of the initial puncture has varied from 50 to 95 per cent of patients (Tandon, 1978). The CSF protein also may be normal early in the disease; in advanced stages, spinal subarachnoid block may ensue, with the development of xanthochromic fluid which may have a protein level greater than 1.0 gm/dl.

**TABLE 7–5 Cerebrospinal Fluid Findings on Hospital Admission
in 35 Patients With Tuberculous Meningitis**

		Total	Died	Mortality Rate (Per Cent)
Leukocyte count	<50	3	1 ⎫	20
(per mm³)	51–200	12	2 ⎬	
	201–1,000	19	7 ⎫	40
	>1,000	1	1 ⎭	
Polymorphonuclear cells	0	5	2 ⎫	28
(per cent)	1–25	20	5 ⎬	
	26–50	5	1 ⎫	
	51–75	4	3 ⎬	40
	>75	1	0 ⎭	
Glucose (mg/dl)	0–20	14	5	36
	21–40	12	4	33
	41–60	7	1	
	>60	2	1	
Protein (mg/dl)	0–50	5	3 ⎫	33
	51–100	7	1 ⎭	
	101–200	13	4	31
	>200	10	3	30
Acid-fast	Positive	7	1	
bacilli smear	Negative	25	10	
	Unknown	3	0	
Tubercle bacilli	Positive	26	8	
culture	Negative	8	3	
	Unknown	1	0	

(From Hinman, 1967)

Hemorrhagic CSF has been recorded in rare cases of tuberculous meningitis attributed to fibrinoid degeneration of cortical or meningeal blood vessels (Tandon, 1978). The traditional view that the CSF chloride (see Chapter 6) is specifically depressed in tuberculous meningitis has proved incorrect; the low CSF chloride reflects only the low plasma chloride that often accompanies the disease. There is no diagnostic specificity to the CSF chloride level, and its measurement has been abandoned. The bromide partition test (see Chapter 6), which was viewed as having some value in differentiating the various lymphocytic meningitides from tuberculous meningitis, has recently been reassessed by Rangan and Virmani (1976). It appears to lack sufficient sensitivity or specificity to warrant its use.

Fungal Infections of the Nervous System

The common fungal diseases of the nervous system include cryptococcosis, coccidioidomycosis, candidiasis, and blastomycosis. However, a broad range of other fungi has been reported to involve the nervous system (Fetter *et al.*, 1967;

Rippon, 1978). Neurological involvement is usually characterized by signs of meningitis and cerebritis. There is considerable overlap in the CSF changes associated with both the common and the rare fungal infections. Their differentiation depends upon identification with the appropriate cultures and upon specific immune reactions, usually a complement fixation test (Henry, 1979). The CSF findings in the more common fungal diseases are summarized here.

Cryptococcosis (Torulosis)

The central nervous system manifestations of infection with *Cryptococcus neoformans* are quite variable. The fungus may produce meningitis, meningoencephalitis, or an intracranial mass lesion due to single or multiple granulomas. It often simulates tuberculous meningitis. However, the clinical course is strikingly variable. Fulminant cases may terminate in death within two weeks, or, rarely, the illness may be a very indolent meningeal infection, waxing and waning over many years without treatment.

Weenink and Bruyn (1978) analyzed the literature regarding the natural history of the disease in 465 patients. The CSF changes often parallel the variations in the pattern of the disease. The intracranial pressure is often elevated. The fluid is usually clear, but it may be cloudy and slightly *viscous* when large numbers of yeasts are present. The cell count may be only minimally elevated in some patients despite the presence of many yeasts within the fluid. In most patients, the cell count is moderately elevated, but it rarely exceeds 800 cells per mm^3 (Fetter *et al.*, 1967). The protein is usually elevated, ranging from normal levels to as high as 500 mg or more per dl. The glucose levels are usually depressed to levels between 10 and 40 mg per dl, but normal levels also are seen early in the illness or with localized cerebral granulomas.

The yeast cells may be observed in the CSF in most cases of meningitis, and they are often very numerous. They may be confused with small mononuclear cells and included in the cell count by the unwary observer unless India ink is added to the spinal fluid prior to counting. It is essential that well-filtered India ink be used in these studies to avoid artifacts. The capsules of the yeast are readily seen as transparent halos around spherical or budding cells in such preparations. Carmine stains may also reveal the clear halo that is pathognomonic of the encapsulated yeast. Cryptococci are the only encapsulated fungi that invade the nervous system, and their presence in CSF is usually sufficient for diagnosis. Cultures of the yeast are most readily obtained using agar culture media containing glucose, such as Sabouraud's glucose agar (Weenink and Bruyn, 1978; Henry, 1979). The yeast is virulent for white mice when injected intracerebrally.

An earlier recommendation that the presence of alcohol in the CSF served as a useful index of cryptococcal infection was considered invalid by Wilson *et al.* (1967). The presence of cryptococcal antigen in the CSF is reported to be a reliable guide to diagnosis. In some patients, the detection of the antigen may be the sole means of establishing diagnosis during life. Snow and Dismukes (1975) concluded that if the cryptococcal antigen is present in the CSF in a titer equal to or greater than 1:8 in suspected cases, antifungal therapy should be initiated.

Coccidioidomycosis

Coccidioidomycosis, a systemic fungal infection prevalent only in California, the southwestern United States, Mexico, and Central and South America, is responsible for a subacute or chronic meningitis, often associated with an obstructive hydrocephalus and multiple cerebral granulomas (Ajello, 1977; Goldstein and Lawrence, 1978). The meningeal signs may be minimal or absent despite abnormalities in the CSF, and the pressure is often acutely elevated. It may be reduced late in the course of the disease because of the development of spinal block.

The protein is minimally elevated in 90 per cent of cases early in the course of the illness, but major elevations from 100 to 300 mg per dl and above are observed later. The CSF glucose level, with a normal blood glucose, is usually between 20 and 40 mg per dl. However, early in the disease a normal glucose level is commonly noted. The leukocytic count is variable; it may be below 50 per mm^3 or up to 200 per mm^3 early in the illness; elevations up to several thousand per mm^3 are seen later. In the early stages polymorphonuclear granulocytes predominate; later the response is chiefly mononuclear. Occasionally, an eosinophilia of up to 11 per cent of about 500 white cells has been observed (Pappagianis and Crane, 1977).

The presence of complement fixing antibody to *C. immitis* in the CSF, regardless of the titer, is a very reliable clinical means of diagnosing meningitis because false positive tests are rare. Titers between 1:2 and 1:512 have been recorded in most cases. Pappagianis and Crane (1977) reported a positive complement fixation test in 93 per cent of 47 cases. Recent modifications in the test have reduced the incidence of false negative CSF results to 5 per cent (Goldstein and Lawrence, 1978). Data are lacking regarding the relationship between the antibody titer in CSF and serum in various stages of the illness.

Ventricular, cisternal, and lumbar fluids have been shown to be quite different in patients with coccidioidal meningitis. Thus, the ventricular fluid may have a nearly normal composition despite marked changes in the lumbar fluid. The ventricular fluid may have no complement fixing antibody and a normal glucose level, despite a high titer and a very depressed glucose level in the lumbar fluid. This indicates that the composition of the fluid reflects the degree of inflammatory changes in the adjacent tissue. The ependyma may be spared, despite marked leptomeningeal disease, and the changes in the cisternal fluid may be more abnormal than in lumbar fluid. Ventricular fluid, often obtained from an Ommaya reservoir, may be very misleading as an index to the activity of the disease (Goldstein *et al.*, 1972). Amphotericin B treatment is generally continued as long as complement fixing antibodies are still present in the lumbar fluid. The pleocytosis induced by the intrathecal administration of amphotericin B may make a subsequent cell count an uncertain guide to the activity of the disease.

Candidiasis

Candida infection of the nervous system has been associated with only about 5 of the 80 species of yeast-like fungi (Tveten, 1978). *Candida albicans* has been the causative agent in most cases which present as a subacute meningitis. Black (1970) reviewed 42 patients with intracranial infection by *Candida;* 27 had meningitis, and 15 had direct invasion of the brain with the formation of multiple abscesses and granulomas. The fluid was usually clear and colorless, but it was slightly opalescent and xanthochromic in long-standing cases. Yeast was observed in the CSF sediment; India ink preparations revealed it to be nonencapsulated in contrast to *Torula*.

In general, there is not a close correlation between the clinical findings and the changes in the fluid (Tveten, 1978). A slight to moderate pleocytosis is most common, but cell counts of up to 2000 per mm³ have occurred. The pleocytosis is mixed and predominantly polymorphonuclear in acute forms of the disease; it is mononuclear in more chronic infections (DeVita *et al.*, 1966). The protein level has ranged between 50 and 200 mg/dl in most cases, but levels as high as 940 mg/dl have been reported. An increase in CSF gamma globulins was reported in some cases. The CSF glucose level was reduced in about two thirds of the cases.

Blastomycosis

In North American blastomycosis, the central nervous system was involved in only 6.1 per cent of 668 cases reported in the last 30 years (Leers, 1978). Chronic meningitis and microabscesses were the most common pathological findings. Intracranial hypertension was usually observed. The causative fungus, *Blastomyces dermatiditis,* was rarely seen in the fluid or recovered by culture. Often the diagnosis was not made ante mortem without finding the fungus in biopsies from brain, liver, or skin. With central nervous system involvement, the CSF protein content was generally increased and the glucose content usually normal. There was usually a mixed leukocytic pleocytosis in the fluid.

Viral Meningitis and Encephalitis

The CSF findings are similar in viral encephalitis and meningitis. Their differentiation depends upon clinical features; in many cases there is clinical evidence of involvement of both the meninges and the parenchyma, warranting the use of the term "meningoencephalitis." In *aseptic meningitis* there is an inflammatory CSF without evidence of purulent meningitis. Detailed clinical and laboratory studies are essential to distinguish the various forms of viral meningoencephalitis from infections due to pyogenic bacteria, particularly when antibiotic treatment may have obscured the typical granulocytic response and depressed glucose levels. Tuberculosis, the various fungi, the protozoal diseases, carcinomatous meningitis, and granulomatous diseases such as sarcoidosis also must be differentiated from viral meningoencephalitis. *Mycoplasma pneumoniae* rarely causes a nonviral encephalitis or meningitis, clinically similar to that caused by the viral agents.

The acute viral meningitides and encephalitides are caused by heterogeneous viruses. Table 7–6 lists the major viruses that have been incriminated in these disorders. It should be noted that even the outstanding diagnostic laboratories of the Center for Disease Control at Atlanta in 1976 could not establish the cause of the encephalitis in 71 per cent of the diagnosed cases (Ho, 1978).

PRESSURE.   The CSF pressure is normal or increased in the various meningoencephalitides. There are no specific correlations with either the etiological

TABLE 7–6 Viruses Responsible for Meningitis and Encephalitis

DNA Viruses
HERPESVIRUSES
    Herpes simplex virus, Type 1 and 2
    B virus
    Varicella-zoster virus
    Cytomegalovirus
    Epstein-Barr virus
ADENOVIRUSES
POXVIRUSES
    Variola and vaccinia
PAPOVAVIRUSES
RNA Viruses
MYXOVIRUSES
    Influenza virus
    Parainfluenza virus
PARAMYXOVIRUSES
    Mumps virus
    Rubeola (measles) virus
RHABDOVIRUSES
    Rabies
ARENAVIRUSES
    Lymphocytic choriomeningitis virus
PICORNAVIRUSES
    Enteroviruses
        Polioviruses, Types 1, 2, 3
        Coxsackie A virus, Types 1–23
        Coxsackie B virus, Types 1–6
        ECHO virus, Types 1–32
    Rhinoviruses
TOGA VIRUSES
    Non-Arthropod-Borne
        Rubella virus
    Arthropod-Borne
        Togavirus A
            Eastern equine encephalitis virus
            Venezuelan equine encephalitis virus
            Western equine encephalitis virus
        Togavirus B
            Dengue virus
            St. Louis encephalitis virus
            Murray Valley encephalitis virus
            Japanese B encephalitis virus
            Russian Spring-summer encephalitis virus
            Yellow fever virus
        Bunyamera Group C
            California encephalitis virus

agent or the clinical syndrome. During the acute phase, with fever, dramatic meningeal signs, and an inflammatory fluid, elevations from 200 mm to 400 mm or more are common. Herpes simplex encephalitis may be responsible for marked intracranial hypertension because of its predilection for causing focal cerebritis and edema in the temporal lobes with mass effects.

CELL COUNT. The cellular response is generally greatest in patients with predominant signs of meningeal irritation. Patients with signs chiefly suggestive of parenchymatous disease without signs of meningeal involvement often have very few cells present in the CSF, 5 to 10 per mm³, or no increase in cell count. The differential cell count is predominantly lymphocytic and mononuclear in type. However, in the most acute stages of viral meningitis, polymorphonuclear granulocytes may predominate. When this occurs, it may be difficult to differentiate between a viral and a bacterial cause, particularly with a partially treated bacterial meningitis. The total cell count may be increased to levels of 1000 white cells per mm³ and more. In lymphocytic choriomeningitis, counts as high as 3000 per mm³ have been reported, and such high counts suggest this viral agent.

PROTEIN.   The protein level is usually mildly increased to 50 to 80 mg/dl in many cases of viral meningitis. However, both normal protein levels and increased levels, 80 to 200 mg/dl and higher, are not unusual. The electrophoretic analyses of the CSF reveal either the pattern of increased entry of plasma protein or a mild or moderate increase in immunoglobulin (IgA and IgG) content. Table 7–3 (page 258) summarizes such changes in IgM, IgA, and IgG content. No specific correlations have been determined between the protein level and the viral agent, the prognosis, or the changes in immunoglobulin level.

GLUCOSE.   The CSF glucose is characteristically normal in most cases of viral meningoencephalitides. However, there are definite exceptions to this generalization. Wilfert (1969) reported that 25 per cent of patients with mumps meningoencephalitis had CSF glucose levels between 20 and 40 mg/dl. Uncommonly, a depressed glucose level has also been described in herpes simplex encephalitis (Illis and Gostling, 1972; Sarubbi *et al.*, 1973). A depression in the CSF glucose has been rarely reported in herpes zoster meningoencephalitis (Wolf, 1974). While the clinician needs to be aware of these exceptions, depressed glucose levels should not be presumed to be due to these viral infections except by exclusion of the more common causes of hypoglycorrhachia. See Table 6–11 (p. 212).

Cytomegalic Inclusion Disease

The neurologic and systemic manifestations of cytomegalic inclusion disease are quite diverse; they include meningitis, encephalitis, acute polyneuritis, labyrinthitis, and idiopathic facial paralysis (Dorfman, 1978). In many cases of meningoencephalitis, the CSF revealed nonspecific changes of an aseptic meningitis. The CSF changes in patients with acute polyneuropathy are indistinguishable from the findings in other cases of acute polyneuritis; that is, the protein level is elevated in most cases, ranging as high as 360 mg/dl without a significant pleocytosis.

Rabies

In a recent review, Atanasiu and Gamet (1978) described the CSF findings in rabies as follows: the CSF is generally under increased pressure; the cell count may be normal, or there may be a mild pleocytosis with as many as 125 mononuclear cells per mm³; the protein may be slightly increased; and the glucose is normal. Thus, the CSF findings in rabies are similar to those in most cases of benign forms of meningoencephalitis.

Herpes Simplex Encephalitis

Although there are no pathognomonic changes in the CSF in herpes simplex encephalitis, the fluid is abnormal in most cases. Illis and Gostling (1972) analyzed the CSF changes in 131 reported cases. The fluid had a normal cell count and protein level on first examination in 10 per cent of the cases. This relatively high incidence of a normal fluid is disquieting, because it serves to delay early diagnosis, which would facilitate the use of antiviral agents. At first puncture, the total cell count was usually 50 to 100 cells per mm^3. In 10 of 131 cases, the cell count was between 1000 and 3000 per mm^3. The cell count was predominantly lymphocytic, though in the early stages polymorphonuclear leukocytes were at times "numerous."

The total white cell count in the CSF tended to rise with the length of the illness, but this tendency was less marked than the rise of protein as the illness progressed. The relationship between the cellular reaction and the protein level was not linear. The finding of red blood cells in the CSF in the absence of a traumatic puncture was not unusual. The authors concluded that in about 40 per cent of the cases red cells were found on the first examination; in about 11 per cent xanthochromia was noted. Red cells and xanthochromia, when present, serve to distinguish herpes simplex encephalitis from most other forms of viral encephalitis. The differentiation between subarachnoid bleeding and a traumatic lumbar puncture is imperative in such cases.

At first examination, the protein level was moderately raised, between 50 and 90 mg/dl in half the cases; it was within normal limits in about 25 per cent of the cases, and between 90 and 410 mg/dl in about 25 per cent of the cases. There was a distinct tendency for the protein level to increase with time after the onset of the encephalitis. The CSF glucose was moderately reduced in a small number of cases; this occurrence has rarely been reported in other forms of encephalitis except for mumps and herpes zoster. Of 224 patients with herpes encephalitis, 46 per cent had signs of meningeal irritation that usually appeared 4 to 11 days after the onset of encephalitis. The overall mortality in cases of herpes encephalitis was 70 per cent, independently of the age of the patient.

Although patients with herpes encephalitis associated with intracranial hypertension and evidence of subarachnoid hemorrhage are very seriously ill, the CSF changes have *not* been shown to have specific prognostic significance in any given patient. An increased CSF level of gamma globulin has been seen in some cases; its precise incidence and the time of its occurrence have not been well defined.

Mollaret's Meningitis

Mollaret's benign recurrent aseptic meningitis is a rare disorder characterized by recurrent attacks of fever and signs of meningeal irritation. The attacks generally last several days and are separated by symptom-free intervals which may last for weeks, months, or years. The disease persists for an average of 3 to 5 years; the number of attacks varies greatly, with an average of 5, although dozens of attacks have been recorded in individual patients (Frederiks and Bruyn, 1978). During the attacks, there is a pleocytosis and some elevation of the CSF protein (usually 70 to 100 mg/dl), but the glucose level has usually remained normal. According to the review by Frederiks and Bruyn (1978), the cell count during an attack ranged from 200 to several thousand per mm^3. Most cells have been mononuclear, but a granulocytic response as high as 35 per cent has also been noted. The presence of some large endothelial cells during the few days of the attack has been emphasized (Mollaret, 1977); however, they rapidly disappeared, and their presence was not considered essential for the diagnosis. A rise in the gamma globulin level has been reported in a few cases. Studies to establish an etiology have thus far been unrewarding.

Nervous System Complications of Varicella-Zoster Virus

The neurological complications of varicella-zoster virus infections include meningoencephalitis, acute cerebellar ataxia, cranial neuropathies, myelitis, polyradiculitis, and polyneuritis (McKendall and Klawans, 1978). Johnson and Milbourn (1970) analyzed the CSF findings in 52 patients having varicella with meningoencephalitis and with the syndrome of acute cerebellar ataxia. The CSF showed a predominantly lymphocytic pleocytosis ranging from 0 to 2795 cells per mm^3; 80 per cent of the patients had fewer than 100 cells. The pleocytosis was somewhat greater in patients with meningoencephalitis than in those with acute cerebellar ataxia. The protein levels were normal or mildly elevated; levels between 100 and 175 mg/dl were uncommon. Similar CSF changes have been reported with myelitis. A low-grade pleocytosis was a common finding in acute segmental herpes zoster; counts as high as 600 per mm^3 were noted in over one half of the patients (Thomas and Howard, 1972). Such findings are in accord with the pathological evidence of inflammation involving the spinal ganglion, anterior and posterior nerve roots, adjacent leptomeninges, and spinal cord. Varicella-zoster antigen was demonstrated in CSF cells by indirect immunofluorescent staining in 9 of 11 cases of herpes zoster (Peters et al., 1979). This technique may prove useful in establishing the diagnosis.

Poliomyelitis

The CSF findings in 115 cases of acute poliomyelitis were thoroughly analyzed by Merritt and Fremont-Smith (1938). The pressure varied between 60 and 600 mm; it was less than 150 mm in one third of the patients, between 150 and 200 mm in one third, and greater than 200 mm in the remaining third. Only 2 patients had a pressure greater than 300 mm. Intracranial hypertension was found most often in patients with paralytic respiratory insufficiency, which presumably was responsible for hypercarbia.

The cell count varied greatly with the stage of the disease. It was highest in the *preparalytic stage,* when it averaged 185 white cells per mm^3. During the preparalytic stage until less than seven days after the onset of paralysis, cell counts below 10 per mm^3 occurred in only 2 per cent of the patients. There were more than 300 cells in only 7 per cent and more than 500 cells in only 3 of the 115 cases. The average count fell to 50 cells per mm^3 one week and to 5 cells per mm^3 one month after the onset of the paralysis. Polymorphonuclear leukocytes predominated early in the disease in some cases, particularly in the preparalytic stage, but approximately 80 per cent of the cases studied during the first five days of the illness showed a lymphocytic predominance. Red cells were not observed (apart from those induced by needle trauma).

The protein level was normal or moderately increased during the early stages of the illness. In 98 patients studied during the preparalytic stage or less than seven days after the onset of the paralysis, the average protein level was 47 mg/dl, ranging between 12 and 200 mg/dl. It was normal in 60 of the 98 patients and greater than 100 mg/dl in only 4 patients. As the disease progressed, there was generally an increase in the CSF protein level for the first two or three weeks.

The highest protein level recorded in this series of patients was 366 mg/dl. The highest levels were recorded between the twentieth and thirtieth day of the paralytic illness, when the average level was 164 mg/dl. This was followed by a gradual fall. After the second month, most proteins had fallen to normal levels, but persistent elevations were also noted. The mechanism for the delay in onset of the elevated protein content was not established. Merritt and Fremont-Smith (1938) did not observe any relationship between the degree of any CSF abnormality and the presence or severity of paralysis or the site of paralysis when present. A mild elevation in gamma globulin content (midzone colloidal gold curve) was observed in some patients. The glucose levels were normal.

Chemical Meningitis and Spinal Arachnoiditis

Spinal arachnoiditis is an acute, subacute, or chronic disorder in which an inflammatory process involves the spinal cord, the cauda equina, or both. It has been reported as a direct consequence of a spinal injection of an anesthetic agent, an antibiotic or other drug, or a radiographic contrast medium. In some instances, the chemical meningitis was attributed to contamination of the syringe with a detergent. At times the cause of the arachnoiditis cannot be established. Whisler (1978) has reviewed the literature regarding various agents that have been incriminated following their intrathecal injection. These have included procaine, sulfonamides, antibiotics, methotrexate, and corticosteroids in a depot preparation. The various radiographic agents used in myelography have been implicated in several reports. The water soluble contrast medium metrizamide was less likely to induce adhesive arachnoiditis than was oily contrast media (Hansen *et al.*, 1978). Blood in the CSF appears to increase the likelihood of the development of arachnoiditis following injection of radiographic contrast media. This observation is the basis for the admonition to defer the injection of contrast media when there is a bloody tap unless the need is very urgent, as in a case of acute cord compression.

The results of manometric spinal fluid examination may be normal or may give evidence of a partial or complete spinal block. The latter occurs more often with chronic arachnoiditis. In such cases, the initial pressure is usually low or nonobtainable, and the jugular compression test (see Chapter 5) may be mildly or strongly positive. There is almost always a mild or moderate pleocytosis, largely lymphocytic. In acute chemical meningitis, polymorphonuclear granulocytes may predominate, and a mild eosinophilia may also be seen. The protein level is usually increased to a variable degree. In some cases of chemical meningitis due to iodinated albumin, the glucose level has been reduced despite sterile cultures. This suggests that the sterile inflammation induces an increased rate of glycolysis in the adjacent spinal cord.

Barnes and Fish (1972) reported 5 cases of acute chemical meningitis occurring in 50 patients undergoing lumbar cisternography in which radiolabelled serum albumin was used. This was severe enough to cause fever and meningeal signs in the 5 affected patients. The CSF showed a normal to mildly elevated pressure, pleocytosis from 96 to 6400 polymorphonuclear leukocytes, an elevated protein (112 to 550 mg/dl), and in 1 case a glucose of 20 mg per dl. The CSF was sterile. It took about 2 weeks for the CSF to become clear.

EFFECTS OF PNEUMOENCEPHALOGRAPHY. The injection of air for pneumoencephalography into the CSF elicits an inflammatory reaction. The largest number of cells seen 30 minutes later has been 30 per mm^3 (Marrack *et al.*, 1961). These were chiefly mononuclear in type. Up to 300 or more leukocytes per mm^3 were observed several hours after infection. At 24 hours, the cells consisted chiefly of neutrophils, changing to mononuclear cells over the ensuing 48 to 72 hours as the cell counts fell toward normal. Mild elevations in protein commonly persist more than 24 or 48 hours. In the past, the injection of large volumes of air (50 to 80 ml) caused a greater inflammatory response than that observed with the smaller volumes currently used (Bickerstaff, 1951).

Meningism

The syndrome of *meningism* has rarely been referred to in recent clinical literature, although the term was commonly used in the past. It was loosely applied to patients with headache and signs and symptoms of meningeal irritation in the absence of bacterial, fungal, or viral meningitis, i.e., with a normal CSF composition. Merritt and Fremont-Smith's (1938) use of the term included patients with a CSF pleocytosis of up to 18 mononuclear cells per mm^3. Some early reports failed to exclude patients with a parameningeal infection, such as mastoiditis or lateral sinus thrombosis. I would limit the use of the term to describe the syndrome of headache and signs of meningeal irritation in patients with an acute febrile illness, usually viral, in whom the CSF examination reveals a normal cell count, protein level, and glucose level. The CSF pressure is commonly elevated. *Meningism* differs from *meningismus*; the latter refers to the symptoms and signs of meningeal irritation that occurs with meningitis. Meningismus may also be seen with fever and systemic infections without meningeal involvement. Meningism is most often seen in children or young adults, and it often proves diagnostically confusing.

Merritt and Fremont-Smith (1938) described the findings in 70 patients who were considered to have meningism. About half the patients were under the age of 10, and 80 per cent were under the age of 20. The pressure was recorded in 44 patients; in 10 patients it was between 250 and 500 mm. The cell count was normal in 51 of 63 fluids examined. (A slight pleocytosis was noted in 12 instances, ranging between 6 and 18 cells; I believe the diagnosis in these patients is suspect. They probably had a viral meningitis.) The protein level was normal or greatly reduced. The lumbar CSF protein levels were below 10 mg/dl in 7 patients, below 15 mg in 25, and below 20 mg in 43. The only other abnormality described was the frequent occurrence of a reduced CSF chloride level. However, the corresponding serum chloride levels were not reported.

There is no satisfactory explanation for the syndrome. Merritt and

Fremont-Smith (1938) considered acute hypotonicity of the serum to account for it. While an acute episode of inappropriate secretion of antidiuretic hormone (not described until 1957) might have accounted for some cases, the pathophysiology remains obscure. The low CSF protein is probably secondary to the intracranial hypertension, as discussed in Chapter 6. It is possible that an increased rate of CSF formation occurs in some cases, but this is just a speculation for which there is no evidence. It is difficult to assess the frequency of occurrence of the syndrome.

In summary, the diagnosis of *meningism* is one of exclusion. Meningism describes the occurrence of headache, meningeal signs, and a normal CSF commonly under increased pressure, in association with an acute, febrile, systemic illness. It is usually brief in duration, and at times the diagnostic lumbar puncture appears to be therapeutic, i.e., it is followed by prompt improvement in the presenting symptoms.

Infectious Mononucleosis

The incidence of neurological manifestations of infectious mononucleosis has varied greatly in different reports. CSF abnormalities have been observed in as many as 26 per cent of patients in a series of 164 cases (Silverstein, 1978). Symptomatic neurological involvement in other large series has been reported to occur less often, occurring in 5.5 to 7.3 per cent of patients. Gautier-Smith (1965) classified the neurological complications as follows: lymphocytic meningitis, encephalomyelitis, polyneuritis, and mononeuritis. The CSF findings varied corresponding to the type of neurological involvement. With lymphocytic meningitis, intracranial hypertension was noted. Pleocytosis, usually between 10 and 150 lymphocytes per mm^3, was observed in patients with lymphocytic meningitis as well as in patients with encephalomyelitis. Finkel (1965) reported atypical lymphocytes in the CSF identical to those in the peripheral blood. A mild to moderate increase in total protein content has also been observed in patients with meningitis or encephalomyelitis. At times the elevation in protein content has been delayed until the cell count returned to normal in the third or fourth week of the illness. In patients with polyneuritis, the CSF findings were the same as those observed in the idiopathic Guillain-Barré syndrome (see Polyneuritis). Gautier-Smith (1965) did not find the CSF changes to be a reliable guide to the course of the illness.

Behçet's Syndrome

The literature regarding Behçet's syndrome, thoroughly reviewed by Alema (1978), indicates that the rate of neurological involvement has varied between 10 and 25 per cent in different series. In patients with characteristic mucocutaneous (orogenital) lesions and ocular involvement (uveitis), the neurological manifestations have been quite varied. They may simulate multiple sclerosis, with evidence of multifocal involvement of the nervous system, including pyramidal tract and brain stem signs. In some patients, signs of meningoencephalitis predominate. Similarly, the CSF findings were also quite varied. They include most often a mild pleocytosis and elevated protein. Alema (1978) has summarized Gherardi's earlier analysis of 36 patients. The pleocytosis varied between 10 and 200 leukocytes per mm³ in 27 per cent of the patients. The protein alone was elevated in 19 per cent, and there was an increase in both cells and protein in 37 per cent. The gamma globulin (colloidal gold test) was "frequently" elevated, which represents another similarity to the findings in multiple sclerosis and other inflammatory disorders of the nervous system.

Vogt-Koyanagi-Harada Syndrome

The Vogt-Koyanagi-Harada (VKH) syndrome is a rare disorder characterized by inflammation of the uvea, the retinal pigment epithelium, and the meninges. In some patients there is also evidence of encephalitis, involvement of the 2nd and 8th cranial nerves, and hair and skin changes, including poliosis, canities, alopecia, and vitiligo. Manor (1978) has reviewed the clinical and cerebrospinal fluid findings. The most constant abnormal laboratory finding was a CSF pleocytosis in 29 of 36 patients in whom the CSF was examined. Even with no clinical evidence of neurological involvement, pleocytosis was usually present. The pleocytosis ranged between 4 and 700 cells per mm³, mostly lymphocytes. Five of 29 patients had cell counts between 300 and 700 per mm³, and 11 of 29 patients had cell counts that were less than 100 per mm³. The CSF protein content was either normal or slightly increased. An elevated CSF gamma globulin level was reported in some cases, but its frequency has not been established because in most reports (found chiefly in the ophthalmological literature) it was not measured. The CSF pressure was mildly elevated in some cases, but the frequency of this finding is not known. The CSF glucose level was normal, and no specific inflammatory agent or serological responses have been reported.

Subacute Sclerosing Panencephalitis

Subacute sclerosing panencephalitis (SSPE) is a chronic encephalitis associated with the measles virus. The encephalitis is insidious in onset and progresses very slowly; it is a usually fatal disease of childhood and adolescence which runs a course of 3 to 4 years in 80 per cent of cases (Zeman, 1978). A variety of eponyms has been used in the past, including Dawson's disease, and it is likely that a case of "encephalitis periaxialis diffusa" described by Schilder represented a case of SSPE (Lumsden, 1972).

The CSF findings serve as a strong clue to the diagnosis. The CSF pressure is normal, the protein level is normal or slightly increased, and the cell count is usually normal. However, there is a strikingly elevated concentration of the gamma globulin content, composing usually 20 to 50 per cent of the total protein and associated with oligoclonal bands in the immunoglobulin range as demonstrated by agarose gel electrophoresis (Norrby and Vandvik, 1975). These bands were shown to represent antibodies to measles virus, formed within the central nervous system. The CSF findings are analogous to those observed in progressive rubella panencephalitis.

Progressive Rubella Panencephalitis

Progressive rubella panencephalitis (PRP) is a rare chronic progressive encephalitis that occurs subacutely in adolescents and young adults and is associated with rubella virus infection of the brain. Wolinsky (1978) summarized the literature regarding the CSF changes that provide clues to the diagnosis. The fluid is under normal pressure; it usually contains a mild lymphocytic pleocytosis (less than 37 cells per mm^3) and has a mild elevation of protein (60 to 142 mg/dl). The most striking finding is the greatly increased concentration of gamma globulin, composing 35 to 52 per cent of the total protein. Agarose gel electrophoresis reveals an oligoclonal pattern with several distinct bands in the gamma globulin range. These bands have been selectively absorbed by rubella-infected cell packs. Rubella antibody titers, measured with hemagglutination inhibition or complement fixation techniques, have been elevated in both serum and CSF. The concentration ratio of antibody in the two compartments (serum to CSF) has ranged between 8 and 32, in contrast to the immunoglobulin concentration ratio in normal subjects of about 200. The marked elevation in the CSF concentration cannot be attributed to increased entry from the plasma, because the CSF albumin and total protein are little affected. The decreased ratio indicates the local production of the antibody within the central nervous system, where immunoglobulin-containing plasma cells have been demonstrated. Thus, the striking increase in the gamma globulin content serves as a strong clue to the diagnosis in suspected cases. Increases of similar magnitude (35 to 52 per cent) are rarely seen in any other disease apart from subacute sclerosing panencephalitis.

Pertussis Encephalopathy
(Postinfectious and Postimmunization)

While pertussis has become an uncommon disease in the United States, it is still a childhood disease with a high rate of morbidity and mortality, due to an encephalopathy of diverse causes, in countries without universal immunization (Swisher, 1978). Pleocytosis in the CSF is the major laboratory finding according to most published series of cases. Zellweger (1959) noted 5 to 45 cells in 10 of 21 patients, and a mild elevation of protein, as high as 101 mg/dl, in 17 of 21 patients. The cells were almost always lymphocytes. The incidence of CSF pleocytosis was 50 per cent in pertussis encephalopathy with seizures (Celermajer and Brown, 1966).

Leptospirosis and Weil's Disease

The leptospiral infections may cause a variety of neurological syndromes, including meningoencephalitis, aseptic meningitis, and Weil's disease, which is characterized also by hepatitis and icterus. With acute leptospirosis, evidence of meningitis was observed in 68 per cent to 90 per cent of patients in various series (Gsell, 1978). (The continental literature, summarized by Gsell, refers to serous meningitis, pseudotumor, and meningism as manifestations of leptospirosis, usually implying the findings of an aseptic lymphocytic meningitis.) Cargill and Beeson (1947) reported an abnormal CSF in 13 of 14 patients with Weil's disease, 6 of whom had clinical signs of meningitis. In acute leptospirosis, the CSF was usually normal until the 4th or 5th day of illness, when pleocytosis appeared. The cell count then rose with a mild pleocytosis, usually 15 to 100 cells, although much higher counts have been observed. In various series the granulocytes predominated initially, but the cellular response then became lymphocytic. The protein increase was also delayed in onset and then rose to levels as high as 100 mg/dl. An increase in gamma globulin has also been reported. The CSF glucose is also depressed with leptospiral meningitis, with a variable incidence reported. In Weil's disease, subarachnoid hemorrhage has also been documented. Gsell's (1978) recent review provides an excellent bibliography regarding the neurological complications of leptospirosis and the CSF findings therein.

Brucellosis

Brucellosis has heterogeneous effects on the nervous system; it has been responsible for encephalitis, meningitis, vascular syndromes, myelopathy, cranial neuritis, radiculitis, and neuritis (Sahs, 1978). In meningitis, the CSF is cloudy or xanthochromic and, in most reports, under increased pressure. Pleocytosis of 200 to 400 or more cells, elevated protein level, and depressed glucose level have also been observed. As expected, the brucella agglutination titers in the CSF are much lower than in the blood.

Neurosyphilis

In the prepenicillin era, the CSF findings were considered essential for the diagnosis and appropriate management of neurosyphilis. In recent years, the ease of treatment with penicillin has diminished the dependency on the CSF findings, and relatively few recent published data deal with the subject. However, the Center for Disease Control (CDC) in 1976 stated that the CSF examination is "mandatory" in patients with suspected symptomatic neurosyphilis. The CDC stated further that CSF examination is also desirable in patients with syphilis of greater than one year's duration, to exclude asymptomatic neurosyphilis. The CDC also recommended CSF examination in infants with congenital syphilis before treatment and as part of the last follow-up visit after treatment with alternative antibiotics, when penicillin cannot be used because of drug allergy.

In their definitive monograph regarding neurosyphilis in the prepenicillin era, Merritt, Adams, and Solomon (1946) emphasized that knowledge of the CSF findings was essential for the appropriate diagnosis and treatment of the disease. Their extensive data regarding the CSF findings in various stages of the disease compose the most complete information available, and much of the laboratory data presented here is extracted from their work. Similar CSF findings in 770 luetic patients were also described by Locoge and Cumings (1958). The changes in neurosyphilis will be presented in relation to the various forms of the disease: early syphilis (primary and secondary stages), latent period, asymptomatic neurosyphilis, meningeal neurosyphilis (acute or subacute syphilitic meningitis), gumma, meningovascular neurosyphilis, meningovascular syphilis of the spinal cord, paretic neurosyphilis, and tabes dorsalis.

Serological Tests for Syphilis

The serological diagnosis of syphilis depends on the demonstration of antibodies, either (1) the nonspecific, nontreponemal globulin complex called *reagin antibodies,* or (2) the *specific treponemal antibodies.*

The reagin tests depend upon the combination of reagin in the patient's serum with an antigen composed of a suspension of cardiolipin activated by the addition of cholesterol and lecithin. There are two types of reagin tests: flocculation tests and complement fixation tests. The original diagnostic test for syphilis developed by Wassermann was a complement fixation test, as is the Kolmer test, which has also been widely used. The flocculation tests depend on the precipitation of reagin with various colloidal lipid antigens. The Venereal Disease Research Laboratory (VDRL) test developed by the United States Public Health Service, which is perhaps in greatest use as a screening test, employs cardiolipin antigen for either a slide test or a tube test (Storm-Mathisen, 1978). Both qualitative and quantitative tests are available; the response to therapy is indicated by a falling titer measured with a quantitative test. However, sero-resistant cases have a persistent titer despite adequate therapy. Reagin is first detected in the serum about 4 to 6 weeks after infection, or 1 to 3 weeks after appearance of the chancre. Positive reagin tests in CSF are considered to be virtually diagnostic of neurosyphilis in the absence of contamination of the fluid with blood, but a positive test does not differentiate between active or inactive (treated) forms of the disease.

A false positive response may occur with acute bacterial or viral infections and following vaccination for smallpox. Chronic false positive reactions occur with many autoimmune diseases, including systemic lupus erythematosus, thyroiditis, and hemolytic anemia. Leprosy and the various nonvenereal treponemal diseases, such as yaws and pinta, often give positive reagin tests as well (Storm-Mathisen, 1978). The incidence of false positive reactions has been variously estimated at 3 to 40 per cent (Sparling, 1971), making the more specific tests of special importance.

SPECIFIC TREPONEMAL ANTIBODY TESTS. These tests use treponemal antigens and therefore are more specific for luetic infection than are the reagin tests. The Treponema Pallidum Immobilization (TPI) test depends upon the ability of antibodies in the serum of syphilitic patients, in the presence of complement, to inhibit the normal movements of virulent spirochetes. It has been viewed as the standard of specific tests, but it is technically difficult and not generally suitable for routine clinical use. The test becomes positive somewhat later than do the reagin tests in early syphilis; then the TPI generally remains positive permanently despite vigorous antiluetic treatment.

Several fluorescent tests which use dead treponemes are now widely used. These tests use a drop of a virulent suspension of *T. pallidum,* dried and fixed upon a slide, to which is added a sample of the patient's serum. If antibodies are present, the treponemes become coated with a layer of antibody globulin. This is detected by the addition of a fluorescein-labelled antiserum, which unites with the coated treponemes and allows their identification by the appearance of fluorescence with dark field illumination. The initial test, the Fluorescent Treponema Antibody (FIA) test, gave a considerable number of false positive reactions because of the presence in many normal subjects of a "group antibody" to a number of nonpathogenic treponemes.

The Fluorescent Treponemal Antibody Absorption (FTA-ABS) test, now widely used, is an improvement of the former test. It blocks the action of group antibody by dilution of the patient's serum with an extract of Reiter treponemes (nonpathogens), thus leaving only specific antibody free to combine with the antigens of *Treponema pallidum*. The FTA-ABS test has been viewed as the most specific test for luetic infection; it provides a positive result in all diagnostic categories. However, it requires technical skill, and it does not readily provide quantitative data (Sparling, 1971; King and Nicol, 1975; Storm-Mathisen, 1978).

The various serological tests using serum have also been applied to the study of the CSF. A positive reagin test reaction in CSF is generally considered evidence of either asymptomatic or symptomatic neurosyphilis, except that a positive CSF reagin test may be observed in purulent (nonsyphilitic) meningitis, which would allow serum reagin to cross the barrier in sufficient concentration. The normal blood-CSF barrier allows the appearance in CSF of immunoglobulins to only 0.1 per cent to 0.2 per cent of the plasma level.

Although various laboratories have performed either the FTA or the FTA-ABS on CSF, there is little rationale for performing either, because both tests depend upon the presence of circulating immunoglobulins derived from the serum (Traviesa *et al.*, 1978). Thus, while the serum FTA-ABS appears to be highly suited for case detection, there appears to be no place for either routine FTA-ABS or FTA testing of CSF, because the antibody present represents only a dilute serum sample. The report of Jaffe *et al.* (1978) also supports this generalization. (There have been occasional reports of positive CSF tests with a negative plasma test [Kolar and Burkhart, 1977]). These are presumed to represent technical errors.) In patients with symptomatic or asymptomatic neurosyphilis, Wilkenson (1973) found that the CSF FTA-ABS test was positive in 67 per cent of cases, a higher rate than observed with two reagin tests, the VDRL and the Wassermann; however, it is presumed that such patients would all have had positive serum FTA-ABS tests. There seems to be no basis for applying the FTA-ABS test to CSF in clinical practice.

COLLOIDAL GOLD TEST. The colloidal gold test, an empirically developed test for qualitative changes in the CSF proteins (see Chapter 6), differentiated the first-zone, midzone, and end-zone (third-zone) patterns. The three patterns were also termed the paretic, tabetic, and meningitic curves respectively, based on the assumption that the appearance of these patterns correlated with the presence of these diseases, e.g., with general paresis, tabes dorsalis, and a nonluetic inflammatory meningitis (see Chapter 6).

The colloidal gold test is now considered to be outmoded, because it is insensitive to increased gamma globulin when compared with various electrophoretic methods. However, much of the older literature regarding neurosyphilis dealt extensively with the colloidal gold test. In referring to this literature, the term "elevation in gamma globulin" will be substituted for both a first-zone (paretic) gold curve, and a midzone (tabetic) gold curve.

EFFECT OF BLOOD ON CSF SEROLOGICAL REACTIONS.   The effect of a bloody tap upon the serological reactions in CSF has been clarified by Jaffe *et al.* (1978). When blood with a high titer and positive VDRL reaction was diluted with normal CSF, the CSF FTA-ABS test became positive with as few as 2400 red cells per ml. Thus, a false positive CSF serological finding may be obtained with a bloody tap. The minimal number of red cells necessary depends upon the serological titer present in the blood. Davis and Sperry (1979) have determined that the minimal volumes of blood required to turn the various CSF serological tests positive are as follows: Kahn, 30 μl; Wassermann, 10 μl; VDRL, 3 μl; and CSF-FTA, 0.8 μl.

Luetic Syndromes

EARLY SYPHILIS (PRIMARY AND SECONDARY STAGES).   Involvement of the CSF is commonly noted when early syphilis is diagnosed, i.e., during the first six months after the primary infection. The most common abnormality noted is a mild pleocytosis, but an increased protein level, a positive Wassermann reaction, and a slight increase in gamma globulin are also noted. The pleocytosis is generally less than 100 lymphocytes per mm³, although higher cell counts are also observed. The frequency of an abnormal CSF in early syphilis is variable. Merritt *et al.* (1946) summarized the findings in several reports; in some series, as high as 35 per cent of the patients had an abnormal CSF prior to the appearance of a secondary rash; however, a lower incidence of only 9 per cent was also reported. A further increase in the incidence of such changes was reported to occur with the appearance of a secondary rash. These CSF findings often revert to normal during the latent period, after the disappearance of the secondary cutaneous manifestations. Thus, transient abnormalities in the CSF occur frequently with both primary and secondary syphilis.

LATENT PERIOD.   During the latent period, which as a rule has a duration of many years prior to the development of asymptomatic or symptomatic neuro-syphilis, the CSF is normal by definition.

ASYMPTOMATIC NEUROSYPHILIS.   Asymptomatic neurosyphilis is the term applied to patients without clinical signs or symptoms of syphilis of the nervous system but with abnormalities in the CSF attributable to the disease. The incidence of asymptomatic neurosyphilis in untreated cases is greatest in the second or third year of the infection. Thereafter, the occurrence of symptomatic neurosyphilis is likely to increase in the absence of antiluetic treatment.

Merritt *et al.* (1946) described the CSF findings in 200 patients with asymptomatic neurosyphilis, all of whom had received prior antiluetic therapy and had normal neurological examinations. They noted that 37 per cent had a pleocytosis between 5 and 100 white cells; 3 per cent had 100 to 200 white cells. A minor increase in protein content was noted in 40 per cent of the cases, and 82 per cent had a gamma globulin increase. The Wassermann reaction was negative in 16 per cent of these cases. (One wonders how the authors could have made a reliable diagnosis of asymptomatic neurosyphilis without a positive CSF serological finding!). Thus, in asymptomatic neurosyphilis, active inflammation as indicated by a pleocytosis might be either absent or present. They concluded that inflammatory changes in the fluid in patients with presumed asymptomatic neurosyphilis was an indication for additional antiluetic therapy.

Acute or Subacute Syphilitic Meningitis. Merritt *et al.* (1946) described the CSF findings in 80 patients with acute or subacute syphilitic meningitis. The time of occurrence of the luetic meningitis following the primary lesion varied greatly; it was less than one year in about two thirds of the patients, but latent intervals of as many as 20 years were also reported. The CSF pressure was increased to levels above 200 mm in 65 per cent of patients. The cell counts varied in the 80 patients; 40 per cent had a pleocytosis of 500 to 2000 mononuclear cells per mm^3; the balance had counts between 10 and 500 per mm^3. The colloidal gold test result was abnormal in 96 per cent of patients, and the Wassermann reaction was positive in 86 per cent. The glucose content was recorded in 31 patients with acute syphilitic meningitis; it was less than 30 mg/dl in 10 per cent and between 31 and 40 mg/dl in 35 per cent of these patients. The appearance of a few eosinophils in the CSF in meningovascular syphilis has been reported by subsequent investigators (Oehmichen, 1976).

Gumma. Cerebral gumma is rarely seen in contemporary clinical practice. The manifestations in the CSF include intracranial hypertension, increased protein content to a mild or moderate degree, increased CSF gamma globulin content, and a positive Wassermann reaction (Merritt *et al.*, 1946). Thus, the findings simulate those associated with cerebral glioma. The findings in patients with a gumma of the spinal cord are similar to those just listed, except that the pressure is normal, and there may be evidence of spinal subarachnoid hemorrhage.

Meningovascular Syphilis (Cerebrovascular Neurosyphilis). In cerebrovascular neurosyphilis, the clinical signs result from the lesions of ischemic infarction. The CSF findings are dependent upon the degree of meningeal reaction which accompanies the vascular disease. The findings in 42 cases were described by Merritt *et al.* (1946). In the majority of patients, only a minor degree of meningeal involvement was noted. The CSF pressure was normal in 85 per cent of patients. Sixty per cent of patients had a pleocytosis, varying between 11 and 100 cells per mm^3, almost all of which were mononuclear cells. An increase in protein was noted in 66 per cent of patients, varying between 45 and 260 mg/dl; it was greater than 100 mg/dl in 25 per cent. The gamma globulin was increased in 75 per cent of patients. The Wassermann reaction was positive in 81 per cent. The findings in luetic involvement of the spinal cord (meningomyelitis and spinal artery thrombosis) were similar, with the frequent occurrence also of a spinal subarachnoid block.

These data compose perhaps the largest series available of the CSF changes in meningovascular syphilis. However, it is surprising to note the frequency with which the CSF was normal and the Wassermann reaction negative. Although the serological tests of that time were less reliable than today, it is not clear how the authors could make such a specific diagnosis in patients with stroke and a normal CSF! Presumably, such patients presented with stroke and positive blood serological reactions. The patients were studied between 1925 and 1945, prior to the definition of many forms of cerebrovascular disease such as carotid and basilar artery insufficiency and cerebral arteritis. It is probably hazardous and erroneous to make the diagnosis of active cerebrovascular syphilis if the CSF examination is entirely normal.

General Paresis (Paretic Neurosyphilis). While Merritt *et al.* (1946) considered the CSF findings in general paresis to be so constant and characteristic to warrant the use of the term "paretic formula," the findings overlapped considerably with the CSF changes associated with the other forms of neurosyphilis. The typical paretic formula in 100 untreated patients included: (1) a clear fluid under normal or slightly increased pressure; (2) a pleocytosis ranging as high as 175 mononuclear leukocytes per mm^3; (3) an increased protein content, usually between 50 and 100 mg/dl; (4) a marked increase in gamma globulin content (usually a first-zone colloidal gold curve); and (5) a strong positive Wassermann reaction. The cell count was usually between 25 and 75 cells per mm^3. However, in patients with lesser meningeal reactions, 5 to 25 cells per mm^3 and a normal CSF protein content were also observed.

TABETIC NEUROSYPHILIS. The CSF findings in tabes dorsalis depend upon the activity of the disease. According to Merritt *et al.* (1946), the abnormalities in the CSF tended to decrease with the duration of disease; this is not so in paresis. In early tabes, the CSF findings might show the typical tabetic or paretic formula. However, with treatment, the CSF formula reverted to normal, as seen in so-called "burnt-out" tabes, despite the persistence of lighting pains, Charcot's joints, or visceral crises. The only difference between the findings in 100 tabetic patients and those in 100 paretic patients was the higher incidence of a normal cell count (53 per cent) in tabes and the lesser degree of gamma globulin increase, e.g. the presence, more often, of a midzone than a first zone colloidal gold curve. These authors reported that only 72 per cent of patients had a positive Wassermann reaction. It is likely that the more sensitive serological tests available today show a higher incidence of a positive serological reaction.

MODIFIED NEUROSYPHILIS. While the classic categories of neurosyphilis just discussed (tabes dorsalis, general paresis, meningovascular syphilis) are still seen, they have become clinical rarities in advanced countries (British Medical Journal, 2 September 1978). Hooshmand *et al.* (1972) reported on 241 patients diagnosed as having neurosyphilis on the basis of a positive serum FTA-ABS test, with clinical findings and CSF changes in support of the diagnosis. The most common presenting symptoms were seizures, poor vision, stroke, and mental changes. In contrast to the older literature, these workers emphasized that active progression of neurosyphilis may occur in the *absence* of a pleocytosis, they also noted that many patients showed a transient increase in CSF cell count in response to therapy. The report of Joyce-Clarke and Molteno (1978) describes the diagnostic problems associated with modified neurosyphilis. These authors require a "significant" elevation in CSF protein level and positive serological reactions in the CSF, as well as a fall in CSF protein level in response to therapy, to establish the diagnosis of active neurosyphilis. A significant elevation in CSF immunoglobulins is also supportive of the diagnosis.

COMPARISON OF LUMBAR, CISTERNAL, AND VENTRICULAR FLUIDS. Merritt *et al.* (1946) compared the changes in fluid obtained from various loci in a small number of luetic patients. In most cases, the lumbar fluid showed the greatest degree of abnormality and the ventricular fluid the least. The cisternal fluid changes were intermediate.

INFLUENCE OF THERAPY ON CSF ABNORMALITIES. An acute increase in the severity of the meningeal reaction was described with the institution of antiluetic therapy in the prepenicillin era. Similarly, a meningeal Herxheimer's reaction was also documented with the initiation of penicillin treatment by Hooshmand *et al.* (1972). In the prepenicillin era, treatment with a combination of malaria and tryparsamide therapy was associated with a return of the cell count to normal, usually within a year, although relapses were also noted. The precise time course of the disappearance of the cellular changes with various therapeutic penicillin regimens has not been well established.

The protein levels also fell toward normal, although in some cases a persistent elevation was noted. The increase in gamma globulin level was the abnormality most resistant to treatment, and abnormalities of the colloidal gold curve persisted for several years or indefinitely. The Wassermann reaction also reverted to normal very slowly in some patients. Even after 5 years, after presumably adequate therapy, 30 per cent of patients still had strongly positive CSF serological reactions. There is no satisfactory explanation for such seroresistance. There appeared to be no direct correlation between clinical outcome and the rapidity of the reversal of the changes in the fluid; however, the data regarding this issue are sparse (Oxelius *et al.*, 1969).

Parasitic Infections of the Nervous System

Cysticercosis

The CSF changes in cysticercosis of the nervous sytem have been recently reviewed by Trelles and Trelles (1978) and by Latovitzki *et al.* (1978). The intracranial pressure is often increased, particularly with extensive meningeal involvement and in the racemose form of the disease. A low pressure syndrome due to spinal block has also been well documented. The CSF glucose level was depressed in 16 of 99 patients and in 7 of 36 patients, in two reported series. The total protein was often elevated and the gamma globulins increased in 88 per cent of 35 patients. There was often a marked cellular reaction, with mononuclear, polymorphonuclear, and eosinophilic leukocytes. The eosinophilia was usually between 2 and 70 per cent of the total white count. The frequency of CSF eosinophilia has varied between 20 and 77 per cent in several large series of cases. The pleocytosis may improve rapidly with the systemic administration of adrenal steroids.

Trichinosis

Trichinosis has become rather rare in the United States. According to the earlier literature, reviewed by Kramer and Aita (1978), between 10 and 24 per cent of patients had neurological signs and symptoms, which included an encephalitic syndrome as well as aseptic meningitis. The CSF examined in 74 cases of acute trichinosis was normal in 50 per cent, and in 28 per cent, larvae were found. With meningeal involvement, a decreased glucose level was reported. More commonly, the protein and gamma globulin levels were high. The leukocytic pleocytosis included eosinophils as well as polymorphonuclear and mononuclear cells. Red cells and xanthochromia were seen in association with the multiple small hemorrhagic lesions in the cerebrum.

Amebic Infections of the Nervous System

Amebic infections of the nervous sytem have been classified into two major categories: (1) amebic brain abscess or cerebritis due to *Entamoeba histolytica*, usually secondary to a hepatic amebic abscess; and (2) primary amebic meningoencephalitis (PAM) due to "free-living" amebae such as *Naegleria fowleri* and the species of *Acanthamoeba* and *Hartmanella*. Duma (1978) has reviewed the epidemiology and the clinical features of the two types of infection.

AMEBIC BRAIN ABSCESS. The CSF changes in amebic brain abscess or cerebritis due to *Entamoeba histolytica* are analogous to the findings associated with abscess or cerebritis due to pyogenic bacteria. The intracranial pressure is commonly elevated. The cell count varied between 0 and as many as 6600 white cells per mm³, in 5 cases tabulated by Duma (1978). Such high counts generally have been due to a ruptured amebic abscess. The differential cell count varied between predominantly lymphocytic and predominantly granulocytic in type. The glucose level was normal except in one case when it fell to 30 mg/dl. The protein level also varied between normal and 400 mg/dl. Amebae have not been seen in the CSF with *E. histolytica* infection.

PRIMARY AMEBIC MENINGOENCEPHALITIS (PAM). This disease usually presents as an acute febrile meningoencephalitis with diffuse and focal signs of cerebral involvement, commonly meningeal signs and seizures. Chronic cases of PAM have also been reported. Unlike the findings with cerebral amebiasis due to *E. histolytica*, the free-living amebae *Naegleria*, are commonly found on examination of the CSF in PAM. These can be identified by direct observation of the amebae or by their isolation and culture. Direct observation is accomplished by examining an unstained wet preparation of CSF, using a cover slip, or with the hanging drop method, using ordinary light microscopy (Duma *et al.*, 1969). The amebae are seen to be mobile and must be differentiated from mononuclear leukocytes in the fluid. The various stains used for permanent preparations have been reviewed by Duma (1978). The isolation and culture of free-living amebae is easily accomplished. The reader is referred to Singh's (1975) review of the methods currently in use.

The cell count in PAM varies between a slight increase and the presence of gross pus with more than 26,000 white cells per mm³. The cells are predominantly polymorphonuclear granulocytes. Eosinophils usually are *absent*, which distinguishes PAM from nervous sytem infections due to the nematodes. Red cells may be present because of the hemorrhagic necrosis of the brain that occurs in some cases. The glucose level may be normal or depressed to levels lower than 10 mg/dl. The total protein has been elevated to levels as high as 1 gm/dl, according to some reports.

African Trypanosomiasis

The clinical features of African trypanosomiasis (sleeping sickness) have been reviewed by Dumas and Girard (1978). During the meningoencephalitic phase of the disease, which develops insidiously over a period of months or years, *Trypanosoma* may be isolated in the CSF by microscopic examination of the sediment. During the second month of the meningoencephalitis, a mild to moderate pleocytosis has been noted of 10 to 30 white cells per mm³, and later the cell count increases, usually to between 100 and 400 per mm³. Mott cells, monocytes containing PAS positive granules that are commonly seen in the peripheral blood, may also be observed in the CSF. The CSF protein is generally between 60 and 100 mg/dl. CSF electrophoresis reveals a considerable elevation in the gamma globulin; levels ranging up to about 36.5 per cent of the total protein have been described. Increases of this magnitude are rarely seen in other conditions, apart from subacute sclerosing panencephalitis (SSPE) and chronic rubella panencephalitis.

American Trypanosomiasis (Chagas' Disease)

Spina-Franca *et al.* (1978) have recently reviewed the clinical findings in Chagas' disease. The CSF is generally normal in the acute stage of the illness. In the chronic stages, a minor pleocytosis of 5 to 20 mononuclear cells per mm³ has been reported in a few cases.

Filariasis

The neurological complications of filariasis were reviewed by Dumas and Girard (1978). These include several syndromes, including encephalopathy or encephalitis, intracranial hypertension and brain edema, and spinal cord compression. The CSF changes in these various patterns of the disease are quite variable. They include evidence of increased intracranial pressure and subarachnoid hemorrhage, and in some cases a low-grade pleocytosis. There have been no more specific features reported.

Malaria

The very diverse clinical manifestations of cerebral malaria were reviewed by Vietze (1978). The CSF changes are also variable, and they are not characteristic. An increase in pressure is common; there may be slight elevations in cell count and in protein level. Slight xanthochromia has been reported occasionally.

Toxoplasmosis

In Couvreur and Desmont's (1978) review of toxoplasmosis, they reported that the CSF is normal in the chronic phase of the disease. Changes in the CSF are characteristically seen in acute toxoplasmosis (which presents as an encephalopathy without localizing signs, or as a meningoencephalitis, or as a space-occupying lesion (Townsend *et al.*, 1975). The intracranial pressure may be elevated. There is a largely mononuclear pleocytosis, usually minor, 10 to 50 per mm³, but occasionally counts as high as 1000 cells have been reported. An increased percentage of eosinophils has been reported in some cases. The protein content is raised slightly, but massive elevations to levels as high as 800 mg/dl have also been reported. An increase in gamma globulin level has also been documented. Toxoplasma in the CSF has also been observed in a few acute cases.

Paragonimiasis

Paragonimiasis is prevalent in the Orient and some parts of Africa and South America. It appears in three different forms: cerebral, spinal, and meningeal paragonimiasis. Oh (1978) has reviewed the spinal fluid changes in the three forms of the disease. The findings were similar to those associated with other parasitic granulomas, with a variable incidence of intracranial hypertension, xanthochromia, elevated protein, and a mixed pleocytosis with a variable incidence of eosinophilia. The gamma globulins were commonly elevated.

Brain Tumor

The changes in the CSF associated with brain tumor vary greatly with tumor type, location, and stage of the illness. In the early literature, the CSF with brain tumor was almost always described as abnormal (Sayk, 1974). Diagnosis earlier in the course of the illness is now more frequent because of the increased awareness of physicians and the availability of modern diagnostic techniques. Thus, it is no longer true that the most common CSF findings at the time of diagnosis are intracranial hypertension and a greatly elevated CSF protein, for these changes often are absent early in the course of primary or secondary neoplasms. In current practice, examination of the CSF, especially of its cellular elements and glucose concentration, is of major importance in the diagnosis of neoplastic involvement of the brain and meninges. While a variety of enzyme assays have been abnormal in cases of brain tumor, to date none of these has proved sufficiently diagnostic to warrant their use in clinical practice (see Chapter 6). Intracranial hypertension associated with brain tumor has been reviewed in Chapter 4 and will not be discussed further here.

Appearance

The CSF is usually clear in appearance. Xanthochromia occurs secondary to a high CSF protein or to bleeding. In the absence of bleeding, faint xanthochromia is usually noted when the CSF protein exceeds about 150 mg/dl. The pigmentation is due to the presence of sufficient bilirubin; both free and conjugated bilirubin are albumin-bound and are derived from the serum. This occurs chiefly with large, malignant tumors such as metastatic tumors or glioblastoma which have caused a major defect in the permeability of the endothelial cell barrier, or with tumors located in the CSF pathways such as acoustic neuroma or intraventricular tumors. The tumors most likely to be responsible for subarachnoid hemorrhage include melanoma among the metastatic tumors, and oligodendroglioma among the primary tumors. To these should be added rare primary tumors of the choroid plexus, which also may be responsible for intraventricular bleeding.

Melanin pigmentation of the CSF, associated with extensive involvement of the leptomeninges in metastatic melanoma, has been observed rarely. This occurs also with melanoblastomatosis of the meninges, a rare malignancy which appears to arise from the melanin-pigmented pial cells normally overlying the medulla. Melanin in phagocytic cells in the meninges or in the CSF sediment can be differentiated from hemosiderin by failure of the melanin pigment to stain with Prussian blue (Sayk, 1974).

Rarely, there is clouding of the CSF due to a very heavy pleocytosis, which occurs occasionally with leptomeningeal carcinomatosis or with a necrotic glioblastoma multiforme that has invaded the ventricular wall. Rarely, the CSF appears *viscous* as it drips from the needle, but the hyperviscosity cannot be explained by the degree of pleocytosis or by the protein present. The protein may be only mildly (50 to 70 mg/dl) or moderately (70 to 100 mg/dl) elevated. Such viscosity may be due to diffuse meningeal infiltration with mucin-producing adenocarcinoma, usually metastatic from the gastrointestinal tract. The presence of mucin can be established by staining a dried sample of the CSF with mucicarmine.

Cytological Studies

Brain tumors may be associated with a leukocytic pleocytosis as well as with malignant cells in the fluid. Cells are usually found when tumors are close to the ventricular surface or infiltrate the leptomeninges. In a study of heterogeneous brain tumors, Merritt and Fremont-Smith (1938) reported that most patients had a normal cell count, although occasionally a moderate or marked pleocytosis was recorded. This occurred most often with malignant gliomas, in which white cell counts as high as 337 per mm³ were noted. They also refer to individual case reports of glioblastoma in the older literature describing high cell counts, ranging between 300 and 7000 cells per mm³, predominantly polymorphonuclear leukocytes. These were associated with large necrotic tumors involving the corpus callosum or ventricular walls, or both.

The recent description of large numbers of macrophages within primary brain tumors indicates that the tumor mass serves as a repository and source for the inflammatory cells found in the CSF (Morantz *et al.*, 1979). Sayk (1974) reviewed the cell counts in 305 cases of brain tumor. The highest average counts were found in medulloblastoma, 36 ± 4 (SD) cells per mm³. The cell count was 20 ± 6.5 in metastatic tumor and 16 ± 11 in cerebral glioma. There was little difference in cell count with the various types of tumor.

Improved techniques for cytomorphology using CSF have provided a valuable diagnostic aid (see Chapter 6). This has proved true particularly with primary and secondary tumors that infiltrate the leptomeninges and in the management of meningeal leukemia (El-Batata, 1968; Oehmichen, 1976; Balhuizen *et al.*, 1978). There has been considerable variation in the literature regarding the percentage of positive cytological findings with various techniques, with figures ranging between 7 and 50 per cent. The higher success rates were obtained when cyst fluids were included in the study.

Balhuizen *et al.* (1978) summarized their experience with 262 primary and metastatic tumors. They used a modification of Sayk's sedimentation chamber, which they favored because structure is preserved and only small volumes (1 to 2 ml) are required. With primary brain tumor, lumbar CSF cytological findings were positive preoperatively in about 15 per cent of cases. The figures were higher with ependymomas than with low-grade astrocytomas. Postoperatively, cytological findings from a greater percentage of fluids were positive. The success rate was higher using ventricular fluid than with lumbar fluid. The findings from cytological examination in 64 cases of cerebral metastatic tumors were positive in 20 per cent of cases. The cytological findings were positive in 29 of 37 cases with leptomeningeal carcinomatosis or sarcomatosis. Thus, cytological studies are an important diagnostic aid. (See the later discussion of meningeal carcinomatosis.) There is uncertainty regarding the optimal technique for cyto-morphology. Contrasting views regarding the choice of technique for cyto-morphology are discussed in Chapter 6.

Protein

An increase in protein concentration is the most common abnormal CSF finding associated with brain tumor. It occurs as a consequence of increased endothelial cell permeability, which is often observed also with isotope encephalography or contrast-enhanced computed tomography. However, the CSF protein level in some patients is a more sensitive indicator of increased endothelial cell permeability than brain scans or computed tomograms. Thus, an elevated CSF protein may be observed with normal radiographic and isotopic studies. This occurs with various neoplasms, particularly those invading the ventricular system or the subarachnoid space, including acoustic neuroma, meningeal carcinoma, and intraventricular tumors. With infiltrative tumors of the hemispheres or brain stem with few features of malignancy, like low-grade astrocytomas, the CSF protein is more likely to be normal than with highly malignant glioblastomas, which are very vascular because of extensive endothelial cell proliferation. In patients with a cerebello-pontine angle syndrome, the occurrence of a CSF protein greater than 200 mg/dl favors the presence of a neurofibroma (neurilemoma) over meningioma, presumably because the endothelial cells of the former tumor are more permeable to protein than are those of meningioma. The protein content of lumbar CSF at first puncture in 182 cases of brain tumor, reported by Merritt and Fremont-Smith (1938), is tabulated in Table 7–7.

TABLE 7–7   The Protein Content of the Lumbar Cerebrospinal Fluid in 182 Cases of Brain Tumor

Location and Type of Tumor	Lumbar Cerebrospinal Fluid Protein Content (Mg per Dl)					
	Under 45	45–100	100–200	200–500	500–1500	Total
Supratentorial						
Glioma of cerebral hemisphere	23	27	15	5	1	71
Glioma of third ventricle	0	1	0	1	1	3
Glioma of corpus callosum	0	4	0	3	0	7
Meningioma	4	7	4	0	0	15
Metastatic and other tumors of cerebrum	10	13	5	2	0	30
Pituitary and suprasellar tumor	2	3	0	0	0	5
Subtentorial						
Acoustic neuroma	0	2	3	11	0	16
Other cerebellopontine angle tumors	2	1	2	1	0	6
Glioma of cerebellum or fourth ventricle	12	7	3	1	0	23
Glioma of brain stem	3	2	0	1	0	6
Total	56	67	32	25	2	182
Per cent	31	37	17	14	1	100

(After Merritt and Fremont-Smith, 1938)

Electrophoretic studies of CSF proteins in brain tumor have most characteristically shown patterns reflecting increased amounts of plasma proteins. However, in some cases, there has been an increase of variable magnitude in the gamma globulin content of the fluid. Castaigne *et al.* (1972) reported that 34 per cent of 102 patients with heterogeneous brain tumors had an elevated CSF gamma globulin. This was also recognized in the older literature; with the use of colloidal gold tests, first-zone and mid-zone colloidal reactions were observed occasionally (Sayk, 1974). However, the data regarding the elevated gamma globulin were not corrected for the entry of serum protein; there is uncertainty about the frequency of increased immunoglobulin synthesis within the brain in cases of brain tumor.

Protein Content of Ventricular and Lumbar Fluids

In the past, clinicians depended greatly upon the ventriculographic findings in their diagnostic evaluation of patients with mass lesions. A comparison of the ventricular and lumbar fluid proteins was considered to be diagnostically useful. In a study of 94 brain tumor cases, Merritt and Fremont-Smith (1938) compared the protein content of fluids obtained by a combined puncture of these loci, or by a puncture of the lateral ventricles within a few days of the lumbar puncture.

The possible ventricular fluid findings and their significance were interpreted as follows: (1) Normal protein content in the fluids from both lateral ventricles with increased lumbar CSF protein indicated that the tumor was in the posterior fossa (cerebellar hemisphere, fourth ventricle, or cerebellopontine angle). (2) An increased protein content in the fluid from only one lateral ventricle indicated that the tumor was on the side with the increased protein content. (3) An increased protein content in the fluid from both lateral ventricles indicated that the tumor was midline in location (corpus callosum, third ventricle) or that there were multiple metastatic tumors.

Glucose

The concentration of glucose is normal in patients with brain tumor, except that low CSF glucose levels occur in patients with carcinomatous meningitis. The presence of a low glucose level in patients with brain tumor is reliable evidence of extensive meningeal involvement with tumor (assuming that infection has been excluded). (See discussion of carcinomatous meningitis.)

Enzymes

The many enzymes that have been assayed in CSF are reviewed in Chapter 6. Enzyme levels have been commonly elevated in patients with malignant brain tumors, reflecting increased entry from the serum or their derivation from the tumor or from the infiltrated and compressed brain. While increased enzyme levels of every species assayed have been associated with highly malignant tumors, no specific correlations between enzyme level and tumor type have been established. The lack of specificity of the enzyme assays has limited their usefulness in clinical practice. At present, enzyme analyses are considered to be only of investigative interest.

Other Substances

There has been interest in the assay of other substances in the CSF that might be valuable in the diagnosis of brain tumor. These have included *desmosterol, polyamines, fibronectin, lipids,* and *pituitary hormones.* See the discussion of these constituents in Chapter 6.

Benign Intracranial Hypertension

The differential diagnosis of benign intracranial hypertension (BIH) and the multiple etiological factors associated with the syndrome were discussed in Chapter 4. The diagnosis of BIH, by definition, depends upon the demonstration of intracranial hypertension by lumbar puncture. While it is generally stated that the composition of the CSF is normal in patients with BIH, it is noteworthy that the CSF protein is commonly *reduced* in this syndrome. (The pathogenesis of a low CSF protein was discussed in Chapter 6.) Greer (1968) reported the CSF protein levels in a heterogeneous series of 105 patients; in 43 patients, the CSF protein level was less than 20 mg/dl. No other abnormalities in the fluid have been reported. While occasionally a mildly elevated protein, 50 to 70 mg/dl, has been noted in patients with presumed BIH, elevations of the protein level or a pleocytosis should warn the clinician that the diagnosis of BIH is doubtful and that the intracranial hypertension is probably symptomatic of a chronic meningeal disorder, inflammatory or neoplastic in nature.

Tumors and Other Diseases of the Spinal Cord

The changes in the CSF associated with spinal cord tumors vary with tumor type and location and with the stage of the illness. The literature regarding the incidence and location of different tumor types has been reviewed in detail by Guidetti and Fortuna (1975). In a review of 4674 cases, about 20 per cent were intramedullary in location (chiefly glioma and ependymoma). About 50 per cent were divided equally into meningioma and neurilemoma (neurofibroma), and the balance were miscellaneous tumors.

Spinal Subarachnoid Hemorrhage

The most frequent cause of spinal subarachnoid hemorrhage with a spinal cord tumor is spinal angioma. Hemorrhage in cases of a primary spinal tumor is a rare occurrence. Such hemorrhages have usually arisen in tumors involving the terminal portion of the cord, or cauda equina. In 28 such cases, 16 were ependymomas and 6 were neurinomas of the cauda equina; 6 tumors, including astrocytomas and ependymomas, were located within the substance of the cord (Runnels and Hanberg, 1974; Guidetti and Fortuna, 1975).

Manometric Studies

When tumors of the cord, conus, and cauda equina reach sufficient size, they obstruct the subarachnoid space and give rise to spinal block. The

Queckenstedt test and particularly cuff manometrics are useful in establishing the presence of such obstructive lesions (see discussion of spinal block in Chapter 5). However, these manometric tests do not differentiate between intramedullary and extramedullary lesions. At a relatively early stage of the disease, the manometric finding of a partial or total spinal block suggests an extramedullary tumor, because intramedullary tumors tend to grow longitudinally and obstruct the flow of CSF later. Tumors of the cervical or lumbar region obstruct the CSF flow later than tumors of the thoracic region, because the spinal canal is wider in the former regions. Inability to obtain fluid at several lumbar levels suggests the presence of a huge tumor of the conus or cauda equina filling the lumbar canal.

The hazards of lumbar puncture below the level of a complete spinal block have been discussed in Chapter 5. The drainage of fluid in such cases may aggravate the degree of cord compression and impaction, resulting in further neurological deficit. Quantitative electromanometry, developed by Gilland (1964) and by Lakke (1975), has elucidated the hydrodynamics of spinal block, but these techniques are suitable chiefly for clinical investigation. In clinical practice, information obtained by contrast myelography has usually obviated the use of cuff manometrics in the diagnosis of spinal cord tumor. However, the findings obtained with manometry can provide valuable information in diagnosing patients in whom myelography is contraindicated, or in evaluating the response to treatment (see Chapter 5).

Intracranial Hypertension

The occurrence of papilledema and intracranial hypertension as a consequence of a spinal cord tumor is rare (Teng *et al.*, 1960; Glasauer, 1964; Arseni and Maretsis, 1967; Buchsbaum and Gallo, 1969; Mittal *et al.*, 1970; Ridsdale and Moseley, 1978). The pathogenesis of this disorder was discussed in some detail in Chapter 4. The nature of the spinal tumor and its location were analyzed by Menzel in 38 reported cases of tumor which produced papilledema (Schliack and Stille, 1975). Half the tumors were located in the lumbar region; the rest were in the thoracic or thoracolumbar region, with only a few in the cervical region. Papilledema also occurred with tumors at the foramen magnum, probably causing CSF obstruction within the posterior fossa. About half the tumors were ependymomas, 5 were neurofibromas (neurinomas), and 4 were meningiomas. Thus, the distribution of tumor types responsible for intracranial hypertension was similar to the usual range of spinal cord tumors. The tumors were variable in size, extending over 1 to 7 vertebral bodies. There was no particular age predominance or any specific clinical features.

Cellular Response

The change in cell count with cord tumors and other diseases of the spinal cord has been reviewed by Laterre (1975) and summarized in Table 7–8. The common occurrence of a low-grade mononuclear pleocytosis is notable, but this finding lacks diagnostic specificity. Cytomorphology is of particular importance in the differential diagnosis of chronic meningeal syndromes, including leukemia and carcinomatous meningitis. The cytological findings with primary and

**TABLE 7–8   Total Protein Content and Cell Count in
Tumors and Other Diseases of the Spinal Cord**

| | | NUMBER OF CASES | | | | |
| | *Number* | *Protein (mg/dl)* | | | *Cells (mm³)* | |
DIAGNOSIS	*of Cases*	*< 50*	*50–100*	*> 100*	*< 10*	*> 10*
Meningioma, neurinoma	31	5	7	19	25	6
Intramedullary tumor	17	6	3	8	14	3
Extradural (sarcoma, metastatic tumor)	25	6	4	15	20	5
Syringomyelia and congenital malformation (Arnold-Chiari malformation)	59	49	9	1	53	6
Cervical spondylosis with myelopathy	193	158	32	3	188	5
Multiple sclerosis	598	513	82	3	481	117
ALS	83	72	11		82	1
Lumbar disc	350	295	52	3	343	7

(After Laterre, 1975)

metastatic tumors of the spinal cord are similar to the findings with intracranial tumors. (See discussion of tumor cells in Chapter 6.)

Protein

The increase in CSF protein content observed with cord tumors and other diseases of the spinal cord has been reviewed by Laterre (1975) and summarized in Table 7–8. Although there are no specific correlations between tumor type and location and protein level, a few generalizations can be stated. Froin's syndrome, with clotting of the CSF sample, is more likely to occur with complete block in the lumbar sac than in the cervical region, independently of the tumor type. A complete block due to tumor (or spondylosis) in the cervical region, as revealed by myelography, may be associated with only a minor elevation in protein. The occurrence of a higher CSF protein below a cord tumor than above it has long been recognized.

Hill *et al.* (1959) studied the protein concentration and composition from fluid above and below a spinal block as well as from the ventricular system. Electrophoretic analyses showed that the albumin percentage composition relative to the globulin content was increased as the total protein increased progressively. This is analogous to the increasing percentage of albumin observed along the CSF pathway in normal subjects. While increased entry of protein from the serum is considered to be responsible (as discussed in Chapter 6), a decreased rate of bulk flow removal of proteins also affects the concentration of the various proteins when there is a spinal block. No data are available regarding the quantitative importance of each mechanism.

Cervical Spondylosis

The findings in cervical spondylosis with myelopathy listed in Table 7–8 are noteworthy. A spinal fluid protein above 100 mg/dl was very unusual, occurring in only 3 of 193 cases. Similarly, a cell count greater than 10 per mm³ was also unusual, occurring in only 5 of 193 cases. Such elevations should alert the clinician to other diagnostic possibilities.

Lumbar Disc Disease

The CSF is usually normal in lumbar disc disease unless the disc herniation is large enough to encroach upon the spinal canal. In Laterre's (1975) review, 295 of 350 patients had a normal protein level, and 52 patients had a protein level greater than 100 mg/dl. Thus, such protein elevations should alert the clinician to other diagnostic possibilities. It is noteworthy that herniated discs may rarely be large enough to cause complete spinal block. Cell counts greater than 10 are unusual, occurring in only 7 of 350 cases (see Table 7–8).

Spinal Angiomas

Aminoff (1976) reviewed the clinical findings in 60 patients with spinal angiomas. Manometric evidence of obstruction in the subarachnoid space was found in only 1 of 17 patients in whom the response to the Queckenstedt test had been recorded. The CSF protein was more than 50 mg/dl in 35 (70 per cent) of the 50 patients without subarachnoid hemorrhage. The highest value was 520 mg/dl. The white cell count was increased, ranging from 6 to 50 cells per mm³ in 11 cases, and in 3 cases this was the sole CSF abnormality. In 4 patients with a pleocytosis, the fluid had been examined soon after an acute episode of an increased deficit. These observations were in accord with previously published cases.

Syringomyelia

The various forms of syringomyelia and their pathogenesis have been discussed by Barnett *et al.* (1973). The CSF changes depend upon the presence or absence of spinal block. In the absence of block, the lumbar protein is often normal or mildly elevated (see Table 7–8). Limited data are available regarding the protein level in fluid from the syrinx compared to fluid from the cistern and the lumbar region. A highly elevated protein in fluid from the syrinx favors the presence of an associated neoplasm. In some cases, the protein level of the syrinx level is lower than in the lumbar fluid and close to the ventricular or cisternal level. Gardner (1965) considered such cases to be examples of syringohydromelia, when the syrinx was in continuity with the fourth ventricle.

Meningeal Carcinomatosis

The clinical presentation of meningeal carcinomatosis is variable, and the diagnosis depends upon the demonstration of malignant cells in the CSF. The clinical terminology also includes *carcinomatous meningitis* and *diffuse meningeal neoplasia*. Antemortem diagnosis is facilitated by the availability of improved cytomorphological techniques. (The technical advances in cytomorphology were reviewed in Chapter 6.) The CSF findings were described by Berg (1953), Fischer-Williams *et al.* (1955), Dinsdale and Taghavy (1964), Parsons (1972), and others. The report of Olson *et al.* (1974) summarized the CSF findings in 47 patients with meningeal carcinomatosis diagnosed over a four-year period. In this series, patients with leptomeningeal spread from primary brain tumors (e.g., glioblastoma, medulloblastoma) and meningeal leukemia were excluded. The primary sites of the meningeal metastases, in decreasing incidence, were: (1) breast carcinoma, (2) lymphomas (lymphosarcoma, reticulum cell sarcoma, Hodgkin's disease), (3) lung carcinoma (epidermoid, adenocarcinoma, oat cell), and (4) adenocarcinoma of the pancreas. This series approximates the distribution in other reports in which a wide variety of tumor types were implicated.

Early in the course of carcinomatous meningitis, the lumbar CSF pressure is normal. At various times in the course of the illness, the pressures ranged between 90 and 550 mm in the 47 cases of Olson *et al.* (1974), but in more than half the patients it was below 150 mm on first lumbar puncture. (Low pressures are seen in patients with complete spinal block, which occurs late in the course of the illness.) The white blood cell count ranged from 0 to 500 per mm³, and the differential count revealed 0 to 95 per cent polymorphonuclear cells in these patients. The protein ranged between 24 and 1200 mg/dl. It was normal in 12 of 47 patients on first puncture, and the protein remained within normal limits in 4 of the patients on subsequent puncture.

Olson *et al.* (1974) stated that "in no instance was hypoglycorrhachia the only abnormal CSF finding" in the series of 47 patients. In contrast, I have observed this in 2 patients with meningeal melanomatosis. (The patients had a normal total white cell count, but cytomorphological studies were not performed.) Malignant cells were found in 21 of the 47 cases on first puncture; with repeated taps, malignant cells were observed in 80 per cent of the cases by use of the Papanicolaou stain on the sediment. In the latter study, the cytocentrifuge was used. It is possible that the frequency of positive cytological findings would have been increased by the use of a sedimentation technique or one of the filtration techniques described in Chapter 6 (Gondos and King, 1976). These CSF findings are similar to those reported by Sayk (1974), although that author omitted the diagnostic importance of a depressed glucose level in such cases. The presence of malignant cells in CSF does not necessarily establish the diagnosis of carcinomatous meningitis (diffuse meningeal neoplasia). Malignant cells are often found in the CSF of patients with brain tumors, particularly those involving the ventricular wall or the cortex, as discussed earlier (Oehmichen, 1976; Balhuizen *et al.*, 1978). However, a low CSF glucose level is a localizing finding in such cases, because its occurrence reflects *diffuse* meningeal involvement rather than focal cerebral or meningeal metastases.

There has been speculation about the mechanism of the low CSF glucose in meningeal carcinomatosis (see Chapter 6). The factors to be considered include: (1) increased glucose utilization by malignant cells in the leptomeninges, (2) increased glucose utilization by cerebral tissue adjacent to the CSF, and (3) a defect of glucose entry into the CSF. Evidence for increased glycolysis is based on the observation that CSF lactate levels are increased in such cases. This finding has not been systematically studied, but it has been observed often. Evidence for a defect in glucose entry was obtained in 2 patients with carcinomatous meningitis (Fishman, 1963). The intravenous administration of 50 per cent glucose (0.9 gm per kg) failed to increase the CSF lumbar glucose level 30 to 70 mg/dl above the resting level, as observed in normal subjects. Additional data are needed to elucidate the quantitative importance of the several factors that contribute to a low CSF glucose in carcinomatous meningitis.

Several biochemical "markers" in the CSF of cancer patients have been assessed in patients with meningeal carcinomatosis. These included β-glucuronidase, carcinoembryonic antigen (CEA), acid phosphatase, and chorionic gonadotropin (Schold *et al.*, 1978). These assays may prove useful for diagnosis and for monitoring treatment in patients with metastatic disease to the brain and meninges.

Meningeal Sarcoidosis

Involvement of the central nervous system in sarcoidosis is an uncommon complication of the disease. The neurological manifestations include multiple cranial nerve palsies, signs of hypothalamic involvement, hydrocephalus, and signs of meningitis. Gaines *et al.* (1970) reviewed the world literature and summarized the CSF findings in 57 patients with neurological symptoms. Of these, 41 (72 per cent) had a pleocytosis, 40 (70 per cent) had an increased protein level, and 10 (18 per cent) had a decreased glucose level. The range of changes was not given. Delaney's (1977) review of 23 cases provided analogous data.

The pleocytosis is usually between 10 and 100 mononuclear cells. The protein elevations are generally between 50 and 200 mg/dl. The glucose levels usually range between 30 and 40 mg/dl. Patients with obvious meningeal signs, hydrocephalus, and multiple cranial nerve palsies are more likely to have an abnormal CSF. A low CSF glucose strongly favors the presence of diffuse meningeal sarcoidosis. Patients with restricted hypothalamic sarcoid are more likely to have a normal CSF examination. The clinical manifestations of meningeal sarcoidosis are quite similar to the findings in meningeal carcinomatosis, and their differentiation depends upon detailed cytomorphological studies of the CSF. In sarcoid meningitis, the pleocytosis consists almost entirely of mononuclear inflammatory cells.

Lymphomatoid granulomatosis: This rare lymphoreticular proliferative and granulomatous disease, predominantly involves the lungs. The kidneys, skin, and central nervous system are also frequently affected. Saito (1978) has summarized the CSF findings in a patient with neurological involvement. The CSF protein content was elevated to a level of 375 mg/dl in association with a glucose level of 24 mg/dl and a pleocytosis of 225 mononuclear cells per mm^3. These cells were chiefly reticular cells with one or more ameboid protrusions of the cytoplasmic membrane. The differentiated plasma cells were also present, as were small numbers of lymphocytes, neutrophils, and red blood cells. The cellular changes were more striking in the cisternal than in the lumbar fluid. Thus, the findings simulate the findings in sarcoidosis, meningeal lymphoma and other diffuse meningeal neoplasms.

Head Injury

The changes in the CSF associated with head injury depend upon the absence or presence of cerebral contusion, compression, and ischemia. In uncomplicated cerebral concussion, the CSF is normal. With cerebral contusion, a variable degree of subarachnoid bleeding is apparent. The induced chemical meningitis and leukocytic pleocytosis of a subarachnoid block must be differentiated from a secondary bacterial meningitis as a result of a basilar skull fracture. The changes in the CSF and their time course following subarachnoid hemorrhage have been discussed in Chapter 6.

Intracranial hypertension in 160 patients with severe head injury was studied systematically by Miller *et al.* (1977), using monitoring techniques in an intensive care unit. Twenty-eight of the 160 cases had a low normal intracranial pressure on admission (10 mm Hg or less), and the balance had variable degrees of increased pressure. No differences were noted in the intracranial pressures recorded in various categories of head injury (acute epidural or subdural hematoma, acute intracranial hematoma, or diffuse brain injury). The morbidity and mortality were higher in patients with severe and sustained degrees of intracranial hypertension.

Studies of acid-base balance and lactate levels in patients with head injury have revealed patterns indicative of CSF metabolic acidosis and systemic respiratory alkalosis (Zupping, 1970). King *et al.* (1974) studied sequentially CSF and arterial lactate, pH, pCO_2, bicarbonate, and pO_2 levels in 17 patients with uncomplicated head injury. Lactate was markedly elevated in both fluids for the first 3 days after injury; the elevation persisted thereafter in the CSF. This finding is attributable to cerebral ischemia and edema. Zupping (1970) studied 45 patients with severe head injuries, which included acute and chronic intracerebral hematomas. The CSF metabolic acidosis was most pronounced in deeply comatose and moribund patients. There was a good correlation between the changes in CSF bicarbonate and lactate (see discussion of acid-base balance in Chapter 6).

Subdural Hematoma

The CSF findings in 50 cases of subdural hematoma were analyzed by Merritt and Fremont-Smith (1938). In 37 patients (74 per cent), the lumbar CSF pressure was greater than 200 mm. In 26 patients (50 per cent), the CSF revealed evidence of subarachnoid bleeding, indicating the presence also of cerebral contusion. The CSF protein was normal in patients without evidence of subarachnoid bleeding. Plum and Posner (1972) reported the CSF findings in 51 patients. Half had a normal CSF, and the other half had a protein level greater than 50 mg/dl, giving evidence of subarachnoid bleeding.

Cerebrovascular Disease

The CSF examination is very useful in the differential diagnosis of the various forms of cerebrovascular disease. The changes in the CSF associated with stroke are well illustrated by Merritt and Fremont-Smith's (1938) analysis of 121 autopsy-proven cases, including 70 of cerebral hemorrhage and 51 of cerebral thrombosis. In the latter group, known embolic lesions originating in the heart were excluded. Patients with evidence of neurosyphilis were also excluded from the analysis. The major observations of Merritt and Fremont-

Smith (1938) will be summarized presently. Their data, referred to as the Boston series, were derived from the largest series of diagnoses confirmed by autopsy. More recently, Sornas *et al.* (1972) studied the cytological changes following stroke in 116 patients. Lumbar punctures were performed within 3 days of onset, and the tap was repeated at 2 to 3 day intervals for a week and at weekly intervals therafter. These data are referred to as the Lund series. Many of these patients survived the stroke and thus differ from the fatal cases of the Boston series.

Cerebral Hemorrhage

The data from the Boston series will be summarized first. The CSF pressure at first puncture was increased above 200 mm in 57 per cent, above 300 mm in 38 per cent, and above 400 mm in 19 per cent of the cases. In almost half these fatal cases, the patients had a normal intracranial pressure, which indicates that it is a poor index of prognosis. It is of special interest that 20 per cent of the patients had a clear fluid and the rest had varying degrees of pigmentation attributable to blood and its products. (The origin and significance of these pigments in CSF following subarachnoid hemorrhage were discussed in Chapter 6.)

Fluids grossly bloody to the naked eye contained several thousand to many hundreds of thousands of red cells per mm^3. (See discussion of CSF appearance in Chapter 6.) While the initial proportion of white cells to red cells was the same as that in blood, there was a progressive increase in the absolute number of white cells and their proportion to the red cells, reflecting the meningeal reaction induced by blood. The precise temporal relationships between the number of red cells and the relative increase in white cell count was not described. In addition, with necrosis of the ventricular wall secondary to hemorrhage adjacent to the ventricle, an even greater leukocytic response was introduced. Cell counts as high as 1900 and 3600 leukocytes per mm^3, largely polymorphonuclear cells, were observed in such cases.

The bloody fluids had an increase in protein content which was initially proportional to the red cell count but which was then elevated out of proportion to the cell count, reflecting an increased influx of serum proteins across the disrupted blood-brain barrier. The protein levels varied between 40 and 2200 mg/dl. (The occurrence of a depressed glucose level in subarachnoid hemorrhage was discussed in Chapter 6.)

In the Lund series, 16 patients with intracerebral hematoma were studied. They also showed a polymorphonuclear response that was greater than that observed with ischemic strokes. Four patients had a mild pleocytosis, and 4 others had a considerable pleocytosis (700, 900, 4600, and 21,000 polymorphonuclear leukocytes respectively). The maximal granulocytic response occurred on the third or fourth day after onset. A polymorphonuclear reaction on the first day favored the presence of an intracerebral hematoma.

Lee *et al.* (1975) found that 25 per cent of 16 patients with autopsy-verified intracerebral hemorrhage had a clear fluid. However, the lumbar punctures were performed within 24 hours in 3 cases and within 48 hours in the fourth. Thus, a delayed appearance of blood in the lumbar sac with intracerebral hemorrhage might explain the clear fluid in such cases.

When there is a bloody CSF, it may be useful to correct the polymorphonuclear cell count for the white cells that have entered the CSF from the blood. A formula for such correction has been described by Sornas *et al.* (1972). (See Chapter 6.)

Cerebral Thrombosis

The intracranial pressure was usually normal or only slightly elevated in the 51 patients reported by Merritt and Fremont-Smith (1938). These pressures were greater than 200 mm in 21 per cent of these autopsy-proven cases; in 4 per cent the pressure was between 300 mm and 400 mm. The occurrence of intracranial hypertension in these fatal cases reflected extensive cerebral infarction and edema. In 51 fatal cases, 46 patients had a clear fluid, 4 had a xanthochromic fluid, and 1 had blood-tinged fluid. Thus, about 10 per cent of the cases were associated with hemorrhagic infarction, which was reflected in the fluid.

The white cell count in 7 of the 51 patients was between 6 and 67 cells per mm^3; the rest were normal. The relationship between the degree of pleocytosis and the time after the onset of the stroke was not worked out, nor were other forms of arteritis (cranial arteritis or granulomatous angitis) apart from neurosyphilis, excluded. The protein content was normal in half the patients, and in only 2 patients was it over 100 mg/dl. (It is not clear whether other causes of increased CSF protein such as myxedema or diabetic polyneuropathy were excluded in these patients.)

In the Lund series, serial punctures after ischemic stroke revealed a minor leukocytic response, which was maximal during the first seven days. The white count was usually normal by the end of the second week.

Cerebral Embolism

The CSF changes associated with cerebral embolism are generally indistinguishable from those associated with cerebral thrombosis. In 13 patients of the Boston series with nonseptic embolism, the cell count was normal in 10; in 3 there was a slight pleocytosis, with a high of 45 white cells per mm^3. It seems certain that among the autopsy-proven cases of cerebral thrombosis just described, there were included significant numbers of emboli from the carotid system. (The carotid arteries in the neck were not examined at autopsy in the 1930's.) The CSF findings associated with septic embolism due to subacute bacterial endocarditis are discussed later.

In summary, the use of the CSF findings in the differential diagnosis of cerebral thrombosis, embolism, and hemorrhage is limited. In the Boston series, 20 per cent of the patients with cerebral hemorrhage had a clear fluid at the first puncture, and 10 per cent of the patients with cerebral thrombosis had a xanthochromic or slightly bloody fluid. The fact that a clear CSF does not exclude a cerebral hemorrhage or a hemorrhagic infarction must be considered in the decision to institute anticoagulant therapy. Computed tomography indicates the presence of intrahemispheric blood with great clarity, although the limits of its sensitivity to very small hemorrhages have not been established. A polymorphonuclear reaction (10 to 1000 per mm^3) occurs with an intracerebral hematoma, but it is also compatible with extensive infarction of cerebral tissue adjacent to the CSF and with the wide range of inflammatory disorders.

Cerebral Arteritis

Giant Cell (Temporal) Arteritis

The neurological manifestations of giant cell (temporal) arteritis are diverse, and the CSF findings are also variable. The CSF is usually normal in patients when the disease is manifested chiefly in the external carotid arteries. However, when the cerebral vasculature is involved, abnormalities of the CSF have been noted, not surprisingly. The pressure is usually normal. The CSF protein may be increased to a level as high as several hundred mg/dl, with few if any cells. Occasionally, pleocytosis has been reported, with counts as high as 650 white cells per mm³, including both lymphocytes and polymorphonuclear granulocytes. The CSF glucose levels have been normal in the available reports (Hamilton et al., 1971).

Granulomatous Angitis

Granulomatous angitis is a rare necrotizing vasculitis confined primarily to the central nervous system (Faer et al., 1977; Jellinger, 1977). Vincent (1977) summarized the CSF findings in 18 reported cases and found the CSF pressure to be increased in some patients. In 15 of 18 cases, the CSF protein ranged between 75 and 560 mg/dl, but in 3 cases it was normal. The cell count varied between 25 and 176 per mm³, and the cells were largely lymphocytic in 15 cases. In 3 cases the cell count was probably normal. Evidence for mild subarachnoid bleeding was observed in a few cases; in these a decreased CSF glucose was seen. The CSF gamma globulin was increased in some patients, but this was not reported by most authors. I have observed oligoclonal bands in a typical case of granulomatous arteritis. The observation that 3 of 18 reported patients had normal CSF examination results indicates the difficulty of diagnosis.

Bacterial Endocarditis

The incidence of neurological complication in bacterial endocarditis was 39 per cent in the recent studies by Pruitt et al. (1978). The neurological manifestations were diverse and included cerebral embolism, subarachnoid and intracerebral hemorrhage, and seizures. The patients had a wide variety of infectious agents, including streptococci, staphylococci, hemophilus, enterobacteria, and candida. The CSF findings in the 69 patients examined were also diverse. In 21 of the 69 patients (30 per cent), the CSF was normal, but in 19 patients (28 per cent) the fluid was purulent (demonstrating a polymorphonuclear leukocytic pleocytosis), with a high protein content and a reduced glucose content. In 17 patients (25 per cent), the fluid was aseptic (predominantly lymphocytic pleocytosis), with a normal glucose level and a normal or slightly elevated protein level. In 9 patients (13 per cent), the fluid was hemorrhagic (more than 200 red cells per mm³ in all tubes).

Cultures were positive in only 11 of the 69 patients, and in each of these the fluid was purulent. There was a close correlation between the CSF findings and the infecting organism. Virulent organisms such as S. aureus, Streptococcus pneumoniae, and enteric gram-negative rods were frequently associated with a purulent fluid. Conversely, a relatively nonvirulent organism such as S. viridans was usually associated with a normal or aseptic CSF.

Congestive Heart Failure

The intracranial pressure is characteristically elevated in cases of severe congestive heart failure. Harrison (1934) and Friedfeld and Fishberg (1934) studied the venous pressure and CSF pressure in such cases; they showed that the intracranial hypertension was secondary to increased central venous pressure and that both returned toward normal with the administration of digitalis. Merritt and Fremont-Smith (1938) reported a series of 32 patients with congestive heart failure with CSF pressures ranging between 185 and 500 mm; about 50 per cent of the patients had a pressure of 300 mm or greater.

While the increased intracranial pressure in these cases was attributable to increased central venous pressure, additional contributing factors were the severity of the respiratory acidosis and the degree of cerebral hypoxia associated with heart failure. Both acidosis and hypoxia cause acute cerebral vasodilation and increased cerebral blood flow and thereby intracranial hypertension. However, the quantitative importance of each of the three factors — central venous pressure, acidosis, and hypoxia — in such cases has not been delineated. The CSF cell count and total protein content were normal in these patients. I am unaware of any further studies of this problem since the publications of Harrison (1934), Friedfeld and Fishberg (1934), and Merritt and Fremont-Smith (1938).

Eclampsia and Pregnancy

The CSF is abnormal in most patients with eclampsia. In the early literature, Spellman (1922) reported that 50 per cent of 68 patients had intracranial hypertension and 25 per cent had bloody CSF. More recently, Morrison et al. (1972) and Fish et al. (1972) reported the findings in a group of 21 patients with eclampsia. The CSF protein was elevated in 18 of 21 cases, averaging 78 mg/dl, with a range of 42 to 200 mg/dl. The fluid was grossly bloody in 6 patients, with pink or turbid fluid due to red cells in all but 1 of the others. Red cells were found in 20 of the 21 cases; the CSF glucose was normal. The CSF uric acid was elevated in all cases; the mean was 1.9 mg/dl (range 1.0 to 2.8), compared to a normal mean of 0.3 mg/dl. This increase reflected the elevated plasma uric acid level, which was highly elevated in all cases; mean serum level was 8.6 mg/dl (range 4.8 to 12.2). In normal pregnancy, the CSF composition is normal (Davis, 1979).

CSF Pressure in Labor

The changes in CSF pressure during labor have been studied with isovolumetric strain gauge transducers. Marx *et al.* (1961) reported their findings in 20 normal women during labor. In supine women during the first stage of labor, pressures ranged from 160 to 350 mm water, with an average of 285 mm. During uterine contractions, the CSF pressure ranged from 110 to 390 mm above the resting level. Hopkins *et al.* (1965) obtained similar data in their study of labor.

Uremia

Meningeal signs, pleocytosis, and alteration of the blood-CSF barrier occur in patients with uremia of diverse origin (Madonick *et al.*, 1950; Locke *et al.*, 1961; Funder and Wieth, 1967). In the reported studies, it has been difficult to relate the CSF changes to the various clinical manifestations or to the cause of the uremia. In one report, almost one third of the uremic patients examined had nuchal rigidity as well as Kernig's sign; about half these patients were also shown to have pleocytosis (Madonick *et al.*, 1950). The intracranial pressure was commonly elevated, but it is not clear how often this was a reflection of congestive heart failure and increased central venous pressure. In another series, about 10 per cent of the uremic patients studied had more than 5 leukocytes per mm^3 (ranging from 7 to 600) in the CSF. The severity of the pleocytosis bore no relation to the degree of azotemia (Schreiner and Maher, 1961). Cell counts greater than 50 per mm^3 favor the presence of neuropathological changes apart from the uremia, such as stroke and opportunistic infection.

The concentration of urea in normal CSF is slightly less than in serum; the CSF/serum concentration ratio is about 0.9 (Bradbury *et al.*, 1963). In patients with uremia, with serum urea levels in the range of 300 to 500 mg/dl, the CSF/serum concentration ratio remained unchanged. With hemodialysis, however, the concentration ratio was elevated, ranging from 1.0 to 4.0, for 12 to 24 hours after the onset of dialysis; i.e., the serum urea fell more rapidly than the CSF urea (Funder and Wieth, 1967). Cerebral dysfunction during dialysis (the "dysequilibrium syndrome") is probably caused by delayed clearance of urea and other osmotically active solutes from the central nervous system, with the creation of a transient osmotic difference, which favors intracellular fluid accumulation in the brain and increased CSF pressure (Arieff *et al.*, 1973).

Schreiner and Maher (1961) found that 30 of 52 uremic patients had CSF protein levels greater than 60 mg/dl; 19 exceeded 80 mg, and 11 were over 100 mg/dl. Elevations of CSF protein may be reduced to the normal range during the immediate posthemodialysis period. The increase in protein content is dependent upon an alteration in the permeability properties of capillary endothelial cells in brain, the mechanism of which is not known (Fishman, 1970; Raskin and Fishman, 1976).

The mechanism of uremic twitching was carefully pursued by Harrison *et al.* (1936) and Harrison and Mason (1937) over 40 years ago. In experimental canine uremic encephalopathy, they found that the occurrence of twitching correlated better with the phosphate levels in the CSF than with those in the serum. Large intravenous doses of phosphate produced twitching, with a delay that correlated with the time of elevation of the CSF phosphate. Furthermore, intracisternal injection of phosphate caused more severe twitching. The effect of the administration of phosphate on the ionized calcium and magnesium was not determined.

More recently, in 17 patients with uremia, it was noted that although ratios of CSF to serum phosphate were widely dispersed and not significantly different from those in control patients, the five patients with twitching had CSF phosphate levels higher than 3.8 mg/dl; none of the other 12 uremic patients achieved levels greater than 3.3 mg/dl, and twitching was not evident in any of them (Freeman *et al.*, 1962). However, Harrison *et al.* (1936) had already pointed out that increased CSF phosphate cannot be the sole cause of twitching, because this phenomenon was observed despite normal serum and CSF levels of this anion. More data regarding cerebral phosphate, calcium, and magnesium metabolism in cases of uremia are needed to clarify the role of phosphate as a uremic neurotoxin.

Hepatic Encephalopathy

The intracranial pressure is usually normal in patients with chronic hepatic encephalopathy; however, in a fulminant hepatic failure (FHF), brain edema is a common occurrence. Ware *et al.* (1971) reported edema in 16 of 32 patients with FHF studied at autopsy, and 4 of these had cerebellar or uncal herniation or both. The cause of the FHF was acute viral or toxic hepatitis; cases of Reye's syndrome were not included. While life-threatening intracranial hypertension is a feature of Reye's syndrome, the CSF is otherwise normal in this disorder (De Vivo and Keating, 1976).

The major changes in the CSF associated with hepatic encephalopathy are elevations in the concentration of ammonia, glutamine, and alpha-ketoglutaramate (Walshe, 1951; Gilon *et al.*, 1953; Caeser, 1962; Brandstetter and Barzilai, 1960; Muting *et al.*, 1968; Hourani *et al.*, 1971; Plum, 1971; Duffy *et al.*, 1974). (These constituents were reviewed in Chapter 6.) In clinical practice, an elevation in the glutamine level is the most useful diagnostic finding. Hourani *et al.* (1971) reported the CSF glutamine levels in 86 patients as follows: normal subjects 12.6 ± 5.1 mg/dl; patients with liver disease, 21.6 ± 6.2 mg/dl; patients with hepatic encephalopathy, 40.3 ± 14 mg/dl. Figure 7–1 illustrates the CSF glutamine levels in patients with hepatic encephalopathy and liver disease, and in control subjects (Plum, 1971). The data illustrate the close but imperfect correlation between glutamine level and hepatic encephalopathy. The changes in ammonia and alpha-ketoglutaramate in hepatic encephalopathy parallel the changes in glutamine level, but the technical ease with which glutamine is measured compared to the other two compounds favors its use as the most suitable diagnostic test. (See Chapter 6.)

The CSF protein is often elevated in patients with hepatic coma. Dillon and Schenker (1972) reviewed the CSF findings in 70 patients with hepatic coma and found the protein increased (levels not given) in 20 per cent of cases. On the other hand, Amatuzio *et al.* (1953) found the CSF protein elevated in 11 consecutive patients with hepatic coma. Adams and Foley (1953) described the CSF in 25 patients with hepatic coma in whom the CSF protein values were not elevated despite faint xanthochromia in those with high serum bilirubin levels. The discrepancy regarding the CSF protein in the several reports is not

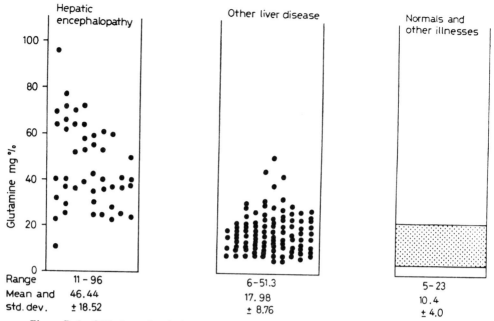

Figure 7-1   CSF glutamine in hepatic encephalopathy, liver disease, and controls (from Plum, 1971). The original data are from Gilon *et al.* (1953). Brandstetter and Barzilai (1960), and Caesar (1962); the means are calculated from the total. Controls include both healthy subjects and patients in coma from non-liver causes.

explained. It is not clear, in the various reports, whether there was any correlation between the elevated CSF protein content in hepatic encephalopathy and the presence of alcoholic neuropathy or the depth of coma. In summary, it seems necessary to consider other causes of an elevated CSF protein in patients with hepatic encephalopathy before assuming the change is attributable to hepatic failure, although the latter has been observed.

Diabetic Ketoacidosis

The CSF and blood were studied in six patients with diabetic ketoacidosis before and 4 to 9 hours after treatment, by Ohman *et al.* (1971). On admission, the patients were comatose or obtunded. The CSF pressure was lower than 120 mm in each case. Despite the systemic metabolic acidosis, the mean blood pH was 7.09 and the CSF pH was normal, 7.35, on admission. There was a minor fall in the CSF pH with treatment, reminiscent of the paradoxical pH changes discussed in Chapters 4 and 6. This finding suggested that bicarbonate therapy would have aggravated the CSF acidosis and might have had deleterious effects. The concentration of β-hydroxybutyrate in blood and CSF fell with treatment. Acetoacetate fell in the blood but was unchanged in the CSF. The mean blood glucose levels fell from 596 to 232 mg/dl, and the CSF glucose levels fell from 374 to 274 mg/dl; i.e., the CSF level was higher than the blood level with treatment. The greater CSF osmolality was viewed as a reason for caution against the excessively rapid correction of blood hyperosmolality.

Systemic Lupus Erythematosus

The heterogeneous neurological manifestations of systemic lupus erythematosus (SLE) include encephalopathy, seizures, focal signs of cerebral dysfunction, myelopathy, and peripheral neuropathy. Johnson and Richardson (1968) reviewed the literature regarding the CSF findings in 88 well-annotated cases of neurological involvement. In 42 patients (44 per cent), the protein content was greater than 50 mg/dl, but protein levels in excess of 100 mg/dl were seldom seen except in patients with neuropathy or myelopathy. In 28 patients (32 per cent), the white cell count was greater than 5 per mm^3; in only 9 patients was there a pleocytosis in excess of 50 cells, in the absence of bacterial or fungal meningitis. Intracranial hypertension has also been observed rarely (Bettman *et al.*, 1968, Silberberg and Laties, 1973).

In a few isolated cases, to which Johnson and Richardson (1968) refer, there was a polymorphonuclear pleocytosis in the absence of apparent infection, but in most cases the cellular response was lymphocytic. The clinician should be alert to the possibility of opportunistic infections in such cases. There has been a single reported case in which LE cells were observed in the CSF, but these occurred in association with subarachnoid hemorrhage (Nosanchuk and Kim, 1976). LE cells in the CSF have not been described in other reports of central nervous system lupus. It is of interest that spinal fluid abnormalities in the absence of neurological signs have been observed, including an increase in protein and a lymphocytic pleocytosis. The CSF glucose is usually normal in SLE, but reduced levels have been reported in patients with transverse myelopathy due to lupus (Andrianakos *et al.*, 1975).

The literature is controversial regarding the immunoglobulins in the CSF of patients with central nervous system lupus. No specific changes have been noted in most cases, although mild elevations in gamma globulin have been observed occasionally. However, Levin *et al.* (1972) reported that the mean level for IgG was significantly *low* in patients with active CNS disease, with a return to normal levels following remission. This observation requires further substantiation. It is of interest that Atkins *et al.* (1971), using an immunofluorescent technique, observed an increased deposit of gamma globulin in the choroid plexus of two patients with lupus; this was not true of control subjects.

The measurement in CSF of antinuclear antibodies, free DNA, and complement and its components has been carried out in patients with central nervous system lupus. Petz and colleagues (1971) found abnormally low CSF levels of complement fraction C4 in patients with neurological involvement, whereas the CSF levels were normal in lupus patients without evidence of neurological disease. The low values were interpreted as evidence that an immune reaction occurred in the central nervous system in such patients. They also reported that C4 was unstable in CSF even when stored at −50° C. This instability has limited its application to routine clinical diagnosis.

Rheumatoid Arthritis

The CSF findings in rheumatoid arthritis were systematically studied by Ludwig *et al.* (1943) in 101 patients. In this series, 59 patients suffered from peripheral joint disease alone, and 42 patients had spondylitis with or without peripheral joint involvement. The CSF was normal except for increased protein levels, abnormal colloidal gold curves, or a combination of the two. Twelve per cent of the 59 patients with peripheral joint involvement and 38 per cent of the patients with spondylitis had such abnormalities. Fifteen of the 16 patients with increased cerebrospinal fluid protein levels had presumed spondylitis, which suggested a relation between an elevated protein level and the presence of arthritis in the spinal articulations. It is not clear whether any of these patients had an associated herniated disc. Rheumatoid meningitis is a very rare complication.

Rheumatoid Meningitis

Rheumatoid pachymeningitis is a rare complication of rheumatoid arthritis and may give rise to spinal cord compression. Markenson *et al.* (1979) have reported such a case, which responded to surgical decompression and steroid therapy. There were a very high protein level and a depressed glucose level below the point of the block. Differences in cell count, protein level, and glucose content between lumbar and cisternal fluid indicated that the disease process was localized. There were elevated immunoglobulins and low molecular weight IgM and immune complexes in the loculated CSF below the block, implicating an immune reaction in the pathogenesis of the meningeal disease, probably similar to the inflammatory processes involving other organs in rheumatoid arthritis.

Multiple Sclerosis

The extensive literature regarding the CSF changes in multiple sclerosis has been reviewed in great detail by Tourtellotte (1970) and by Lumsden (1972). This section summarizes the older literature and emphasizes some of the newer data. The reader should consult those two reviews for additional details about the older literature. The CSF changes can be epitomized as follows. The CSF may be entirely normal according to current methods, or it may show a variety of changes. The abnormalities found in the CSF in patients with multiple sclerosis may include a mononuclear pleocytosis, an increase in protein, and an increase in the immunoglobulins. The intracranial pressure is almost always normal, and glucose is not affected. These changes will be described in further detail separately.

Cellular Changes

The increased number of mononuclear leukocytes in the CSF of patients with multiple sclerosis is in accord with the pathology of the disease. Their presence reflects cellular infiltrates found in the regions of acute and chronic demyelinating lesions in the white matter of the brain and spinal cord. The data obtained from several large groups of patients with multiple sclerosis reveal a normal cell count in about two thirds of cases and a low level of pleocytosis in the lumbar CSF in about one third of cases. The findings in the series of Freedman and Merritt (1950), Yahr *et al.* (1954), Tourtellotte (1970), and McAlpine *et al.* (1972) are quite similar. Lumsden's (1972) data are summarized in Table 7–9. Tourtellotte (1970) concluded that the total white count was less than 16 per mm^3 in 95 per cent of patients. The cellular responses are lymphocytic or mononuclear, and Tourtellotte (1970) has stated that a polymorphonuclear pleocytosis of greater than 0.5 per cent is rare. While there is occasional mention of a slight increase in the number of eosinophils (Kolar and Zeman, 1968; Bosch and Oehmichen, 1978), most authors have not reported this finding. Several authors, using a sedimentation technique for cytomorphology, have emphasized the presence of an increased number of plasma cells (Kolar and Zeman, 1968; Oehmichen, 1976). However, most workers, using centrifugation or filtration for cytomorphology, have not differentiated between mononuclear cells, large and small lymphocytes, and plasma cells. Tourtellotte (1970) could not confirm the presence of an increased number of plasma cells in his study of 106 patients with multiple sclerosis. While a mononuclear pleocytosis greater than 50 mononuclear cells per mm^3 has rarely been observed, such an increase should alert the clinician to a possible error in diagnosis and to the consideration of other diagnostic possibilities.

It is generally held by clinicians that there is a relatively greater incidence of pleocytosis during an exacerbation than in periods of remission. However, diagnostic lumbar punctures have most often been performed during a period of exacerbation, and it has proved difficult to validate this impression. Thus, Tourtellotte (1970) compared 50 patients with recent relapse to 56 patients not in relapse and found that 40 per cent of patients during a clinical exacerbation had a cellular increase (greater than 5 cells per mm^3), whereas 32 per cent of the patients not in relapse had a similar increase; i.e., a difference in the incidence (or severity) of the pleocytosis could *not* be shown.

Several reports have shown a positive correlation between a CSF pleocytosis and an increase in the gamma globulin content. Thus, all fluids with 20 or more white cells per mm^3 had an increased gamma globulin content, as did the fluids of 85 per cent of patients with 5 to 20 white cells (Yahr *et al.*, 1954). Similarly, Harter *et al.* (1962) confirmed this observation by showing that 17 per cent of 653 patients with moderately elevated gamma globulin levels had a pleocytosis, and 45 per cent of 294 patients with considerably elevated gamma globulin levels had a pleocytosis. Tourtellotte (1970) also concluded that there was a correlation between the intensity of the abnormal increase in gamma globulin and the degree of elevation of the cell count. However, he found no evidence of an

**TABLE 7–9   CSF Cell Counts in Multiple Sclerosis:
513 Consecutive Patients**

Cell Count (per mm^3)	Number of Cases	Percentage of Cases
0–5	387	75.4
6–10	74	14.4
11–20	41	8.0
21–40	9	1.75
50	1	
61	1	

(From Lumsden, 1972)

increased number of plasma cells in the CSF sediment, which supported his view that the increased CSF immunoglobulins are derived from regions of demyelination in the brain and/or spinal cord where such cells aggregate.

Total Protein

The total protein concentration in CSF is within normal limits in two thirds of patients with multiple sclerosis and mildly or moderately increased in the other third. The reports of Freedman and Merritt (1950), Yahr *et al.* (1954), Gilland (1965), Tourtellotte (1970) and Lumsden *et al.* (1972) support this generalization. The published data have not established a correlation between an elevation of total protein and the clinical activity of the disease. It is clear that a CSF protein level in excess of 100 mg/dl is very atypical; it should warn the physician that the diagnosis of multiple sclerosis is in doubt or that perhaps an additional neurological disease is present. The increase in CSF protein content occurs because of increased endothelial cell permeability associated with demyelinative lesions. This conclusion is supported by the appearance of focal areas of low density, observed with computed tomography, and particularly by the demonstration of focal enhancement following the injection of radiocontrast media (Weinstein *et al.*, 1978). No specific changes have been defined in any of the various proteins constituting the CSF total protein, apart from the gamma globulins and immunoglobulins.

Gamma Globulins and Immunoglobulins

The various gamma globulins and immunoglobulins in normal CSF and their origin were discussed in Chapter 6. The CSF gamma globulin concentration in normal subjects is about 1/300 of that in the serum, from which it is derived. However, in multiple sclerosis, the CSF gamma globulin content is increased preferentially (the serum level is unaffected), reflecting increased immunoglobulin production within the central nervous system (Kabat *et al.*, 1942; Frick and Scheid-Seydel, 1958; Cutler *et al.*, 1970; Tourtellotte, 1970). This mechanism was supported by Lowenthal's (1964) demonstration of increased amounts of gamma globulin in extracts of brain affected by multiple sclerosis and by the analogous studies of Tourtellotte (1970) and colleagues, which support the hypothesis that the CSF serves as a sink for immunoglobulins formed within the region of demyelinative lesions. The use of the IgG-albumin index, which corrects the CSF IgG level for the contribution of IgG derived from the blood, was described in Chapter 6. Table 7–10 provides representative values obtained by a variety of methods in patients with multiple sclerosis and other neurological diseases. The optimal way of expressing a quantitative increase in IgG was also discussed in Chapter 6, i.e., the use of total protein, albumin, transferrin, or alpha$_2$ macroglobulin levels as the denominator to which the IgG level is referred. It was concluded that the decision would depend upon a laboratory's accuracy, sensitivity, and reproducibility in its assay. The use of total protein or albumin levels probably meets these requirements most often.

Tourtellotte (1975) provided a calculation for estimating the rate of CSF immunoglobulin production that may prove useful in the serial study of a single patient (see Chapter 6). In a survey of the literature, Tourtellotte (1970)

TABLE 7–10   Percentage of Abnormal Immunoglobulin Findings in the Cerebrospinal Fluid in Multiple Sclerosis (MS) and Other Neurological Diseases (OND)

IMMUNOGLOBULIN DETERMINATION	MS	OND	REFERENCES
Oligoclonal bands on agar	95	2	Link, 1973
Oligoclonal bands on agar	79	4	Laterre *et al.*, 1970
Oligoclonal bands on agarose	98	16	Link, 1973
Oligoclonal bands on cellulose	41	15	Castaigne *et al.*, 1976
IgG quotient (with albumin)	88	18	Olsson and Pettersson, 1976
IgG β–globulin ratio	93	18	Vandvik and Skrede, 1973
Percentage of IgG in total protein	73	16	Link and Muller, 1971
Percentage of IgG in total protein	80	41	Castaigne *et al.*, 1972

(From Thompson, 1977)

reviewed the reported range of normal CSF gamma globulin values and the percentage of multiple sclerosis patients with elevated values. Thirty-six reports, involving more than 3000 patients, revealed that the upper normal limit of CSF gamma globulin varies substantially. In most reports when electrophoretic separation or immunochemical precipitation was used, the upper limit was between 11 and 13 per cent of the total protein. Clinicians are strongly advised to ascertain that their clinical laboratory has clearly defined its upper limit of normal because of the inherent variations in the methods commonly used. In most reports, an elevated CSF gamma globulin level (more than 2 [SD] above the mean) was observed in 60 to 80 per cent of patients with a clinical diagnosis of multiple sclerosis.

No consistent correlations have been reported between the degree of elevation of the immunoglobulins and the stage or activity of the disease. Thus, some patients with fulminating multiple sclerosis may have normal immunoglobulin levels; other patients with rather minor clinical evidence of the disease may have a striking increase in the immunoglobulin level. These discrepancies may be resolved by improved techniques.

Oligoclonal Bands

The demonstration by agarose gel electrophoresis of oligoclonal bands in the gamma globulins in various inflammatory disorders of the nervous system was discussed in Chapter 6 (see Figure 6–4). Their presence has been demonstrated in 79 per cent (Laterre *et al.*, 1970) to more than 90 per cent of patients with multiple sclerosis (Thompson, 1977; Johnson and Nelson, 1977). (See Figure 7–10.) While they correlate well with an increased IgG level, oligoclonal bands are of special value because they are present more often than an elevated IgG level in patients with multiple sclerosis. While the bands partly represent antibodies to various viral antigens, their relationship to the pathogenesis of the disease is not known (Norrby and Vandvik, 1975; Booe *et al.*, 1972; Forghani *et al.*, 1978, Norrby, 1978). It is important to note that oligoclonal bands present in the serum of patients with monoclonal gammopathies are detected in the CSF. Thus the presence of CSF bands favors the diagnosis of multiple sclerosis only if they have not originated from the serum. *The serum should be studied in all cases with CSF bands to exclude this possibility.* Changes in the other proteins in CSF were discussed in Chapter 6.

Kappa/Lambda Ratio

The kappa/lambda light chain ratios in the CSF (see Chapter 6) have been measured in patients with multiple sclerosis by Link and Zettervall (1970); Vandvik (1977); and Eickhoff and Heipertz (1978). An increase in the kappa/lambda ratio was observed in patients with multiple sclerosis as well as with a variety of the inflammatory disorders, from a ratio of about 1.0 in normal CSF to levels of about 2.3 in multiple sclerosis. At present, the assay is an investigative procedure that may elucidate immunological aspects of inflammatory disorders of the nervous system.

Myelin Basic Protein

The assay of myelin basic protein and of antibodies to myelin basic protein in CSF was discussed in Chapter 6 (Whitaker, 1977; Cohen *et al.*, 1976; Panitch *et al.*, 1980). Their increase in multiple sclerosis is of great theoretical interest. To date, however, assay of myelin basic protein has not been shown to be as useful in diagnosis as the measurement of IgG and the demonstration of oligoclonal bands.

Colloidal Reactions in Multiple Sclerosis

The colloidal gold tests and other colloidal reactions that have served as indicators of qualitative changes in the CSF proteins were discussed in Chapter 6. They have been replaced by more specific qualitative tests for the immunoglobulins present in multiple sclerosis and other inflammatory disorders of the nervous system. In the past, the incidence of an abnormal colloidal gold test result has varied between 44 and 71 per cent in cases of multiple sclerosis (Freedman and Merritt, 1950). The abnormalities have included first- and second-zone elevations, with a value of 2 or more. The greater incidence of a positive test result obtained by modern methods for the direct measurement of the immunoglobulins has clearly outmoded the colloidal gold test.

Myelinotoxic Activity of CSF

The ability of unconcentrated CSF from about 60 per cent of patients with multiple sclerosis to cause myelin lesions in the optic nerve of tadpoles was reported by Tabira *et al.* (1977). The responsible factor appears to be coupled with the presence of IgG and oligoclonal bands (Stendahl-Brodin *et al.*, 1979). The role of this myelinotoxic factor in the pathogenesis of multiple sclerosis is not known.

Viral Antibodies in CSF

Measurement of antibodies in serum and CSF has suggested local production of viral antibodies in the nervous system of patients with multiple sclerosis.

The viruses implicated in most studies have been measles, rubella, mumps, and vaccinia (Norrby *et al.*, 1974; Vandvik and Degne, 1975; Haire, 1977; Arnadottir *et al.*, 1979). No correlation has been observed between antibody production and the clinical phase of the disease. The antibody activities have been variably selective; in some patients viral antibodies present in high concentration in the serum might be present in or absent from the CSF. Arnadottir *et al.* (1979) suggest that the CSF viral antibodies reflect alterations in the immune system rather than a specific etiologic role of these viruses in multiple sclerosis. The role of the antibodies and the immune responses of patients with multiple sclerosis warrant further study.

CSF Sediment

The electron microscopic study by Herndon and Kasckow (1978) of the sediment obtained after ultracentrifugation of CSF from patients with multiple sclerosis and progressive multifocal leukoencephalopathy has revealed extra-cellular myelin fragments, recognized by their characteristic alternation of major dense lines and intraperiod lines. These fragments were seen in CSF from patients in exacerbation, with evidence of disease involving areas other than the optic nerves. The authors suggested that the myelin destruction in these two diseases results in the release of myelin fragments and other degradation products into the extracellular fluid and their subsequent passage directly into the CSF.

Other Constituents

There has been extraordinary interest in establishing specific biochemical changes in the CSF that might serve as reliable indicators of multiple sclerosis and of other diseases of the nervous system. All the constituents of CSF summarized in Chapter 6 have been determined in multiple sclerosis. None of the changes reported, including assays of the various lipid fractions and enzymes, have had sufficient reliability to warrant their use in clinical practice.

Optic Neuritis

Optic neuritis commonly occurs as an initial or early manifestation of multiple sclerosis. However, optic neuritis also occurs as a distinct illness separable from multiple sclerosis; long-term followup reveals no evidence of recurrent neurological involvement. A wide variation has been reported, between 11 and 76 per cent, in the concurrence of the two diseases (Stendahl *et al.*, 1976). Efforts have been made to identify the two diagnostic entities on the basis of the CSF findings. The following have been studied: CSF total protein content, immunoglobulins, oligoclonal bands, kappa and lambda antigenic determinants, and mononuclear pleocytosis (Perkin and Rose, 1979).

Sandberg and Bynke (1973) reported the CSF findings in 25 patients with acute monosymptomatic optic neuritis. The most common finding was a mononuclear leukocytosis in 60 per cent of cases, ranging between 5.6 and 29.4

cells per mm³. The protein content was elevated in 6 of the 25 cases, ranging between 45 and 65 mg/dl in 4 cases and elevated to 84 and 137 mg/dl in 2. The IgG level was elevated in 4 of the 25 cases, and in 6 cases there were oligoclonal bands. Evidence of multiple sclerosis developed in only 3 of the 25 patients during a short period of followup, and these had abnormal fluids.

Sandberg-Wollheim (1975) did a prospective study of 61 patients with acute monosymptomatic optic neuritis. Fifty-one per cent had a mononuclear pleocytosis, 18 per cent had an elevated IgG level, and 41 per cent had oligoclonal bands. It was concluded that there are no reliable predictive findings in the CSF to indicate those patients likely to develop multiple sclerosis and those likely to have monosymptomatic optic neuritis. However, it seems likely that the presence of an elevated IgG or oligoclonal bands favors the likelihood of multiple sclerosis over optic neuritis, although the former diagnosis should not be made on the basis of the CSF findings unless the clinical findings are indicative of multiple lesions in "time and anatomical space."

Acute Disseminated Encephalomyelitis

A heterogeneous group of disorders is included in the category of acute disseminated encephalomyelitis. The diagnosis of acute multiple sclerosis is sometimes used for such cases in the absence of any precipitating illness. When the syndrome occurs after specific infections, such as varicella, measles, rubella, mumps, scarlet fever, or pertussis, it has been termed parainfectious encephalomyelitis. The CSF findings in encephalomyelitis following varicella-zoster infection were described earlier.

In measles encephalomyelitis, a variable pleocytosis was reported in 466 cases by Miller *et al.* (1956). Lymphocytes predominated, but during the first few days "appreciable" numbers of polymorphonuclear leukocytes were noted. The cell count reached its highest level during the first few days and then rapidly declined. About 20 per cent of patients had a normal cell count. Most patients had cell counts between 50 and 150 per mm³. About 10 per cent of patients had cell counts greater than 200 per mm³. Eight of 466 patients had cell counts between 800 and 1500 per mm³. The protein level did not vary directly with the cell count and usually tended to decline much more slowly. A protein level greater than 100 mg/dl was unusual.

The CSF findings are similar in patients with parainfectious encephalomyelitis due to rubella. Miller *et al.* reported that 20 per cent of 58 patients had a normal cell count and most patients had a cell count between 20 and 100 lymphocytes per mm³. Rarely, cell counts between 200 and 400 per mm³ were observed. The protein level was usually between 60 and 80 mg/dl. The highest level observed was 160 mg/dl in a fluid with a normal cell count. The pressure was elevated in about half the cases.

In 24 cases of mumps parainfectious encephalomyelitis, the cell count was elevated in 18 patients to levels between 11 and 700 per mm³, with 90 to 99 per cent lymphocytes. The protein content was usually elevated, but not above 100 mg/dl (Miller *et al.*, 1956). Similar findings were noted in cases of mumps myelitis. While an increase in CSF immunoglobulins would be expected, its incidence is not known.

Amyotrophic Lateral Sclerosis

The findings in 33 cases of amyotrophic lateral sclerosis, progressive muscular atrophy, and progressive bulbar palsy were reported by Merritt and Fremont-Smith (1938). In 4 of the 33 patients, the cell count was slightly increased to between 5 and 12 mononuclear cells per mm³. The protein content was greater than 45 mg/dl in 12 patients between 75 and 95 mg/dl in 3 patients. There were no differences in the CSF findings in the various clinical forms of amyotrophic lateral sclerosis. The qualitative globulin (Pándy's) test was positive in one third of the patients. Roboz Einstein and Macrae (1968) reported a minor increase in gamma globulin in 3 of 11 patients. Laterre (1975) summarized the findings in 83 cases, as noted in Table 7–7. A protein content in excess of 100 mg/dl and cell counts in excess of 10 per mm³ should alert the clinician to another pathological process. Decreased levels of glutamic acid, homovanillic acid and 5-hydroxyindoleacetic acid have been reported, but these changes lack diagnostic specificity, they have been reported also in parkinsonism and other diseases (Bruck, 1966, Mendell et al. 1971, Tabbador et al. 1978).

Subacute Combined Degeneration (Pernicious Anemia)

The CSF findings in 50 patients with pernicious anemia and signs of spinal cord degeneration were reported by Merritt and Fremont-Smith (1938). The intracranial pressure was normal in 46 patients; 4 patients had 6 to 8 mononuclear cells per mm³. The protein level was normal in 39 patients; in 11 it was between 45 and 95 mg/dl. The colloidal gold test results and the CSF glucose levels were normal.

Acute Idiopathic Polyneuritis (Guillain-Barré Syndrome)

A highly elevated CSF protein in the absence of a pleocytosis (albuminocytological dissociation) was once considered characteristic of acute idiopathic polyneuritis (Guillain, 1936). Subsequent analyses of many cases revealed considerable variation in the degree of protein elevation and in the number of cells present.

Marshall (1963) reviewed the CSF findings in 34 cases. Most of the examinations were done in the first 21 days of the illness; a few cases were studied between day 21 and day 42. In 27 cases the cell count was less than 5 per mm³; in 3 it was under 15, in 2 under 25, and in 2 the counts were 50 and 46 respectively. In 1 case, on day 11 of the illness there were 24 cells per mm³ and 85 mg/dl of protein, and on day 30 there were 0 cells and 140 mg/dl of protein. Seven of the 34 patients had a normal CSF protein content. The time of the lumbar puncture was of importance; thus, in one patient the protein level was normal on day 4 of the illness but rose to 140 mg/dl on day 16. In another case, the protein rose from 330 to 1000 mg/dl between day 2 and day 7. Marshall's

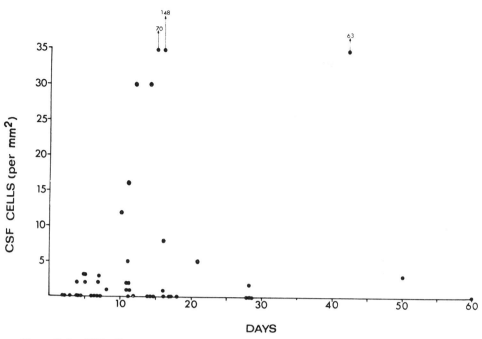

Figure 7-2   CSF cell count in acute idiopathic polyneuritis at intervals after onset of symptoms (from McLeod *et al.*, 1976).

data suggested that the maximum elevation of protein occurred between day 4 and day 18.

The CSF findings in 49 patients were analyzed by McLeod *et al.* (1976) from 2 to 65 days after the onset of symptoms. The protein was less than 40 mg/dl in 12 patients. In most cases, the cell concentration was 3 per mm³ or less, but in 7 cases it was elevated between 3 and 30 per mm³, and in 3 cases it was 70, 148, and 63 cells per mm³, respectively. The data are summarized in Figures 7–2 and 7–3. The figures illustrate the variability in the CSF findings. Though the maximal cellular responses were noted between 10 and 20 days after the onset of symptoms, one exceptional pleocytosis of 63 cells was noted 42 days after the onset of the illness. Although the maximal protein elevations were noted between 10 and 20 days after onset, there was an exception with a protein level of 640 mg/dl noted on day 5.

It is of special interest that the protein concentration in the cisternal fluid may be normal or slightly increased despite marked elevation of the lumbar fluid protein. Aring (1945) described 3 cases in which the lumbar and cisternal fluid proteins were as follows: 330 and 14 mg/dl, 380 and 88 mg/dl, and 1400 and 82 mg/dl. These findings are compatible with the hypothesis that the increased CSF protein is derived largely from the capillaries of the spinal roots as they traverse the subarachnoid space.

An extensive literature supports the involvement of an immunological disorder in the pathogenesis of the Guillain-Barré syndrome (Asbury *et al.*, 1969, Link, 1973). This was suggested by the increased CSF gamma globulins in the

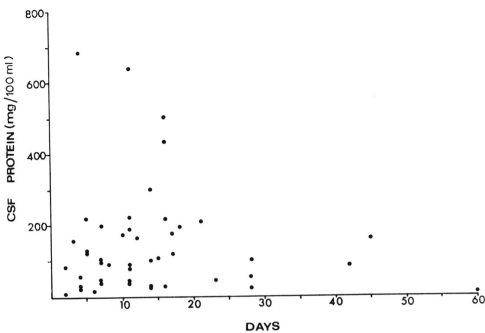

Figure 7–3 CSF protein concentration in acute idiopathic polyneuritis at intervals after onset of symptoms (McLeod *et al.*, 1976).

CSF of many patients (Dencker *et al.*, 1964). Many of the early reports failed to distinguish between increased entry of serum globulins into the CSF as a result of the increased total protein, and the synthesis of immunoglobulins within the central nervous system. Link (1973) reported increased concentration in the CSF of IgA and IgM, less frequently of IgG, expressed as a percentage of the total protein concentration. The serum levels of the three immunoglobulins were normal. Oligoclonal bands were demonstrated in the serum and CSF of 8 of 12 patients. The concentrations of the three immunoglobulins appeared to be elevated most often early in the course of the illness. The kappa/lambda ratios in CSF and serum were normal, about 1.0, in the 12 patients. The changes in the immunoglobulins did not appear to correlate with the severity of the illness.

Intracranial Hypertension and Polyneuritis

Although the intracranial pressure is characteristically normal in the Guillain-Barré syndrome, the occurrence of papilledema and intracranial hypertension is a well-recognized complication. Morley and Reynolds (1966) reviewed the literature and found 27 published cases to which they added another 4 cases. The peak age incidence was 20 to 40 years (like most cases), and there was no sex difference. The duration of the illness ranged from 4 months to 2 years, with an average of 10 months, and in 5 cases the disease was recurrent.

The range of the CSF proteins was quite variable. In 4 patients, the protein was less than 200 mg/dl; in 8 patients, the protein was between 200 and 400 mg/dl; and in the other 16 patients, it was greater than 400 mg/dl. None of these features appeared to differ from the range of findings in polyneuritis uncomplicated by intracranial hypertension.

The pathogenesis of this syndrome was discussed in Chapter 4. There are analogies between it and the syndrome of intracranial hypertension observed with spinal cord tumors (Ridsdale and Moseley, 1978). To recapitulate, the elevated CSF protein *per se* does not appear to be responsible for the intracranial hypertension. It seems more likely that a defect in the giant vesicular transport system of the arachnoid villi may be responsible for the defect in CSF absorption and for the intracranial hypertension.

The CSF findings in other forms of polyneuritis are similar to those of the idiopathic form of the disease; they include postdiphtheritic polyneuritis and polyneuritis due to infectious mononucleosis, porphyria, or a specific infection such as the acute exanthems.

Brachial Plexus Neuropathy

Brachial plexus neuropathy has been described under a variety of names, including acute brachial neuritis, brachial plexitis, neuralgic amyotrophy, the syndrome of Parsonage and Turner, and others. Tsairis *et al.* (1972) reviewed the natural history of the disorder in 99 patients, in 35 of whom lumbar puncture was performed 1 week to 6 months after the onset of symptoms. The CSF was examined within 3 weeks after the onset in 20 patients. In 1 patient with infectious mononucleosis, there was a "mild" increase in protein and "slight" pleocytosis. In 3 patients, the protein level was between 50 and 60 mg/dl (normal < 45 mg/dl). The CSF examination, including the gamma globulin in 16 patients, was otherwise normal.

Diabetic Neuropathy

The elevation of CSF protein in patients with diabetic neuropathy is well established (Rundles, 1945; Madonick *et al.*, 1952). However, in most cases, the literature has failed to delineate the clinical features of the diabetic neuropathy, including its distribution and severity.

The elevated CSF protein in patients with diabetic neuropathy was studied by Ives (1957). In a series of 370 diabetic patients, 64 patients had signs or symptoms of peripheral neuropathy. Of these, 68 per cent (44 cases) had an elevated CSF protein level. The total protein content varied from 51 mg/dl to 224 mg/dl, with an average of 77 mg/dl. This was similar to the findings reported by Joslin *et al.* (1959) in a series of 157 diabetic patients, of whom 72 per cent had an elevated protein level, the highest being 440 mg/dl. An elevated CSF protein has been noted in almost every case of diabetic amyotrophy (Bruyn and Garland, 1970).

Few correlations have been established between the degree of protein elevation and the clinical aspects of diabetic neuropathy. Ives (1957) noted no correlation with the duration of illness, the presence of retinopathy, or renal disease, although other authors have reported a correlation between the protein elevation and the severity of the neuropathy (Joslin *et al.*, 1959; Kutt *et al.*, 1960). I would recommend caution in attributing an elevated CSF protein (greater than 60 mg/dl) to diabetes mellitus unless there is objective evidence of peripheral neuropathy, either sensory or sensorimotor in type; i.e., in its absence another cause is likely.

Kutt *et al.* (1960) reported that the CSF electrophoretic patterns in diabetic neuropathy showed an increase in the alpha$_2$ globulin content. The corresponding serum levels were not described, and the origin and significance of the change are unclear. Diabetic patients have been reported to have increased CSF levels of sorbitol and fructose (Wray and Winegrad, 1966). The correlation between such changes and the occurrence and severity of complications such as diabetic neuropathy is not known. The relationship of the CSF glucose level to the blood level was discussed in Chapter 6. The cell count is normal in diabetic peripheral neuropathy.

Hereditary Neuropathies and Myelopathies

An increased CSF protein is also common in various hereditary neuropathies and myelopathies, including Charcot-Marie-Tooth disease, Dejerine-Sottas hypertrophic polyneuritis, amyloid neuropathy, Friedreich's ataxia and other spinocerebellar degenerations, and metachromatic leukodystrophy. The levels observed are usually between 50 and 200 mg/dl. The mechanism of the increased protein has not been elucidated. Presumably, the capillaries of the nerve roots are more permeable to proteins. The electrophoretic findings reveal "transudative" patterns, i.e., increased amounts of serum proteins (see Chapter 6).

Refsum's Disease

Refsum's disease, a genetic disorder, has been termed "phytanic acid storage disease." Among its cardinal clinical features are retinitis pigmentosa, chronic polyneuropathy, cerebellar ataxia, and an elevated CSF protein content. Refsum (1975) reported that the CSF protein is elevated in practically all cases and that the cell count is normal. The protein levels are usually in the range of 100 to 700 mg/dl; higher levels have been reported. A correlation between the clinical severity and the protein concentration was observed, particularly in cases with spontaneous remissions and exacerbations as well as in patients in whom clinical improvement was produced with a diet low in phytanic acid.

Paraneoplastic Syndromes

The various paraneoplastic syndromes include the heterogeneous neurological disorders that occur with a systemic malignancy in the absence of metastatic disease. While the term "remote effects of cancer on the nervous system" has become popular since the monograph of Brain and Norris (1965), "paraneoplastic syndromes" is preferred because the neurological disorder often antedates the appearance of the malignancy. In addition, in no case has a malignant tumor yet been shown to *cause* the neurological disorder. The paraneoplastic disorders of the nervous system include (a) progressive multifocal leukoencephalopathy, (b) subacute cerebellar degeneration, (c) carcinomatous neuropathy, and (d) central pontine myelinolysis.

Progressive Multifocal Leukoencephalopathy

This subacute disease of white matter occurs with a variety of systemic malignancies, chiefly the lymphoproliferative disorders, Hodgkin's disease, the leukemias, and sarcoidosis. The illness has been seen in these diseases and occasionally in apparently healthy people. The presence of papovavirus within the oligodendroglial nuclei established the disease as one of the slow virus diseases of the nervous system. The CSF in most cases has been entirely normal. Richardson (1961) commented on 2 cases with a slight elevation in pressure, 275 mm and 200 mm respectively. In 2 other cases, a slight increase in cells was described, 2 to 25 white cells per mm^3; in 2 other cases, there was a slight rise in protein content. Oligoclonal bands have not been described. Thus, the CSF examination is of little value in making the diagnosis.

Subacute Cerebellar Degeneration

This syndrome is seen with a variety of primary neoplasms, and the neurological findings may appear before or after the appearance of the neoplasm. Brain and Wilkinson (1965) described the CSF findings in 11 cases. The cells were normal in 9 and increased in 2 cases, with 11 and 20 mononuclear cells per mm^3 respectively. The protein level was normal in 7 and increased in 4 cases (from 60 to 120 mg/dl). The gamma globulins were increased in 6 cases (abnormal colloidal gold curve). Thus, the CSF examination may be normal or show minor changes compatible with evidence suggestive of an inflammatory process.

Carcinomatous Polyneuropathy

Croft *et al.* (1976) reviewed the CSF findings in carcinomatous peripheral neuropathy and reported that 14 of 19 patients had an elevated protein content. Levels between 100 and 360 mg/dl were seen in 8 of the cases. Abnormalities of the colloidal gold test, including first-zone and midzone elevations, were seen in several cases. The cell counts were normal, 6 or fewer cells per mm^3.

Central Pontine Myelinolysis

Central pontine myelinolysis (CPM) occurs most often in patients with chronic alcoholism, malnutrition, severe burns, renal insufficiency, and systemic malignancies. McCormick and Danneel (1967) reviewed the findings in 66 reported cases. Of these, the lumbar puncture findings in 21 patients were reported as follows: normal in 11, elevated pressure in 6, elevated protein in 5, mildly elevated mononuclear cell count in 4. The associated diseases could probably account for such CSF abnormalities when present. The observation that the CSF was normal in half the cases is of diagnostic interest. Changes in the CSF immunoglobulins have not been reported.

Parkinsonism

The usual clinical indices in the CSF of patients with idiopathic parkinsonism are normal, including pressure, cell count, total protein, and protein electrophoresis. Any such abnormality found in parkinsonism strongly suggests another pathological process. The presence of oligoclonal bands has been reported in two patients with post-encephalitic parkinsonism (Williams *et al.*, 1979). This finding may help differentiate post-encephalitic from idiopathic cases. The CSF amino acids, enzymes, and metabolites of dopamine and serotonin have also been investigated. There are inconsistent reports of changes in the CSF amino acids. Gerstenbrand (1966) reported that the CSF glutamic acid was significantly reduced in Parkinson's disease. However, the specificity of this finding is dubious, because similar reductions were observed in Huntington's chorea and amyotrophic lateral sclerosis (Bruck, 1966). Van Sande *et al.* (1970) reported that 15 amino acids were increased in parkinsonism, but this was not confirmed by Gjessing *et al.* (1974). A reduction in CSF gamma aminobutyric acid (GABA) was reported in parkinsonism, but similar levels were found in Huntington's chorea, schizophrenia, and tardive dyskinesia (Faull *et al.*, 1978).

The acid metabolites of dopamine and serotonin (homovanillic acid and 5-hydroxyindoleacetic acid) were discussed in Chapter 6. Both metabolites are decreased in the ventricular fluid (Papeschi *et al.*, 1972) and lumbar fluid (Chase and Ng, 1972). However, the decrease is not considered specific for this disorder, because similar changes were found in amyotrophic lateral sclerosis (Mendell *et al.*, 1971; Tabbador *et al.* 1978). The concentration of 3-methoxy-4-hydroxy-phenylethylene glycol (3-MHPG), the metabolite of norepinephrine, is normal in the CSF of patients with parkinsonism (Gordon and Oliver, 1971). To date, assay of the biogenic amines in the CSF have not been shown to have any diagnostic specificity for parkinsonism.

Huntington's Chorea

The usual clinical indices in the CSF are normal in Huntington's chorea, including protein content, protein electrophoresis, cell count, and glucose content. The biogenic amines have been studied extensively. Chase *et al.* (1972) found normal levels of 5-HIAA in the CSF of patients with Huntington's chorea. Homovanillic acid (HVA) was reported to be decreased in severe chorea by Curzon *et al.* (1972). The influence of ventricular enlargement *per se* upon the concentration of HVA in ventricular fluid has not been defined. Aquilonius *et al.* (1972) reported a decreased choline level in the CSF of Huntington patients. These observations and others suggest alterations in the several biogenic amines, but the changes reported have not been shown to have diagnostic specificity. The concentration of GABA was reduced about 50 per cent in Huntington's chorea, and low levels *may* be present in patients at risk prior to the onset of symptoms (Manyam *et al.*, 1978). However, Faull *et al.* (1978), using a very sensitive method (mass spectrometer), found overlapping CSF GABA levels in Huntington's chorea, the psychoses, and tardive dyskinesia. At present, no specific changes in the CSF of patients with Huntington's chorea have been established.

Wilson's Disease

The CSF is usually normal in early Wilson's disease. Rarely, the meninges have been described as thickened and infiltrated with macrophages. There is a case report of a patient with moderate elevations of the CSF cell count, 112 lymphocytes per mm^3, and a protein content of 101 mg/dl (Bennett and Harbilas, 1967).

Sydenham's Chorea

The CSF was entirely normal in 14 patients (Merritt and Fremont-Smith, 1938).

Tay-Sachs Disease

The CSF findings in 11 children with Tay-Sachs disease were described by Tourtellotte *et al.* (1965). Their ages varied between 13 and 46 months. The CSF white cell count was normal, but "foam cells" were found in 4 of 6 infants in whom a specific search was made. These were described as very large cells, usually between 20 and 40 microns in diameter, with a vacuolated, foamy-appearing cytoplasm. Some of the cells appeared to have a granular cytoplasm; others appeared nongranular. Both were considered to probably represent large lipomacrophages. The data suggested that older patients, probably with more severe disease, had a higher percentage of foam cells. The greatest number (71 per cent) of foam cells was seen in the oldest child, although the total cell count remained within normal limits. The frequency of their occurrence in other lipidoses is unknown.

The CSF protein content was normal in all the infants. However, the total CSF lipids were increased in 8 of 11 patients studied. The oldest child had the most abnormal "lipid profile." No specific changes in the CSF lipids were detected; i.e., the total phospholipids, sphingolipids, and cholesterol were all increased. The difficulties in measuring minute amounts of lipid in CSF has limited, to date, the usefulness of such assays in clinical diagnosis. Improved assay methods such as gas-liquid chromatography may make such assays more feasible. Aronson *et al.* (1958) reported elevated CSF enzymes (aldolase, phosphohexose isomerase, glutamic-oxaloacetic transaminase, and lactic dehydrogenase) early in the course of the illness, but the specificity of this finding has not been established further.

Alzheimer's Disease and Related Disorders

The presenile and senile dementias that are considered to comprise Alzheimer's disease are characteristically associated with a normal CSF examination. A minimal increase in CSF protein content is occasionally observed, 50 to 70 mg/dl. However, if there are further increases in protein content, a pleocytosis, or an increase in immunoglobulins, then other diagnoses are likely. The wide range of constituents described in Chapter 6 have not been shown to be significantly altered in Alzheimer's disease. The CSF is similarly normal in the other organic dementias, including Pick's disease, supranuclear palsy, and the subacute dementias such as Jakob-Creutzfeldt disease.

Epilepsy

The CSF is normal in idiopathic epilepsy. Any abnormality in cell count or protein level indicates a pathological process adjacent to the CSF pathways. Merritt and Fremont-Smith's (1938) review of about 800 patients with epilepsy supports this generalization. Acute elevation in intracranial pressure was observed during major seizures. This occurs secondary to an acute increase in cerebral blood flow associated with increased cerebral metabolism. An increase in CSF lactate and primary acidosis of the CSF have been described following severe convulsions, reflecting a marked increase in cerebral glycolysis (Brooks and Adams, 1975). Following a grand mal seizure the CSF is usually normal if head injury has not occurred. However, following idiopathic status epilepticus, a minor pleocytosis, 5 to 30 leukocytes per mm^3, is not unusual. The pathogenesis of this change, its frequency, and its duration are not known.

Narcolepsy and Cataplexy

The CSF in narcolepsy and cataplexy is normal in terms of the usual clinical tests — cell count, total protein, electrophoresis, and glucose content. Parkes *et al.* (1974) studied the homovanillic acid (HVA), 5-hydroxy-indoleacetic acid (5-HIAA), and amino acid composition of the CSF in 20 patients with narcolepsy. No significant changes in serotonin, tryptophan, or 5-HIAA concentrations were observed. A significant fall in HVA levels and low aspartate concentrations were observed. The significance of these reported changes is not known.

Psychiatric Disorders

The CSF is normal in patients with schizophrenia and manic-depressive illness. Abnormalities of pressure, cell count, glucose level, or protein content can not be attributed to these psychoses. A burgeoning literature in the last decade has dealt with the search for abnormalities of the biogenic amines in the lumbar CSF of patients with the gamut of psychiatric illnesses, including autism, schizophrenia, and manic-depressive illness. The data have been summarized in Chapter 6 (see Biogenic Amines). The data have been conflicting and inconsistent. None of the suspected biochemical changes have been shown as yet to be diagnostically useful in the study of psychiatric illness. Several factors pose technical difficulties for the clinical investigator: the lumbar CSF is at a distance from the cerebrum, the cerebral metabolites are difficult to measure in great dilution, and CSF from suitable control subjects is difficult to obtain.

Migraine

Few data are available regarding the CSF changes associated with migraine. While the CSF is normal between migraine attacks, abnormal findings have been reported during or shortly after an attack of hemiplegic migraine. The CSF was normal in all 22 patients in Bradshaw and Parson's (1965) series. However, Whitty (1953) states that the CSF was abnormal in 5 of 7 patients; in 2 the protein was elevated, and in 3 a slight pleocytosis was noted. Symonds (1952) reported a CSF cell count of 185 polymorphonuclear cells in a patient with familial hemiplegic migraine and Whitty (1953) described a patient with a lymphocyte count of 40. I have seen a slight pleocytosis, 5 to 15 mononuclear cells per mm³, in several patients within a day of a severe migraine attack. It is a clinical impression that a pleocytosis and a minor protein elevation tend to occur with attacks of great severity and particularly when associated with signs of focal ischemia. Considering the great frequency of migraine, there is a paucity of data available on this point.

The concentration of gamma aminobutyric acid (GABA) and cyclic AMP has been measured in the CSF of patients with migraine (Welch *et al.*, 1976). Elevated levels of both compounds were observed. GABA was elevated in the CSF of all patients studied during a migraine attack but not in those with asymptomatic migraine or tension headache. Cyclic AMP was elevated in patients studied during or within 48 hours of a migraine attack. Similar changes were noted in patients with recent ischemic strokes.

Kearns-Sayre Syndrome

This curious syndrome is characterized by progressive external ophthalmoplegia, atypical pigmentary degeneration of the retina, and heart block. In many cases there is evidence of widespread neurological disorder, including cerebral, cerebellar, auditory, and vestibular dysfunction. The clinical features and CSF findings have been analyzed by Berenberg *et al.* (1977). CSF protein content was determined in 35 cases. It was greater than 70 mg/dl in all but one case, and between 100 and 400 mg/dl in 20 cases. The CSF gamma globulin was 13 per cent or more in 7 of 11 patients evaluated. This apparent increase was probably a reflection of the increase in total protein. The serum protein electrophoreses were not described. No other CSF abnormalities have been reported.

Myxedema and Hyperthyroidism

Elevation of the spinal fluid protein is commonly noted in myxedema (Bronsky et al., 1958; Nickel and Frame, 1958; Bloomer et al., 1960). Levels between 100 and 340 mg/dl were reported in 12 of 27 patients, although values may also be normal (Bronsky et al., 1958). Myxedema may result in an increased permeability of the blood-CSF barrier analogous to the changes in brain permeability shown in hypothyroid rats (Raskin and Fishman, 1966). It is not known whether myxedema interferes with the function of the arachnoid villi. It is possible that the acid mucopolysaccharides that accumulate in the connective tissue in myxedema also infiltrate the arachnoid villi and dura. An increase in both serum and CSF gamma globulin content has been observed in some patients. At times, only the spinal fluid gamma globulin was elevated with a normal total protein content (Nickel and Frame, 1958). It is likely (but not established) that the increase in CSF gamma globulin reflects only an increase in the serum level. There is no correlation between the degree of protein elevation and the clinical status of the patient, although the protein returns to normal with thyroid therapy. An elevation in CSF pressure above 250 mm was noted in some cases by Thompson et al. (1929). The origin of the elevation is uncertain. The spinal fluid is otherwise not remarkable.

The spinal fluid in hyperthyroidism is within normal limits, apart from the level of spinal fluid protein which is low normal or lower than normal, below 15 mg/dl in some cases (Merritt and Fremont-Smith, 1938). In 15 patients, the average protein level was 24 mg/dl and rose to 37 mg/dl after subtotal thyroidectomy (Thompson and Alexander, 1930). It is possible that the spinal fluid pulsations are increased in hyperthyroidism despite normal mean CSF pressures; this might produce more rapid bulk flow absorption of the fluid and thus induce a reduction in protein concentration.

Hypoparathyroidism

The syndrome of pseudotumor cerebri has been rarely reported as a manifestation of hypoparathyroidism (Bronsky et al., 1958). The CSF pressure was elevated to levels as high as 460 mm. The protein content was increased in some cases. The calcium content of the spinal fluid was slightly depressed, but to a lesser degree than the serum level. The spinal fluid changes reverted to normal with therapy. The pathogenesis of these changes is not understood.

Lead Encephalopathy

Lead encephalopathy is a manifestation of lead poisoning in infants and children. Rarely, with serious intoxication, it has been found in adults. The CSF findings include increased pressure and protein concentration, frequently accompanied by a mononuclear pleocytosis of 30 to 100 cells per mm^3. The CSF changes have caused the condition to be confused with viral or tuberculous meningitis (Ludwig, 1977).

Bromide Intoxication

Perkins (1950) reviewed the CSF findings in 21 patients with bromide intoxication. The CSF protein content was elevated in two thirds of the patients, ranging between 46 and 142 mg/dl. The protein levels returned to normal by the time the patients had recovered. There were no other significant changes. The mechanism whereby bromidism might be responsible for such an increase is not clear. No data are available regarding the effects of the bromide ion on the permeability of the blood-brain barrier.

BIBLIOGRAPHY

Aber, G. M.: Studies of the inter-relationship between cerebrospinal fluid and plasma amino acid concentration in normal individuals. J. Neurochem. 29:291–297, 1977.

Abouleish, E., de la Vega, S., Blendinger, I. et al.: Longterm follow up of epidural blood patch. Anesth. Analg. 54:459–463, 1975.

Adams, J. E. and Prawirohardjo, S.: Fate of red blood cells injected into cerebrospinal fluid pathways. Neurology (Minneap.) 9:561–564, 1959.

Adams, R. D., Fisher, C. M., Hakim, S. et al.: Symptomatic occult hydrocephalus with "normal" cerebrospinal-fluid pressure. N. Engl. J. Med. 273:117–126, 1965.

Adams, R. D. and Foley, J. M.: The neurologic disorder associated with liver disease. Res. Publ. Assoc. Res. Nerv. Ment. Dis. 32:198–237, 1953.

Adolph, R. J., Fukusumi, H. and Fowler, N. O.: Origin of cerebrospinal fluid pulsations. Am. J. Physiol. 212:840–846, 1967.

Afifi, A. M.: Myeloma cells in the cerebrospinal fluid in plasma cell neoplasia. J. Neurol. Neurosurg. Psychiatry. 37:1162–1165, 1974.

Agarwal, G. C., Berman, B. M. and Stark, L.: A lumped parameter model of the cerebrospinal fluid system. IEEE Trans. Biomed. Eng. 16:45–53, 1965.

Aizenstein, M. L. and Korf, J.: On the elimination of centrally formed 5-hydroxyindoleacetic acid by cerebrospinal fluid and urine. J. Neurochem. 32:1227–1233, 1979.

Ajello, L. (ed.): Coccidioidomycosis: Current Clinical and Diagnostic Status. Miami, Symposia Specialists Medical Books, 1977.

Alami, S. Y. and Afifi, A. K.: Cerebrospinal fluid examination. In Race, G. J. (ed.): Laboratory Medicine. Hagerstown, Harper and Row, 1976.

Alema, G.: Behçet's disease. In Vinken, P. J. and Bruyn, G. W. (eds.): Handbook of Clinical Neurology. Vol. 34. Amsterdam, Elsevier/North Holland, 1978, pp. 475–512.

Alksne, J. F. and Lovings, E. T.: Functional ultrastructure of the arachnoid villus. Arch. Neurol. 27:371–377, 1972.

Alksne, J. F. and Lovings, E. T.: The role of the arachnoid villus in the removal of red blood cells from the subarachnoid space. An electron microscope study in the dog. J. Neurosurg. 36:192–200, 1972.

Allen, J., Sheremata, W., Cosgrove, J. B. et al.: Cerebrospinal fluid T and B lymphocytes kinetics related to exacerbations of multiple sclerosis. Neurology (Minneap.) 25:352, 1975. (Abstract)

Almen, T.: Toxicity of radio contrast agents. In Knolfel, P. K. (ed.): Radio Contrast Agents. Vol. 2. Oxford, Pergamon, 1971, pp. 443–550.

Amatuzio, D. S., Weber, L. J. and Nesbitt, S.: Bilirubin and protein in the cerebrospinal fluid of jaundiced patients with severe liver disease with and without hepatic coma. J. Lab. Clin. Med. 41:615–618, 1953.

Ames, A., Akanone, M. and Endo, S.: Na, K, Ca, Mg and Cl concentrations in choroid plexus fluid and cisternal fluid compared with plasma ultrafiltrate. J. Neurophysiol. 27:672–681, 1964.

Ames, A., III, Higashi, K. and Nesbett, F. B.: Relation of potassium concentration in choroid plexus fluid to that in plasma. J. Physiol. 181:506–515, 1965.

Ames, A., III, Higashi, K. and Nesbett, F. B.: Effects of PCO_2 acetezolamide and ouabain on composition of choroid plexus fluid. J. Physiol. 181:516–524, 1965.

Ames, A., III, Sakanous, M. and Endo, S.: Na, K, Ca, Mg and Cl concentrations in choroid plexus fluid and cisternal fluid compared with plasma ultrafiltrate. J. Neurophysiol. 27:672–681, 1964.

Aminoff, M. J.: Spinal Angiomas. Oxford, Blackwell Scientific Publications, 1976, pp. 65–66.

Anderson, D. C., Greenwood, R., Fishman, M. et al.: Acute infantile hemiplegia with cerebrospinal fluid eosinophilic pleocytosis. Unusual case of visceral larva migrans. J. Pediatr. 86:245–247, 1975.

Andersson, H. and Roos, B. E.: 5-Hydroxyindoleacetic acid in cerebrospinal fluid of hydrocephalic children. Acta Paediatr. Scand. (Stockh.) 58:601–608, 1969.

327

Andreoli, T. E., Grantham, J. J. and Rector, F. C. Jr. (eds.): Disturbances in Body Fluid Osmolality. Bethesda, American Physiological Society, 1977.

Andrianakos, A. A., Duffy, J., Suzuki, M. et al.: Transverse myelopathy in systemic lupus erythematosus. Ann. Intern. Med. 83:616–624, 1975.

Antoni, N.: Pressure curves from the cerebrospinal fluid. Acta Med. Scand. Suppl. 170:439–462, 1946.

Aquilonius, S. M. and Eckern, S. A.: Choline acetyltransferase in human cerebrospinal fluid: Non-enzymatically and enzymatically catalyzed acetylcholine synthesis. J. Neurochem. 27:317–318, 1976.

Aquilónius, S. M., Nystrom, B., Schuberth, J. and Sundwall, A.: Cerebrospinal fluid choline in extrapyramidal disorders. J. Neurol. Neurosurg. Psychiatry. 35:720–725, 1972.

Arieff, A. I., Guisado, R. and Lazarowitz, V. C.: Pathophysiology of hyperosmolar states. In Andreoli, T. E., Grantham, J. J. and Rector, F. C., Jr. (eds.): Disturbances in Body Fluid Osmolality. Bethesda, American Physiological Society, 1977, pp. 227–250.

Arieff, A. I. and Kleeman, C. R.: Studies on mechanisms of cerebral edema in diabetic comas. J. Clin. Invest. 52:571–583, 1973.

Arieff, A. I., Llack, F. and Massry, S. G.: Neurological manifestations and morbidity of hyponatremia: Correlation with brain water and electrolytes. Medicine 55:121–129, 1976.

Arieff, A. I. and Massry, S.: Calcium metabolism of brain in acute renal failure. J. Clin. Invest. 53:387–392, 1974.

Arieff, A. I., Massry, S. G., Barrientos, A. et al.: Brain water and electrolyte metabolism in uremia: Effects of slow and rapid hemodialysis. Kidney Int. 4:177–187, 1973.

Aring, C. D.: Infectious polyneuritis. Clinics 4:262–274, 1945.

Arnadottir, T., Reunanen, M., Meurman, O. et al.: Measles and rubella virus antibodies in patients with multiple sclerosis. A longitudinal study of serum and CSF specimens by radioimmunoassay. Arch. Neurol. 36:261–265, 1979.

Aronson, S. M., Saifer, A., Perle, G. and Volk, B. W.: Cerebrospinal fluid enzymes in central nervous system lipidoses (with particular reference to amaurotic idiocy). Proc. Soc. Exp. Biol. Med. 97:331–334, 1958.

Arseni, C. and Maretsis, M.: Tumors of the lower spinal cord associated with increased intracranial pressure and papilledema. J. Neurosurg. 27:105–110, 1967.

Asberg, M., Traskman, L. and Thoren, P.: 5-HIAA in the cerebrospinal fluid: A biochemical suicide predictor? Arch. Gen. Psychiatry 33:1193–1197, 1976.

Asbury, A. K., Arnason, B. G. and Adams, R. D.: The inflammatory lesion in idiopathic polyneuritis. Medicine 48:173–215, 1969.

Ashcroft, G. W. and Sharman, D. F.: 5-Hydroxyindoles in human cerebrospinal fluids. Nature 186:1050–1051, 1960.

Assies, J., Schellekens, A. P. M. and Touber, J. L.: Prolactin in human cerebrospinal fluid. J. Clin. Endocrinol. Metab. 46:576–586, 1978.

Association for Research in Nervous and Mental Disease. Research Publications Vol. 14. The Human Cerebrospinal Fluid. New York, Hoeber, 1924.

Atanasiu, P. and Gamet, A.: Rabies. In Vinken, P. J. and Bruyn, G. W. (eds.): Handbook of Clinical Neurology. Vol. 34. Amsterdam, Elsevier/North Holland, 1978, pp. 235–275.

Atkins, C., Kondon, J., Quismorio, F. P. et al.: The choroidal plexus in systemic lupus erythematosus (SLE). Arthritis Rheum. 14:148, 1971. (Abstract)

Atkinson, J. R. and Ward, A. A., Jr.: Effect of diamox on intracranial pressure and blood volume. Neurology (Minneap.) 8:45–50, 1958.

Axelrod, L.: Glucocorticoid therapy. Medicine 55:39–65, 1976.

Ayala, G.: Die Physiopathologie der Mechanik des Liquor cerebrospinalis und der Rachidealquotient. Mschr. Psychiatr. Neurol. 58:65–101, 1925.

Ayala, G.: Uber der diagnostischen Wert des Liquordruckes und einen Apparat zu seiner Messung. Ztschr. Ges. Neurol. Psychiatr. 34:430–431, 1923.

Ayer, J. B.: Puncture of cisterna magna. Arch. Neurol. Psychiatr. 4:529–541, 1920.

Ayer, J. B.: Puncture of the cisterna magna. Report on 1,985 punctures. J.A.M.A. 81:358–360, 1923.

Baethmann, A., Oettinger, W., Rothenfusser, W. et al.: Biochemical aspects of cerebral edema. In Mrsulja, B. B., Rakic, L. M., Klatzo, I., and Spatz, M. (eds.): Pathophysiology of Cerebral Energy Metabolism. New York, Plenum, 1979.

Bagley, C., Jr.: Functional and organic alterations following the introduction of blood into the cerebrospinal fluid. Res. Publ. Assoc. Res. Nerv. Ment. Dis. 8:217–244, 1929.

Bakay, L.: The Blood-Brain Barrier with Special Regard to the Use of Radioactive Isotopes. Springfield, Illinois, Charles C Thomas, 1956.

Bakay, L., Crawford, J. D., and White, J. C.: The effects of intravenous fluids on cerebrospinal fluid pressure. Surg. Gynecol. Obstet. 99:48–53, 1954.

Bakay, L. and Lee, J. C.: Cerebral Edema. Springfield, Illinois, Charles C Thomas, 1965.

Baker, H., Frank, O., Fennelly, J. J. et al.: A method for assaying thiamine status in man and animals. Am. J. Clin. Nutr. 14:197–201, 1964.

Baker, A. S., Ojemann, R. G., and Swartz, M. N. et al.: Spinal epidural abscess. N. Engl. J. Med. 293:463–468, 1975.

Bakke, O. M., Guldberg, H. C. and Schreiner, A.: Acid monoamine metabolites of cerebrospinal fluid in meningitis and encephalitis. Acta Neurol. Scand. 50:146–152, 1974.

Balhuizen, J. C., Bots, G. T. A. M., Schaberg, A. et al.: Value of cerebrospinal fluid cytology for the diagnosis of malignancies in the central nervous system. J. Neurosurg. 48:747–753, 1978.

Ballenger, J. C., Post, R. M., Sternberg, D. E. et al.: Headaches after lumbar puncture and insensitivity to pain in psychiatric patients. N. Engl. J. Med. 301:110, 1979.

Baltch, A. and Osborne, W.: Inquiry into causes of lowered spinal fluid sugar content. *In vivo* and *in vitro* observations. J. Lab. Clin. Med. 49:882–889, 1957.

Bamford, C., Sibley, W. and Laguna, J.: Anesthesia in multiple sclerosis. Can. J. Neurol. Sci. 5:41–44, 1978.

Bammer, H.: Cerebrospinal fluid complement and multiple sclerosis. Deutsch Z. Nervenheilk. 188:271–288, 1966.

Bannister, R., Gilford, E. and Kocen, R.: Isotope encephalography in the diagnosis of dementia due to communicating hydrocephalus. Lancet 2:1014–1017, 1967.

Baringer, J. R.: A simplified procedure for spinal fluid cytology. Arch. Neurol. 22:305–308, 1970.

Barlow, C. F.: Clinical aspects of the blood-brain barrier. Ann. Rev. Med. 15:187–202, 1964.

Barlow, C. F., Domek, N. S., Goldberg, M. A. and Roth, L. J.: Extracellular brain space measured by S³⁵ sulfate. Arch. Neurol. 5:1–2, 110, 1961.

Barnes, B. and Fish, M.: Chemical meningitis as a complication of isotope cisternography. Neurology 22:83–91, 1972.

Barnett, H. J., Foster, J. B. and Hudgson, P. Syringomyelia. Philadelphia, W. B. Saunders, 1973.

Barrett, D. L. and King, E. B.: Comparison of cellular recovery rates and morphologic detail obtained using membrane filter and cytocentrifuge techniques. Acta Cytol. 20:174–180, 1976.

Barrows, L. J., Hunter, F. T. and Banker, B. Q.: The nature and clinical significance of pigments in the cerebrospinal fluid. Brain 78:59–80, 1955.

Bartter, F. C. and Schwartz, W. B.: The syndrome of inappropriate secretion of anti-diuretic hormone. Am. J. Med. 42:790–806, 1967.

Bass, N. H. and Lundborg, P.: Postnatal development of bulk flow in the cerebrospinal fluid system of the albino rat. Clearance of carboxyl (¹⁴C) inulin after intrathecal infusion. Brain Res. 52:323–332, 1973.

Batnitsky, S., Keucher, T. R., Mealey, J. et al.: Iatrogenic intraspinal epidermoid tumors. J.A.M.A. 237:148–150, 1977.

Bazan, N. G.: Free arachidonic acid and other lipids in the nervous system during early ischemia and after electroshock. In Porcellat, G., Amaducci, C. and Galli, C. (eds.): Function and Metabolism of Phospholipids in the Central and Peripheral Nervous System. Vol. 72. New York, Plenum Press, 1976, pp. 317–335.

Beatty, H. N. and Oppenheimer, S.: Cerebrospinal fluid lactic dehydrogenase and its isoenzymes in infections of the central nervous system. N. Engl. J. Med. 297:1197–1202, 1968.

Becht, F. C.: Studies on the CSF. Am. J. Physiol. 51:1–125, 1920.

Becker, N. W. and Sutton, C. H.: Histochemistry of choroid plexus. In Netsky, M. G. and Shuangshoti, S. (eds.): The Choroid Plexus in Health and Disease. Charlottesville, University of Virginia Press, 1975, pp. 113–150.

Bedford, T. H. B.: The effect of prolonged occlusion of the external jugular veins on the cerebrospinal fluid and the torcular venous pressure in the dog. Brain 59:324–336, 1936.

Beggs, J. L. and Waggener, J. D.: Transendothelial vesicular transport of protein following compression injury to the spinal cord. Lab. Invest. 34:428–439, 1976.

Bekaert, J. and Demeester, G.: Influence of the potassium concentration of the blood on the potassium level of the cerebrospinal fluid. Exper. Med. Surg. 12:480–501, 1954.

Beks, J. W. F., Bosch, D. A. and Brock, M. (eds.): Intracranial Pressure III. New York, Springer-Verlag, 1976.

Bell, E. G., Subramanian, G., McAfee, J. G. and Ross, G. S.: Radiopharmaceuticals for cisternography. In Harbert, J. C. (ed.): Cisternography and Hydrocephalus. A Symposium. Springfield, Illinois, Charles C Thomas, 1972, pp. 161–171.

Bell, W. E., Joynt, R. J. and Sahs, A. L.: Low spinal fluid pressure syndromes. Neurology (Minneap.) 10:512–521, 1960.

Bell, W. E. and McCormick, W. F.: Increased Intracranial Pressure in Children. 2nd Ed. Philadelphia, W. B. Saunders, 1978.

Benabid, A. L., de Rougemont, J. and Barge, M.: La pression intracrânienne. II. Vérification expérimental d'un modèle mathématique. J. Physiol. (Paris) 70:41–59, 1975.

Bennett, M. V. L.: Electrical impedance of brain surfaces. Brain Res. 15:584–590, 1969.

Bennett, R. A. and Harbilas, E.: Wilson's disease with aseptic meningitis and penicillamine-related cheilosis. Arch. Intern. Med. 120:374–376, 1967.

Benson, D. F., LeMay, M., Patten, D. H. et al.: Diagnosis of normal pressure hydrocephalus. N. Engl. J. Med. 283:609–615, 1970.

Bercaw, B. J. and Greer, M.: Transport of intrathecal ^{131}I RISA in benign intracranial hypertension. Neurology 20:787–790, 1970.

Berenberg, R. A., Pellock, J. M., DiMauro, S. et al.: Lumping or Splitting? "Ophthalmoplegia-Plus" or Kearns-Sayre Syndrome? Ann. Neurol. 1:37–54, 1977.

Berg, L.: Hypoglycorrhachia of non-infectious origin: Diffuse meningeal neoplasia. Neurology 3:811–824, 1953.

Berg, L., Rosomoff, H. L., Aronson, N. et al.: The syndrome of increased intracranial pressure without localizing signs. Arch. Neurol. Psychiat. 74:498–505, 1955.

Bergmann, L., Dencker, S. J., Johanssohn, B. G. and Svennerholm, L.: Cerebrospinal fluid gamma globulins in subacute sclerosing leucoencephalitis. J. Neurochem. 15:781–785, 1968.

Bering, E. A.: Water exchange of the central nervous system and cerebrospinal fluid. J. Neurosurg. 9:275–287, 1952.

Bering, E. A., Jr.: Choroid plexus and arterial pulsation of cerebrospinal fluid. Demonstration of the choroid plexus as a cerebrospinal fluid pump. Arch. Neurol. Psychiat. 73:165–172, 1955.

Bering, E. A. Jr.: Problems of the dynamics of the cerebrospinal fluid with particular reference to the formation of cerebrospinal fluid and its relationship to cerebral metabolism. Clin. Neurosurg. 5:77–98, 1958.

Bering, E. A., Jr.: Circulation of the cerebrospinal fluid. Demonstration of the choroid plexuses as the generator of the force for flow of fluid and ventricular enlargement. J. Neurosurg. 19:405–413, 1962.

Bering, E. A., Jr. and Salibi, B.: Production of hydrocephalus by increased cephalic venous pressure. Arch. Neurol. Psychiat. 81:693–698, 1959.

Bering, E. A., Jr., and Sato, O.: Hydrocephalus: changes in formation and absorption of cerebrospinal fluid within the cerebral ventricles. J. Neurosurg. 20:1050–1063, 1963.

Berlin, R. D.: Purines: Active transport by isolated choroid plexus. Science 163:1194–1195, 1969.

Berman, L. B., Lapham, L. W., and Pastore, E.: Jaundice and xanthochromia of the spinal fluid. J. Lab. Clin. Med. 44:273–279, 1954.

Berry, J. F., Logothetis, J. and Boris, M.: Determination of the fatty acid of cerebrospinal fluid by gas-liquid chromatography. Neurology 15:1089–1094, 1965.

Bessman, A. N., Alman, R. W., Hayes, G. J. et al.: The differential rates of diffusion of nitrous oxide into the cerebrospinal fluid. J. Lab. Clin. Med. 40:851–859, 1952.

Bettman, J. W., Daroff, R. B., Sanders, M. D. and Hoyt, W. F.: Papilledema and asymptomatic intracranial hypertension in systemic lupus erythematosus. Arch. Ophthalmol. 80:189–193, 1968.

Betz, A. L., Csejtey, J. and Goldstein, G. W.: Hexose transport and phosphorylation by capillaries isolated from rat brain. Am. J. Physiol. 236:C96–C102, 1979.

Betz, A. L. and Goldstein, G. W.: Polarity of the blood-brain barrier: Neutral amino acid transport into isolated brain capillaries. Science 202:225–227, 1978.

Betz, E.: Cerebral blood flow: its measurement and regulation. Physiol. Rev. 52:595–630, 1972.

Bickerstaff, E. R.: Changes in the cerebrospinal fluid after pneumoencephalography. Lancet 1:1209–1210, 1951.

Bingham, W. G., Paul, S. E., and Sastry, K. S. S.: Effect of steroid on enzyme response to cold injury in rat brain. Neurology 2:111–121, 1971.

Birzis, L., Carter, C. H. and Maren, T. H.: Effect of acetazolamide on CSF pressure and electrolytes in hydrocephalus. Neurology (Minneap.) 8:522–528, 1958.

Bito, L. Z.: Blood-brain barrier; Evidence for active cation transport between blood and the extracellular fluid of brain. Science 165:81–83, 1969.

Bito, L. Z., Davson, H. and Fenstermacher, J. D. (eds.): The Ocular and Cerebrospinal Fluids. New York, Academic Press, 1977.

Bito, L. Z., Davson, H. and Hollingsworth, J.: Facilitated transport of prostaglandins across the blood-cerebrospinal fluid and blood-brain barriers. J. Physiol. (Lond.) 256:273–285, 1976.

Bito, L. Z. and Myers, R. E.: The ontogenesis of haematoencephalic cation transport processes in the rhesus monkey. J. Physiol. (Lond.) 208:153–170, 1970.

Bito, L. Z. and Wallenstein, M. C.: Transport of prostaglandins across the blood-brain and blood-aqueous barriers and the physiological significance of these absorptive transport processes. In Bito, L. Z., Davson, H. and Fenstermacher, J. D. (eds.): The Ocular and Cerebrospinal Fluids. New York, Academic Press, 1977.

Black, J. T.: Cerebral candidiasis: Case report of brain abscess secondary to Candida albicans and review of literature. J. Neurol. Neurosurg. Psychiat. 33:864–870, 1970.

Black, P. M., Callahan, L. V. and Kornblith, P. L.: Tissue cultures from cerebrospinal fluid specimens in the study of human brain tumors. J. Neurosurg. 49:697–704, 1978.

Bland, R. D., Lister, R. C. and Ries, J. P.: Cerebrospinal fluid lactic acid level and pH in meningitis. Am. J. Dis. Child. 128:151–156, 1974.

Blasberg, R. G., Patlak, C. and Fenstermacher, J. D.: Intrathecal chemotherapy: Brain tissue profiles after ventriculo-cisternal perfusion. J. Pharmacol. Exper. Ther. 195:73–83, 1975.

Bleich, H. L., Berkman, P. M. and Schwartz, W. B.: The response of cerebrospinal fluid composition to sustained hypercapnia. J. Clin. Invest. 43:11–16, 1964.

Bloomer, H. A., Papadopoulos, N. M. and McLane, J. E.: Cerebrospinal fluid gamma globulin concentration in myxedema. J. Clin. Endocrinol. Metab. 20:869–874, 1960.

Boddie, H. G., Banna, M. and Bradley, W. G.: "Benign" intracranial hypertension: A survey of the clinical and radiological features and long-term prognosis. Brain 97:313–326, 1974.

Booe, I., Tourtellotte, W. W., and Brandes, D. W.: Brain and measles-specific immunoglobulin G in cerebrospinal fluid of patients with subacute sclerosing panencephalitis. Neurology (Minneap.) 26:377, 1976 (abstract).

Booij, J.: Pre-albumin in the cerebrospinal fluid. In Ariens-Kappers. J. (ed.): Progress in Neurobiology. Amsterdam, Elsevier, 1956, p. 164.

Boreus, L. D. and Sundstrom, B.: Intracranial hypertension in a child during treatment with nalidixic acid. Br. Med. J. 2:744–745, 1967.

Borgesen, S. E., Gjerris, F. and Sorensen, S.: The resistance to cerebrospinal fluid absorption in humans. Acta Neurol. Scand. 57:85–96, 1978.

Borgesen, S. E., Gjerris, F. and Sorenson, S. C.: Intracranial pressure and conductance to outflow of cerebrospinal fluid in normal pressure hydrocephalus. J. Neurosurg. 50:489–493, 1979.

Bosch, I. and Oehmichen, M.: Eosinophilic granulocytes in cerebrospinal fluid: analysis of 94 cerebrospinal fluid specimens and review of the literature. J. Neurol. 219:93–105, 1978.

Bourke, R. S., Kimelberg, H. K., Daze, M. A. et al.: Studies on the formation of astroglial swelling and its inhibition by clinically useful agents. In Popp, A. J. et al. (eds.): Neural Trauma. New York, Raven Press, 1979, pp. 95–113.

Bourke, R. S. and Nelson, K. M.: Further studies on the K^+-dependent swelling of the primate cerebral cortex in vivo: The enzymatic basis of the K^+-dependent transport of chloride. J. Neurochem. 19:663–685, 1972.

Bourke, R. S. and Nelson, K. M.: Studies on the site of medicated transport of chloride from blood into cerebrospinal fluid: effects of acetazolamide. J. Neurochem. 19:1225–1232, 1972.

Bowen, J. C., Fleming, W. H. and Thompson, J. C.: Increased gastric release following central nervous system injury. Surgery 75:720–724, 1974.

Bowers, M. B., Jr., Heninger, G. R. and Gerbode, F.: Cerebrospinal fluid, 5-hydroxyindoleacetic acid and homovanillic acid in psychiatric patients. Int. J. Neuropharmacol. 8:255–262, 1969.

Bradbury, M.: The Concept of a Blood-Brain Barrier. Chichester, John Wiley and Sons, 1979.

Bradbury, M. W. B. and Bronsted, H. E.: Sodium-dependent transport of sugars and iodide from the cerebral ventricles of the rabbit. J. Physiol. (Lond.) 234:127–143, 1973.

Bradbury, M. W. B. and Davson, H.: The transport potassium between blood, cerebrospinal fluid and brain. J. Physiol. (Lond.) 181:151–174, 1965.

Bradbury, M. W. B. and Kleeman, C. R.: Stability of the potassium content of cerebrospinal fluid and brain. Am. J. Physiol. 213:519–528, 1967.

Bradbury, M. W. B. and Kleeman, C. R.: The effect of chronic osmotic disturbance on the concentrations of cations in cerebrospinal fluid. J. Physiol. 204:181–193, 1969.

Bradbury, M. W. B., Stubbs, J., Hughes, I. E. and Parker, P.: The distribution of potassium, sodium, chloride and urea between lumbar cerebrospinal fluid and blood serum in human subjects. Clin. Sci. 25:97–105, 1963.

Bradford, F. K. and Johnson, P. C., Jr.: Passage of intact iron-labeled erythrocytes from subarachnoid space to systemic circulation in dogs. J. Neurosurg. 19:332–336, 1962.

Bradley, K. C.: Cerebrospinal fluid pressure. J. Neurol. Neurosurg. Psychiatry 33:387–397, 1970.

Bradley, R. D. and Semple, S. J. G.: A comparison of certain acid-base characteristics of arterial blood, jugular venous blood and cerebrospinal fluid in man, and the effect on them of some acute and chronic acid-base disturbances. J. Physiol. (Lond.) 160:381–391, 1962.

Bradshaw, P. and Parsons, M.: Hemiplegic migraine, a clinical study. Q. J. Med. 34:65–85, 1965.

Braham, J., Sarova-Pinhas, I., Front, D. et al.: A simple CSF manometric test for adult hydrocephalus associated with dementia. A comparison with radioisotope encephalography. Eur. Neurol. 5:294–302, 1971.

Brain, W. R. and Norris, F., Jr. (eds.): The Remote Effects of Cancer on the Nervous System. New York, Grune and Stratton, 1965.

Brain, W. R. and Wilkinson, M.: Subacute cerebellar degeneration in patients with carcinoma. In Brain, W. R. and Norris, F., Jr. (eds.): The Remote Effects of Cancer on the Nervous System. New York, Grune and Stratton, 1965, pp. 17–23.

Brandstetter, S. and Barzilai, D.: Glutamine estimation in CSF in liver disease. Am. J. Dig. Dis. 5:945–960, 1960.

Bray, P. F. and Herbst, J. J.: Pseudotumor cerebri as a sign of "catch-up" growth in cystic fibrosis. Am. J. Dis. Child. 126:78–79, 1973.

Brightman, M. W.: Ultrastructural characteristics of adult choroid plexus. Relation to the blood-cerebrospinal fluid barrier to proteins. In Netsky, M. G. and Shuangshoti, S. (eds.): The Choroid Plexus in Health and Disease. Charlottesville, University of Virginia Press, 1975, pp. 86–112.

Brightman, M. W.: Morphology of blood-brain interfaces. In Bito, L. Z., Davson, H., Fenstermacher, J. D. (eds.): The Ocular and Cerebrospinal Fluids. New York, Academic Press, 1977, pp. 1–25.

Brightman, M. W., Klatzo, I., Olsson, Y. and Reese, T. S.: The blood-brain barrier to proteins under normal and pathological conditions. J. Neurol. Sci. 10:215–239, 1970.

Brightman, M. W., Prescott, L. and Reese, T. S.: Intercellular junctions of special ependyma. In Knigge, K. M. et al. (eds.): Brain-Endocrine Interaction II. The Ventricular System in Neuroendocrine Mechanisms. Basel, S. Karger, 1975, pp. 146–165.

Brightman, M. W. and Reese, T. S.: Junctions between intimately opposed cell membranes in the vertebrate brain. J. Cell Biol. 40:648–677, 1969.

Briseid, K., Falkum, A., Qvigstad, E. K. et al.: Arginine esterase in cerebrospinal fluid and pro-arginine esterase in plasma from patients with migraine. Acta Neurol. Scand. 54:301–311, 1976.

Brisman, R.: Pioneer studies on the circulation of the cerebrospinal fluid with particular reference to studies by Richard Lower in 1669. J. Neurosurg. 32:1–4, 1970.

Brock, M. and Dietz, H. (eds.): Intracranial Pressure. Experimental and Clinical Aspects. Berlin, Springer-Verlag, 1972.

Brock, M., Fieschi, C., Ingvar, D. H. et al. (eds.): Cerebral Blood Flow. Berlin, Springer-Verlag, 1969.

Brock, M., Furuse, M., Weber, R. et al.: Brain tissue pressure gradients. In Lundberg, N., Ponten, U. and Brock, M. (eds.): Intracranial Pressure. Berlin, Springer-Verlag, 1965, pp. 215–217.

Brocker, R. J.: Technique to avoid spinal tap headache. J.A.M.A. 168:261–267, 1958.

Broman, T.: The Permeability of the Cerebrospinal Vessels in Normal and Pathological Conditions. Copenhagen, A. Munskgaard, 1949.

Broman, T., Radner, S., and Svanberg, L.: The duration of experimental disturbance in the cerebrovascular permeability due to circumscribed gross damage of the brain. Acta Psychiat. Neurol. 24:167–173, 1949.

Bromley, L. L., Craig, J. D. and Kessell, A. W. L.: Infected intervertebral disc after lumbar puncture. Br. M. J. 1:132–133, 1949.

Bronsky, D., Kushner, D. S., Dubin, A. et al.: Idiopathic hypoparathyroidism and pseudohypoparathyroidism: Case reports and review of the literature. Medicine 37:317–352, 1958.

Bronsky, D., Shrifter, H., De La Huerge, J. et al.: Cerebrospinal fluid proteins in myxedema with special reference to electrophoretic partition. J. Clin. Endocrinol. Metab. 18:470–476, 1958.

Brook, I., Bricknell, K. S., Overturf, G. D. et al.: Measurement of lactic acid in cerebrospinal fluid of patients with infections of the cerebral nervous system. J. Infect. Dis. 137:384–390, 1978.

Brooks, B. R. and Adams, R. D.: Cerebrospinal fluid acid-base and lactate changes after seizures in unanesthetized man. Neurology 25:935–942, 1975.

Brooks, B. R., Engel, W. K. and Sode, J.: Blood-to-cerebrospinal fluid barrier for cyclic adenosine monophosphate in man. Arch. Neurol. 34:468–469, 1977.

Brooks, C., McC., Kao, F. F. and Lloyd, B. B. (eds.): Cerebrospinal Fluid and the Regulation of Ventilation. Oxford, Blackwell Scientific Publications, 1965.

Browder, J. and Meyers, R.: Behaviour of the systemic blood pressure, pulse rate and spinal fluid pressure associated with acute changes in intracranial pressure artificially produced. Arch. Surg. 36:1–19, 1938.

Brown, J. K.: Lumbar puncture and its hazards. Dev. Med. Child. Neurol. 18:803–816, 1976.

Bruce, D. A., Langfitt, T. W., Miller, T. D., et al.: Regional cerebral blood flow, intracranial pressure and brain metabolism in comatose subjects. J. Neurosurg. 38:131–144, 1973.

Bruck, H.: Aminosaurebestimmunogen in serum und liquor bei degenerativen. Krankh. Wien. Z. Nervenheilk. Suppl. 1:149–154, 1966.

Bruyn, G. W., and Garland, H.: Neuropathies of endocrine origin. In Vinken, P. J. and Bruyn, G. W. (eds.): Handbook of Clinical Neurology. Vol. 8. Amsterdam, Elsevier, 1970, pp. 29–72.

Buchsbaum, H. W. and Gallo, A. E., Jr.: Polyneuritis, papilledema, and lumboperitoneal shunt. Arch. Neurol. 21:253–257, 1969.

Budka, H., Guseo, A., Jellinger, K. et al.: Intermittent meningitic reaction with severe basophilia and eosinophilia in CNS leukaemia. A special type of hypersensitivity. J. Neurol. Sci. 28:459–468, 1976.

Buhlman, A., Scheitlin, W. and Rossier, P. H.: Die Beziehungen zwischen Blut und Liquor cerebrospinalis bei Strorungen das Saure-Basen-Gleichgewichtes. Schweiz. Med. Wschr. 93:427–432, 1963.

Buhrley, L. E. and Reed, D. J.: The effect of furosemide on sodium-22 uptake into cerebrospinal fluid and brain. Exp. Brain Res. 14:503–510, 1972.

Bulgar, R. J., Schrier, R. W., Arend, W. P. and Swanson, A. G.: Spinal fluid acidosis and the diagnosis of pulmonary encephalopathy. N. Engl. J. Med. 274:433–437, 1966.

Bullock, L. T., Gregersen, M. I. and Kinney, R.: The use of hypertonic sucrose solution intravenously to reduce cerebrospinal fluid pressure without a secondary rise. Am. J. Physiol. 112:82–96, 1935.

Bunge, M. A., Bunge, R. P. and Ris, H.: Ultrastructural study of remyelination in an experimental lesion in adult cat spinal cord. J. Biophys. Biochem. Cytol. 10:67–94, 1961.

Bunge, R. P., Bunge, M. A. and Ris, H.: Electron microscopic study of demyelination in an experimentally induced lesion in adult cat spinal cord. J. Biophys. Biochem. Cytol. 7:685–696, 1960.

Bunnag, T., Comer, D. S., Punyagupta, S.: Eosinophilic myeloencephalitis caused by *Ghathostoma spinigerum*. Neuropathology of nine cases. J. Neurol. Sci. 10:419–434, 1970.

Burrows, G.: On Disorders of the Cerebral Circulation. London, Longman, 1846.

Buryakova, A. V. and Sytinsky, I. A.: Amino acid composition of cerebrospinal fluid in acute neuroinfections in children. Arch. Neurol. 32:28–31, 1975.

Butler, W. T., Alling, D. W., Spickard, A. and Utz, J. P.: Diagnostic and prognostic value of clinical and laboratory findings in crytpococcal meningitis. A follow-up study of forty patients. N. Engl. J. Med. 270:59–67, 1964.

Byers, R. K.: To tap or not to tap. Pediatrics 51:561, 1973.

Byrom, F. B.: The pathogenesis of hypertensive encephalopathy and its relation to the malignant phase of hypertension: experimental evidence from the hypertensive rat. Lancet 2:201–211, 1954.

Caesar, J.: Levels of glutamine and ammonia and the pH of cerebrospinal fluid and plasma in patients with liver disease. Clin. Sci. 22:33–41, 1962.

Calabrese, V. P., Selhorst, J. B. and Harbison, J. W.: Cerebrospinal fluid infusion test in pseudotumor cerebri. Ann. Neurol. 4:173, 1978. (Abstract)

Caldareli, M., Di Rocco, C. and Rossi, G. F.: Lumbar subarachnoid infusion test in paediatric neurosurgery. Devel. Med. Child. Neurol. 21:71–82, 1979.

Cantore, G., Guidetti, B. and Virno, M.: Oral glycerol for the reduction of intracranial pressure. J. Neurosurg. 21:278–283, 1964.

Carey, M. E., Chau, S. W. and French, L. A.: Experience with brain abscesses. J. Neurosurg. 36:1–9, 1972.

Cargill, W. H. and Beeson, P. B.: Value of spinal fluid examination as diagnostic procedure in Weil's disease. Ann. Intern. Med. 27:396–400, 1947.

Carlsson, C. and Dencker, S. J.: Cerebrospinal fluid uric acid in alcoholics. Acta Neurol. Scand. 49:39–46, 1973.

Carmichael, E., Doupe, J. and Williams, D. L.: The cerebrospinal fluid pressure of man in the erect posture. J. Physiol. 91:186–201, 1937.

Castaigne, P., Lhermitte, F., Schuller, E. et al.: Etude électrophorétique des protéines du liquid céphalo-rachidien dans 104 cas de tumeurs du nevraxe. Rev. Neurol. 127:505–515, 1972.

Castaigne, P., Lhermitte, F., Schuller, E. et al.: Oligoclonal aspect of gamma-globulins in CSF: Diagnostic value. In Field, E. J., Bell, T. M. and Carnegie, P. R. (eds.): Multiple Sclerosis: Progress in Research. Amsterdam, North Holland, 1972, pp. 152–158.

Caveness, W. F., Carsten, A. L., Roisin, L. and Schade, J. P.: Pathogenesis of x-irradiation effects in the monkey cerebral cortex. Brain Res. 7:1–120, 1968.

Celermajer, J. M. and Brown, J.: The neurological complications of pertussis. Med. J. Aust. 1:1006–1069, 1966.

Center for Disease Control, Syphilis: Recommended treatment schedules, 1976. Ann. Intern. Med. 85:94–96, 1976.

Chan, P. H. and Fishman, R. A.: Effects of hyperosmolality on release of neurotransmitter amino acids from rat brain slices. J. Neurochem. 29:179–181, 1977.

Chan, P. H. and Fishman, R. A.: Brain edema: Induction in cortical slices by polyunsaturated fatty acids. Science 201:358–360, 1978.

Chan, P. H. and Fishman, R. A.: Elevation of rat brain amino acids, ammonia and idiogenic osmoles induced by hyperosmolality. Brain Res. 161:293–302, 1979.

Chan, P. H., Fishman, R. A., Lee, J. L. et al.: Effects of excitatory neurotransmitter amino acids on swelling of rat brain cortical slices. J. Neurochem., 1980 (in press).

Chan, P. H., Wong, Y. P. and Fishman, R. A.: Hyperosmolality induced GABA release from cat brain slices: studies of calcium dependency and sources of release. J. Neurochem. 30:1363–1368, 1978.

334 BIBLIOGRAPHY

Chaplin, E. R., Schlueter, M. A., Phibbs, R. H. et al.: Fetal hemoglobin in the diagnosis of neonatal subarachnoid hemorrhage. Pediatrics 58:751–754, 1976.

Chapman, L. and Wolff, H. G.: Property of cerebrospinal fluid associated with disturbed metabolism of the central nervous system. Science 128:1208–1209, 1958.

Chapman, L. F. and Wolff, H. G.: Studies of proteolytic enzymes in CSF. Capacity of incubated mixtures of CSF and plasma proteins to form vasodilator substances that contract the isolated rat uterus. A.M.A. Arch. Intern. Med. 103:86–94, 1959.

Chartrand, S. A. and Cho, C. T.: Persistent pleocytosis in bacterial meningitis. J. Pediatr. 88:424–426, 1976.

Chase, T. N. et al.: CSF monoamine catabolites in drug-induced extrapyramidal disorders. Neuropharmacology 9:265–268, 1970.

Chase, T. N., Gordon, E. K. and Ng, L. K. Y.: Norepinephrine metabolism in the central nervous system of man: Studies using 3-methyoxy-4-hydroxyphenylethylene glycol levels in cerebrospinal fluid. J. Neurochem. 21:581–587, 1973.

Chase, T. N. and Ng, L. K. Y.: Central monoamine metabolism in Parkinson's disease. Arch. Neurol. 27:486–491, 1972.

Chase, T. N., Watanabe, A. M., Brodie, K. H. et al.: Huntington's chorea. Effect of serotonin depletion. Arch. Neurol. 26:282–284, 1972.

Chen, J. H.: Measurement of gonadotropin in cerebrospinal fluid. N. Engl. J. Med. 297:114, 1977. (Letter)

Christy, N. P. and Fishman, R. A.: Studies of the blood-cerebrospinal fluid barrier to cortisol in the dog. J. Clin. Invest. 40:1997–2006, 1961.

Chutkow, J. H. and Meyers, S.: Chemical changes in the cerebrospinal fluid and brain in magnesium deficiency. Neurology 18:963–974, 1968.

Clark, R. M., Capra, N. F. and Halsey, J. F. Jr.: Method for measuring brain tissue pressure response to alterations in pCO_2, systemic blood pressure and middle cerebral artery occlusion. J. Neurosurg. 43:1–8, 1975.

Clarke, E., and O'Malley, C. D.: The Human Brain and Spinal Cord. Berkeley, University of California Press, 1968.

Clasen, R. A., Pandolfi, S. and Casey, D.: Furosemide and pentobarbital in cryogenic cerebral injury and edema. Neurology 24:642–648, 1974.

Clasen, R. A., Pandolfi, S., and Hass, G. M.: Vital staining, serum albumin and the blood-brain barrier. J. Neuropathol Exp. Neurol. 29:266–284, 1970.

Clements, R. S. J., Morrison, A. D. and Blumenthal, S. A.: Increased cerebrospinal fluid pressure during treatment of diabetic ketosis. Lancet 2:671–675, 1971.

Clendenon, N. R., Allen, N., Ito, T. et al.: Response of lysosomal hydrolases of dog spinal cord and cerebrospinal fluid to experimental trauma. Neurology 28:78–84, 1978.

Coben, L. A. and Smith, K. R.: Iodide transfer at four cerebrospinal fluid sites in the dog: Evidence for spinal iodide carrier transport. Exp. Neurol. 23:76–90, 1969.

Coblenz, J. J., Mattis, S., Zingessen, L. H. et al.: Presenile dementia. Clinical aspects and evaluation of cerebrospinal fluid dynamics. Arch Neurol. 29:299–308, 1973.

Cockrill, J. R.: Non-electrolytes: Their distribution between the blood and cerebrospinal fluid. Arch. Neurol. Psychiat. 25:1297–1305, 1931.

Cohen, D. J., Shaywitz, B. A., Johnson, W. T. et al.: Biogenic amines in autistic and atypical children: Cerebrospinal fluid measures of homovanillic acid and 5-hydroxyindoleacetic acid. Arch. Gen. Psychiat. 31:845–853, 1974.

Cohen, F. L.: Conus medullaris syndrome following multiple intrathecal corticosteroid injections. Arch. Neurol. 36:228–231, 1979.

Cohen, H.: The magnesium content of the cerebrospinal and other body fluids. Q. J. Med. 20:173–186, 1927.

Cohen, S. R., Herndon, R. M. and McKhann, G. M.: Radio-immunoassay of myelin basic protein in spinal fluid. N. Engl. J. Med. 295:1455–1457, 1976.

Cohn, W. E. and Murayama, M. M.: A study with radioactive isotopes of the permeability of the blood-cerebrospinal fluid barrier to ions. Am. J. Physiol. 140:47–64, 1943.

Colling, K. G. and Rossiter, R. J.: Alkaline and acid phosphatase in cerebrospinal fluid. Data for normal fluids and fluids from patients with meningitis, poliomyelitis, or syphilis. Canad. J. Res. 28:56–68, 1950.

Controni, G., Rodriguez, W. J., Hicks, J. M. et al.: Cerebrospinal fluid latic acid levels in meningitis. J. Pediat. 91:379–384, 1977.

Coonrod, J. D. and Drennan, D. P.: Pneumococcal pneumonia: capsular polysaccharide antigenemia and antibody responses. Ann. Intern. Med. 84:254–260, 1976.

Cooper, A. J., Beaty, H. N., Oppenheimer, S. I. et al.: Studies on the pathogenesis of meningitis, VII. Glucose transport and spiral fluid production experimental pneumococcal meningitis. J. Lab. Clin. Med. 71:473–483, 1968.

Cooper, E. R. A.: Nerves of the meninges and the choroid plexus. Acta Anat. (Basel) 33:298–318, 1958.

Cooper, E. S., Lechner, E. and Bellet, S.: Relation between serum and cerebrospinal fluid electrolytes under normal and abnormal conditions. Am. J. Med. 18:613–621, 1955.

Coppen, A. J. and Russell, G. F. M.: Effect of intravenous acetazolamide on cerebrospinal fluid pressure. Lancet 2:926–927, 1957.

Corning, J. L.: Spinal anesthesia and local medication of the cord. N. Y. State Med. J. 42:483–485, 1885.

Cory, H. T., Lascelles, P. T., Millard, B. J. et al.: Measure of prostaglandin F_2 in human cerebrospinal fluid by single ion monitoring. Biomed. Mass Spectrom. 3:117–121, 1976.

Cosgrove, J. B. and Agius, P.: Studies in multiple sclerosis. II. Comparison of the beta-gamma globulin ratio, gamma globulin elevation and first zone colloidal gold curve in the cerebrospinal fluid. Neurology 16:197–204, 1966.

Couvreur, J. and Desmonts, G.: Toxoplasmosis. In Vinken, P. J. and Bruyn, G. W. (eds.): Handbook of Clinical Neurology. Vol. 35. Amsterdam, North Holland, 1978, pp. 115–141.

Cowie, J., Lambie, A. T. and Robson, J. S.: The influence of extracorporeal dialysis on the acid-base composition of blood and cerebrospinal fluid. Clin. Sci. 23:397–407, 1962.

Cramer, H., Ng, L. K. Y. and Chase, T. N.: Adenosine 3'-5'-monophosphate in cerebrospinal fluid: Effects of drugs and neurologic disease. Arch. Neurol. 29:197–199, 1973.

Croft, P. B., Urich, H. and Wilkinson, M.: Peripheral neuropathy of sensorimotor type associated with malignant disease. Brain 90:31–66, 1967.

Crone, C.: Facilitated transfer of glucose from blood into brain tissue. J. Physiol. 181:103–113, 1965.

Cronquist, S. and Lundberg, N.: Regional cerebral blood flow in intracranial tumours with special reference to cases with intracranial hypertension. International Symposium on CSF and CBF. Lund and Copenhagen, May 1968. Scand. J. Clin. Lab. Invest. Suppl. 102.

Cross, H. E.: Examination of cerebrospinal fluid in fat embolism. Arch. Intern. Med. 115:470–474, 1965.

Cserr, H. F.: Physiology of the choroid plexus. Physiol. Rev. 51:273–311, 1971.

Cserr, H. F., Cooper, D. N. and Milhorat, T. H.: Flow of cerebral interstitial fluid as indicated by the removal of extracellular markers from rat caudate nucleus. In The Ocular and Cerebrospinal Fluids. Academic Press, New York, 1977, pp. 461–474.

Cserr, H. F. et al. (eds): Fluid Environment of the Brain: Proceedings. Symposium held at the Mount Desert Island Biological Laboratory, Salisbury Cove, Maine, Sept. 1974.

Cumings, J. N.: Biochemical aspects of motor neuron disease. Proc. R. Soc. Med. 55:1023–1024, 1962.

Cuneo, R. A., Caronna, J. J., Pitts, L. et al.: Upward transtentorial herniation. Seven cases and a literature review. Arch. Neurol. 36:618–623, 1979.

Curl, F. D. and Pollay, M.: Transport of water and electrolytes between brain and ventricular fluid in the rabbit. Exp. Neurol. 20:558–574, 1968.

Curzon, G., Gumpert, J. and Sharpe, D.: Amine metabolites in the cerebrospinal fluid in Huntington's chorea. J. Neurol. Neurosurg. Psychiatry 35:514–519, 1972.

Cushing, H.: Some experimental and clinical observations concerning states of increased intracranial tension. Am. J. Med. Sci. 124:375–400. 1902.

Cushing, H.: Studies on cerebrospinal fluid. J. Med. Res. 31:1–19, 1914.

Cushing, H.: The Third Circulation. London, Oxford University Press, 1926.

Cushing, H.: Peptic ulcers and the interbrain. Surg. Gynecol. Obstet. 55:1–34, 1932.

Cushing, H. and Goetsch, E.: Concerning the secretion of the infundibular lobe of the pituitary body and its presence in the cerebrospinal fluid. Am. J. Physiol. 27:60–86, 1910.

Cutler, R. W. P. and Barlow, C. F.: The effect of hypercapnia on brain permeability to protein. Arch. Neurol. 14:54–63, 1966.

Cutler, R. W. P., Lorenzo, A. V. and Barlow, C. F.: Sulfate and iodide in brain. The influence of cerebrospinal fluid. Arch. Neurol. 18:316–323, 1968.

Cutler, R. W. P., Merler, E. and Hammerstad, J.: Production of antibody by the central nervous system in subacute sclerosing panencephalitis. Neurology (Minneap.) 18:129–132, 1968.

Cutler, R. W. P., Page, L., Galicich, J. and Watters, G. V.: Formation and absorption of cerebrospinal fluid in man. Brain 91:707–720, 1968.

Cutler, R. W. P., Watters, G. V. and Hammerstad, J. P.: The origin and turnover of cerebrospinal fluid albumin and gamma globulin in man. J. Neurol. Sci. 10:259–268, 1970.

Czaky, T. Z.: Choroid plexus. In Lajtha, A. (ed.): Handbook of Neurochemistry. Vol. 2. New York, Plenum Press, 1969, pp. 49–69.

D'Alessio, D. J.: Wolff's Headache and Other Head Pain. 3rd Edition. New York, Oxford University Press, 1972.

Dandy, W. E.: Experimental hydrocephalus. Ann. Surg. 70:129–142, 1919.

Dandy, W. E.: Intracranial pressure without brain tumor, diagnosis and treatment. Ann. Surg. 106:492–513, 1937.

Dandy, W. E. and Blackfan, K. D.: Internal hydrocephalus. An experimental, clinical and pathological study. Amer. J. Dis. Child. 8:406–482, 1914.

Dardenne, G., Dereymaeker, A. and Lacheron, J. M.: Cerebrospinal fluid pressure and pulsality. An experimental study of circulatory and respiratory influences in normal and hydrocephalic dogs. Eur. Neurol. 2:193–216, 1969.

Dattner, B. and Thomas, E. W.: Bilateral abducens palsy following lumbar puncture. N.Y. State J. Med. 41:1660–1662, 1941.

Davidoff, L. M. and Dyke, C. G.: A presentation of a series of cases of serous meningitis. J. Nerv. Ment. Dis. 83:700–705, 1936.

Davidson, D., Pullar, I. A., Mawdsley, C. et al.: Monoamine metabolites in CSF in multiple sclerosis. J. Neurol. Neurosurg. Psychiat. 40:741–745, 1977.

Davidson, N.: Neurotransmitter Amino Acids. New York, Academic Press, 1976, 179 pages.

Davies, D. G.: Cerebrospinal fluid sampling technique and Astrup pH and PCO_2 values. J. Appl. Physiol. 40:123–125, 1976.

Davis, L. E.: Normal laboratory values of CSF during pregnancy. Arch. Neurol. 36:443, 1979.

Davis, L. E. and Sperry, S.: The CSF-FTA test and the significance of blood contamination. Ann. Neurol. 6:68–69, 1979.

Davison, A. N., Humphrey, J. H., Liversedge, A. L. et al. (eds.): Multiple Sclerosis Research. Amsterdam, Elsevier, 1975.

Davson, H.: Physiology of the Ocular and Cerebrospinal Fluids. London, Churchill, 1956.

Davson, H.: Physiology of the Cerebrospinal Fluid. London, Churchill, 1967, 445 pages.

Davson, H.: The blood-brain barrier. In Bourne, G. H. (ed.): The Structure and Function of Nervous Tissue. Vol. 4. New York, Academic Press, 1972, pp. 321–445.

Davson, H.: The blood-brain barrier. J. Physiol. 255:1–28, 1976.

Davson, H., Domer, F. R. and Hollingsworth, J. R.: The mechanism of drainage of the cerebrospinal fluid. Brain 96:329–336, 1973.

Davson, H. and Hollingsworth, J. R.: Active transport of ^{131}I across the blood-brain barrier. J. Physiol. (Lond.) 233:327–347, 1973.

Davson, H., Hollingsworth, J. R. and Segal, M. D.: The mechanism of drainage of the cerebrospinal fluid. Brain 93:665–678, 1970.

Davson, H., Kleeman, C. R., and Levin, E.: Quantitative studies of the passage of different substrates out of the cerebrospinal fluid. J. Physiol. 161:126–142, 1962.

Davson, H. and Luck, C. P.: The effect of acetazolamide on the chemical composition of the aqueous humour and cerebrospinal fluid of some mammalian species and on the rate of turnover of [24]Na in these fluids. J. Physiol. (Lond.) 137:279–293, 1957.

Davson, H. and Segal, M. B.: The effects of some inhibitors and accelerators of sodium transport in the turnover of [22]Na in the cerebrospinal fluid and the brain. J. Physiol. (Lond.) 209:131–153, 1970.

Davson, H. and Welch, K.: The relations of blood, brain and cerebrospinal fluid. In Siesjo, B. K. and Sorensen, S. C. (eds.): Ion Homeostasis of the Brain. Alfred Benzon Symposium III. New York, Academic Press, 1971, pp. 9–21.

Dayan, A. D. and Stokes, M. I.: Rapid diagnosis of encephalitis by immunofluorescent examination of cerebrospinal-fluid cells. Lancet 1:177–179, 1973.

Decker, C. F., Aras, A. and Decker, L. E.: Determination of magnesium and calcium in cerebrospinal fluid by atomic absorption spectroscopy. Anal. Biochem. 8:344–348, 1964.

Degne, M., Dahl, H. and Vandvik, B.: Interferon in the serum and cerebrospinal fluid in patients with multiple sclerosis and other neurological disorders. Acta Neurol. Scand. 53:152–160, 1976.

Delaney, J. F.: Spinal fluid aluminum levels in patients with Alzheimer disease. Ann. Neurol. 5:580–581, 1979.

Delaney, P.: Neurological manifestations in sarcoidosis. Review of the literature with a report of 23 cases. Ann. Intern. Med. 87:336–345, 1977.

DeLange, S. D.: Progressive hydrocephalus. In Vinken, P. J. and Bruyn, G. W. (eds.): Handbook of Clinical Neurology. Vol. 30. Amsterdam, Elsevier, 1977, pp. 525–564.

Delfs, E.: Quantitative chorionic gonadotropin: Prognostic value in hydatidiform mole and chorion-epithelioma. Obstet. Gynecol. 9:1–24, 1957.

Delpech, B. and Lichtblau, F.: Étude quantitative des immunoglobulines G et de l'albumine du liquide céphalo-rachidien. Clin. Chim. Acta 37:15–23, 1972.

Demopoulos, H. B., Flamm, E. S., Seligman, M. L. et al.: Antioxidant effects of barbiturates in model membranes undergoing free radical change. In Ingvar, D. H. and Lassen, N. A. (eds.): Cerebral Function Metabolism and Circulation. Acta Neurol. Scand. (Suppl. 64) 56:152–153, 1977.

Demopoulos, H. B., Milvy, P., Kakari, S. et al.: Molecular aspects of membrane structure in cerebral edema. In Reulen, H. J. (ed.): Steroids and Brain Edema. Berlin, Springer-Verlag, 1972, pp. 29–39.

Dempsey, J. A., Forster, H. V. and DoRico, G. A.: Ventilatory acclimatization to moderate hypoxemia in man. The role of spinal fluid (H+). J. Clin. Invest. 53:1091–1100, 1974.

Dencker, S. J.: Variation of total cerebrospinal fluid proteins and cells with sex and age. World Neurol. 3:778–780, 1962.

Dencker, S. J.: Quantification of individual CSF proteins by immune precipitation in agar gel. J. Neurochem. 16:465–466, 1969.

Dencker, S. J., Malm, U., Ross, B. E. and Werdinius, B.: Acid monoamine metabolites of cerebrospinal fluid in mental depression and mania. J. Neurochem. 13:1445–1548, 1966.

Dencker, S. J. and Swahn, B.: Clinical Value of Protein Analysis in Cerebrospinal Fluid. A Micro-Immunoelectrophoretic Study. Lund Universitets Arsskrift N. F. Avd. 2, Bd. 57, Nr. 10. Lund, Gleerup, 1961.

Dencker, S. J. and Swahn, B.: The diagnostic value of lipoprotein determinations in cerebrospinal fluid. Acta Psychiat. Scand. 36:325–336, 1961.

Dencker, S. J., Swahn, B. and Ursing, B.: Protein pattern of cerebrospinal fluid during the course of acute polyradiculoneuropathy. Acta Med. Scand. 175:499–506, 1964.

Den Hartog Jager, W. A.: Cytopathology of the cerebrospinal fluid with the sedimentation technique after Sayk. J. Neurol. Sci. 9:155–177, 1969.

Denny-Brown, D.: The changing pattern of neurologic medicine. N. Engl. J. Med. 246:839–846, 1952.

Deonna, T. and Guignard, J. P.: Acute intracranial hypertension after nalidixic acid administration. Arch. Dis. Child. 49:743–74, 1974.

Derakhshen, I. and Kaufman, B.: Subdural effusion of cerebrospinal fluid after lumbar puncture. Arch. Neurol. 29:127, 1973.

Dereux, J., Vandehaute, A. and Deheck, M.: Arachnoidite apparue au cours d'un traitement par les injections sous-arachnoïdiennes d'hydrocortisone. Rev. Neurol. 94:301–304, 1956.

Desgnez, P. and Traverse, P. M. (eds.): Transport functions of Plasma Proteins. Amsterdam, Elsevier, 1966.

DeVita, V. T., 2d, Utz, J. P., Williams, T. et al.: *Candida* meningitis. Arch. Intern. Med. 117:527–535, 1966.

De Vivo, D.: Reye syndrome: A metabolic response to an acute mitochondrial insult? Neurology 28:105–108, 1978.

De Vivo, D. and Keating, J. P.: Reye's syndrome. Adv. Pediatr. 22:175–229, 1976.

Dewhurst, K.: The composition of the cerebrospinal fluid in the neurosyphilitic psychoses. Acta Neurol. Scand. 45:119–123, 1969.

Diamond, I.: Bilirubin encephalopathy (kernicterus). In Goldensohn, E. S. and Appel, S. H. (eds.): Scientific Approaches to Clinical Neurology. Philadelphia, Lea and Febiger, 1977, pp. 1212–1231.

Diamond, I. and Schmid, R.: Experimental bilirubin encephalopathy: The mode of entry of bilirubin-^{14}C into the central nervous system. J. Clin. Invest. 45:678–689, 1966.

Diamond, J. H. and Bossert, W. H.: Standing-gradient osmotic flow: A mechanism for coupling of water and solute transport in epithelia. J. Gen. Physiol. 50:2061–2083, 1967.

Di Bona, G. F.: Neural control of renal function. Fed. Proc. 37:1191–1219, 1978.

Di Chiro, G.: Unintentional spinal cord arteriography: A warning. Radiology 112:231–233, 1974.

Di Chiro, G., Ashburn, W. L. et al.: Radioisotope encephalocisternography and encephaloventriculography. J. Neurosurg. 36:127–132, 1972.

Di Chiro, G., Reames, P. M. and Matthews, W. B.: RISA-ventriculography and RISA-cisternography. Neurology 14:185–191, 1964.

Dickinson, J. C. and Hamilton, P. B.: The free amino acids of human spinal fluid determined by ion exchange chromatography. J. Neurochem. 13:1179–1187, 1966.

Dila, C. F. and Pappius, H. M.: Cerebral water and electrolytes: An experimental mode of inappropriate secretion of antidiuretic hormone. Arch. Neurol. 26:85–90, 1972.

Dillon, D. and Schenker, S.: Cerebrospinal fluid protein. Concentration in hepatic coma. J.A.M.A. 221:507, 1972. (Letter)

Dimant, J. and Grob, D.: Electrocardiographic changes and myocardial damage in patients with acute cerebrovascular accidents. Stroke 8:448–455, 1977.

DiMattio, J., Hochwald, G. M., Malhan, C. and Wald, A.: Effects of changes in serum osmolarity on bulk flow of fluid into cerebral ventricles and on brain water content. Pfluegers Arch. 359:253–264, 1975.

Dinsdale, H. B. and Taghavy, A.: Carcinomatosis of the meninges. Can. Med. Assoc. J. 90:505–512, 1964.

Dixon, W. E. and Halliburton, W. D.: The cerebrospinal fluid. I. Secretion of the fluid. J. Physiol. 47:215–242, 1913.

Dodge, P. R., Crawford, J. D. A. and Probst, J. H.: Studies in experimental water intoxication. Arch. Neurol. 3:513–529, 1960.

Dohrmann, G. J.: The choroid plexus: A historical review. Brain Res. 18:197–218, 1970.

Domer, F. R.: Effects of diuretics on cerebrospinal fluid formation and potassium movement. Exp. Neurol. 24:54–64, 1969.

Dorfman, L. J.: Cytomegalic inclusion disease. In Vinken, P. J. and Bruyn, G. W. (eds.): Handbook of Clinical Neurology. Vol. 34. Amsterdam, Elsevier/North Holland, 1978, pp. 209–233.

Dotzauer, G. and Naeve, W.: Der portmortale Liquordruck. Deutsch Z. Ges. Gerichtl. Med. 52:273–282, 1962.

Drewinko, B., Sullivan, M. P. and Martin, T.: Use of the cytocentrifuge in the diagnosis of meningeal leukemia. Cancer 31:1331–1336, 1973.

Dripps, R. D. and Vandam, L. D.: Hazards of lumbar puncture. J.A.M.A. 147:1118–1121, 1951.

Dripps, R. D. and Vandam, L. D.: Longterm follow up of patients who received 10,098 spinal anesthetics: Failure to discover major neurological sequelae. J.A.M.A. 156:1486–1491, 1954.

D'Souza, E., Mandal, B. K., Hooper, J. et al.: Lactic acid concentration in cerebrospinal fluid and differential diagnosis of meningitis. Lancet 2:579–580, 1978.

DuBoulay, G. H.: Pulsatile movements in the CSF pathways. Br. J. Radiol. 39:255–262, 1966.

DuBoulay, G., O'Connell, J. E. A., Currie, J. et al.: Further investigations on pulsatile movements in the cerebrospinal fluid pathways. Acta Radiol. 13:496–523, 1972.

Ducker, T. B.: Increased intracranial pressure in pulmonary edema. Part I. Clinical study of eleven patients. J. Neurosurg. 28:112–117, 1968.

Ducos, R., Donoso, J., Weickhardt, U. et al.: Sedimentation versus cytocentrifugation in the cytologic study of craniospinal fluid. Cancer 43:1479–1482, 1979.

Duffy, G. P.: Lumbar puncture in the presence of raised intracranial pressure. Br. Med. J. 1:407–409, 1969.

Duffy, T. E., Vergara, F. and Plum, F.: α-Ketoglutaramate in hepatic encephalopathy. In Plum, F. (ed.): Brain Dysfunction in Metabolic Disorders. Res. Publ. Assoc. Res. Nerv. Ment. Dis. 53:39–52, 1974.

Dufresne, J. J.: Praktische Zytologische Liquors. Basel, Ciba-Geigy, 1973.

Duma, R. J.: Amoebic infections of the nervous system. In Vinken, P. J. and Bruyn, G. W. (eds.): Handbook of Clinical Neurology. Vol. 35. Amsterdam, North Holland, 1978, pp. 25–65.

Duma, R. J., Ferrell, H. W., Nelson, C. E. et al.: Primary amebic meningoencephalitis. N. Engl. J. Med. 281:1315–1323, 1969.

Dumas, M. and Girard, P. L.: Human African trypanosomiasis (sleeping sickness). In Vinken, P. J. and Bruyn, G. W. (eds.): Handbook of Clinical Neurology. Vol. 35. Amsterdam, North Holland, 1978, pp. 67–83.

Dumas, M. and Girard, P. L.: Filariasis of the nervous system. In Vinken, P. J. and Bruyn, G. W. (eds.): Handbook of Clinical Neurology. Vol. 35. Amsterdam, North Holland, 1978, pp. 161–173.

Dunbar, H. G., Guthrie, T. C. and Karpell, B.: A study of the cerebrospinal fluid pulse wave. Arch. Neurol. 14:624–630, 1966.

Dunn, D., Dhopesh, V. and Mobini, J.: Spinal subdural hematoma: a possible hazard of lumbar puncture in an alcoholic. J.A.M.A. 241:1712–1713, 1979.

Dunsker, S. B., Torres-Reyes, E. and Peden, J. C.: Pseudotumor cerebri associated with idiopathic cryofibrinogenemia. Arch. Neurol 23:120–127, 1970.

Dupont, J. R., Van Wart, C. S. and Kraintz, L.: The clearance of major components of whole blood from cerebrospinal fluid following simulated subarachnoid hemorrhage. J. Neuropathol. Exp. Neurol 20:450–455, 1961.

Duvoisin, R. C. and Dettbarn, W. D.: Cerebrospinal fluid acetylcholine in man. Neurology 17:1077–1081, 1967.

Dyken, P. R.: Cerebrospinal fluid cytology: Practical clinical usefulness. Neurology 25:210–217, 1975.

Edelson, R. N., Chernik, N. L. and Posner, J. B.: Spinal subdural hematomas complicating lumbar puncture: occurrence in thrombocytopenic patients. Arch. Neurol. 31:134–137, 1974.

Ehrlich, P.: Das Sauerstoff-Bedurfhis des Organismus. Eine Farbenanalytische Studie. Berlin, 1885 (cited in Friedemann, 1942).

Eickhoff, K. and Heipertz, R.: Determination of immunoglobulin content of CSF based on light chain characteristics. Ann. Neurol. 3:509–512, 1978.

Eisenberg, H. M., McComb, J. G. and Lorenzo, A. V.: Cerebrospinal fluid overproduction and hydrocephalus associated with choroid plexus papilloma. J. Neurosurg. 40:381–385, 1974.

Ekbom, K., Greitz, T. and Kugelberg, E.: Hydrocephalus due to ectasia of the basilar artery. J. Neurol. Sci. 8:465–477, 1969.

Ekstedt, J.: CSF hydrodynamic studies in man. 1. Method of constant pressure CSF infusion. J. Neurol. Neurosurg. Psychiatry 40:105–115, 1977.

El-Batata, M.: Cytology of cerebrospinal fluid in the diagnosis of malignancy. J. Neurosurg. 28:317–326, 1968.

Ellington, E. and Margolis, G.: Block of arachnoid villus by subarachnoid hemorrhage. J. Neurosurg. 30:651–657, 1969.

Elliott, K. A. C. and Jasper, H.: Measurement of experimentally induced brain swelling and shrinkage. Am. J. Physiol. 157:122–129, 1949.

Elman, R.: Spinal arachnoid granulations with special reference to the cerebrospinal fluid. Bull. Johns Hopkins Hosp. 34:99–104, 1923.

Enevoldsen, G. M. and Jensen, F. T.: Autoregulation and CO_2 responses of cerebral blood flow in patients with acute severe head injury. J. Neurosurg. 48:689–703, 1978.

Enna, S. J., Stern, L. Z., Wastek, A. J. et al.: Cerebrospinal fluid gammaaminobutyric acid variations in neurological disorders. Arch. Neurol. 34:683–685, 1977.

Estanol, B. V., Loyo, M. V., Matoes, J. H. et al.: Cardiac arrhythmias in experimental subarachnoid hemorrhage. Stroke 8:440–447, 1977.

Estanol, B. V. and Martin, O. S.: Cardiac arrhythmias and sudden death in subarachnoid hemorrhage. Stroke 6:382–386, 1975.

Evans, D. I. K., O'Rourke, C. and Jones, P. M.: The cerebrospinal fluid in acute leukemia of childhood: Studies with the cytocentrifuge. J. Clin. Pathol. 27:226–230, 1974.

Evans, J. P., Espey, F. F., Kristoff, F. V. et al.: Experimental and clinical observations on rising intracranial pressure. Arch. Surg. 63:107–114, 1951.

Evans, R. J. C. and McElwain, T. J.: Eosinophilic meningitis in Hodgkin's disease. Br. J. Clin. Pract. 23:382–384, 1969.

Faer, M. J., Mead, J. H. and Lynch, R. D.: Cerebral granulomatous angitis: case report and literature review. A. J. R. 129:463–467, 1977.

Fauci, A. S.: Glucocorticosteroid therapy: mechanism of action and clinical considerations. Ann. Intern. Med. 84:304–315, 1976.

Faull, K. F., Do Amaral, J. R., Berger, P. A. et al.: Mass spectrometric identification and selected ion monitoring quantitation of gamma-amino-butyric acid (GABA) in human lumbar cerebrospinal fluid. J. Neurochem. 31:1119–1122, 1978.

Faupel, G., Reulen, H. J., Muller, D. et al.: Double blind study on the effects of steroids on severe closed head injury. In Pappius, H. M. and Feindel, W. (eds.): Dynamics of Brain Edema. New York, Springer-Verlag, 1976, pp. 337–343.

Fay, T.: A new test for the diagnosis of certain headaches, the cephalgiogram. Dis. Nerv. Syst. 1:312–315, 1940.

Feldberg, W. and Fleischhauer, K.: Penetration of bromphenol blue from the perfused cerebral ventricles into the brain tissue. J. Physiol. 150:451–462, 1960.

Feldman, W. F.: Relation of concentrations of bacteria and bacterial antigen in cerebrospinal fluid to prognosis in patients with bacterial meningitis. N. Engl. J. Med. 296:433–435, 1977.

Felgenhauer, K.: Protein size and cerebrospinal fluid composition. Klin. Wochenschr. 52:1158–1164, 1974.

Fencl, V., Vale, R., Jr. and Broch, J. A.: Respiration and cerebral blood flow in metabolic acidosis and alkalosis in humans. J. Appl. Physiol. 27:67–76, 1969.

Fender, F. A. and MacKenzie, A. S.: Effect of albumin solution on cerebrospinal fluid pressure. Arch Neurol. Psychiat. 59:529–531, 1948.

Ferry, D. J., Gooding, R., Stanefer, J. C. et al.: Effect of Pantopaque myelography on cerebrospinal fluid fractions. J. Neurosurg. 38:167–171, 1973.

Fetter, B. F., Klintworth, G. K. and Wilson, S. H.: Mycoses of the Central Nervous System. Baltimore, Williams and Wilkins, 1967.

Fieschi, C., Battistini, N., Beduschi, A. et al.: Regional cerebral blood flow and intraventricular pressure in acute head injuries. J. Neurol. Neurosurg. Psychiatry 37:1378–1388, 1974.

Findlay, L. and Kemp, R. H.: Osteomyelitis of the spine following lumbar puncture. Arch. Dis. Child. 18:102–105, 1943.

Finkel, H. E.: Infectious mononucleosis encephalitis. Am. J. Med. Sci. 249:425–427, 1965.

Firemark, H., Barlow, C. F. and Roth, L. J.: The entry, accumulation and binding of diphenylhydantoin-2-C^{14} in brain. Int. J. Neuropharmacol. 2:25–38, 1963.

Fischer, G. W., Brenz, R. W., Alden, E. R. et al.: Lumbar puncture and meningitis. Am. J. Dis. Child. 129:590–592, 1975.

Fischer-Williams, M., Bosanquet, F. D. and Daniel, P. M.: Carcinomatosis of the meninges: A report of three cases. Brain 78:42–58, 1955.

Fish, S. A., Morrison, J. C., Bucovaz, E. T. et al.: Cerebral spinal fluid studies in eclampsia. Am. J. Obstet. Gynecol. 112:502–512, 1972.

Fisher, R. G., Pomeroy, J. and Henry, J. P.: The free amino acids in adult human cerebrospinal fluid. Acta Neurol. Scand. 44:619–630, 1968.

Fisher, V. J. and Christiansen, L. C.: Cerebrospinal fluid acid-base balance during a changing ventilatory state in man. J. Appl. Physiol. 18:712–716, 1963.

Fishman, R. A.: Failure of intracranial pressure-volume change to influence renal function. J. Clin. Invest. 32:847–850, 1953.

Fishman, R. A.: Effects of isotonic intravenous solutions on normal and increased intracranial pressure. Arch. Neurol. & Psychiat 70:350–360, 1953.

Fishman, R. A.: Exchange of albumin between plasma and cerebrospinal fluid. Am. J. Physiol. 175–96–98, 1953.

Fishman, R. A.: Factors influencing the exchange of sodium between plasma and cerebrospinal fluid. J. Clin. Invest. 38:1698–1708, 1959.

Fishman, R. A.: Studies of the transport of sugars between blood and cerebrospinal fluid in normal states and in meningeal carcinomatosis. Trans. Am. Neurol. Assoc. 88:114–118, 1963.

Fishman, R. A.: Carrier transport of glucose between blood and cerebrospinal fluid. Am. J. Physiol. 206:836–844, 1964.

Fishman, R. A.: Neurological manifestations of magnesium metabolism. Arch. Neurol. 12:562–569, 1965.

Fishman, R. A.: Carrier transport and the concentration of glucose in cerebrospinal fluid in meningeal diseases. Ann. Intern. Med. 63:153–155, 1965. (Editorial)

Fishman, R. A.: Occult hydrocephalus. N. Engl. J. Med. 274:466–467, 1966. (Letter to the Editor)

Fishman, R. A.: The blood brain and CSF barriers to penicillin and related organic acids. Arch. Neurol. 15:113–124, 1966.

Fishman, R. A.: Permeability changes in experimental uremic encephalopathy. Arch. Intern. Med. 126:835–837, 1970.

Fishman, R. A.: Cerebrospinal fluid. In Baker, A. B. and Baker, L. H. (eds.): Clinical Neurology. New York, Harper and Row, 1971.

Fishman, R. A.: Cell volume, pumps and neurologic function: Brain's adaptation to osmotic stress. In Plum, F. (ed.): Brain Dysfunction in Metabolic Disorders. Res. Publ. Assoc. Res. Nerv. Ment. Dis. 53:159–171, 1974.

Fishman, R. A.: Brain edema: N. Engl. J. Med. 273:706–711, 1975.

Fishman, R. A.: Neurological manifestations of hyponatremia. In Vinken, P. J. and Bruyn, G. W. (eds.): Handbook of Clinical Neurology. Vol. 28. Amsterdam, North Holland, 1976, pp. 495–505.

Fishman, R. A., Chan, P. H., Lee, J. L. et al.: Effects of superoxide free radicals on the induction of brain edema. Neurology 29:546, 1979. (Abstract)

Fishman, R. A. and Christy, N. P.: Fate of adrenal cortical steroids following intrathecal injections. Neurology 15:1–6, 1965.

Fishman, R. A., Cowen, D. and Silberman, M.: Intracranial venous thrombosis during the first trimester of pregnancy. Neurology 7:217–220, 1957.

Fishman, R. A. and Greer, M.: Changes in the cerebrum associated with experimental obstructive hydrocephalus. Arch. Neurol. 8:156–161, 1963.

Fishman, R. A., Ransohoff, J. and Osserman, E. F.: Factors influencing the concentration gradient of protein in cerebrospinal fluid. J. Clin. Invest. 37:1419–1424, 1958.

Fishman, R. A. and Raskin, N. H.: Experimental uremic encephalopathy: Permeability and electrolyte metabolism of brain and other tissues. Arch. Neurol. 17:10–21, 1967.

Fishman, R. A., Reiner, M. and Chan, P. H.: Metabolic changes associated with iso-osmotic regulation in brain cortex slices. J. Neurochem. 28:1061–1067, 1977a.

Fishman, R. A., Sligar, K. and Hake, R. B.: Effects of leukocytes on brain metabolism in granulocytic brain edema. Ann. Neurol. 2:89–94, 1977b.

Fitch, W., Barker, J., McDowall, D. G. and Jennett, W. B.: The effects of methoxyflurane on cerebrospinal fluid pressure in patients with and without intracranial space occupying lesions. Br. J. Anaesth. 41:564–574, 1969.

Fitch, W. and McDowall, D. G.: Effect of halothane on intracranial pressure gradients in the presence of intracranial space occupying lesions. Br. J. Anaesth. 43:904–912, 1971.

Fitz-Hugh, G. S., Robins, R. B. and Craddock, W. D.: Increased intracranial pressure complicating unilateral neck dissection. Laryngoscope 76:893–906, 1966.

Flamm, E. S., Demopoulos, H. B., Seligman, M. L. et al.: Free radicals in cerebral ischemia. Stroke 9:445–447, 1978.

Flamm, E. S., Demopoulos, H. B., Seligman, M. L. et al.: Barbiturates and free radicals. In Popp, A. J. et al. (eds.): Neural Trauma. New York, Raven Press, 1979, pp. 289–296.

Fleischer, H. S., Rudman, D. R., Fresh, C. B. et al.: Concentrations of 3',5' cyclic adenosine monophosphate in ventricular CSF of patients following severe head trauma. J. Neurosurg. 47:517–524, 1977.

Flexner, L. B.: The chemistry and nature of the cerebrospinal fluid. Physiol. Rev. 14:161–187, 1934.

Fog, M.: The relationship between the blood pressure and the tonic regulation of the pial arteries. J. Neurol. Psychiat. 1:187–197, 1938.

Foldes, F. F. and Arrowood, J. G.: Changes in cerebrospinal fluid pressure under the influence of continuous subarachnoidal infusion of normal saline. J. Clin. Invest. 27:346–351, 1948.

Foley, J.: Benign forms of intracranial hypertension — "toxic" and "otitic" hydrocephalus. Brain 78:1–41, 1955.

Foley, K. M. and Posner, J. B.: Does pseudotumor cerebri cause the empty sella syndrome? Neurology 25:565–569, 1975.

Foltz, E. L. and Ward, A. A., Jr.: Communicating hydrocephalus from subarachnoid bleeding. J. Neurosurg. 13:546–566, 1956.

Forbes, H. S.: The cerebral circulation. Observation and measurement of pial vessels. Arch. Neurol. Psychiat. 19:751–761, 1938.

Ford, D. H.: Blood-brain barrier: A regulatory mechanism. Rev. Neurosci. 2:1–42, 1976.

Forghani, B., Cremer, N. E., Johnson, K. P. et al.: Viral antibodies in cerebrospinal fluid of multiple sclerosis and control patients: Comparison between radioimmunoassay and conventional techniques. J. Clin. Microbiol. 7:63–69, 1978.

Fourth International Symposium on Intracranial Pressure. Berlin, Springer-Verlag, 1979. (in press)

Fraschini, F., Muller, E. and Zanoboni, A.: Post-mortem increase of potassium in human cerebrospinal fluid. Nature 198:1208, 1963.

Frederiks, J. A. M. and Bruyn, G. W.: Mollaret's meningitis. In Vinken, P. J. and Bruyn, G. W. (eds.): Handbook of Clinical Neurology. Vol. 34. Amsterdam, Elseview/North Holland, 1978, pp. 545–552.

Freedman, D. A. and Merritt, H. H.: The cerebrospinal fluid in multiple sclerosis. Res. Pub. Assoc. Res. Nerv. Ment. Dis. 28:428–439, 1950.

Freeman, J. and Ingvar, D. H.: Elimination by hypoxia of cerebral blood flow, autoregulation and EEG relationship. Exp. Brain Res. 5:61–71, 1968.

Freeman, R. B., Sheff, M. F., Maher, J. F. et al.: The blood-cerebrospinal fluid barrier in uremia. Ann. Intern. Med. 56:233–240, 1962.

Fremont-Smith, F. and Forbes, H. S.: Intraocular and intracranial pressure. Arch. Neurol. Psychiat. 18:550–555, 1927.

Fremont-Smith, F. and Merritt, H. H.: Relationship of arterial blood pressure to cerebrospinal fluid pressure in man. Arch. Neurol. Psychiat. 30:1309–1317, 1933.

Frick, E. and Scheid-Seydel, L.: Untersuchungen mit J131-markiertem γ-globulin zur frage der abstammung der liquoreiweisskorper. Klin. Wochenschr. 36:857–865, 1958.

Fridovich, I.: Superoxide dismutases. Ann. Rev. Biochem. 44:147–159, 1975.

Friedfeld, L. and Fishberg, A. M.: The relation of the cerebrospinal and venous pressures in heart failure. J. Clin. Invest. 13:495–501, 1934.

Friedman, A. and Levinson, A.: Cerebrospinal fluid inorganic phosphorus in normal and pathologic conditions. Arch. Neurol. Psychiat. 74:424–440, 1955.

Friedman, H. S. and Rubin, M. A.: Clinical significance of the magnesium:calcium ratio. Technic for the determination of magnesium and calcium in biologic fluids. Clin. Chem. 1:125–133, 1955.

Friedemann, U.: Blood-brain barrier. Physiol. Rev. 22:125–145, 1942.

Froin, G.: Inflammations méningées avec réaction chromatique, fibrineuse et cytologique du liquid céphalo-rachidien. Gaz. Hôp. (Paris), 1903.

Froin, G., and Foy, G.: Syndrome de coagulation massive au cours d'une meningite; action novice d'une injection sous-arachnoidienne de collargol. Lancette Francaise: Gaz. Hop. (Paris), 81:1587–1592, 1908.

Froman, C. and Crampton-Smith, A.: Metabolic acidosis of the cerebrospinal fluid associated with subarachnoid hemorrhage. Lancet 1:965–967.

Fumagalli, R. and Paoletti, P.: Sterol test for human brain tumors: Relationship with different oncotypes. Neurology 21:1149–1156, 1971.

Funder, J. and Wieth, J. O.: Changes in cerebrospinal fluid composition following hemodialysis. Scand. J. Clin. Lab. Invest. 19:301–312, 1967.

Gaines, J. D., Eckman, P. B. and Remington, J. S.: Low CSF glucose level in sarcoidosis involving the central nervous system. Arch. Intern. Med. 125:333–336, 1970.

Galbraith, J. and Sullivan, J. H.: Decompression of the perioptic meninges for relief of papilledema. Am. J. Opthalmol. 76:687–692, 1973.

Galicich, J. H. and French, L. A.: Use of dexamethasone in the treatment of cerebral edema resulting from brain tumors and brain surgery. Am. Practit. 12:169–174, 1961.

Galicich, J. H., French, L. A. and Melby, J. C.: Use of dexamethasone in the treatment of cerebral edema associated with brain tumors. Lancet 81:46–53, 1961.

Ganshirt, H.: Die sauerstoffdruck im liquor cerebrospinalis. Wien Med. Wochenschr. 116:953–957, 1966.

Garcia-Bengochea, F.: The effect of cortisone on cerebrospinal fluid production in castrated adult cats. Neurology 16:512–514, 1966.

Garcia-Bunuel, L. and Garcia-Bunuel, V. M.: Enzymic determination of free myoinsoitol in human cerebrospinal fluid and plasma. J. Lab. Clin. Med. 64:461–468, 1964.

Gardner, W. J.: Hydrodynamic mechanisms of syringomyelia: Its relationship to myocele. J. Neurol. Neurosurg. Psychiatry 28:247–259, 1965.

Garelis, E., Young, S. N., Lal, S. et al.: Monoamine metabolites in lumbar CSF: The question of their origin in relation to clinical studies. Brain Res. 79:1–8, 1974.

Garfield, J.: Brain abscesses and focal suppurative infections. In Vinken, P. J. and Bruyn, G. W. (eds.): Handbook of Clinical Neurology. Vol. 33. Amsterdam, Elsevier/North Holland Biomedical Press, 1978, pp. 107–147.

Gautier-Smith, P. C.: Neurological complications of glandular fever. Brain 88:323–334, 1965.

Gellman, M.: Injury to intervertebral discs during spinal puncture. J. Bone Joint Surg. 22:980–985, 1940.

Gerstenbrand, F. Uber aminosaurebest immungen in serum und liquor bei extrapyramidalen krankheitsbildern. Wien. Z. Nervenheilk. (Suppl. 1):130–135, 1966.

Geschwind, N.: The mechanisms of normal pressure hydrocephalus. J. Neurol. Sci. 7:481–493, 1968.

Gilland, O.: CSF dynamic diagnosis of spinal block III: An equation for block influence on cisterno-lumbar electromanometrics. Acta Neurol. Scand. 41:Suppl. 13:47–74, 1964.

Gilland, O.: Multiple sclerosis classification scheme integrating clinical and CSF findings. Acta Neurol. Scand. 41:Suppl. 13:563–575, 1965.

Gilland, O.: CSF dynamic diagnosis of spinal block VI. Reliability of combined cisterno-lumbar electromanometrics. Acta Neurol. Scand. 42:Suppl. 21:1–43, 1966.

Gilland, O.: Lumbar cerebrospinal fluid total protein in healthy subjects. Acta Neurol. Scand. 43:526–529, 1967.

Gilles, F. H. and Davidson, R. I.: Communicating hydrocephalus associated with deficient dysplastic parasaggital arachnoidal granulatomas. J. Neurosurg. 35:421–426, 1971.

Gilon, E., Szeinberg, A., Tauman, G. et al.: Glutamine estimation in cerebrospinal fluid of cases of liver cirrhosis and hepatic coma. J. Lab. Clin. Med. 53:713–719, 1953.

Gius, J. A. and Grier, D. H.: Venous adaptation following bilateral radical neck dissection with excision of the jugular veins. Surgery 28:305–319, 1950.

Gjessing, L. R., Gjesdahl, P., Dietrichson, P. et. al.: Free amino acids in the cerebrospinal fluid in old age and in Parkinson's disease. Eur. Neurol. 12:33–37, 1974.

Gjessing, L. R., Gjesdahl, P. and Sjaastad, O.: The free amino acids in human cerebrospinal fluid. J. Neurochem. 19:1807–1808, 1972.

Glasauer, F. E.: Thoracic and lumbar intraspinal tumors associated with increased intracranial pressure. J. Neuro. Neurosurg. Psychiatry 27:451–458, 1964.

Glaser, G. H.: Brain dysfunction in uremia. In Plum, F. (ed.): Brain Dysfunction in Metabolic Disorders. Res. Publ. Assoc. Res. Nerv. Ment. Dis. 53:173–199, 1974.

Glass, J. P., Melamed, M., Chernik, N. C. and Posner, J. B.: Malignant cells in cerebrospinal fluid (CSF): The meaning of a positive CSF cytology. Neurology 29:1369–1375, 1979.

Glasser, L., Payne, C. and Corrigan, J. J.: The in vivo development of plasma cells: A morphologic study of human cerebrospinal fluid. Neurology 27:448–459, 1977.

Goldensohn, E. S., Whitehead, R. W., Parry, T. M. et. al.: Studies on diffusion respiration. IX. Effect of diffusion respiration and high concentration of CO_2 on cerebrospinal fluid pressure of anesthetized dogs. Am. J. Physiol. 165:334–340, 1951.

Goldman, E. E. 1913 (cited in Friedemann, 1942).

Goldring, S. and Hanford, C. G.: Effect of leukocytes and bacteria on glucose contents of the CSF in meningitis. Proc. Soc. Exp. Biol. Med. 75:669–672, 1950.

Goldstein, D. J. and Cubeddu, L. X.: Dopamine-beta-hydroxylase activity in human cerebrospinal fluid. J. Neurochem. 26:193–195, 1976.

Goldstein, E. and Lawrence, R. M.: Coccidiomycosis of the central nervous system. In Vinken, P. J. and Bruyn, G. W. (eds.): Handbook of Clinical Neurology. Vol. 35. Amsterdam, North Holland, 1978, pp. 443–457.

Goldstein, E., Winship, M. S. and Pappagianis, D.: Ventricular fluid and the management of coccidioidal meningitis. Ann. Intern. Med. 77:243–246, 1972.

Goldstein, G. W.: Relation of potassium transport to oxidative metabolism in isolated brain capillaries. J. Physiol. 286:185–196, 1979.

Goldstein, G. W., Romoff, M., Bogin, F. et al.: Relationship between the concentrations of calcium and phosphorus in blood and cerebrospinal fluid. J. Clin. Endocrinol. Metab. 49:58–62, 1979.

Goldstein, G. W., Wolinsky, J. S., Csejtey, J. et. al.: Isolation of metabolically active capillaries from rat brain. J. Neurochem. 25:715–717, 1975.

Goldstein, G. W., Wolinsky, J. S. and Csejtey, J.: Isolated brain capillaries: a model for the study of lead encephalopathy. Ann. Neurol. 1:235–239, 1977.

Goldstein, N. P., McKenzie, R. B. and McGuckin, W. F.: Changes in cerebrospinal fluid of patients with multiple sclerosis after treatment with intrathecal methylprednisolone acetate: A preliminary report. Proc. Mayo Clin. 37:657–668, 1962.

Gomez, D. G., Potts, D. G., Deonarine, V. and Reilly, K. F.: Effect of pressure gradient changes on the morphology of arachnoid villi and granulations of the monkey. Lab. Invest. 26:648–657, 1973.

Gondos, B. and King, E. P.: Cerebrospinal fluid cytology: diagnostic accuracy and comparison of different techniques. Acta Cytol. 20:542–547, 1976.

Gooddy, W., Hamilton, E. I. and Williams, T. R.: Spark-source mass spectrometry in the investigation of neurological disease. II. Element levels in brain, cerebrospinal fluid and blood: Some observations on their abundance and significance. Brain 98:65–70, 1975.

Gooddy, W., Williams, T. R. and Nicholas, D.: Spark-source mass spectrometry in the investigation of neurological disease. I. Multi-element analysis in blood and cerebrospinal fluid. Brain 97:327–336, 1974.

Gordon, E.: The acid base balance and oxygen tension of the cerebrospinal fluid and their implications for the treatment of patients with brain lesion. Acta Anaesthesiol. Scand. (Suppl.) 39:1–36, 1971.

Gordon, E. K. and Oliver, J.: 3-Methoxy-4-hydroxyphenylethylene glycol in human cerebrospinal fluid. Clin. Chim. Acta 35:145–150, 1971.

Gordon, M. J., Skillman, J. J., Zervas, N. T. et al.: Divergent nature of gastric mucosal permeability and gastric acid secretion in sick patients with general surgical and neurological disease. Ann. Surg. 178:285–294, 1973.

Gottfries, C. G., Gottfries, I., Johansson, B. et al.: Acid monoamine metabolites in human cerebrospinal fluid and their relations to age and sex. Neuropharmacology 10:665–672, 1971.

Gottfries, C. G., Gottfries, I. and Roos, B. E.: Homovanillic acid and 5-hydroxyindoleacetic acid in the cerebrospinal fluid of patients with senile dementia, presenile dementia and Parkinsonism. J. Neurochem. 16:1341–1345, 1969.

Grant, D. N.: Benign intracranial hypertension: A review of 79 cases in infancy and childhood. Arch. Dis. Child. 46:651–655, 1971.

Grant, W. T. and Cone, W. V.: Graduated jugular compression in the lumbar manometric test for spinal subarachnoid block. Arch. Neurol. Psychiat. 32:1194–1201, 1934.

Grantham, J. J.: Pathophysiology of hypo-osmolar conditions: A cellular perspective. In Andreoli, T. H., Grantham, J. J., and Rector, F. C. Jr. (eds.): Disturbances in Body Fluid Osmolality. Bethesda, American Physiological Society, 1977, pp. 217–225.

Gray, H.: History of lumbar puncture (rachicentesis): The operation and the idea. Arch. Neurol. Psychiat. 6:61–69, 1921.

Graziani, L. J., Escriva, A. and Katzman, R.: Exchange of calcium between blood, brain and cerebrospinal fluid. Am. J. Physiol. 208:1058–1064, 1965.

Graziani, L. J., Kaplan, R. K., Escriva, A. et al.: Calcium flux into CSF during ventricular and ventriculocisternal perfusion. Am. J. Physiol. 213:629–636, 1967.

Green, J. B., Oldewurtel, H. A. and Forster, F. M.: Glutamic oxalacetic transaminase (GOT) and lactic dehydrogenase (LDH) activities. Neurology (Minneap.) 9:540–544, 1959.

Green, J. B., Papadopoulos, N., Cevallos, W., Forster, F. M. and Hess, W. C.: The cholesterol and cholesterol ester content of cerebrospinal fluid in patients with multiple sclerosis and other neurological diseases. J. Neurol. Neurosurg. Psychiatry 22:117–119, 1959.

Green, J. B. and Perry, M.: Leucine-amino-peptidase activity in CSF. Neurology (Minneap.) 13:924–926, 1963.

Greenberg, D. M., Aird, R. B. and Balter, M. D., et al.: A study with radioactive isotopes of permeability of blood-CSF barrier to ions. Am. J. Physiol. 140:47–64, 1943.

Greenfield, J. G. and Carmichael, E. A.: The Cerebro-spinal Fluid in Clinical Diagnosis. London, Macmillan, 1925.

Greenlee, J. E. and Mandell, G. L.: Neurological manifestations of infective endocarditis. A review. Stroke 4:958–963, 1973.

Greensher, J., Mofenson, H. C., Borofsky, L. G. et al.: Lumbar puncture in the neonate: A simplified technique. J. Pediatr. 78:1034–1035, 1971.

Greer, M.: Management of benign intracranial hypertension (pseudotumor cerebri). Clin. Neurosurg. 15:161–174, 1968.

Greitz, T.: Effect of brain distention on cerebral circulation. Lancet 1:863–865, 1969.

Greitz, T. V., Grepe, A. O., Kalmer, M. S. et al.: Pre- and postoperative evaluation of cerebral blood flow in low-pressure hydrocephalus. J. Neurosurg. 31:644–651, 1969.

Grubb, R. L., Jr., Raichle, M. E., Eichling, J. O. et al.: Effects of subarachnoid hemorrhage on cerebral blood volume, blood flow, and oxygen utilization in humans. J. Neurosurg. 46:446–453, 1977.

Grubb, R. L., Raichle, M. E., Phelps, M. E. et al.: Effects of increased intracranial pressure on cerebral blood volume, blood flow, and oxygen utilization in monkeys. J. Neurosurg. 43:388–398, 1975.

Gsell, O. R.: Leptospiroses and relapsing fever. In Vinken, P. J. and Bruyn, G. W. (eds.): Handbook of Clinical Neurology. Vol. 33. Amsterdam, Elsevier/North Holland Biomedical Press, 1978, pp. 395–419.

Guidetti, B. and Fortuna, A.: Differential diagnosis of intramedullary and extramedullary tumours.

In Vinken, P. J. and Bruyn, G. W. (eds.): Handbook of Clinical Neurology. Vol. 19. Amsterdam, North Holland, 1975, pp. 51–75.

Guidetti, B., Guiffre, R., and Gambacorta, F.: Followup study of 100 cases of pseudotumor cerebri. Acta Neurochir. 18:259–267, 1968.

Guido, L. J. and Patterson, R. H.: Neurological deficits secondary to intraoperative CSF drainage: Successful resolution with an epidural blood patch. J. Neurosurg. 45:348–351, 1976.

Guillain, G.: Radiculoneuritis with acellular hyperalbuminosis of the cerebrospinal fluid. Arch. Neurol. Psychiat. 36:975–990, 1936.

Guillaume, J. and Janny, P.: Manométrie intracrannienne continue; intérêt de la méthode et premiers résultats. Rev. Neurol. (Paris) 84:131–142, 1951.

Guinane, J. E.: Cerebrospinal fluid pulse pressure and brain compliance in adult cats. Neurology 25:559–564, 1975.

Guisado, R., Arieff, A. I. and Massry, S. G.: Effects of glycerol infusion on brain water and electrolytes. Am. J. Physiol. 227:865–872, 1974.

Guisado, R., Arieff, A. I. and Massry, S. G.: Effects of glycerol administration on experimental brain edema. Neurology 26:69–75, 1976.

Guthrie, T. C., Dunbar, H. S. and Karpell, B.: Ventricular size and chronic increased intracranial venous pressure in the dog. J. Neurosurg. 33:407–414, 1970.

Gutierrez, Y., Friede, R. L. and Kaliney, W. J.: Agenesis of arachnoid granulations and its relationship to communicating hydrocephalus. J. Neurosurg. 43:553–558, 1975.

Haerer, A. F.: Citrate and alpha-ketoglutarate in cerebrospinal fluid and blood. Neurology 21:1059–1065, 1971.

Hagen, G. A. and Elliott, W. J.: Transport of thyroid hormones in serum and cerebrospinal fluid. J. Clin. Endocrinol. Metab. 37:415–422, 1973.

Hagnevik, K., Gordon, E., Lins, L. E. et al.: Glycerol induced hemolysis with hemoglobinuria and acute renal failure. Lancet 1:75–77, 1974.

Haire, M.: Significance of virus antibodies in multiple sclerosis. Br. Med. Bull. 33:40–44, 1977.

Hakim, S.: Algunas observaciones sobre la presion del LCR. Sindrome hidrocefalico en el adulto con "presion normal" del LCR. Thesis No 957, Javeriana University School of Medicine, Bogotá, Colombia, 1964.

Hakim, S.: Biomechanics of hydrocephalus. In Harbert, J. C. (ed.): Cisternography and Hydrocephalus. A Symposium. Springfield, Illinois, Charles C Thomas, 1972, pp. 25–54.

Hakim, S.: Considerations on the physics of hydrocephalus and its treatment. In Bito, L. Z., Davson, H. and Fenstermacher, J. D. (eds.): The Ocular and Cerebrospinal Fluids. New York, Academic Press, 1977, pp. 391–399.

Hakim, S. and Adams, R. D.: The special clinical problem of symptomatic hydrocephalus with normal cerebrospinal fluid pressure. Observations on cerebrospinal fluid hemodynamics. J. Neurol. Sci. 2:307–327, 1965.

Hamilton, C. R., Shelley, W. M. and Tumulty, P. A.: Giant cell arteritis: Including temporal arteritis and polymyalgia rheumatica. Medicine 50:1–27, 1971.

Hamilton, W. F., Woodbury, R. A. and Harper, H. T.: Arterial, cerebrospinal and venous pressures in man during cough and strain. Am. J. Physiol. 141:42–50, 1944.

Hammerstad, J. P., Lorenzo, A. V. and Cutler, R. W. P.: Iodide transport from the spinal subarachnoid fluid in the cat. Am. J. Physiol. 216:353–358, 1969.

Hansen, E. B. Fahrenkrug, A. and Praestholm, J.: Late meningeal effects of myelographic contrast media with special reference to metrizamide. Br. J. Radiol. 51:321–327, 1978.

Hansen, H. H.: The cyto-centrifuge and cerebrospinal fluid cytology. Acta Cytol. 18:259–262, 1974.

Hansen, J. M. and Siersback-Nielsen, K.: Cerebrospinal fluid thyroxine. J. Clin. Endocrinol. Metab. 29:1023–1026, 1969.

Hanson, H. A., Johansson, B. and Blomstrand, C.: Ultrastructural studies on cerebrovascular permeability in acute hypertension. Acta Neuropathol. 32:187–198, 1975.

Harbert, J. C.: Radionuclide cisternography. Semin. Nucl. Med. 1:90–106, 1971.

Harbert, J. C. (ed.): Cisternography and Hydrocephalus. A Symposium. Springfield, Illinois, Charles C Thomas, 1972.

Harker, L. A. and Slichter, S. J.: Bleeding time as a screening test to evaluate platelet function. N. Engl. J. Med. 287:155–158, 1972.

Harper, A. M.: Autoregulation of cerebral blood flow: influence of the arterial blood pressure on the blood flow through the cerebral cortex. J. Neurol. Neurosurg. Psychiatry 29:398–403, 1966.

Harper, M., Jennett, B., Miller, D. and Rowan, J. (eds.): Blood Flow and Metabolism in the Brain. London, Churchill Livingstone, 1975.

Harris, A. A., Sokalski, S. J. and Levin, S.: Pneumococcal meningitis. In Vinken, P. J. and Bruyn, G. W. (eds.): Handbook of Clinical Neurology. Vol. 33. Amsterdam, North Holland, 1978, pp. 35–52.

Harris, W. H. and Sonnenblick, E. H.: A study of calcium and magnesium in the cerebrospinal fluid. Yale J. Biol. Med. 27:297–303, 1955.

Harrison, W. B., Jr.: Cisternal pressure in congestive heart failure and its bearing on orthopnea. J. Clin. Invest. 12:1075–1081, 1933.

Harrison, T. R. and Mason, M. F.: The pathogenesis of the uremia syndrome. Medicine 16:1–44, 1937.

Harrison, T. R., Mason, M. F. and Resnik, H.: Observations on the mechanism of muscular twitchings in uremia. J. Clin. Invest. 15:463–464, 1936.

Harrison, W. G., Jr.: Cerebrospinal fluid pressure and venous pressure in cardiac failure and the effect of spinal drainage in the treatment of cardiac decompensation. Arch. Intern. Med. 53:782–791, 1934.

Harter, D. H., Yahr, M. D. and Kabat, E. A.: Neurological diseases with elevation of cerebrospinal fluid gamma globulin: a critical review. Trans. Am. Neurol. Assoc. 87:210–212, 1962.

Hassin, G. B., Oldberg, E. and Tinsley, M.: Changes in the brain in plexectomized dogs: with comments on the cerebrospinal fluid. Arch. Neurol. Psychiatr. 38:1224–1239, 1937.

Hatfalvi, B. I.: The dynamics of post spinal headache. Headache 17:64–66, 1977.

Haymaker, W. and Kernohan, J. W.: Landry-Guillain-Barré syndrome: Clinicopathologic report of 50 fatal cases and a critique of the literature. Medicine 28:59–141, 1949.

Hedley-Whyte, E. T., Lorenzo, V. A., and Hsu, D. W.: The role of arteries and endothelial vesicles in breakdown of the blood-brain barrier with drug induced seizures. J. Neuropathol. Exp. Neurol. 35:331, 1976. (Abstract)

Heiblim, D. I., Evans, H. E., Glass, L. et al.: Amino acid concentrations in cerebrospinal fluid. Arch. Neurol. 35:765–768, 1978.

Heipertz, R., Eickhoff, K. and Karstens, K. H.: Cerebrospinal fluid concentrations of magnesium and inorganic phosphate in epilepsy. J. Neurol. Sci. 41:55–60, 1979.

Heisey, S. R., Held, D. and Pappenheimer, J. R.: Bulk flow and diffusion in the cerebrospinal fluid system of the goat. Am. J. Physiol. 203:775–781, 1962.

Held, D., Fencl, V. and Pappenheimer, J. R.: Electrical potential of cerebrospinal fluid. J. Neurophysiol. 27:942–959, 1964.

Hellstrom, B. and Kjellin, K. G.: The diagnostic value of spectrophotometry of the CSF in the newborn period. Devel. Med. Child. Neurol. 13:789–797, 1971.

Helrich, M., Papper, E. M., Brodie, B. B., Fink, M. and Rovenstine, E. A.: The rate of intrathecal procaine and the spinal fluid level required for surgical anesthesia. J. Pharmacol. Exper. Therap. 100:78–82, 1950.

Hempel, K. J. and Elmohamed, A.: Anatomical variation of the dura mater and the dural venous sinuses. In Vinken, P. J. and Bruyn, G. W. (eds.): Handbook of Clinical Neurology. Vol. 30. Amsterdam, North Holland, 1977, pp. 415–429.

Henry, J. B.: Clinical Diagnosis and Management by Laboratory Methods. 16th Edition. Philadelphia, W. B. Saunders, 1979.

Herbert, F. K.: The total and diffusible calcium of serum and the calcium of cerebrospinal fluid in human cases of hypocalcaemia and hypercalcaemia. J. Biochem. 27:1987–1991, 1934.

Herndon, R. M. and Johnson, M.: A method for the electron microscopic study of cerebrospinal fluid sediment. J. Neuropathol. Exp. Neurol. 29:320–330, 1970.

Herndon, R. M. and Kasckow, J.: Electron microscopic studies of cerebrospinal fluid sediment in demyelinating disease. Ann. Neurol. 4:515–524, 1978.

Hill, N. C., Goldstein, N. P., McKenzie, B. F. et al.: Cerebrospinal fluid proteins, glycoproteins, and lipoproteins in obstructive lesions of the central nervous system. Brain 82:581–593, 1959.

Hinman, A. R.: Tuberculous meningitis at Cleveland Metropolitan General Hospital, 1959–1963. Am. Rev. Respir. Dis. 95:670–673, 1967.

Hinman, R. C. and Magee, K. R.: Guillain-Barré syndrome with slow progressive onset and persistent elevation of spinal fluid protein. Ann. Intern. Med. 67:1007–1012, 1967.

Hirano, A., Ghatak, N. R., Becker, N. H., et al.: A comparison of the fine structures of small blood vessels in intracranial and retroperitoneal malignant lymphomas. Acta Neuropathol. 27:93–104, 1974.

Hirano, A., Zimmerman, H. M. and Levine, S.: Intramyelinic and extracellular spaces in tri-ethyl tin intoxication. J. Neuropath. Exp. Neurol. 27:571–580, 1968.

Ho, M.: Acute viral encephalitis. In Vinken, P. J. and Bruyn, G. W. (eds.): Handbook of Clinical Neurology. Amsterdam, North Holland, 1978, pp. 63–82.

Hochwald, G. M.: Influx of serum proteins and their concentration in spinal fluid along the neuraxis. J. Neurol. Sci. 10:269–278, 1970.

Hochwald, G. M., Lux, W. E., Jr., Sahar, A. and Ransohoff, J.: Experimental hydrocephalus. Changes in cerebrospinal fluid dynamics as a function of time. Arch. Neurol. 26:120–129, 1972.

Hochwald, G. M., Sahar, A., Sadik, A. L. and Ransohoff, J.: Cerebrospinal fluid protection and histological observations in animals with experimental obstructive hydrocephalus. Exp. Neurol. 25:190–199, 1969.

Hochwald, G. M. and Thorbecke, G. J.: Use of an antiserum against cerebrospinal fluid in demonstration of trace proteins in biological fluids. Proc. Soc. Exp. Biol. Med. 109:91–95, 1962.

Hochwald, G. M., Wald, A. and Malhan, C.: The sink action of cerebrospinal fluid volume flow. Effect on brain water content. Arch. Neurol. 33:339–344, 1976.

Hochwald, G. M. and Wallenstein, M.: Exchange of albumin between blood, cerebrospinal fluid, and brain in the cat. Am. J. Physiol. 212:1199–1204, 1967.

Hochwald, G. M., Wallenstein, M. C. and Mathews, E. S.: Exchange of proteins between blood and spinal subarachnoid fluid. Am. J. Physiol. 217:348–353, 1969.

Hoedt-Rasmussen, K., Skinhoj, E., Paulson, O. et al.: Regional cerebral blood flow in acute apoplexy. Arch. Neurol. 17:271–281, 1967.

Hoff, J. and Barber, R.: Transcerebral mantle pressure in normal pressure hydrocephalus. Arch. Neurol. 31:101–105, 1974.

Hoff, J. T. and Reis, D. J.: Localization of regions mediating the Cushing response in CNS of cat. Arch. Neurol. 23:228—240, 1970.

Hoff, J. T., Smith, A. L., Hankinson, H. L. et al.: Barbiturate protection from cerebral infarction in primates. Stroke 6:28–33, 1975.

Holliday, M. A., Kalayci, M. N. and Harrah, J.: Factors that limit brain volume changes in response to acute and sustained hyper- and hyponatrema. J. Clin. Invest. 47:1916–1928, 1968.

Hong, S. L. and Levine, L.: Inhibition of arachidonic acid release from cells as the biochemical action of anti-inflammatory corticosteroids. Proc. Natl. Acad. Sci. U.S.A. 73:1730–1734, 1976.

Hooshmand, H.: Pseudotumor cerebri: Treatment with dexamethasone. Neurology 22:451, 1972. (Abstract)

Hooshmand, H., Escobar, M. R. and Kopf, S. W.: Neurosyphilis. A study of 241 patients. J.A.M.A. 219:726–729, 1972.

Hopkins, E. L., Hendricks, C. H. and Cibils, L. H.: Cerebrospinal fluid pressure in labor. Am. J. Obstet. Gynecol. 93:907–916, 1965.

Horbein, T. F. and Sorensen, S. C.: DC potential difference between different cerebrospinal fluid sites and blood in dogs. Am. J. Physiol. 223:415–419, 1972.

Hossman, K. A.: Development and resolution of ischemic brain swelling. In Pappius, H. M. and Feindel, W. (eds.): Dynamics of Brain Edema. New York, Springer-Verlag, 1976, pp. 219–227.

Hossman, K. A. and Olsson, Y.: The effect of transient cerebral ischemia on the vascular permeability to protein tracers. Acta Neuropathol. 18:103–112, 1971.

Hossman, K. A. and Olsson, Y.: Influence of ischemia on the passage of protein tracers across capillaries in certain blood-brain barrier injuries. Acta Neuropathol. 18:113–122, 1971.

Hourani, B. T., Hamlin, E. M. and Reynolds, T. B.: Cerebrospinal fluid glutamine as a measure of hepatic encephalopathy. Arch. Intern. Med. 127:1033–1036, 1971.

Huang, C. T. and Lyons, H. A.: The maintenance of acid-base balance between cerebrospinal fluid and arterial blood in patients with chronic respiratory disorders. Clin. Sci. 31:273–284, 1966.

Huckman, M. S., Fox, J. S., Ramsey, R. G. and Penn, R. D.: Computed tomography in the diagnosis of pseudotumor cerebri. Radiology 119:593–597, 1976.

Hug, C. C.: Transport of narcotic analgesics by choroid plexus and kidney tissue in vitro. Biochem. Pharmacol. 16:345–359, 1967.

Hughson, W.: A note on the relationship of cerebrospinal and intralabyrinthine pressures. Am. J. Physiol. 101:396–407, 1932.

Hull, H. F. and Morrow, G.: Glucorrhea revisited. Prolonged promulgation of another plastic pearl. J.A.M.A. 234:1052–1053, 1975.

Hulme, A. and Cooper, R.: Cerebral blood flow during sleep in patients with raised intracranial pressure. Prog. Brain Res. 30:77–81, 1968.

Humoller, F. L., Mahler, D. M. and Parker, M. M.: Distribution of amino acids between plasma and spinal fluid. Int. J. Neuropsychiat. 2:293–297, 1966.

Hunter, G. and Smith, H. V.: Calcium and magnesium in human cerebrospinal fluid. Nature (London) 186:161–162, 1960.

Hussey, F., Schanzer, B. and Katzman, R.: A simple constant-infusion manometric test for measurement of CSF absorption. II. Clinical studies. Neurology (Minneap.) 20:665–680, 1970.

Huttenlocher, P. R.: Treatment of hydrocephalus with acetazolamide. J. Pediat. 66:1023–1030, 1965.

Illingworth, D. R. and Glover, J.: The composition of lipids in cerebrospinal fluid of children and adults. J. Neurochem. 18:769–776, 1971.

Illis, L. S. and Gostling, J. V.: Herpes simplex encephalitis. Bristol, Scientechnica, Triangle West, 1972, pp. 40–45.

Iivanainen, M. and Taskinen, E.: Differential cellular increase in cerebrospinal fluid after encephalography in mentally retarded patients. J. Neurol. Neurosurg. Psychiatry 37:1252–1258, 1974.

Ingvar, D. H. and Lassen, N. A. (eds.): Cerebral function, metabolism and circulation. Acta Neurol. Scand. Suppl. 64. Vol. 56, 1977.

Ingvar, D. H., Lassen, N. A., Siesjo, B. K. and Skinhoj, E.: Cerebral blood flow and cerebrospinal fluid. 3rd International Symposium. Scand. J. Clin. Lab. Invest. 22 (Suppl. 102), 1968.

Ivers, R. R., McKenzie, B. F., McGuckin, W. F. and Goldstein, N. P.: Spinal fluid gamma globulin in multiple sclerosis and other neurologic diseases. J.A.M.A. 176:515–519, 1961.

Ives, E. R.: Protein content in the cerebrospinal fluid of diabetic patients. Bull. Los Angeles Neurol. Soc. 22:95–111, 1957.

Jackson, I. J. and Snodgrass, S. R.: Peritoneal shunts in treatment of hydrocephalus and increased intracranial pressure. J. Neurosurg. 12:216–222, 1955.

Jaffe, H. W., Larsen, S. H., Peters, M. et al.: Tests for treponemal antibody in CSF. Arch. Intern. Med. 138:252–255, 1978.

Jakupcevic, M., Lackovic, Z., Stefoski, D. and Bulat, M.: Nonhomogenous distribution of 5-hydroxyindoleacetic acid and homovanillic acid in the lumbar CSF of man. J. Neurol. Sci. 31:165–171, 1977.

James, A. E., Jr., New, P. F. J., Heinz, E. R. et al.: A cisternographic classification of hydrocephalus. Am. J. Roentgenol. Radium Ther. Nucl. Med. 115:39–49, 1972.

James, H. E., Langfitt, T. W., Kumar, V. S. et al.: Treatment of intracranial hypertension. Analysis of 105 consecutive recordings of intracranial pressure. Acta Neurochir. 36:189–200, 1977.

Jarnum, S., Lorenzen, I. and Skinhoj, E.: Cisternal fluid oxygen tension in man. Neurology 14:703–707, 1964.

Javid, M. and Settlage, P.: Effect of urea on cerebrospinal fluid pressure in human subjects. J.A.M.A. 160:943–949, 1956.

Jeffcoate, W. J., McLoughlin, L., Hope, J. et al.: Beta-endorphin in human cerebrospinal fluid. Lancet 2:119–121, 1978.

Jefferson, A.: A clinical correlation between encephalopathy and papilloedema in Addison's disease. J. Neurol. Neurosurg. Psychiatry 19:21–27, 1956.

Jellinger, K.: Giant cell granulomatous angitis of the central nervous system. J. Neurol. 215:175–190, 1977.

Jeppsson, P. G.: Studies on the blood-brain barrier in hypothermia. Acta Neurol. Scand. 38 (Suppl. 160):1–229, 1962.

Jimerson, D. C., Post, R. M., Carman, J. S. et al.: CSF calcium: Clinical correlates in affective illness and schizophrenia. Biol. Psychiatry 14:37–51, 1979.

Johansson, B.: Brain barrier pathology in acute arterial hypertension. In Levi, G., Battistin, H. and Lajtha, A. (eds.): Advances in Experimental Medicine and Biology. Vol. 69. Transport Phenomena in the Nervous System. New York, Plenum Press, 1976.

Johnson, I., Gilday, D. C., Paterson, A. and Hendrick, E. B.: The definition of a reduced CSF absorption syndrome: (clinical and experimental studies). In Lundberg, N., Ponten, U. and Brock, M. (eds.): Intracranial Pressure II. Berlin, Springer-Verlag, 1975, pp. 50–53.

Johnston, I. and Paterson, A.: Benign intracranial hypertension: I. Diagnosis and prognosis. II. Pressure and circulation. Brain 97:289–300, 301–312, 1975.

Johnson, K. P. and Nelson, B. T.: Multiple sclerosis. Diagnostic usefulness of cerebrospinal fluid. Arch. Neurol. 2:425–431, 1977.

Johnson, R. and Milbourn, P. E.: Central nervous system manifestations of chicken pox. Can. Med. Assoc. J. 102:831–834, 1970.

Johnson, R. T. and Johnson, K. P.: Hydrocephalus as a sequela of experimental myxovirus infections. Exp. Mol. Pathol. 10:68–80, 1969.

Johnson, R. T. and Richardson, E. P.: Neurological manifestations of systemic lupus erythematosus. Medicine 47:337–369, 1968.

Johnston, I. H. and Jennett, B.: The place of continuous intracranial pressure monitoring in neurosurgical practice. Acta Neurochir. 29:53–63, 1973.

Johnston, I. H. and Rowan, J. O.: Raised intracranial pressure and cerebral blood flow. Intracranial pressure gradients and regional cerebral blood flow. J. Neurol. Neurosurg. Psychiatry 37:585–592, 1974.

Jones, M. D. and Newton, T. H.: Inadvertent extra-arachnoid injections in myelography. Radiology 80:818–822, 1963.

Jordan, R. M., Kendall, J. W., Seaich, J. L. et al.: Cerebrospinal fluid hormone concentration in the evaluation of pituitary tumors. Ann. Intern. Med. 85:49–55, 1976.

Jordan, R. M., McDonald, S. D., Stevens, E. A. et al.: Cerebrospinal fluid prolactin. A reevaluation. Arch. Intern. Med. 139:208–211, 1979.

Joslin, E. P., Root, H. F., White, P. et al.: The Treatment of Diabetes Mellitus. Philadelphia, Lea and Febiger, 1959.

Joyce-Clarke, N. and Molteno, A. C. B.: Modified neurosyphilis in the Cape Peninsula. S. Afr. Med. J. 53:10–14, 1978.

Kabat, E. A., Moore, D. H. and Landow, H.: An electrophoretic study of the protein components in cerebrospinal fluid and their relationship to the serum proteins. J. Clin. Invest. 21:571–577, 1942.

Kalbag, R. M. and Woolf, A. L.: Cerebral Venous Thrombosis. London, Oxford University Press, 1967.

Kam-Hansen, S.: Reduced number of active T cells in cerebrospinal fluid in multiple sclerosis. Neurology 29:897–899, 1979.

Kam-Hansen, S., Fryden, A. and Link, H.: B and T lymphocytes in cerebrospinal fluid and blood in multiple sclerosis, optic neuritis and mumps meningitis. Acta Neurol. Scand. 58:95–103, 1978.

Kaplan, A.: Electrophoresis of cerebrospinal fluid proteins. Am. J. Med. Sci. 253:549–555, 1967.

Kaplan, L. and Kennedy, F.: The effect of head posture on the manometrics of the cerebrospinal fluid in cervical lesions. A new diagnostic test. Brain 73:337–345, 1950.

Karch, S. B.: Upper gastrointestinal bleeding as a complication of intracranial disease. J. Neurosurg. 37:27–29, 1972.

Kassan, S. S. and Kagen, L. J.: Elevated levels of cerebrospinal fluid guanosine 3,5-cyclic monophosphate (c-GMP) in systemic lupus erythematosus. Am. J. Med. 64:732–741, 1978.

Katzenellenbogen, S.: The Cerebrospinal Fluid and its Relations to the Blood: A physiological and clinical study. Baltimore, Johns Hopkins Press, 1935.

Katzman, R.: Maintenance of a constant brain extracellular potassium. Fed. Proc. 35:1244–1247, 1976.

Katzman, R., Aleu, F. and Wilson, C.: Further observations on tri-ethyl tin edema. Arch. Neurol. 9:178–187, 1963.

Katzman, R., Clasen, R., Klatzo, I. et al.: Report of Joint Committee for Stroke Resources. IV. Brain edema in stroke. Stroke 8:509–540, 1977.

Katzman, R., Fishman, R. A. and Goldensohn, E. S.: Glutamic-oxaloacetic transaminase activity in spinal fluid. Neurology (Minneap.) 7:853–855, 1957.

Katzman, R. and Hussey, F.: A simple constant-infusion manometric test for measurement of CSF absorption. I. Rationale and method. Neurology (Minneap.) 20:534–544, 1970.

Katzman, R. and Pappius, H. M.: Brain Electrolytes and Fluid Metabolism. Baltimore, Williams and Wilkins, 1973.

Katzman, R. and Schimmel, H.: Water movement. In Lajtha, A. (ed.): Handbook of Neurochemistry. Vol. 2. New York, Plenum Press, 1969, pp. 11–22.

Kaufman, D. M., Miller, M. H. and Steigbigel, N. H.: Subdural empyema. Analysis of 17 recent cases and review of the literature. Medicine 54:485–498, 1975.

Kaufmann, G. E. and Clark, K.: Continuous simultaneous monitoring of intraventricular and cervical subarachnoid cerebrospinal fluid pressure to indicate development of cerebral or tonsillar herniation. J. Neurosurg. 33:145–150, 1970.

Kawamura, Y., Meyer, J. S., Hiromoto, H. et al.: Neurogenic control of cerebral blood flow in the baboon. Effects of the cholinergic inhibitory agent, atropine, on cerebral autoregulation and vasomotor reactivity to changes in Pa CO_2. J. Neurosurg. 43:676–688, 1975.

Keats, A. S. and Mithoefer, J. C.: The mechanism of increased intracranial pressure induced by morphine. N. Engl. J. Med. 252:1110–1113, 1955.

Kellie, G.: An account of the appearances observed in the dissection of two or three individuals presumed to have perished in the storm of the 3rd, and whose bodies were discovered in the vicinity of Leith on the morning of the 4th, November 1821 with some reflections on the pathology of the brain. Trans. Edinb. Med. Chir. Soc. 1:84–169, 1824.

Kemeny, A., Boldizsar, H. and Pethes, G.: The distribution of cations in plasma and cerebrospinal fluid following infusion of solutions of salts of sodium, potassium, magnesium and calcium. J. Neurochem. 7:218–227, 1961.

Kennedy, C. and Sokoloff, L.: An adaptation of the nitrous oxide method to the study of the cerebral circulation in children: normal values for cerebral blood flow and cerebral metabolic rate in childhood. J. Clin. Invest. 36:1130–1137, 1957.

Kennedy, D. H. and Falton, R. J.: Tuberculous meningitis. J.A.M.A. 241:264–268, 1979.

Kennedy, F., Effron, A. S. and Perry, G.: The grave spinal cord paralyses caused by spinal anesthesia. Surg. Gynecol. Obstet. 91:385–398, 1950.

Kessler, L. A. and Cheek, W. R.: Eosinophilia of the cerebrospinal fluid of non-infectious origin: Report of 2 cases. Neurology 9:371–374, 1959.

Kety, S. S. and Schmidt, C. F.: The determination of cerebral blood flow in man by the use of nitrous oxide in low concentrations. Am. J. Physiol. 143:53–66, 1945.

Kety, S. S. and Schmidt, C. F.: The nitrous oxide method for the quantitative determination of cerebral blood flow in man: theory, procedure and normal values. J. Clin. Invest. 27:476–483, 1948.

Kety, S. S., Shenkin, H. A. and Schmidt, C. F.: The effects of increased intracranial pressure on cerebral circulatory effects in man. J. Clin. Invest. 27:493–499, 1948.

Key, E. A. H. and Retzius, G.: Anatomie des Nervensystems und des Bindegewebes. Stockholm, 1875.

Kibler, R. F., Couch, R. S. C. and Crompton, M. R.: Hydrocephalus in the adult following spontaneous subarachnoid hemorrhage. Brain 84:45–61, 1961.

Kinal, M. E.: Hydrocephalus and the dural venous sinuses. J. Neurosurg. 19:155–200, 1962.

Kindley, A. D. and Harris, F.: Repeat lumbar puncture in the diagnosis of meningitis. Arch. Dis. Child. 73:590–592, 1978.

King, A. and Nicol, C.: Venereal Diseases. 3rd Edition. London, Balliere Tindall, 1975.

King, D. K., Loh, K. K., Ayala, A. G. and Gamble, J. F.: Eosinophilic meningitis and lymphomatous meningitis. Ann. Intern. Med. 82:228, 1975. (Letter)

King, L. R., McLaurin, R. L. and Knowles, H. C. Jr.: Acid-base balance and arterial and CSF lactate levels following human head injury. J. Neurosurg. 40:617–625, 1974.

Kiser, J. L. and Kendig, J. H.: Intracranial suppuration. A review of 139 consecutive cases, with electron microscopic observation in 3. J. Neurosurg. 20:494–511, 1963.

Kjallquist, A. N., Lundenberg, N. and Ponten, V.: Respiratory and cardiovascular changes during rapid spontaneous variations of ventricular fluid pressure in patients with intracranial hypertension. Acta Neurol. Scand. 10:291–317, 1964.

Kjellin, K. G.: Determination of the iron content in the cerebrospinal fluid. J. Neurochem. 13:413–421, 1966.

Kjellin, K. G.: Bilirubin compounds in the CSF. J. Neurol. Sci. 13:161–173, 1971.

Kjellin, K. G. and Soderstrom, C. E.: Diagnostic significance of CSF spectrophotometry in cerebrovascular diseases. J. Neurol. Sci. 23:359–369, 1974.

Klatzo, I.: Neuropathological aspects of brain edema. J. Neuropathol. Exp. Neurol. 26:1–14, 1967.

Klatzo, I. and Seitelberger, F.: Brain Edema. New York, Springer-Verlag, 1967.

Klockars, M., Reitamo, S., Webber, T. et al.: Cerebrospinal fluid lysozyme in bacterial and viral meningitis. Acta Med. Scand. 203:71–74, 1978.

Knigge, K. M., Scott, D. E., Kobayashi, H. et al. (eds.): Brain-Endocrine Interaction. II. Basel, S. Karger, 1975.

Knopp, L. M., Atkinson, J. R. and Ward, A. A., Jr.: The effect of diamox on cerebrospinal fluid pressure of cat and monkey. Neurology (Minneap.) 7:119–123, 1957.

Kocen, R. S. and Parsons, M.: Neurological complications of tuberculosis. Some unusual manifestations. Q. J. Med. 39:17–30, 1970.

Koch-Weser, J. and Gilmore, F. B.: Benign intracranial hypertension in an adult after tetracycline therapy. J.A.M.A. 200:345–347, 1967.

Kofman, S., Garvin, J. S., Nagamani, D. et al.: Treatment of cerebral metastases from breast cancer with prednisolone. J.A.M.A. 163:1473–1479, 1957.

Kolar, O. J. and Burkhart, J. E.: Neurosyphilis. Br. J. Vener. Dis. 53:221–225, 1977.

Kolar, O. J. and Zeman, W.: Spinal fluid cytomorphology. Description of apparatus, technique, and findings. Arch. Neurol. 18:44–51, 1968.

Kolar, O. J., Zeman, W., Ciembroniewicz, F. et al.: Uber die Bedutung der eosinophilen Leukocyten bei neurologischen Krankheiten. Wien. Z. Nervenheilk. 27:97–106, 1969.

Kolmel, H. W.: Atlas of Cerebrospinal Fluid Cells. Berlin, Springer-Verlag, 1976.

Kontos, H. A., Wei, E. P., Navari, R. M. et al.: Responses of cerebral arteries and arterioles to acute hypotension and hypertension. Am. J. Physiol. 234:371–383, 1978.

Korein, J., Cravioto, H. and Leicach, M.: Reevaluation of lumbar puncture. A study of 129 patients with papilledema or intracranial hypertension. Neurology 9:290–297, 1959.

Korf, J. and van Praag, H. M.: Amine metabolisms in the human brain. Further evaluation of the probenecid test. Brain Res. 35:221–230, 1971.

Kormorowski, R. A., Farmer, S. G., Hanson, G. A. et al.: Cerebrospinal fluid lactic acid in diagnosis of meningitis. J. Clin. Microbiol. 8:89–92, 1978.

Koster, H., Shapiro, A. and Leifensohn, A.: Concentration of procaine in cerebrospinal fluid of human beings after subarachnoid injection. Arch. Surg. 37:603–608, 1938.

Kovach, A. G. and Sandor, P.: Cerebral blood flow and brain function during hypotension and shock. Annu. Rev. Physiol. 38:571–596, 1976.

Kramer, M. D. and Aita, J. F.: Trichinosis. In Vinken, P. J. and Bruyn, G. W. (eds.): Handbook of Clinical Neurology. Vol. 35 Amsterdam, North Holland, 1978, pp. 267–290.

Krentz, M. J. and Dyken, P. R.: Cerebrospinal fluid cytomorphology. Sedimentation vs. filtration. Arch. Neurol. 26:253–257, 1972.

Krieg, A. F.: Cerebrospinal fluid and other body fluids. In Henry, J. B. (ed.): Clinical Diagnosis and Management by Laboratory Methods. 16th Ed. Philadelphia, W. B. Saunders, 1979, pp. 635–657.

Kronholm, V. and Lintrup, J.: Spectrophotometric investigations of the cerebrospinal fluid in the near ultraviolet region. Acta Psychiat. Scand. 35:314–329, 1960.

Kuberski, T.: Eosinophils in the cerebrospinal fluid. Ann. Intern. Med. 91:70–75, 1979.

Kunkle, E. C.: Acetylcholine in the mechanism of headaches of the migraine type. Arch. Neurol. Psychiat. 81:135–141, 1959.

Kunkle, E. C., Ray, B. S. and Wolff, H. G.: Experimental studies on headache: Analysis of the headache associated with changes in intracranial pressure. Arch. Neurol. Psychiat. 49:323–358, 1943.

Kutt, H., Hurwitz, J. L., Ginsburg, S. M. et al.: CSF proteins in diabetes mellitus. Arch. Neurol. 4:31–36, 1961.

Kutt, H., Hurwitz, L. J., Ginsburg, S. M. et al.: Cerebrospinal fluid protein in diabetes mellitus. Arch. Neurol. 4:43–48, 1961.

Kutt, H., McDowell, F., Chapman, L. et al.: Abnormal protein fractions of cerebrospinal fluid demonstrated by starch gel electrophoresis Neurology (Minneap.) 10:1064–1067, 1960.

Kuusela, P., Vaheri, A., Palo, J. et al.: Demonstration of fibronectin in human cerebrospinal fluid. J. Lab. Clin. Med. 92:595–601, 1978.

Kyle, R. A. and Greipp, P. R.: The laboratory investigation of monoclonal gammopathies. Proc. Mayo Clin. 53:719–739, 1978.

Laitinen, L.: Origin of arterial pulsations of cerebrospinal fluid. Acta Neurol. Scand. 44:168–176, 1968.

Lajtha, A. and Ford, D. H. (eds.): Progress in Brain Research. Vol. 29. Brain Barrier Systems. Amsterdam, Elsevier, 1968.

Lakke, J. P. W.: Detection of obstruction of the spinal canal by CSF manometry. In Vinken, P. J. and Bruyn, G. W. (eds.) Handbook of Clinical Neurology. Vol. 19. Amsterdam, North Holland, 1975, pp. 91–123.

Lakke, J. P. W. and Teelken, A. W.: Amino acid abnormalities in cerebrospinal fluid of patients with Parkinsonian and extrapyramidal disorders. Neurology 26:489–495, 1976.

Lange, C.: Über die Ausflockung von Goldsol durch Liquor cerebrospinalis. Veroffentl. Hufeland, Gesellsch. Berl. 2:21–33, 1913.

Langfitt, T. W.: Clinical methods for monitoring intracranial pressure and measuring cerebral blood flow. Clin. Neurosurg. 22:302–320, 1975.

Langfitt, T. W., Kassell, N. F. and Weinstein, J. D.: Cerebral blood flow with intracranial hypertension. Neurology 18:761–773, 1965.

Langfitt, T. W., McHenry, L. C., Reivich, M. and Wollman, H. (eds.): Cerebral Circulation and Metabolism. Berlin, Springer-Verlag, 1975.

Larson, G. M., Schall, G. L. and DiChiro, G.: The unsuccessful injection in cisternography: Incidence, cause and appearance. In Harbert, J. C. (ed.): Cisternography and Hydrocephalus. A Symposium. Springfield, Illinois, Charles C Thomas, 1972, pp. 153–171.

Larsson, O., Marinovich, N. and Barber, K.: Double-blind trial of glycerol therapy in early stroke. Lancet 1:832–834, 1976.

Lassen, N. A.: Cerebral blood flow and oxygen consumption in man. Physiol. Rev. 39:183–238, 1959.

Lassen, N. A.: Control of cerebral circulation in health and disease. Circ. Res. 34:749–760, 1974.

Lassen, N. A.: Luxury-perfusion syndrome and its possible relation to acute metabolic acidosis localized within the brain. Lancet 2:1113–1115, 1966.

Lassen, N. A.: Neurogenic control of cerebral circulation. In Langfitt, T., McHenry, L., Reivich, M. and Wollman, H. (eds.): Cerebral Circulation and Metabolism. Berlin, Springer-Verlag, 1975.

Lassen, N. A. and Agnoli, A.: The upper limit of autoregulation of cerebral blood flow — on the pathogenesis of hypertensive encephalopathy. Scand. J. Clin. Lab. Invest. 30:113–116, 1972.

Lassen, N. A., Hoedt-Rasmussen, K., Sorensen, S. C. et al.: Regional cerebral blood flow in man determined by krypton. Neurology 13:719–727, 1963.

Laterre, E. C.: Les Protéines du Liquide Céphalo-rachidien à L'état Normal et Pathologique. Bruxelles, Editions Arscia, Paris, Librairie Maloine, 1965, pp. 148–161.

Laterre, E. C.: Cerebrospinal fluid. In Vinken, P. J. and Bruyn, G. W. (eds.): Handbook of Clinical Neurology. Vol. 19. Amsterdam, North Holland, 1975, pp. 125–138.

Laterre, E. C., Callewaert, A., Heremans, J. F. et al.: Electrophoretic morphology of gamma globulins in cerebrospinal fluid of multiple sclerosis and other diseases of the nervous system. Neurology (Minneap.) 20:982–990, 1970.

Latovitzki, N., Abrams, G., Clark, C. et al.: Cerebral cysticercosis. Neurology 28:838–841, 1978.

Laurell, C. B.: Electroimmunoassay. Scand. J. Clin. Lab. Invest. 29 Suppl. 124:21–37, 1972.

Laursen, H. and Westergaard, E.: Enhanced permeability to horseradish peroxidase across cerebral vessels in the rat after portocaval anastomosis. Neuropath. Appl. Neurobiol. 3:29–43, 1977.

Lee, J. C.: Evolution in the concept of the blood-brain barrier phenomenon. In Zimmerman, H. W. (ed.): Progress in Neuropathology. New York, Grune and Stratton, 1971, pp. 84–145.

Lee, M. C., Heaney, L. M., Jacobson, R. L. et al.: Cerebrospinal fluid in cerebral hemorrhage and infarction. Stroke 6:638–641, 1975.

Leers, W. D.: North American blastomycosis. In Vinken, P. J. and Bruyn, G. W. (eds.): Handbook of Clinical Neurology. Vol. 35. Amsterdam, North Holland, 1978, pp. 401–411.

Lehrer, G. M.: Beta-glucuronidase in CSF of patients with diseases of the nervous system. Trans. Am. Neurol. Assoc. 88:56–68, 1963.

LeMay, M. and New, P. F., Jr.: Radiological diagnosis of occult normal-pressure hydrocephalus. Radiology 96:347–358, 1970.

Lempert, J., Meltzer, P. E., Wever, E. G. et al.: Structure and function of the cochlear aqueduct. Arch. Otolaryngol. 55:134–145, 1952.

Leusen, I.: The influence of calcium, potassium and magnesium ions in cerebrospinal fluid on vasomotor system. J. Physiol. (Lond.) 110:319–329, 1949.

Leusen, I.: Regulation of cerebrospinal fluid composition with reference to breathing. Physiol. Rev. 52:1–56, 1972.

Levin, A. S., Fredenberg, H. H., Petz, L. D. et al.: IgG levels in cerebrospinal fluid of patients with central nervous system manifestations of systemic lupus erythematosus. Clin. Immunol. Immunopathol. 1:1–5, 1972.

Levin, F.: Are the terms blood-brain barrier and brain capillary permeability synonymous? In Bito, L. Z., Davson, H. and Fenstermacher, J. (eds.): The Ocular and Cerebrospinal Fluids. New York, Academic Press, 1977, pp. 191–199.

Levin, S., Harris, A. A. and Sokalski, S. J.: Bacterial meningitis. In Vinken, P. J. and Bruyn, G. W. (eds.): Handbook of Clinical Neurology. Vol. 33. Amsterdam, Elsevier/North Holland Biomedical Press, 1978, pp. 1–20.

Levinson, A.: History of cerebrospinal fluid. Am. J. Syphilis 2:267–275, 1918.

Levinson, A.: Cerebrospinal Fluid in Health and Disease, 3rd Ed. St. Louis, C. V. Mosby, 1929.

Lewin, E.: Epileptogenic cortical foci induced with ouabain. Sodium, potassium, water content and sodium-potassium-activated ATPase activity. Exp. Neurol. 30:172–177, 1971.

Lindeman, J., Muller, W. K., Vesteeg, J. et al.: Rapid diagnosis of meningoencephalitis, encephalitis. Immunofluorescent examination of fresh and in vitro cultured cerebrospinal fluid cells. Neurology (Minneap.) 24:143–148, 1974.

Lindvall, M., Edvinsson, L. and Owman, C.: Sympathetic nervous control of cerebrospinal fluid production from the choroid plexus. Science 201:176–178, 1978.

Link, H.: Immunoglobulin G and low molecular weight proteins in human cerebrospinal fluid. Acta Neurol. Scand. 43 (Suppl. 28), 1967.

Link, H.: Comparison of electrophoresis on agar gel and agarose gel in the evaluation of gamma-globulin abnormalities in cerebrospinal fluid and serum in multiple sclerosis. Clin. Chim. Acta 46:383–389, 1973.

Link, H.: Immunoglobulin abnormalities in the Guillain-Barré syndrome. J. Neurol. Sci. 18:11–23, 1973.

Link, H.: Demonstration of oligoclonal immunoglobulin G in Guillain-Barré syndrome. Acta Neurol. Scand. 52:111–120, 1975.

Link, H. and Muller, R.: Immunoglobulins in multiple sclerosis and infections of the nervous system. Arch. Neurol. 25:326–344, 1971.

Link, H., Norrby, E. and Olsson, J. E.: Immunoglobulins and measles antibodies in optic neuritis. N. Engl. J. Med. 289:1103–1107, 1973.

Link, H., Norrby, E. and Olsson, J. E.: Immunoglobulin abnormalities and measles antibody response in chronic myelopathy. Arch. Neurol. 33:26–32, 1976.

Link, H. and Olsson, J. E.: Beta-trace protein concentration in CSF in neurological disorders. Acta Neurol. Scand. 48:57–68, 1972.

Link, H. and Tibbling, G.: Principles of albumin and IgG analysed in neurological disorders. III. Evaluation of IgG synthesis within the central nervous system in multiple sclerosis. Scand. J. Clin. Lab. Invest. 37:385–401, 1977.

Link, H. and Zettervall, O.: Multiple sclerosis. Disturbed kappa:lambda chain ratio of immunoglobulin G in cerebrospinal fluid. Clin. Exp. Immunol. 6:435–438, 1970.

Link, H., Zettervall, O. and Blemou, G.: Individual cerebrospinal fluid (CSF) proteins in the evaluation of increased CSF total protein. J. Neurol. 203:119–132, 1972.

Locke, S., Merrill, J. P. and Tyler, H. R.: Neurologic complications of uremia. Arch. Intern. Med. 108:519–530, 1961.

Lockwood, A. H.: Acute and chronic hyperosmolality. Arch. Neurol. 32:62–64, 1975.

Locoge, M. and Cumings, J. N.: Cerebrospinal fluid in various diseases. Br. Med. J. 1:618–620, 1958.

Loeb, J.: The hyperosmolar state. N. Engl. J. Med. 290:1184–1187, 1974.

Loeschke, H. H.: DC potentials between CSF and blood. In Siesjo, B. K. and Sorensen, S. C. (eds.): Ion Homeostasis of the Brain. Alfred Benzon Symposium III. New York, Academic Press, 1971, pp. 77–96.

Lofgren, J.: Effects of variations in arterial pressure and arterial carbon dioxide tension on the cerebrospinal fluid pressure volume relationships. Acta Neurol. Scand. 49:586–598, 1973.

Lofgren, J. and Zwetnow, N. W.: Cranial and spinal components of the cerebrospinal fluid pressure volume curve. Acta Neurol. Scand. 49:575–585, 1973.

Loman, J.: Components of cerebrospinal fluid pressure as affected by changes in posture. Acta Neurol. Psychiat. 31:679–681, 1934.

Loman, J. and Meyerson, A.: Studies in the dynamics of the human cranio-vertebral cavity. Am. J. Psychiat. 92:791–815, 1935.

Lombaert, A. and Carton, H.: Benign intracranial hypertension due to A-hypervitaminosis in adults and adolescents. Eur. Neurol. 14:340–350, 1976.

Long, D.: Capillary ultrastructure and the blood-brain barrier in human malignant brain tumours. J. Neurosurg. 32:127–144, 1970.

Long, D. M., Maxwell, R. and Choi, K. S.: A new therapy regimen for brain edema. In Pappius, H. M. and Feindel, W. (eds.): Dynamics of Brain Edema. New York, Springer-Verlag, 1976, pp. 293–300.

Lord, R. A., Dupree, E., Goldblum, R. M. et al.: Cerebrospinal fluid IgM in the absence of serum-IgM in combined immunodeficiency. Lancet 2:528–529, 1973.

Lorenzo, A. V.: Factors governing the composition of the cerebrospinal fluid. In Bito, L. Z., Davson, H. and Fenstermacher, J. D. (eds.): The Ocular and Cerebrospinal Fluids. (Fogarty International Center Symposium.) Exp. Eye Res. 25 (Suppl.) 205–228, 1977.

Lorenzo, A. V. and Bresnan, M. J.: Deficit in cerebrospinal fluid absorption in patients with symptoms of normal pressure hydrocephalus. Devel. Med. Child. Neurol. Suppl. 15. 29:35–41, 1973.

Lorenzo, A. V., Bresnan, M. J. and Barlow, C. F.: Cerebrospinal fluid absorption deficit in normal pressure hydrocephalus. Arch. Neurol. 30:387–393, 1974.

Lorenzo, A. V. and Cutler, R. W. P.: Amino acid transport by choroid plexus in vitro. J. Neurochem. 16:577–585, 1969.

Lorenzo, A. V., Hammerstad, J. P. and Cutler, R. W. P.: Cerebrospinal fluid formation and absorption and transport of iodide and sulfate from the spinal subarachnoid space. J. Neurol. Sci. 10:247–258, 1970.

Lorenzo, A. V., Hedley-Whyte, E. T., Eisenberg, H. M. and Hsu, D. W.: Increased penetration of horseradish peroxidase across the blood-brain barrier induced by Metrazol seizures. Brain Res. 88:136–140, 1975.

Lorenzo, A. V., Page, K. K. and Watters, G. V.: Relationship between cerebrospinal fluid formation, absorption and pressure in human hydrocephalus. Brain 93:679–692, 1970.

Low, N. L., Schneider, J. and Carter, S.: Polyneuritis in children. Pediatrics 22:972–990, 1958.

Lowenthal, A.: Agar Gel Electrophoresis in Neurology. Amsterdam, Elsevier, 1964.

Lowenthal, A.: Enzymes du liquide céphalo-rachidien. In Schmidt, R. M. (ed.): Der Liquor Cerebrospinalis. Berlin, VEB Verlag Volk und Gesundheit, 1968.

Lowenthal, A., Noppe, M., Gheuens, J. et al.: Alpha-albumin (glial fibrillary acidic protein) in normal and pathological human brain and cerebrospinal fluid. J. Neurol. 219:87–91, 1978.

Lucas, J. T., Ducker, T. B. and Perot, P. L.: Adverse reactions to intrathecal saline injection for control of pain. J. Neurosurg. 42:557–561, 1975.

Ludwig, A. O., Short, C. L. and Bauer, W.: Rheumatoid arthritis as a cause of increased cerebrospinal fluid protein. N. Engl. J. Med. 228:306–310, 1943.

Ludwig, G. D.: Lead posioning. In Goldensohn, E. S. and Appel, S. H. (eds.): Scientific Approaches to Clinical Neurology. Philadelphia, Lea and Febiger, 1977, pp. 1346–1373.

Lumsden, C.: The clinical pathology of multiple sclerosis. Part III. In McAlpine, D., Lumsden, C. and Acheson, E. D. (eds.): Multiple Sclerosis: A Reappraisal. 2nd Ed. London, Churchill Livingstone, 1972, pp. 311–621.

Lund-Andersen, H.: Transport of glucose from blood to brain. Physiol. Rev. 59:305–352, 1979.

Lundberg, N.: Continuous recording and control of ventricular fluid pressure in neurosurgical practice. Acta Psychiatr. Scand. Suppl. 149 Vol. 36, 1960.

Lundberg, N., Cronquist, S. and Kjallquist, A.: Clinical investigations on inter-relations between intracranial pressure and intracranial hemodynamics. Prog. Brain Res. 30:69–81, 1968.

Lundberg, N., Ponten, U. and Brock, M. (eds.): Intracranial Pressure II. New York, Springer-Verlag, 1975.

Lundberg, N. and West, K. A.: Leakage as a source of error in measurement of the cerebrospinal fluid pressure by lumbar puncture. Acta Neurol. Scand. Suppl. 3:115–120, 1965.

Lups, S. and Haan, A. M. F. H.: The Cerebrospinal Fluid. Amsterdam, Elsevier, 1954.

Lysak, W. R. and Svien, H. J.: Long term follow up on patients with diagnosis of pseudotumor cerebri. J. Neurosurg. 25:284–287, 1966.

MacGee, E. E.: Cerebrospinal fluid fistula. Chapter 9. In Vinken, P. J. and Bruyn, G. W. (eds.): Handbook of Clinical Neurology. Vol. 24. New York, American Elsevier, 1976. pp. 183–199.

MacKnight, A. D. C. and Leaf, A.: Regulation of cellular volume. Physiol. Rev. 57:510–573, 1977.

MacNab, B. H.: The development of the knowledge and treatment of hyrocephalus. In Hydrocephalus and Spina Bifida. London, National Spastics Society, 1966.

Madonick, M. J., Berke, K. and Schiffer, I.: Pleocytosis and meningeal signs in uremia: report on sixty-two cases. Arch. Neurol. Psychiat. 64:431–436, 1950.

Madonick, M. J. and Margolis, J.: Protein content of spinal fluid in diabetes mellitus. Report on 100 cases. Arch. Neurol. Psychiat. 68:641–644, 1952.

Magee, K. R. and DeJong, R. N.: Paralytic brachial neuritis: Discussion of clinical features with review of 23 cases. J.A.M.A. 174:1258–1262, 1960.

Malloy, J. J. and Low, F. N.: Scanning electron microscopy of the subarachnoid space in the dog. J. Comp. Neurol. 167:257–283, 1976.

Manfredi, F.: Acid-base relations between serum and cerebrospinal fluid in man under normal and abnormal conditions. J. Lab. Clin. Med. 59:128–136, 1962.

Mani, K. S. and Townsend, H. R.: The EEG in benign intracranial hypertension. Electroencephalogr. Clin. Neurophysiol. 16:604–610, 1964.

Mann, J. D., Butler, A. B., Rosenthal, J. E. et al.: Regulation of intracranial pressure in rat, dog, and man. Ann. Neurol. 3:156–165, 1978.

Mann, J. D., Johnson, R. N., Butler, A. B. et al.: Impairment of cerebrospinal fluid circulatory dynamics in pseudotumor cerebri and response to steroid treatment (abstract). Neurology 29:550, 1979.

Manno, N. J., Uhlein, A. and Kernohan, A.: Intraspinal epidermoids. J. Neurosurg. 10:754–765, 1962.

Manor, R. S.: Vogt-Koyanagi-Harada syndrome. In Vinken, P. J. and Bruyn, G. W. (eds.): Handbook of Clinical Neurology. Vol. 34. Amsterdam, Elsevier/North Holland, 1978, pp. 513–544.

Manyam, N. V. B., Hare, T. A., Katz, L. et al.: Huntington's disease. Cerebrospinal fluid GABA levels in at-risk individuals. Arch. Neurol. 35:728–730, 1978.

Manz, H. J.: The pathology of cerebral edema. Hum. Pathol. 5:291–313, 1974.

Marchesi, V. and Gowans, J. L.: The migration of lymphocytes through the endothelium of venules in lymph nodes: An electron microscopic study. Proc. Roy. Soc. (Biol.) 159:283–290, 1964.

Maren, T. H.: Carbonic anhydrase: Chemistry, physiology, and inhibition. Physiol. Rev. 47:595–781, 1967.

Maren, T. H.: The effect of acetazolamide on HCO_3 and Cl^- uptake into cerebrospinal fluid of cat and dogfish. In Siesjo, B. K. and Sorensen, S. C. (eds.): Ion Homeostasis of the Brain. Alfred Benzon Symposium III. New York, Academic Press, 1971, pp. 290–311.

Maren, T. H.: Bicarbonate formation in cerebrospinal fluid: Role in sodium transport and pH regulation. Am. J. Physiol. 222:885–899, 1972.

Maren, T. H. and Broder, L. S.: The role of carbonic anhydrase in anion secretion into cerebrospinal fluid. J. Pharmacol. Exper. Therap. 172:197–202, 1970.

Margolis, C. Z. and Cook, C. D.: The risk of lumbar puncture in pediatric patients with cardiac and/or pulmonary disease. Pediatrics 51:562–564, 1973.

Markenson, J. A., McDougal, J. S., Tsairis, P. et al.: Rheumatoid meningitis. Ann. Intern. Med. 90:786–789, 1979.

Marley, J. B. and Reynolds, E. H.: Papilledema and the Landry-Guillain-Barré syndrome. Brain 89:205–222, 1966.

Marmarou, A., Shulman, K. and Erlich, S.: An evaluation of static and dynamic properties of tissue pressure catheters. In Lundberg, N., Ponten, U. and Brock, M. (eds.): Intracranial Pressure. Berlin, Springer-Verlag, 1975, pp. 211–213.

Marmarou, A., Shulman, K. and Rosende, R. M.: A nonlinear analysis of the cerebrospinal fluid system and intracranial pressure dynamics. J. Neurosurg. 49:332–344, 1978.

Maroon, J. C. and Mealy, J., Jr.: Benign intracranial hypertension: Sequel to tetracycline therapy in a child. J.A.M.A. 216:1479–1480, 1971.

Marrack, D., Marks, V. and Couch, R. S.: Changes in the lumbar cerebro-spinal fluid during air encephalography. Br. J. Radiol. 34:635–639, 1961.

Marshall, J.: The Landry-Guillain-Barré syndrome. Brain 86:55–66, 1963.

Marshall, L. F., Shapiro, H. M., Rauscher, A. et al.: Pentobarbital therapy for intracranial hypertension in metabolic coma. Reyes Syndrome. Crit. Care Med. 6:1–5, 1978.

Marshall, L. F., Shapiro, H. M. and Smith, R. W.: Barbiturate treatment of intracranial hypertensive states. In Popp, A. J. et al.(eds.): Neural Trauma. New York, Raven Press, 1979, pp. 347–351.

Marshall, W. J., Jackson, J. L. F. and Langfitt, T. W.: Brain swelling caused by trauma and arterial hypertension: hemodynamic aspects. Arch. Neurol. 21:545–553, 1969.

Marton, L. J.: Polyamines and brain tumors. In Modern Concepts in Brain Tumor Therapy. Natl. Cancer Inst. Monogr. 46:127–131, 1976.

Marton, L. J., Edwards, E. S., Levin, V. A., et al.: Predictive value of cerebrospinal fluid polyamines in medulloblastoma. Cancer Res. 39:993–998, 1979.

Marton, L. J., Heby, O., Levin, V. A. et al.: The relationship of polyamines in cerebrospinal fluid to the presence of central nervous system tumors. Cancer Res. 36:973–977, 1976.

Marx, G. F., Zemaitis, M. T. and Orkin, L. R.: Cerebrospinal fluid pressure during labor and obstretical anesthesia. Anesthesiology 22:348–354, 1961.

Masdeu, J. C., Breuer, A. C. and Schoene, W. C.: Spinal subarachnoid hematomas: clue to a source of bleeding in traumatic lumbar puncture. Neurology 29:872–876, 1979.

Masserman, J. H.: Cerebrospinal hydrodynamics. IV. Clinical experimental studies. Arch. Neurol. Psychiat. 32:523–553, 1934.

Masserman, J. H.: Cerebrospinal hydrodynamics. Studies of the volume elasticity of the human ventriculo-subarachnoid system. J. Comp. Neurol. 61:543–552, 1935.

Mathew, N. T., Meyer, J. S. and Ott, E. O.: Increased cerebral blood volume in benign intracranial hypertension. Neurology (Minneap.) 25:646–649, 1975.

Mathew, N. T., Meyer, J. S., Rivera, V. M. et al.: Double-blind evaluation of glycerol therapy in acute cerebral infarction. Lancet 2:1327–1329, 1972.

Mathies, A. W. Jr.: Influenza meningitis (hemophilus influenzae). In Vinken, P. J. and Bruyn, G. W. (eds.): Handbook of Clinical Neurology, Vol. 33. Amsterdam, Elsevier/North Holland, 1978, pp. 53–59.

Matsuda, M., Yoneda, S., Handa, H. et al.: Cerebral hemodynamic changes during plateau waves in brain-tumor patients. J. Neurosurg. 50:483–488, 1979.

Matthews, W. F. and Frommeyer, W. B., Jr.: The *in vitro* behaviour of erythrocytes in human cerebrospinal fluid. J. Lab. Clin. Med. 45:508–515, 1955.

McArdle, B. and Zilkha, K. J.: The phospholipid composition of cerebrospinal fluid in neurological disorders. Brain 85:389–402, 1962.

McCance, R. A. and Watchorn, E.: Inorganic constituents of cerebrospinal fluid. I. Calcium and magnesium. Q. J. Med. 24:371–379, 1931.

McCarthy, K. D. and Reed, D. J.: The effect of acetazolamide and furosemide on cerebrospinal fluid production and choroid plexus carbonic anhydrase activity. J. Pharmacol. Exper. Therap. 189:194–201, 1974.

McCormick, W. F. and Danneel, C. M.: Central pontine myelinolysis. Arch. Intern. Med. 119:444–477, 1967.

McCracken, G. H. and Sarff, L. D.: Endotoxin in cerebrospinal fluid. J.A.M.A. 289:931–934, 1973.

McDowell, M. E., Wolf, A. V. and Steer, A.: Osmotic volumes of distribution. Idiogenic changes in osmotic pressure associated with administration of hypertonic solutions. Am. J. Physiol. 180:545–558, 1955.

McGale, E. H. F., Pye, I. F., Stonier, C. et al.: Studies of the inter-relationship between cerebrospinal fluid and plasma amino acid concentrations in normal individuals. J. Neurochem. 29:291–298, 1977.

McGillicuddy, J. E., Kindt, G. W., Raisis, J. E. and Miller, C. A.: The relation of cerebral ischemia, hypoxia and hypercarbia to the Cushing response. J. Neurosurg. 48:730–740, 1978.

McGraw, C. P., Alexander, E., Jr., and Howard, G.: Effect of dose and dose schedule on the response of intracranial pressure to mannitol. Surg. Neurol. 10:127–130, 1978.

McHenry, L. C., Jr.: Garrison's History of Neurology. Springfield, Illinois, Charles C Thomas, 1969.

McHenry, L. C., Jr., Goldberg, H. I., Jaffe, M. E. et al.: Regional cerebral blood flow response to carbon dioxide inhalation in cerebrovascular disease. Arch. Neurol. 27:403–412, 1972.

McKendall, R. R. and Klawans, H. L.: Nervous system complications of varicella-zoster virus. In Vinken, P. J. and Bruyn, G. W. (eds.): Handbook of Clinical Neurology. Vol. 34. Amsterdam, North Holland, 1978, pp. 161–183.

McKhann, G. M.: A cellular approach to neurological disease. Johns Hopkins Med. J. 143:48–57, 1978.

McLaurin, R. L. (ed.): Head Injuries: Second Chicago Symposium on Neural Trauma. New York, Grune and Stratton, 1976.

McLeod, J. G., Walsh, J. C., Prineas, J. W. et al.: Acute idiopathic polyneuritis. J. Neurol. Sci. 27:145–162, 1976.

McQuarrie, I., Hansen, A. E., and Ziegler, M. R.: Studies on the convulsive mechanism in idiopathic hypoparathyroidism. J. Clin. Endocrinol. 1:788–798, 1941.

McQueen, J. D. and Jeanes, L. D.: Dehydration and rehydration of the brain with hypertonic urea and mannitol. J. Neurosurg. 21:118–128, 1964.

Mealey, J.: Fat emulsion as a cause of cloudy cerebrospinal fluid. J.A.M.A. 180:246–248, 1962.

Meberg, A. and Sangstad, O. D.: Hypoxanthine in cerebrospinal fluid in children. Scand. J. Clin. Lab. Invest. 38:437–440, 1978.

Meinig, G., Aulich, A., Wende, S. et al.: The effect of dexamethasone and diuretics on peritumor brain edema: Comparative study of tissue water content and CT. In Pappius, H. M. and Feindel, W. (eds.): Dynamics of Brain Edema. New York, Springer-Verlag, 1976, pp. 301–305.

Meltzer, H. Y. and Stahl, S. M.: The dopamine hypothesis of schizophrenia: A review. Schizophrenia Bull. 2:19–76, 1976.

Mendell, J. R., Chase, T. N. and Engel, W. K.: Amyotropic lateral sclerosis: A study of central monamine metabolism and therapeutic trial of levodopa. Arch. Neurol. 25:320–325, 1971.

Menkes, J. H.: To tap or not to tap. Pediatrics 51:560–561, 1973.

Menkin, V.: Effect of adrenal cortical extract on capillary permeability. Am. J. Physiol. 129:691–697, 1940.

Merritt, H. H., Adams, R. D. and Solomon, H. C.: Neurosyphilis. New York, Oxford University Press, 1946.

Merritt, H. H. and Bauer, W.: The equilibrium between cerebrospinal fluid and blood plasma. III The distribution of calcium and phosphorus between cerebrospinal fluid and blood serum. IV. The calcium content of serum, cerebrospinal fluid, and aqueous humor at different levels of parathyroid activity. J. Biol. Chem. 90:215–246, 1931.

Merritt, H. H. and Fremont-Smith, F.: The Cerebrospinal Fluid. Philadelphia, W. B. Saunders, 1938.

Messert, B. and Wannamaker, B. B.: Reappraisal of the occult hydrocephalus syndrome. Neurology 24:224–231, 1974.

Mestrezat, W.: Le Liquide Céphalo-rachidien Normal et Pathologique. Paris, A. Maloine, 1912.

Metzger, A. L. and Rubenstein, A. H.: Reversible cerebral edema complicating diabetic ketoacidosis. Br. Med. J. 3:746–747, 1970.

Meyer, J. S., Itoh, Y., Okamoto, S. et al.: Circulatory and metabolic effects of glycerol infusion in patients with recent cerebral infarction. Circulation 51:701–712, 1975.

Meyer, J. S., Stoica, E., Pascu, I. et al.: Catecholamine concentrations in CSF and plasma of patients with cerebral infarction and haemorrhage. Brain 96:277–288, 1973.

Meyer, J. S., Welch, K. M. A., Okamoto, S. et al.: Disordered neurotransmitter function. Demonstrator by measurement of nor-epinephrine and 5-hydroxy-triphetamine in CSF of patients with recent cerebral infarction. Brain 97:655–664, 1974.

Michelson, A. M., McCord, J. M. and Fridovich, I. (eds.): Superoxide and Superoxide Dismutases. New York, Academic Press, 1977.

Milhorat, T. H.: Hydrocephalus and the Cerebrospinal Fluid. Baltimore, Williams and Wilkins, 1972.

Milhorat, T. H.: The third circulation revisited. J. Neurosurg. 42:628–645, 1975.

Milhorat, T. H., Clark, R. G., Hammock, M. K. et al.: Structural, ultrastructural and permeability changes in the ependyma and surrounding brain following equilibration in progressive hydrocephalus. Arch. Neurol. 22:397–407, 1970.

Millen, J. W. and Woollam, D. H. M.: The Anatomy of the Cerebrospinal Fluid. London, Oxford University Press, 1962.

Miller, A., Bader, R. A. and Bader, M. E.: The neurologic syndrome due to marked hypercapnia, with papilledema. Am. J. Med. 33:309–318, 1962.

Miller, H. G., Stanton, J. B. and Gibbons, J. L.: Parainfectious encephalomyelitis and related syndromes, a critical review of the neurological complications of certain specific fevers. Q. J. Med. 25:427–505, 1956.

Miller, J. D.: Volume and pressure in the cerebrospinal axis. Clin. Neurosurg. 22:76–105, 1975.

Miller, J. D., Becker, D. P., Ward, J. D. et al.: Significance of intracranial hypertension in severe head injury. J. Neurosurg. 47:503–516, 1977.

Miller, J. D., Garibi, J. and Pickard, J. D.: Induced changes of cerebrospinal fluid volume. Effects during continuous monitoring of ventricular fluid pressure. Arch. Neurol. 28:265–269, 1973.

Miller, J. D. and Leech, P.: Effects of mannitol and steroid therapy on intracranial volume-pressure relationships in patients. J. Neurosurg. 42:274–281, 1975.

Miller, J. K., Hesser, F. and Tompkins, V. N.: Herpes simplex encephalitis: Report of 20 cases. Ann. Intern. Med. 64:92–103, 1966.

Millhouse, O. E.: Lining of the third ventricle in the rat. In Knigge, K. M. et al. (eds.): Brain-Endocrine Interaction. II. The Ventricular System in Neuro-endocrine Mechanisms. Basel, S. Karger, 1975, pp. 9–18.

Miner, L. C. and Reed, D. J.: Composition of fluid obtained from choroid plexus tissue isolated in a chamber *in situ*. J. Physiol. (Lond.) 227:127–139, 1972.

Mingioli, E. S., Strober, W., Tourtellotte, W. W. et al.: Quantitation of IgG, IgA and IgM in the CSF by radioimmunoassay. Neurology (Minneap.) 28:991–995, 1978.

Mitchell, R. A., Carman, C. T., Severinghaus, J. W. et al.: Stability of cerebrospinal fluid pH in chronic acid-base disturbances in blood. J. Appl. Physiol. 20:443–452, 1965a.

Mitchell, R. A., Herbert, D. A. and Carman, C. T.: Acid-base constants and temperature coefficients for cerebrospinal fluid. J. Appl. Physiol. 20:27–30, 1965b.

Mitchell, R. A. and Singer, M. M.: Respiration and cerebrospinal fluid pH in metabolic acidosis and alkalosis. J. Appl. Physiol. 20:905–911, 1965.

Mittal, M. M., Gupta, N. C. and Sharma, M. L.: Spinal epidural meningioma associated with increased intracranial pressure. Neurology 20:818–820, 1970.

Moir, A. T. B., Ashcroft, G. W., Crawford, T. B. B. et al.: Cerebral metabolites in cerebrospinal fluid as a biochemical approach to the brain. Brain 93:357–368, 1970.

Molinari, G. F., Pircher, F., Heyman, A.: Serial brain scanning using Technetium-99 in patients with cerebral infarction. Neurology 17:627–636, 1967.

Mollaret, P.: La meningite endothelio-leucocytaire multi-recurrente benign. Rev. Neurol. 133:225–244, 1977.

Mollgard, K. and Saunders, N. R.: Complex tight junctions of epithelial and of endothelial cells in early foetal brain. J. Neurocytol. 4:453–468, 1975.

Moore, E. W., Strohmeyer, G. W. and Chalmer, T. C.: Distribution of ammonia across the blood-cerebrospinal fluid barrier in patients with hepatic failure. Am. J. Med. 35:350–362, 1963.

Morantz, R. A., Wood, G. W., Foster, M. et al.: Macrophages in experimental and human brain tumors. J. Neurosurg. 50:305–311, 1979.

Morariu, M. A.: Transient spastic paraparesis following abdominal aortography: Management with cerebrospinal fluid lavage. Ann. Neurol. 3:185, 1978 (Letter)

Morley, J. B. and Reynolds, E. H.: Papillaedema and the Landry-Guillain-Barré syndrome. Case reports and a review. Brain 89:205–222, 1966.

Morrison, J. C., Whybrew, D. W., Wiser, W. L. et al.: Laboratory characteristics in toxemia. Obstet. Gynecol. 39:866–872, 1972.

Moseley, J. I., Carton, C. A. and Stern, W. E.: Spectrum of complications in the use of intrathecal fluorescein. J. Neurosurg. 48:765–767, 1978.

Mulley, G., Wilcox, R. G. and Mitchell, J. R. A.: Dexamethasone in acute stroke. Br. Med. J. 2:994–996, 1978.

Munch-Petersen, S.: The copper content in cerebrospinal fluid in adults (and children) with and without sufferings in the central nervous system. Acta Psychiat. Neurol. Scand. 25:251–274, 1950.

Musher, D. M. and Schell, R. F.: False positive gram stains of cerebrospinal fluid. Ann. Intern. Med. 79:603–604, 1973. (Letter)

Muting, D., Heinze, J., Reikowski, J. et al.: Enzymatic ammonia determinations in the blood and cerebrospinal fluid of healthy persons. Clin. Chim. Acta 19:391–395, 1968.

Nabeshima, S., Reese, T. S., Landis, D. M. et al.: Junctions in the meninges and marginal glia. J. Comp. Neurol. 164:127–169, 1975.

Nachum, R., Lipsey, A. and Siegel, S. F.: Rapid detection of gram-negative bacterial meningitis by the limulus lysate test. N. Engl. J. Med. 289:931–934, 1973.

Naidoo, B. T.: The cerebrospinal fluid in the healthy newborn infant. S. Afr. Med. J. 42:933–935, 1968.

Nasralla, M., Gawronska, E. and Hsia, D.: Studies on the relation between serum and spinal fluid bilirubin during early infancy. J. Clin. Invest. 37:1403–1412, 1958.

Naumann, H. N.: Cerebrospinal fluid electrolytes after death. Proc. Soc. Exp. Biol. Med. 98:16–18, 1958.

Navab, M., Mallia, A. K., Kanda, Y. et al.: Rat plasma prealbumin. Isolation and partial characterization. J. Biol. Chem. 252:5100–5106, 1977.

Neblett, C. R., McNeel, D. P., Waltz, T. A. et al.: Effect of cardiac glycosides on human cerebrospinal fluid production. Lancet 2:1008–1009, 1972.

Neches, W. and Platt, M.: Cerebrospinal fluid LDH in 287 children including 53 cases of meningitis of bacterial and non-bacterial etiology. Pediatrics 41:1097–1103, 1968.

Nelson, J. R. and Goodman, S. J.: An evaluation of the cerebrospinal fluid infusion test for hydrocephalus. Neurology (Minneap.) 21:1037–1053, 1971.

Nerenberg, S. T., Prasad, R. and Rothman, M. E.: Cerebrospinal fluid IgG, IgA, IgM, IgD and IgE levels in central nervous system disorders. Neurology 28:988–990, 1978.

Netsky, M. G. and Shuangshoti, S. (eds.): The Choroid Plexus in Health and Disease. Charlottesville, University of Virginia Press, 1975, p. 351.

Neville, B. G. R. and Wilson, J.: Benign intracranial hypertension following corticosteroid withdrawal in childhood. Br. Med. J. 3:554–556, 1970.

Newman, J., Josephson, A. S., Cacatian, A. et al.: Spinal fluid lysozyme in the diagnosis of central nervous system tumors. Lancet Sept. 28:756–757, 1974.

Nickel, S. N. and Frame, B.: Neurological manifestations of myxedema. Neurology 8:511–517, 1958.

Nilsson, K. and Olsson, J.-E.: Analysis for cerebrospinal fluid proteins by isoelectric focusing on polyacrylamide gel: Methodological aspects and normal values, with special reference to the alkaline region. Clin. Chem. 24:1134–1139, 1978.

Nonne, M.: Der pseudotumor cerebri. Neue Deutsche Chir. 10:107, 1914.

Nornes, H., Rootwelt, K. and Sjaastad, O.: Normal pressure hydrocephalus. Eur. Neurol. 9:261–274, 1973.

Norrby, E.: Viral antibodies in multiple sclerosis. Prog. Med. Virol. 24:1–39, 1978.

Norrby, E., Link, H. and Olsson, J. E.: Measles virus antibodies in multiple sclerosis comparison of antibody titers in cerebrospinal fluid and serum. Arch. Neurol. 30:285–292, 1974.

Norrby, E. and Vandvik, B.: Relationship between measles virus-specific antibody activities and oligoclonal IgG in the central nervous system of patients with subacute sclerosing panencephalitis and multiple sclerosis. Med. Microbiol. Immunol. (Berl.) 162:63–72, 1975.

Nosanchuk, J. S. and Kim, C. W.: Lupus erythematosus cells in CSF. J.A.M.A. 263:2883–2884, 1976.

Nye, S. W., Tangchai, P., Sundarakiti, S. et al.: Lesions of the brain in eosinophilic meningitis. Arch. Pathol. 89:9–19, 1970.

Nyland, H. and Waess, A.: Lymphocyte subpopulations in blood and cerebrospinal fluid from patients with acute Guillain-Barré syndrome. Eur. Neurol. 17:247–252, 1978.

Oberchain, T. G. and Stern, W. E.: Continuous pressure monitoring in experimental obstructive hydrocephalus. I. The dynamics of acute ventricular obstruction. Arch. Neurol. 29:287–294, 1973.

Obrador, S.: Cysticercosis cerebri. Acta Neurochir. (Wien) 10:320–364, 1962.

O'Brien, M. D. and Waltz, A. G.: Intracranial pressure gradients caused by experimental cerebral ischemia and edema. Stroke 4:694–698, 1973.

Obrist, W. D., Thompson, H. K., King, C. H. et al.: Determination of regional cerebral blood flow by inhalation of 133 Xenon. Circ. Res. 20:124–135, 1967.

O'Connell, J. E. A.: The vascular factor in intracranial pressure and the maintenance of the CSF circulation. Brain 66:204–228, 1943.

Oehmichen, M.: Cerebrospinal Fluid Cytology: An Introduction and Atlas. Philadelphia, W. B. Saunders, 1976.

Oehmichen, M.: Characterization of mononuclear phagocytes of the human CSF using membrane markers. Acta Cytol. 20:548–552, 1976.

Oehmichen, M. and Gruninger, H.: Cytokinetic studies on the origin of cells of the cerebrospinal fluid. J. Neurol. Sci. 22:165–176, 1974.

Offerhaus, L. and Van Gool, J.: Electrocardiographic changes and tissue catecholamines in experimental subarachnoid hemorrhage. Cardiovasc. Res. 3:433–440, 1969.

Oh, S. J.: *Paragonimus* in the central nervous system. In Vinken, P. J. and Bruyn, G. W. (eds.): Handbook of Clinical Neurology. Vol. 35. Amsterdam, North Holland, 1978.

Ohman, J. L., Jr., Marliss, E. B., Aoki, T. T., et al.: The cerebrospinal fluid in diabetic ketoacidosis. N. Engl. J. Med. 284:283–290, 1971.

Oldendorf, W. H.: Stereospecificity of blood-brain barrier. Permeability to amino acids. Am. J. Physiol. 224:967–969, 1973.

Oldendorf, W. H.: The blood brain barrier. In Bito, L. Z., Davson, H. and Fenstermacher, J. D. (eds.): The Ocular and Cerebrospinal Fluids. New York, Academic Press, 1977, pp. 177–190.

Oldendorf, W. H., Cornford, M. E. and Brown, W. J.: The large apparent work capability of the blood-brain barrier: a study of the mitochondrial content of capillary endothelial cells in brain and other tissues of the rat. Ann. Neurol. 1:409–417, 1977.

Olsen, S.: The brain in uremia. Acta Psychiat. Neurol. Scand. Suppl. 156 36:1–128, 1961.

Olson, M. E., Chernik, N. L. and Posner, J. B.: Infiltration of the leptomeninges by systemic cancer. A clinical and pathological study. Arch. Neurol. 30:122–137, 1974.

Olson, Y., Klatzo, I., Sourander, P. et al.: Blood-brain barrier to albumin in embryonic new born and adult rats. Acta Neuropathol. (Berl.) 10:117–122, 1968.

Olsson, J. E. and Link, H.: Immunoglobulin abnormalities in multiple sclerosis. Arch. Neurol. 28:392–399, 1973.

Olsson, J. E., Link, H. and Muller, R.: Immunoglobulin abnormalities in multiple sclerosis: relation to clinical parameters: disability, duration and age of onset. J. Neurol. Sci. 27:233–245, 1976.

Olsson, J. E. and Pettersson, B.: A comparison between agar gel electrophoresis and CSF serum quotients of IgG and albumin in neurological diseases. Acta Neurol. Scand. 53:308–322, 1976.

Olsson, Y., Crowell, R. M. and Klatzo, I.: The blood-brain barrier to protein tracers in focal cerebral ischemia and infarction caused by occlusion of the middle cerebral artery. Acta Neuropathol. 18:89–102, 1971.

Oppelt, W. W., MacIntyre, I. and Rall, D. P.: Magnesium exchange between blood and cerebrospinal fluid. Am. J. Physiol. 205:959–962, 1963.

Oppelt, W. W., Owens, E. S. and Rall, D. P.: Calcium exchange between blood and cerebrospinal fluid. Life Sci. 2:599–605, 1963.

Oppelt, W. W., Patlak, C. S. and Rall, D. P.: Effect of certain drugs on cerebrospinal fluid production in the dog. Am. J. Physiol. 206:247–250, 1964.

Orlowski, M., Sessa, G. and Green, J. P.: Gamma-glutamyl transpeptidase in brain capillaries: Possible site of a blood-brain barrier for amino acids. Science 184:66–69, 1974.

Ostheimer, G. W., Palahniuk, R. J. and Shnider, S. M.: Epidural blood patch for post-lumbar-puncture headache. Anesthesiology 41:307–308, 1974.

Otila, E.: Studies on the cerebrospinal fluid in premature infants. Acta Paediatr. (Suppl. 8) 35:3–100, 1948.

O'Toole, R. D., Thornton, G. E., Mukherjee, M. K. et al.: Dexamethasone in tuberculous meningitis. Relationship of cerebrospinal fluid effects to therapeutic efficiency. Ann. Intern. Med. 70:39–48, 1969.

Oxelius, V. A., Rorsman, H. and Laurell, A. B.: Immunoglobulins of cerebrospinal fluid in syphilis. Br. J. Vener. Dis. 45:121–125, 1969.

Pallis, C., MacIntyre, I. and Anstall, H.: Some observations on magnesium in cerebrospinal fluid. J. Clin. Pathol. 18:762–764, 1965.

Panitch, A. H., Hooper, C. and Johnson, K. P.: CSF antibody to myelin basic protein in multiple sclerosis and subacute sclerosing panencephalitis. Arch. Neurol. 1980 (in press).

Pape, L. and Katzman, R.: Effects of hydration on blood and cerebrospinal fluid modalities. Proc. Soc. Exp. Biol. Med. 134:430–433, 1970.

Papeschi, R. et al.: The concentration of homovanillic and 5-hydroxyindoleacetic acids in ventricular and lumbar CSF. Studies in patients with extrapyramidal disorders, epilepsy, and other diseases. Neurology 22:1151–1159, 1972.

Pappagianis, D. and Crane, R.: Survival in coccidiodal meningitis since introduction of amphotericin B. In Ajello, L. (ed.): Coccidiodomycosis: Current Clinical and Diagnostic Status. Miami, Symposia Specialists Medical Books, 1977, pp. 222–236.

Pappenheimer, J. R., Fencl, V., Karnovsky, M. et al.: Peptides in cerebrospinal fluid and their relation to sleep and activity. Res. Publ. Assoc. Res. Nerv. Ment. Dis. 53:201–210, 1974.

Pappenheimer, J. R., Heisey, S. R. and Jordan, E. F.: Active transport of diodrast and phenolsulfonphthalein from cerebrospinal fluid to blood. Am. J. Physiol. 200:1–10, 1961.

Pappenheimer, J. R., Heisey, S. R., Jordon, E. F. et al.: Perfusion of the cerebral ventricular system in unanesthetized goats. Am. J. Physiol. 203:763–774, 1962.

Pappius, H. M. and Dayes, L. A.: Hypertonic urea: Its effects on the distribution of water and electrolytes in normal and edematous brain tissue. Arch. Neurol. 13:395–402, 1965.

Pappius, H. M. and Feindel, W. (eds.): Dynamics of Brain Edema. New York, Springer-Verlag, 1976.

Pardridge, W. M. and Oldendorf, W. H.: Transport of metabolic substrates through the blood-brain barrier. J. Neurochem. 28:5–12, 1977.

Parkes, J. D., Fenton, G., Struthers, G. et al.: Narcolepsy and cataplexy. Clinical features, treatment and cerebrospinal fluid findings. Q. J. Med. 43:525–536, 1974.

Parsons, M.: The spinal form of carcinomatous meningitis. Q. J. Med. 41:509–518, 1972.

Partin, J. C., Partin, J. S., Schubert, W. et al.: Brain ultrastructure in Reye's syndrome. J. Neuropathol. Exp. Neurol. 34:425–444, 1975.

Patel, Y. C., Rao, K. and Reichlin, S.: Somatostatin in human cerebrospinal fluid. N. Engl. J. Med. 296:529–533, 1977.

Patrick, B. S., Smith, R. R. and Bailey, T. O.: Aseptic meningitis due to spontaneous rupture of craniopharyngioma cyst. Case Report. J. Neurosurg. 41:387–390, 1974.

Patten, B. M.: How much blood makes the cerebrospinal fluid bloody? J.A.M.A. 206:378, 1968. (Letter)

Patten, B. M., Harati, Y., Acosta, L. et al.: Free amino acid levels in amyotrophic lateral sclerosis. Ann. Neurol 4:305–309, 1978.

Pauli, H. G., Vorburger, C. and Reubi, F.: Chronic derangements of cerebrospinal fluid acid-base components in man. J. Appl. Physiol. 17:993–998, 1962.

Paulson, G. W.: Low value for protein in the spinal fluid of leukemic patients. Confin. Neurol. 30:337–340, 1968.

Paulson, G. W. and Stickney, D.: Cerebrospinal fluid after death. Confin. Neurol. 33:149–162, 1971.

Pedersen, H. F.: Cerebrospinal fluid cholesterol and phospholipids in multiple sclerosis. Acta Neurol. Scand. 50:171–182, 1974.

Perel, J. M., Levitt, M. and Dunner, D. L.: Plasma and cerebrospinal fluid probenecid concentrations as related to accumulation of acidic biogenic amines metabolites in man. Psychopharmacologia 35:83–90, 1974.

Perkin, G. D. and Rose, F. C.: Optic Neuritis and Its Differential Diagnosis. New York, Oxford University Press, 1979.

Perkins, H. A.: Bromide intoxication. Arch. Intern. Med. 85:783–794, 1950.

Perry, T. L. and Hansen, S.: Is GABA detectable in human CSF? J. Neurochem. 27:1537–1538, 1976.

Perry, T. L., Hansen, S. and Kennedy, J.: CSF amino acids and plasma-CSF amino acid ratios in adults. J. Neurochem. 24:587–589, 1975.

Perry, T. L., Hansen, S., Stedman, D. and Love, D.: Homocarnosine in human cerebrospinal fluid: an age-dependent phenomenon. J. Neurochem. 15:1203–1206, 1968.

Perry, T. L. and Jones, R. T.: The amino acid content of human cerebrospinal fluid in normal individuals and in mental defectives. J. Clin. Invest. 40:1363–1372, 1961.

Peters, A. C. B., Versteeg, J., Bots, G. et al.: Nervous system complications of herpes zoster: immunofluorescent demonstration of varicella-zoster antigen in CSF cells. J. Neurol. Neurosurg. Psychiatry. 42:452–457, 1979.

Petersdorf, R. G. and Harter, D.: The fall in cerebrospinal fluid sugar in meningitis. Arch. Neurol 4:21–30, 1961.

Petersdorf, R. G., Swarner, D. R. and Garcia, H.: Studies on the pathogenesis of meningitis during pneumococcal bacteremia. J. Clin. Invest. 41:320–327, 1962.

Petito, C. K.: Early and late mechanism of increased vascular permeability following experimental cerebral infarction. J. Neuropathol. Exp. Neurol. 38:222–234, 1979.

Petito, C. K., Schaefer, J. A. and Plum, F.: Ultrastructural characteristics of the brain and blood-brain barrier in experimental seizures. Brain Res. 127:251–267, 1977.

Petz, L. D., Sharp, G. C. and Cooper, N. R.: Serum and cerebral spinal fluid complement and serum antibodies in systemic lupus erythematosus. Medicine 50:259–275, 1971.

Pickering, G. W.: Lumbar puncture headaches. Brain 71:274–280, 1948.

Pilz, H.: Die Lipide des Normallen und Pathologischen Liquor Cerebrospinalis. New York, Springer-Verlag, 1970.

Plotz, C. M., Knowleton, A. I. and Ragan, C.: The natural history of Cushing's syndrome. Am. J. Med. 13:597–614, 1952.

Plum, C. M.: The cholesterol content of cerebrospinal fluid with special regard to the occurrence in cases with multiple sclerosis. Acta Psychiat. Neurol. Scand. 35 (Suppl. 148):79–100, 1960.

Plum, C. M.: Free amino acid levels in the cerebrospinal fluid of normal humans and their variations in cases of epilepsy and Spielmayer-Vogt-Batten disease. J. Neurochem. 23:595–600, 1974.

Plum, C. M. and Fog, T.: Studies in multiple sclerosis. IV. The cholinesterase activity of cerebrospinal fluid. Acta Psychiat. Neurol. Scand. 35 (Suppl. 148):28–40, 1960.

Plum, F.: The CSF in hepatic encephalopathy. Exp. Biol. Med. 4:34–41, 1971.

Plum, F. and Posner, J. B.: Diagnosis of Stupor and Coma. 2nd Ed. Philadelphia, F. A. Davis, 1972, p. 286.

Plum, F. and Price, R. W.: Acid-base balance of cisternal and lumbar cerebrospinal fluid. N. Engl. J. Med. 289–1346–1350, 1973.

Plum, F. and Siesjo, B. K.: Review Article: Recent advances in CSF physiology. Anesthesiology, 42:708–730, 1975.

Pollack, L. J. and Boshes, B.: Cerebrospinal fluid pressure. Arch. Neurol. Psychiat. 36:931–974, 1936.

Pollay, M.: Formation of cerebrospinal fluid. Relation of studies of isolated choroid plexus to the standing gradient hypothesis. J. Neurosurg. 42:665–673, 1978.

Pollay, M. and Curl, F.: Secretion of CSF by the ventricular ependyma of the rabbit. Am. J. Physiol. 213:1031–1038, 1967.

Pollay, M., Stevens, A., Estrada, E. et al.: Extracorporeal perfusion of choroid plexus. J. Appl. Physiol. 32:612–617, 1972.

Porter, J. C., Ben-Jonathon, N., Oliver, C. et al.: Secretion of releasing hormones and their transport from CSF to hypophyseal portal blood. In Knigge, K. M. et al. (eds.): Brain-Endocrine Interaction II. The Ventricular System in Neuroendocrine Mechanisms. Basel, S. Karger, 1975, pp. 295–305.

Posner, J. B. and Plum, F.: Independence of blood and cerebrospinal fluid lactate. Arch. Neurol. 16:492–496, 1967.

Posner, J. B. and Plum, F.: Spinal fluid pH and neurologic symptoms in systemic acidosis. N. Engl. J. Med. 277:605–613, 1967.

Posner, J. B., Swanson, A. G. and Plum, F.: Acid-base balance and cerebrospinal fluid. Arch. Neurol. 12:479–496, 1965.

Post, R. M., Fink, E., Carpenter, W. T. and Goodwin, F. K.: Cerebrospinal fluid amine metabolites in acute schizophrenia. Arch. Gen. Psychiatry 32:1063–1069, 1975.

Post, R. M., Lake, C. R., Jimerson, D. C. et al.: Cerebrospinal fluid norepinephrine in affective illness. Am. J. Psychiat. 135:907–912, 1978.

Potts, D. G. and Gomez, D. C.: Radiological studies of cerebrospinal fluid and hydrocephalus. In Bito, L. Z., Davson, H. and Fenstermacher, J. D. (eds.): The Ocular and Cerebrospinal Fluids. New York, Academic Press, 1977, pp. 377–385.

Potts, D. G., Reilly, K. F. and Deonarine, V.: Morphology of the arachnoid villi and granulations. Radiology 105:333–341, 1972.

Prados, M., Strowger, B. and Feindel, W.: Studies on cerebral edema II: Reaction of the brain to the exposure of air; physiologic changes. Arch. Neurol. Psychiat. 54:290–300, 1945.

Press, E. M.: A comparative study of cerebrospinal fluid and serum proteins in multiple sclerosis with special reference to the Lange colloidal gold reaction. Biochem. J. 63:367–373, 1956.

Prockop, L. D.: Hyperglycemia, polyol accumulation, and increased intracranial pressure. Arch. Neurol. 25:126–140, 1971.

Prockop, L. D. and Fishman, R. A.: Experimental pneumococcal meninges: Permeability changes influencing the concentration of sugars and micromolecules in cerebrospinal fluid. Arch. Neurol. 19:449–463, 1968.

Prockop, L. D., Schanker, L. S. and Brodie, B. B.: Passage of lipid-insoluble substances from cerebrospinal fluid to blood. J. Pharmacol. Exper. Therap. 135:266–270, 1962.

Pruitt, A. A., Rubin, R. H., Karchmer, A. W. et al.: Neurologic complications of bacterial endocarditis. Medicine 57:329–345, 1978.

Punyagupta, S., Juttijudata, P. and Bunnag, T.: Eosinophilic meningitis in Thailand. Clinical studies of 484 typical cases probably caused by *Angiostrongylus cantonensis*. Am. J. Trop. Med. Hyg. 24:921–931, 1975.

Purves, M. J.: The Physiology of the Cerebral Circulation. London, Cambridge University Press, 1972.

Queckenstedt, H.: Zur Diagnose der Rückenmarkskopression. Deutsch Z. Nervenheilk. 15:325, 1916.

Quincke, H.: Die Lumbarpunktion des Hydrocephalus. Klin. Wochenschr. 28:929–933, 965–968, 1891.

Rabin, E. Z., Weinberger, V. and Tattrie, B.: Ribonuclease activity of human cerebrospinal fluid. Can. J. Neurol. Sci. 4:125–130, 1977.

Rafaelsen, O. J., Lyngsoe, J. and Deckert, T.: Insulin activity of spinal fluid. Diabetologia 2:216, 1966. (Abstract)

Raichle, M. E., Eichling, J. O., Straatmann, M. D. et al.: Blood-brain barrier permeability of ^{11}C-labeled alcohols and ^{15}O-labeled water. Am. J. Physiol. 230:543–552, 1976.

Raichle, M. E., Grubb, R. L., Jr., Phelps, M. E. et al.: Cerebral hemodynamics and metabolism in pseudotumor cerebri. Ann. Neurol. 4:104–111, 1978.

Raichle, M. E., Hartman, B. K., Eichling, J. O. et al.: Central noradrenergic regulation of cerebral blood flow and vascular permeability. Proc. Natl. Acad. Sci. U.S.A. 72:3726–3730, 1975.

Raisis, J. E., Kindt, G. W., Miller, C. A. et al.: Correlation of ICP with CSF lactate and lactate/pyruvate ratios in hydrocephalus. In Lundberg, N., Ponten, U. and Brock, M. (eds.): Intracranial Pressure II. New York, Springer-Verlag, 1975.

Rall, D. P., Stabenau, J. R. and Zubrod, C. G.: Distribution of drugs between blood and cerebrospinal fluid: General methodology and effect of pH gradients. J. Pharmacol. Exper Therap. 125:185–193, 1959.

Rall, D. P. and Zubrod, C. G.: Mechanisms of drug absorption and excretion— passage of drugs in and out of CSF. Ann. Rev. Pharmacol. 2:109–128, 1962.

Rangan, G. and Virmani, V.: The bromide partition test in tuberculous meningitis: A re-evaluation. Indian J. Med. Res. 64:131–137, 1976.

Rangell, L. and Glassman, F.: Acute spinal epidural abscess as a complication of lumbar puncture. J. Nerv. Ment. Dis. 102:8–18, 1945.

Ransohoff, J., Shulman, K. and Fishman, R. A.: Hydrocephalus — a review of the etiology and treatment. J. Pediatr. 56:399–411, 1960.

Rapoport, S. I.: Blood-Brain Barrier in Physiology and Medicine. New York, Raven Press, 1976.

Raskin, N. H. and Fishman, R. A.: Effects of thyroid on permeability, composition, and electrolyte metabolism of brain and other tissues. Arch. Neurol. 14:21–30, 1966.

Raskin, N. H. and Fishman, R. A.: Neurologic disorders in renal failure. N. Engl. J. Med. 294:143–148, 204–210, 1976.

Rasmussen, T. and Gulati, D. R.: Cortisone in the treatment of post-operative cerebral edema. J. Neurosurg. 19:535–544, 1962.

Ratcheson, R. A. and Ommaya, A. K.: Experience with the subcutaneous cerebrospinal fluid reservoir. N. Engl. J. Med. 279:1025–1031, 1968.

Rawlinson, D. G., Billingham, M. E., Berry, P. F. and Kempson, R. L.: Cytology of the cerebrospinal fluid patients with Hodgkin's disease of malignant lymphoma. Acta Neuropathol. (Berlin) Suppl. VI:187–191, 1975.

Reed, D. J.: The effects of furosemide on cerebrospinal fluid flow. Arch. Int. Pharmacodyn. 178:324–330, 1969.

Reed, D. J. and Woodbury, D. M.: Effect of urea and acetazolamide on brain volume and cerebrospinal fluid pressure. J. Physiol. (Lond.) 164:265–273, 1962.

Reed, D. J. and Woodbury, D. M.: Effect of hypertonic urea on cerebrospinal fluid pressure and brain volume. J. Physiol. (Lond.) 164:252–264, 1964.

Reese, T. S. and Karnovsky, M. J.: Fine structural localization of a blood-brain barrier to exogenous peroxidase. J. Cell Biol. 34:207–217, 1967.

Refsum, S.: Heredopathia atactica polyneuritiformis (Refsum's disease). In Dyck, P. J., Thomas, P. K., and Lambert, E. H. (eds.): Peripheral Neuropathy. Philadelphia, W. B. Saunders, 1975, pp. 868–890.

Rehfield, J. F. and Kruse-Larsen, C.: Gastrin and cholecystokinin in human cerebral fluid. Immunochemical determination of concentrations and molecular heterogeneity. Brain Res. 155:19–26, 1978.

Reimann, A. F. and Anson, B. J.: Vertebral level of termination of the spinal cord with report of a case of sacral cord. Anat. Rec. 88:170–172, 1944.

Reivich, M.: Blood flow metabolism couple in brain. In Plum, F. (ed.): Brain Dysfunction in Metabolic Disorders. Res. Publ. Assoc. Res. Nerv. Ment. Dis. 53:125–140, 1974.

Reulen, H. J., Graham, R., Fenske, A. et al.: The resolution of tissue pressure and bulk flow in the formation and resolution of cold-induced edema. In Pappius, H. M. and Feindel, W. (eds.): Dynamics of Brain Edema. Berlin, Springer-Verlag, 1976, pp. 103–112.

Reulen, H. J. and Kreysch, H. G.: Measurement of brain tissue pressure in cold-induced edema. Acta Neurochir. 29:29–40, 1973.

Reulen, H. J., Tsuyumu, M., Tack, A. et al.: Clearance of edema fluid into cerebrospinal fluid. A mechanism for the resolution of vasogenic brain edema. J. Neurosurg. 48:754–764, 1978.

Richardson, E. P. Jr.: Progressive multifocal leukoencephalopathy. N. Engl. J. Med. 265:815–823, 1961.

Riddoch, G.: Progressive dementia, without headache or changes in the optic discs, due to tumours of the third ventricle. Brain 59:225–233, 1936.

Ridsdale, L. and Moseley, I.: Thoracolumbar intraspinal tumours presenting features of raised intracranial pressure. J. Neurol. Neurosurg. Psychiatry 41:737–745, 1978.

Rieselbach, R. E., DiChiro, G., Freireich, E. J. et al.: Subarachnoid distribution of drugs after lumbar infection. N. Engl. J. Med. 267:1273–1278, 1962.

Rinne, U. K. and Riekkinen, P.: Esterase, peptidase and proteinase activities of human cerebrospinal fluid in multiple sclerosis. Acta Neurol. Scand. 44:156–167, 1968.

Rinne, U. K. and Sonninen, V.: Acid monoamine metabolites in the cerebrospinal fluid of patients with Parkinson's disease. Neurology 22:62–67, 1972.

Rippon, J. W.: Mycosis (pathogenesis and epidemiology). In Vinken, P. J. and Bruyn, G. W. (eds.): Handbook of Clinical Neurology. Vol. 35. Amsterdam, North Holland, 1978, pp. 371–381.

Risberg, J. and Ingvar, D. H.: Regional changes in cerebral blood flow during mental activity. Brain Res. 5:72–78, 1968.

Risberg, J., Lundberg, N. and Ingvar, D. H.: Regional cerebral blood volume during acute transient rise of the intracranial pressure (plateau waves). J. Neurosurg. 31:303–310, 1969.

Riser, M. P.: Le mecanisme de la glycorachie: Contribution á L'étude de la permeabilite meningée. Presse Méd. 35:1457–1459, 1927.

Robinson, R. J., Cutler, R. W. P., Lorenzo, A. U. et al.: Transport of sulfate, thiosulfate and iodide by choroid plexus in vitro. J. Neurochem. 15:1169–1179, 1968.

Roboz, E., Hess, W. C., Di Nella, R. R. et al.: Determination of total lipids, cholesterol and phospholipids in cerebrospinal fluid. J. Lab. Clin. Med. 52:158–162, 1958.

Roboz Einstein, E. and Macrae, D.: Spinal fluid analysis in amyotrophic lateral sclerosis. In Norris, F. H., Jr. and Kurland, L. T. (eds.): Motor Neuron Diseases: Research on Amyotrophic Lateral Sclerosis and Related Disorders. Vol. II. New York, Grune and Stratton, 1968, pp. 175–178.

Rodbard, S. and Saiki, H.: Mechanism of the pressor response to increased intracranial pressure. Am. J. Physiol. 168:234–244, 1952.

Rodda, R. and Denny-Brown, D.: The cerebral arterioles in experimental hypertension. II. The development of arteriolar necrosis. Am. J. Pathol. 49:365–381, 1966.

Rodriguez, E. M.: The cerebrospinal fluid as a pathway in neuroendocrine integration. J. Endocrinol. 71:407–443, 1976.

Ronquist, G., Ericsson, P., Frithz, G. et al.: Malignant brain tumours associated with adenylate kinase in cerebrospinal fluid. Lancet 1:1284–1286, 1977.

Roost, K. T., Pimstone, N. R., Diamond, I. et al.: The formation of cerebrospinal fluid xanthochromia after subarachnoid hemorrhage. Enzymatic conversion of hemoglobin to bilirubin by the arachnoid and choroid plexus. Neurology 22:973–977, 1972.

Rose, A. and Matson, D. D.: Benign intracranial hypertension in children. Pediatrics 39:227–237, 1967.

Rosenblum, M. L., Hoff, J. L., Norman, D. et al.: Decreased mortality from brain abscesses since the advent of computerized tomography. J. Neurosurg. 49:658–668, 1978.

Rosner, M. J. and Becker, D. P.: ICP monitoring: Complications and associated factors. Clin. Neurosurg. 23:494–519, 1976.

Rosomoff, H. L.: Effects of hypothermia and hypertonic urea on distribution of intracranial contents. J. Neurosurg. 18:753–759, 1961.

Rosomoff, H. L., Krieger, A. J. and Kuperman, A. S.: Effects of percutaneous cervical cordotomy on pulmonary function. J. Neurosurg. 31:620–627, 1969.

Ross, S., Rodriguez, W., Controni, G. et al.: Limulus lysate test for gram-negative bacterial meningitis, bedside application. J.A.M.A. 233:1366–1369, 1975.

Rossanda, M. and Gordon, E.: The oxygen tension of cerebrospinal fluid in patients with brain lesion. Acta Anesthesiol. Scand. 14:173–181, 1970.

Rothner, A. D. and Brust, J. C. M.: Pseudotumor cerebri. Report of a familial occurrence. Arch. Neurol. 30:110–111, 1974.

Rottenberg, D. A., Howieson, J. and Deck, M. D. F.: The rate of CSF formation in man: Preliminary observations on metrizamide washout as a measure of CSF bulk flow. Ann. Neurol 2:503–510, 1977.

Rottenberg, D. A., Hurwitz, B. J. and Posner, J. B.: The effect of oral glycerol on intraventricular pressure in man. Neurology 27:600–608, 1977.

Rougemont, J. de., Ames, A. III, Nesbett, F. B. and Hofmann, H. F.: Fluid formed by choroid plexus. A technique for its collection and a comparison of its electrolyte composition with serum and cisternal fluids. J. Neurophysiol. 23:485–495, 1960.

Rowan, J. O. and Johnston, I. H.: Blood pressure response to raised CSF pressure. In Lundberg, N., Ponten, U. and Brock, M. (eds.): Intracranial Pressure II. Berlin, Springer-Verlag, 1975, pp. 298–302.

Royer, P.: Perfusion endocavitaire cérébral. Biol. Méd. (Paris) 39:237–269, 1950.

Rubin, R. C., Henderson, E. S., Ommaya, A. K. et al.: The production of cerebrospinal fluid in man and its modification by acetazolamide. J. Neurosurg. 25:430–436, 1966.

Rudman, D., O'Brien, M. S., McKinney, A. S. et al.: Observations on the cyclic nucleotide concentrations in human cerebrospinal fluid. J. Clin. Endocrinol. Metab. 42:1088–1097, 1976.

Rundles, R. W.: Diabetic neuropathy: General review with a report of 125 cases. Medicine 24:111–160, 1945.

Runnels, J. B. and Hanberg, J. W.: Spontaneous subarachnoid hemorrhage associated with spinal cord tumor. J. Neurosurg. 39:252–254, 1974.

Russell, D. S.: Observations on the Pathology of Hydrocephalus. Medical Research Council Special Report Series, No. 265, London, His Majesty's Stationery Office, 1949, p. 138.

Ryder, H. W., Espey, F. W., Kimball, P. D. et al.: Modification of effect of cerebral blood flow on the CSF pressure by variations in the craniospinal blood volume. Arch. Neurol. Psychiat. 68:170–174, 1952.

Ryder, H. W., Espey, F. F., Kimball, P. D. et al.: Mechanism of the change in cerebrospinal fluid pressure following an induced change in the volume of the fluid space. J. Lab. Clin. Med. 41:428–435, 1953.

Rymer, M. M. and Fishman, R. A.: Protective adaptation of brain to water intoxication. Arch. Neurol. 28:49–54, 1973.

Rytel, M. W.: Rapid diagnostic methods in infectious diseases. Adv. Intern. Med. 20:37–60, 1976.

Sadler, K. and Welch, K.: Concentration of glucose in the new choroidal cerebrospinal fluid of the rabbit. Nature 215:884–885, 1967.

Sahar, A.: Free acetylcholine in the cerebrospinal fluid after brain operations. J. Neurol. Neurosurg. Psychiatry 29:77–79, 1966.

Sahar, A.: The effect of pressure on the production of cerebrospinal fluid by the choroid plexus. J. Neurol. Sci. 16:49–58, 1972.

Sahar, A., Hochwald, G. M. and Ransohoff, J.: Cerebrospinal fluid and cranial sinus pressures. Arch. Neurol. 23:413–418, 1970.

Sahar, A., Hochwald, G. M. and Ransohoff, J.: Experimental hydrocephalus: cerebrospinal fluid formation and ventricular size as a function of intraventricular pressure. J. Neurol. Sci. 11:81–91, 1970.

Sahar, A., Hochwald, G. M. and Ransohoff, J.: Passage of cerebrospinal fluid into cranial venous sinuses in normal and experimental hydrocephalic cats. Exp. Neurol 28:113–122, 1970.

Sahar, A. and Tsipstein, E.: Effects of mannitol and furosemide on the rate of formation of cerebrospinal fluid. Exp. Neurol. 60:584–591, 1978.

Sahs, A. L.: Brucellosis. In Vinken, P. J. and Bruyn, G. W. (eds.): Handbook of Clinical Neurology. Vol. 33. Amsterdam, Elsevier/North Holland Biomedical Press, 1978, pp. 305–326.

Sahs, A. L. and Joynt, R. J.: Brain swelling of unknown cause. Neurology (Minneap.) 6:791–802, 1956.

Saifer, A. and Siegel, H. A.: The photometric determination of the sialic (N-acetylneuraminic) acid distribution in cerebrospinal fluid. J. Lab. Clin. Med. 53:474–483, 1959.

Saito, R.: The cytologic manifestations of lymphatoid granulomatous in cerebrospinal fluid. Acta Cytol. 22:339–343, 1978.

Salminen, S. and Luomanmaki, K.: Distribution of sodium and potassium in serum, cerebrospinal fluid and serum ultrafiltrate in some diseases. Scand. J. Clin. Lab. Invest. 14:425–429, 1962.

Sambrook, M. A., Hutchison, E. C. and Aber, G. M.: Metabolic studies in subarachnoid hemorrhage and strokes. I. Serial changes in acid-base values in blood and cerebrospinal fluid. Brain 96:171–190, 1973.

Ibid.: II. Serial changes in cerebrospinal fluid and plasma urea electrolytes and osmolality. Brain 96:191–202, 1973.

Sampson, D. S. and Clark, K.: A current review of brain abscess. Am. J. Med. 54:201–210, 1978.

Sanborn, G. E., Selhorst, J. B., Calabrese, V. P. et al.: Pseudotumor cerebri and insecticide intoxication. Neurology 29:1222–1227, 1979.

Sandberg, M. and Bynke, H.: Cerebrospinal fluid in 25 cases of optic neuritis. Acta Neurol. Scand. 49:443–452, 1973.

Sandberg-Wollheim, M.: Optic neuritis: Studies on the cerebrospinal fluid in relation to clinical course in 61 patients. Acta Neurol. Scand. 52:167–178, 1975.

Sarff, L. D., Platt, L. H. and McCracken, G. H.: Cerebrospinal fluid evaluation in neonates: Comparison of high-risk infants with and without meningitis. J. Pediatr. 88:473–477, 1976.

Sarubbi, F. A., Jr., Sparling, P. F. and Glezen, W. P.: Herpesvirus hominis encephalitis. Virus isolation from brain biopsy in seven patients and results of therapy. Arch. Neurol. 29:268–273, 1973.

Savage, O.: Speransky's method of spinal pumping in rheumatoid arthritis. Br. Med. J. 1:496–497, March 13, 1948.

Savory, J. and Brody, J. P.: Measurement and diagnostic value of cerebrospinal fluid enzymes. Ann. Clin. Lab. Sci. 9:68–79, 1979.

Sayers, M. P.: Shunt complications. Clin. Neurosurg. 23:393–400, 1976.

Sayk, J.: Cytologie der Cerebrospinalflussigkeit. Wien. Z. Nervenheilk. Suppl. I, 1966, pp. 86–102.

Sayk, J.: The cerebrospinal fluid in brain tumors. In Vinken, P. J. and Bruyn, G. W. (eds.): Handbook of Clinical Neurology. Vol. 16. Amsterdam, North Holland, 1974, pp. 360–417.

Schain, R. J.: Neurohumors and other pharmacologically active substances in cerebrospinal fluid: A review of the literature. Yale J. Biol. Med. 33:15–36, 1960.

Schain, R. J.: Carbonic anhydrase inhibitors in chronic infantile hydrocephalus. Am. J. Dis. Child. 117:621–625, 1969.

Schapira, F.: L'activite aldolasique normale du LCR. Clin. Chim. Acta 7:566–571, 1962.

Schaub, C., Bluet-Pajut, M. T., Szikla, G. et al.: Distribution of growth hormone and thyroid-stimulating hormone in cerebrospinal fluid and pathological compartments of the central nervous system. J. Neurol. Sci. 31:123–131, 1977.

Schettini, A., McKay, L., Majors, R. et al.: Experimental approach for monitoring surface brain pressure. J. Neurosurg. 34:38–47, 1971.

Schliack, H., and Stille, D.: Clinical symptomatology of intraspinal tumours. In Vinken, P. J. and Bruyn, G. W. (eds.): Handbook of Clinical Neurology. Vol. 19. Amsterdam, North Holland, 1975, pp. 23–49.

Schliep, G. and Felgenhauer, K.: The alphamacroglobulin level in cerebrospinal fluid; a parameter for the condition of the blood-CSF barrier. J. Neurol. 207:171–181, 1974.

Schmidt, R. M.: Der Liquor Cerebrospinalis. Berlin, VEB Verlag Volk und Gesundheit, 1968.

Schneck, S. A. and Claman, H. N.: CSF immunoglobulins in multiple sclerosis and other neurological diseases. Arch. Neurol. 20:132–139, 1969.

Schold, C., Fleisher, M., Schwartz, M. et al.: Cerebrospinal fluid biochemical "markers" of central nervous system metastasis. Ann. Neurol. 4:176, 1978.

Schott, G. D. and Holt, D.: Digoxin in benign intracranial hypertension. Lancet 1:358–359, 1974.

Schreiner, G. and Maher, J. F.: Uremia: Biochemistry, Pathogenesis and Treatment. Springfield, Illinois, Charles C Thomas, 1961.

Schrumpf, E. and Bjelke, E.: Vitamin B12 in the serum and the cerebrospinal fluid. Acta Neurol. Scand. 46:243–248, 1970.

Schubert, W. K., Partin, J. C. and Partin, J. S.: Management of Reye's syndrome: Cincinnati experience. In Crocker, J. F. S. (ed.): Reye's Syndrome II. New York, Grune and Stratton, 1979, pp. 155–176.

Schuermann, K. and Reulen, H. J. (eds.): Steroids and Brain Edema. New York, Springer-Verlag, 1972.

Schuller, E., DeLasnerie, N. and Lebow, P.: DNA and RNA antibodies in serum and CSF of multiple sclerosis and subacute sclerosing panencephalitis patients. J. Neurol. Sci. 37:31–36, 1978.

Schultze, H. E. and Heremans, J. F.: Molecular Biology of the Human Proteins. Vol. I. Amsterdam, Elsevier, 1966, pp. 732–761.

Schwab, M.: Das Saure-Basen-Gleichgewich im arteriellen blut und seine beeinsflussung durch carboanhydrase-hemmung. Klin. Wochenschr. 40:1233–1245, 1962.

Schwab, M. and Dammaschke, H.: Atmung, Saure-Basen-Bleichgewicht und Ammoniak/Ammonium in Blut und Liquor cerebrospinalis bei Lebercirrhose. Klin. Wochenschr. 40:184–199, 1962.

Sciarra, D. and Carter, S.: Lumbar puncture headache. J.A.M.A. 148:841–842, 1952.

Sears, E. G.: Nonketotic hyperosmolar hyperglycemia during glycerol therapy for cerebral edema. Neurology 26:89–94, 1976.

Segal, M. B. and Pollay, M.: The secretion of cerebrospinal fluid. In Bito, L. S., Davson, H. and Fenstermacher, J. D. (eds.): The Ocular and Cerebrospinal fluids. London, Academic Press, 1977, pp. 127–148.

Seiler, N.: Assay procedures for polyamines in urine, serum, and cerebrospinal fluid. Clin. Chem. 23:1519–1526, 1977.

Seller, M. J. and Adinolfi, M.: Blood-brain barrier in the human fetus. Lancet 1:1030–1031, 1975.

Sensenbach, W., Madison, L. and Ochs, L.: The effect of ATCH and cortisone on cerebral blood flow and metabolism. J. Clin. Invest. 32:327–380, 1953.

Servo, C., Palo, J. and Pitkanen, E.: Polyols in the cerebrospinal fluid and plasma of neurological, diabetic and uraemic patients. Acta Neurol. Scand. 56:111–116, 1977.

Severinghaus, J. W., Chiodi, H., Eger, E. I. et al.: Cerebral blood flow in man at high altitude: Role of cerebrospinal fluid pH in normalization of flow in chronic hypocapnia. Circ. Res. 19:274–282, 1966.

Severinghaus, J. W., Mitchell, R. A., Richardson, B. W. and Singer, M. M.: Respiratory control at high altitudes suggesting active transport regulation of CSF pH. J. Appl. Physiol. 18:1155–1166, 1963.

Shabo, A. L. and Maxwell, D. S.: The morphology of the arachnoid villi: A light and electromicroscopic study in the monkey. J. Neurosurg. 29:451–463, 1968.

Shabo, A. L. and Maxwell, D. S.: Electron microscopic observations on the fate of particulate matter in the cerebrospinal fluid. J. Neurosurg. 29:464–474, 1968.

Shabo, A. L. and Maxwell, D. S.: The subarachnoid space following the introduction of a foreign protein: An electron microscopic study with peroxidase. J. Neuropathol. Exp. Neurol. 30:506–524, 1971.

Shalit, M. N. and Cotev, S.: Inter-relationship between blood pressure and regional cerebral blood flow in experimental intracranial hypertension. J. Neurosurg. 40:594–602, 1974.

Shapiro, H. M., Wyte, S. R., Harris, A. B. et al.: Acute intraoperative intracranial hypertension in neurological patients: mechanical and pharmacologic factors. Anesthesiology 37:399–405, 1972.

Shapiro, H. M., Wyte, S. R. and Loeser, J.: Barbiturate augmented hypothermia for reduction of persistent intracranial hypertension. J. Neurosurg. 40:90–100, 1974.

Shapiro, W. B., Young, D. F. and Mehta, B. M.: Methotrexate distribution in cerebrospinal fluid after intravenous, ventricular and lumbar injections. N. Engl. J. Med. 293:161–166, 1975.

Shapiro, W. R. and Posner, J. B.: Corticosteroid hormones: effects in an experimental brain tumor. Arch. Neurol. 30:217–221, 1974.

Sharp, M. M., Weller, R. O. and Brice, J. G.: Spinal cord necrosis after intrathecal injection of methylene blue. J. Neurol. Neurosurg. Psychiatry 41:384–386, 1978.

Shaywitz, B. A.: Epidermoid spinal cord tumors and previous lumbar puncture. J. Pediatr. 80:638–640, 1972.

Shaywitz, B. A., Katzman, R. and Escriva, A.: CSF formation and ^{24}Na clearance in normal and hydrocephalic kittens during ventriculocisternal perfusion. Neurology (Minneap.) 19:1159–1168, 1969.

Shenkin, H. A., Goluboff, B. and Haft, H.: The use of mannitol for the reduction of intracranial pressure in intracranial surgery. J. Neurosurgy. 19:897–900, 1962.

Sherwin, A. L., LeBlanc, F. E., and McCann, W. P.: Altered LDH-isoenzymes in brain tumours. Arch. Neurol. 18:311–315, 1968.

Sherwin, A. L., Norns, J. W., and Bulcke, J. A.: Spinal fluid creatine kinase in neurologic disease. Neurology (Minneap.) 19:993–999, 1969.

Shinefield, H. R.: Bacteremia, lumbar puncture and meningitis. Am. J. Dis. Child. 129:547–548, 1975.

Shulman, K. and Ransohoff, J.: Saggital sinus venous pressure in hydrocephalus. J. Neurosurg. 23:169–173, 1965.

Shurtleff, D. B., Kronmal, R. and Foltz, F. C.: Follow-up comparison of hydrocephalus with and without myelomeningocele. J. Neurosurg. 42:61–68, 1975.

Sicard, J. A. and Forestier, J.: Roentgenologic exploration of central nervous system with iodized oil (Lipiodol). Arch. Neurol. Psychiat. 16:420–434, 1956.

Sicuteri, F., Fanciullacci, M., Bavazzano, A., et al.: Kinins and intracranial hemorrhage. Angiology 21:193–210, 1970.

Sidell, A. D. and Daly, D. D.: The electroencephalogram in cases of benign intracranial hypertension. Neurology 11:413–417, 1961.

Siegel, N. J. and Spackman, T. J.: Chronic hypertension with intracranial hypertension and low cerebrospinal fluid concentration of protein. Clin. Pediatr. 11:580–584, 1972.

Siekert, R. G.: Neurological manifestations of infective endocarditis (subacute bacterial endocarditis). In Vinken, P. J. and Bruyn, G. W. (eds.): Handbook of Clinical Neurology. Vol. 33. Amsterdam, Elsevier/North Holland, Biomedical Press, 1978, pp. 469–477.

Siemkowicz, E., Christiansen, I. and Sorensen, S. C.: Changes in cisternal fluid potassium following cardiac arrest. Acta Neurol. Scand. 55:137–144, 1977.

Siemkowicz, E. and Diemer, N. H.: Cytology of human cerebrospinal fluid after cardiac arrest. Acta Neurol. Scand. 57:1–7, 1978.

Siesjo, B. K.: The regulation of cerebrospinal fluid pH. Kidney Int. 1:360–374, 1972.

Siesjo, B. K.: Brain Energy Metabolism. New York, John Wiley and Sons, 1978, p. 607.

Siesjo, B. K. and Sorensen, S. C. (eds.): Ion Homeostasis of the Brain. Alfred Benzon Symposium III. New York, Academic Press, 1971.

Sifontes, J. E., Williams, R. D. B., Lincoln, E. M. et al.: Observations on the effect of induced hyperglycemia on the glucose content of the cerebrospinal fluid in patients with tuberculous meningitis. Am. Rev. Tuberc. 67:732–754, 1953.

Silberberg, D. H. and Laties, A. M.: Increased intracranial pressure in disseminated lupus erythematosus. Arch. Neurol. 29:89–90, 1973.

Silbermann, M. and Fishman, R. A.: Primary (idiopathic) thrombosis of the superior longitudinal sinus. Trans. Am. Neurol. Assoc. 76:164–167, 1951.

Silverstein, A.: EB virus infections of the nervous system. In Vinken, P. J. and Bruyn, G. W. (eds.): Handbook of Clinical Neurology. Vol. 34. Amsterdam, North Holland Publishing Company, 1978, pp. 185–192.

Simmons, R. L., Martin, A. M., Heisterkamp, C. A. et al.: Respiratory insufficiency in combat casualties. 2. Pulmonary edema following head injury. Ann. Surg. 170:39–44, 1969.

Simon, G. and Schröer, H.: The cell-catch procedure. A new method which preserves all cellular elements of spinal-fluid samples. J. Neurosurg. 20:787–792, 1963.

Simon, R. P. and Abele, J. S.: Spinal-fluid pleocytosis estimated by the Tyndall effect. Ann. Intern. Med. 89:75–76, 1978.

Singh, B. N.: Pathogenic and Non-pathogenic Amoebae. New York, John Wiley and Sons, 1975.

Sjaastad, O. and Nordvik, A.: The corpus callosal angle in the diagnosis of cerebral ventricular enlargement. Acta Neurol. Scand. 49:396–406, 1973.

Sjaastad, O., Skalpe, I. O. and Engeset, A.: The width of the temporal horn in the differential diagnosis between pressure hydrocephalus and hydrocephalus ex vacuo. Neurology 19:1087–1093, 1969.

Sjoqvist, O. Beobachtungen über die Liquorsekretion beim Menschen. Zentralbl. Neurochir. 2:8–17, 1937.

Sjostrand, R., Ekstedt, J. and Anggard, E.: Concentration gradients of monoamine metabolites in human cerebrospinal fluid. J. Neurol. Neurosurg. Psychitry 38:666–668, 1975.

Skinhoj, E.: Hemodynamic studies within the brain during migraine. Arch. Neurol. 29:95–98, 1973.

Skinhoj, E. and Strandgaard, S.: Pathogenesis of hypertensive encephalopathy. Lancet 1:461–462, 1973.

Sklar, F. H. and Elashvili, I.: The pressure volume function of brain elasticity. Physiological considerations and clinical applications. J. Neurosurg. 47:670–679, 1977.

Smith, H., Bannister, B. and O'Shea, M. J.: Cerebrospinal fluid immunoglobulins in meningitis. Lancet 2:591–593, 1973.

Snow, R. M. and Dismukes, W. E.: Cryptococcal meningitis. Arch. Intern. Med. 135:1155–1157, 1975.

Soffer, D., Feldman, S. and Alter, M.: Clinical features of the Guillain-Barré syndrome. J. Neurol. Sci. 37:135–143, 1978.

Sokoloff, L.: The actions of drugs upon the cerebral circulation. Pharmacol. Rev. 11:1–85, 1959.

Sokoloff, L.: Relation between physiological function and energy metabolism in the central nervous system. J. Neurochem. 29:13–26, 1977.

Sokolowski, S. J.: A new quantitative technique for the assessment of cerebrospinal fluid absorption in man. J. Neurol. Sci. 23:37–47, 1974.

Sondheimer, F. K., Grossman, H. and Winchester, P.: Suture diastasis following rapid weight gain. Pseudopseudotumor cerebri. Arch. Neurol. 23:314–318, 1970.

Sornas, R.: The cytology of the normal cerebrospinal fluid. Acta Neurol. Scand. 48:313–320, 1972.

Sornas, R., Ostlund, H. and Muller, R.: Cerebrospinal fluid cytology after stroke. Arch. Neurol. 26:489–500, 1972.

Sotos, J. F., Dodge, P. R., Meara, P. et al.: Studies in experimental hypertoxicity: Pathogenesis of the clinical syndrome, biochemical abnormalities and cause of death. Pediatrics 26:525–538, 1960.

Sparling, P. F.: Diagnosis of syphilis. N. Engl. J. Med. 284:642–653, 1971.

Spector, R.: Thiamine transport in the central nervous system. Am. J. Physiol. 230:1101–1107, 1976.

Spector, R.: Vitamin homeostasis in the central nervous system. N. Engl. J. Med. 296:1393–1398, 1977.

Spector, R.: Transport and metabolism of vitamin B6 in rabbit brain and choroid plexus. J. Biol. Chem. 253:2373–2379, 1978.

Spector, R. and Lorenzo, A. V.: Specificity of ascorbic acid transport system of the central nervous system. Am. J. Physiol. 226–1468–1473, 1974.

Spector, R. and Lorenzo, A. V.: Myoinositol transport in the central nervous system. Am. J. Physiol. 228:1510–1518, 1975.

Spector, R. and Lorenzo, A. V.: Folate transport in the central nervous system. Am. J. Physiol. 229:777–782, 1975.

Spencer, W. and Horsley, V.: On the changes produced in the circulation and respiration by increase of the intracranial pressure or tension. Philos. Trans. 182B:201–254, 1892.

Spiegel-Adolf, M., Baird, H. III and Kollias, D.: Lipases in the CSF in various neurological conditions, especially infantile amaurotic idiocy (Tay-Sachs' disease). Confin. Neurol. 17:310–315, 1957.

Spina,-Franca, A.: Biological aspects of neurocysticercosis: alterations of the cerebrospinal fluid. Arq. Neuropsiquiatr. (Sao Paulo) 20:17–30, 1962.

Spina-Franca, A., Libramento, J. A., Bacheschi, A. et al.: Cerebrospinal fluid immunoglobulins in cysticercosis of the central nervous system. Arq. Neuropsiquiatr. 34:40–45, 1976.

Spina-Franca, A. and Mattosinho-Franca, L. C.: American trypanosomiasis (Chagas' disease). In Vinken, P. J. and Bruyn, G. W. (eds.): Handbook of Clinical Neurology. Vol. 35. Amsterdam, North Holland, 1978, pp. 85–114.

Stein, B. M., Fraser, R. A. R. and Tenner, M. S.: Normal pressure hydrocephalus: Complication of posterior fossa surgery in children. Pediatrics 49:50–58, 1972.

Stein, S. C. and Langfitt, T. W.: Normal pressure hydrocephalus. Predicting the results of cerebrospinal fluid shunting. J. Neurosurg. 41:463–470, 1974.

Steinwall, O. and Klatzo, I.: Selective vulnerability of the blood-brain barrier in chemically induced lesions. J. Neuropathol. Exp. Neurol. 25:542–559, 1966.

Stendahl, L., Link, H., Moller, E. et al.: Relationship between genetic markers and oligoclonal IgG in CSF in optic neuritis. J. Neurol. Sci. 27:93–98, 1976.

Stendahl-Brodin, L., Link, H. and Kristensson, K.: Myelinotoxic activity on tadpole optic nerve of cerebrospinal fluid from patients with optic neuritis. Neurology 29:882–886, 1979.

Stern, L. and Gautier, R.: Recherches sur le liquide céphalo-rachidien. I. Les rapports entre le liquide céphalo-rachidien et la circulation sanguine. Arch. Int. Physiol. 17:138–192, 1921.

Stern, W. E., and Coxon, R. V.: Osmolality of brain tissue and its relation to brain bulk. Am. J. Physiol. 206:1–7, 1964.

Stewart-Wallace, A. M.: A biochemical study of cerebral tissue and of changes in cerebral edema. Brain 62:426–438, 1939.

Stoebner, R., Kiser, R. and Alperin, J. B.: Iron deficiency anemia and papilledema: rapid resolution with oral iron therapy. Am. J. Dig. Dis. 15:919–922, 1970.

Storm-Mathisen, A.: Syphilis. In Vinken, P. J. and Bruyn, G. W. (eds): Handbook of Clinical Neurology. Vol. 33. Amsterdam, North Holland, 1978, pp. 337–394.

Strayer, D. R. and Bender, R. A.: Eosinophilic meningitis complicating Hodgkin's disease. A report of a case and review of the literature. Cancer 40:406–409, 1977.

Stutzman, F. L. and Amatuzio, D. S.: A study of serum and cerebrospinal fluid calcium and magnesium in normal humans. Arch. Biochem. 39:271–275, 1952.

Sugar, O.: Central neurological complications of hypoparathyroidism. Arch. Neurol. Psychiatr. 70:86–107, 1953.

Sullivan, H. G., Miller, J. D., Becker D. P. et al.: The physiological basis of intracranial pressure change with progressive epidural brain compression. J. Neurosurg. 47:532–550, 1977.

Summer, K. and Traugott, U.: Liquoreosinophilie nach Myelographie. J. Neurol. 210:127–134, 1975.

Swanson, P. D.: Neurological manifestations of hypernatremia. In Vinken, P. J. and Bruyn, G. W. (eds.): Handbook of Clinical Neurology. Vol. 28. Amsterdam, North Holland, 1976, pp. 443–461.

Swartz, M. N. and Dodge, P. R.: Bacterial meningitis — a review of selected aspects. I. General clinical features, special problems and unusual meningeal reactions mimicking bacterial meningitis. N. Engl. J. Med. 272:725–731, 779–787, 842–848, 898–902, 1965.

Sweet, W. H., Brownell, G. L., Scholl, J. A. et al.: The formation, flow and absorption of cerebrospinal fluid; Newer concepts based on studies with isotopes. Res. Publ. Assoc. Res. Nerv. Ment. Dis. 34:101–159, 1956.

Sweet, W. H. and Locksley, H. B.: Formation, flow and reabsorption of cerebrospinal fluid in man. Proc. Soc. Exp. Biol. Med. 84:397–402, 1953.

Sweet, W. H., Selverstone, B. and Stetten, D.: Studies of formation, flow and absorption of cerebrospinal fluid. II. Studies with heavy water in the normal man. American College of Surgeons Surgical Forum. Philadelphia, W. B. Saunders, 1950, pp. 376–381.

Swisher, C. N.: Neurological sequelae to pertussis infection and immunization. In Vinken, P. J. and Bruyn, G. W. (eds.): Handbook of Clinical Neurology. Vol. 33. Amsterdam, Elsevier/North Holland Biomedical Press, 1978, pp. 275–303.

Symon, L., Branston, N. M. and Strong, A. J.: Autoregulation in acute focal ischemia: An experimental study. Stroke 7:547–554, 1976.

Symon, L. and Dorsch, N. W. C.: Use of long term intracranial pressure measurement to assess hydrocephalic patients prior to shunt surgery. J. Neurosurg. 42:258–273, 1975.

Symon, L., Dorsch, N. W. C. and Stephens, R. J.: Pressure waves in so-called normal pressure hydrocephalus. Lancet 2:1291–1292, 1972.

Symonds, C. P.: Otitic hydrocephalus. Brain 54:55–71, 1931.

Symonds, C. P.: Hydrocephalic and focal cerebral symptoms in relation to thrombophlebitis of the dural sinuses and cerebral veins. Brain 60:531–550, 1937.

Symonds, C. P.: Migrainous variants. Trans. Med. Soc. Lond. 67:237–250, 1952.

Sypert, G. W., Leffman, H. and Ojemann, G. A.: Occult normal pressure hydrocephalus manifested by Parkinsonism-dementia complex. Neurology 23:234–238, 1973.

Tabaddor, K., Wolfson, L. I. and Sharpless, N. S.: Ventricular fluid homovanillic acid and 5-hydroxyindoleacetic acid concentrations in patients with movement disorders. Neurology 28:1249–1253, 1978a.

Tabaddor, K., Wolfson, L. I. and Sharpless, N. S.: Diminished ventricular fluid dopamine metabolites in adult onset dystonia. Neurology 28:1254–1258, 1978b.

Tabira, T., Webster, H. de F., and Wray, S. H.: Multiple sclerosis: Cerebrospinal fluid produces myelin lesions in tadpole optic nerves. N. Engl. J. Med. 295:644–649, 1976.

Tabira, T., Webster, H. de F., and Wray, S.: In vivo test for myelinotoxicity of cerebrospinal fluid. Brain Res. 120:103–112, 1977.

Taggart, J. K. and Walker, A. E.: Congenital atresia of the foramens of Luschka and Magendie. Arch. Neurol. Psychiatr. 48:583–612, 1942.

Tandon, P. N.: Tuberculous meningitis. In Vinken, P. J. and Bruyn, G. W. (eds): Handbook of Clinical Neurology. Vol. 33. Amsterdam, Elsevier/North Holland, 1978, pp. 195–262.

Tasker, W. and Chutorian, A. M.: Chronic polyneuritis of childhood. J. Pediatr. 74:699–708, 1969.

Tedeschi, C. G., Walter, C. E., Lepore, T. et al.: An assessment of the cerebrospinal fluid and choroid plexus in relation to systemic fat embolism. Neurology 19:586–590, 1969.

Teng, P., Wagner, J. H. and Buxbaum, M. W.: Giant ependymoma of the spinal cord associated with papilledema. Arch. Neurol. 2:657–662, 1960.

Tennyson, V.: Ultrastructural characteristics of the telencephalic and myelencephalic choroid plexus in fetus of man and rabbit, and a comparison with the adult choroid plexus in rabbit. In Netsky, M. G. and Shuangshoti, S. (eds.): The Choroid Plexus in Health and Disease. Charlottesville, University of Virginia Press, 1975, pp. 36–72.

Tennyson, V. M. and Pappas, G. D.: Ependyma. In Minckler, J. (ed.): Pathology of the Nervous System. Vol. 1. New York, McGraw-Hill, 1968, pp. 518–530.

Terhaag, B., Scherber, A., Schaps, P. et al.: The distribution of lithium into cerebrospinal fluid, brain tissue and bile in man. Int. J. Clin. Pharmacol. 16:333–335, 1978.

Terrenius, L., Wahlstrom, A., Lindstrom, L. et al.: Increased CSF levels of endorphins in chronic psychosis. Neurosci. Lett. 3:157–162, 1976.

Theodore, J. and Robin, E. D.: Speculations on neurogenic pulmonary edema. Am. Rev. Resp. Dis. 113:405–411, 1976.

Thomas, J. E. and Howard, F. M., Jr.: Segmental zoster paresis — a disease profile. Neurology 22:459–466, 1972.

Thompson, E. J.: Laboratory diagnosis of multiple sclerosis: immunological and biochemical aspects. Br. Med. Bull. 33:28–33, 1977.

Thompson, W. O. and Alexander, B.: Exophthalmic goiter: The protein content of the cerebrospinal fluid. Arch. Intern. Med. 45:122–124, 1930.

Thompson, H. G., Jr., Hirschberg, E., Osnos, M. et al.: Evaluation of phosphohexose isomerase activity in CSF in neoplastic disease of the central nervous system. Neurology (Minneap.) 9:545–552, 1959.

Thompson, R. K. and Malina, S.: Dynamic axial brain stem distortion as a mechanism explaining the cardio-respiratory changes in increased intracranial pressure. J. Neurosurg. 16:664–675, 1959.

Tibbling, G., Link, H. and Ohman, S.: Principles of albumin and IgG analyses in neurological disorders. I. Establishment of reference values. Scand. J. Clin. Lab. Invest. 37:385–390, 1977.

Tichy, J., Alling, C., Dencker, S. J. et al.: Fatty acid profiles of cerebrospinal fluid lipids in normals and chronic alcoholics. Scand. J. Clin. Lab. Invest. 25:191–198, 1970.

Tobey, G. J., Jr. and Ayer, J. B.: Dynamic studies of the cerebrospinal fluid in the different diagnosis of lateral sinus thrombosis. Arch. Otolaryngol. 2:50–57, 1925.

Tornheim, P. A., McLaurin, R. L. and Sawaya, R.: Effect of furosemide on experimental traumatic cerebral edema. Neurosurgery 4:48–52, 1979.

Torrey, E. F.: Headaches after lumbar puncture and insensitivity to pain in psychiatric patients. N. Engl. J. Med. 301:110, 1979.

Tourtellotte, W. W.: Cerebrospinal fluid examination in meningoencephalitis. Modern Treatment (Hoeber Medical Division, Harper and Row) 4:879–897, 1967.

Tourtellotte, W. W.: Cerebrospinal fluid in multiple sclerosis. In Vinken, P. J. and Bruyn, G. W. (eds.): Handbook of Clinical Neurology. Vol. 9. Amsterdam, North Holland, 1970, pp. 324–382.

Tourtellotte, W. W.: On cerebrospinal fluid immunoglobulin-G (IgG) quotients in multiple sclerosis and other diseases. A review and a new formula to estimate the amount of IgG synthesized per day by the central nervous system. J. Neurol. Sci. 10:279–304, 1970.

Tourtellotte, W. W.: What is multiple sclerosis: Laboratory criteria for diagnosis. In Davison, A. N., Humphrey, J. H., Liversedge, A. L. et al. (eds.): Multiple Sclerosis Research. Amsterdam, Elsevier, 1975, pp. 9–26.

Tourtellotte, W. W., Allen, R. J., Haerer, A. F. et al.: Study of lipids in cerebrospinal fluid and serum. In Tay-Sachs disease. Arch. Neurol. 12:300–310, 1965.

Tourtellotte, W. W. and Haerer, A. F.: Lipids in cerebrospinal fluid. XII. In multiple sclerosis and retrobulbar neuritis. Arch. Neurol. 20:605–615, 1969.

Tourtellotte, W. W., Haerer, A. F., Heller, G. L. et al.: Post-lumbar Puncture Headaches. Springfield, Illinois, Charles C Thomas, 1964.

Tourtellotte, W. W. and Ma, B. I.: Multiple sclerosis: The blood-brain-barrier and the measurement of de novo central nervous system IgG synthesis. Neurology 28:76–83, 1978.

Tourtellotte, W. W., Metz, L. N., Bryan, E. R., et al.: Spontaneous subarachnoid hemorrhage. Neurology 14:301–306, 1964.

Tourtellotte, W. W., Reinglass, J. L. and Newkirk, T. A.: Cerebral dehydration action of glycerol. Clin. Pharmacol. Ther. 13:159–171, 1972.

Tourtellotte, W. W., Somers, J. F., Parker, J. A. et al.: A study on traumatic lumbar punctures. Neurology 8:129–134, 1958.

Tourtellotte, W. W., Tavolato, B., Parker, J. A. et al.: Cerebrospinal fluid electroimmunodiffusion. Arch. Neurol. 25:345–350, 1971.

Tower, D. B.: Fluids and electrolytes in the central nervous system: Factors affecting their distribution with special reference to excitability and edema. Electroencephalogr. Clin. Neurophysiol. (Suppl.) 31:43–57, 1972.

Tower, D. B. and McEachern, D.: Acetylcholine and neuronal activity; cholinesterase patterns and acetylcholine in cerebrospinal fluids of patients with craniocerebral trauma. Can. J. Res. 27:105–119, 1949.

Towfighi, J. and Gonatas, N. K.: Effects of intracerebral injection of ouabain in adult and developing rats. An ultrastructural and autoradiographic study. Lab. Invest. 28:170–180, 1973.

Townsend, J. J., Wolinsky, J. S., Baringer, J. R. et al.: Acquired toxoplasmosis, a neglected cause of treatable nervous system disease. Arch. Neurol. 32:335–343, 1975.

Townsend, R. E., Prinz, P. N. and Obrist, W. D.: Human cerebral blood flow during sleep and waking. J. Appl. Physiol. 35:620–625, 1973.

Trauner, D., Brown, F., Ganz, E. et al.: Treatment of elevated intracranial pressure in Reye syndrome. Ann. Neurol. 4:275–278, 1978.

Traviesa, D. C., Prystowsky, S. D., Nelson, B. J. et al.: Cerebrospinal fluid findings in asymptomatic patients with reactive serum fluorescent treponemal antibody absorption tests. Ann. Neurol. 4:524–530, 1978.

Trelles, J. O. and Trelles, L.: Cysticercosis of the nervous system. In Vinken, P. J. and Bruyn, G. W. (eds.): Handbook of Clinical Neurology. Vol. 35. Amsterdam, North Holland, 1978, pp. 291–320.

Triedman, H., Fishman, R. A. and Yahr, M. D.: Determination of plasma and cerebrospinal fluid levels of Dilantin in the human. Trans. Am. Neurol. Assoc. 85:166–170, 1960.

Tripathi, B. S. and Tripathi, R. C.: Vacuolar transcellular channels as a drainage pathway for cerebrospinal fluid. J. Physiol. (Lond.) 239:195–206, 1974.

Tripathi, R. C.: Ultrastructure of the arachnoid matter in relation to outflow of cerebrospinal fluid. A new concept. Lancet 2:8–11, 1973.

Tripathi, R. C.: The functional morphology of the outflow systems of ocular and cerebrospinal fluids. In Bito, L. Z., Davson, H. and Fenstermacher, J. D. (eds.): The Ocular and Cerebrospinal Fluids. New York, Academic Press, 1977, pp. 65–116.

Troost, B. T., Walker, J. E. and Cherington, M.: Hypoglycorrhachia associated with subarachnoid hemorrhage. Arch. Neurol. 19:438–442, 1968.

Trotter, J. L., Luzecky, M., Siegel, B. A. et al.: Cerebrospinal fluid infusion test. Identification of artifacts and correlation with cisternography and pneumoencephalography. Neurology 24:181–186, 1974.

Trupp, M.: Stylet injury syndrome. J.A.M.A. 237:2524, 1977.

Tsairis, P., Dyck, P. J. and Mulder, D. W.: Natural history of brachial plexus neuropathy. Arch. Neurol. 27:109–117, 1972.

Tschirgi, R. D.: Protein complexes and the impermeability of the blood-brain barrier to dyes. Am. J. Physiol. 163:756, 1950. (Abstract)

Tschirgi, R. D.: Chemical environment of the central nervous system. In Field, J. (ed.): Handbook of Physiology. Vol. III. Washington, American Physiological Society, 1960, pp. 1865–1890.

Tschirgi, R. D., Frost, R. W. and Taylor, J. L.: Inhibition of cerebrospinal fluid formation by a carbonic anhydrase inhibitor, 2-acetylamino-1, 3,4-thiodiazole-5 sulfonamide (Diamox). Proc. Soc. Exp. Biol. Med. 87:373–376, 1954.

Tugwell, P., Greenwood, B. M. and Warrell, D. A.: Pneumococcal meningitis: A clinical and laboratory study. Q. J. Med. 45:583–601, 1976.

Turner, L.: The structure of arachnoid granulations with observations on their physiological and pathological significance. Ann. R. Coll. Surg. Engl. 29:237–264, 1961.

Tveten, L.: Candidiasis. In Vinken, P. J. and Bruyn, G. W. (eds.): Handbook of Clinical Neurology. Vol. 35. Amsterdam, North Holland, 1978, pp. 413–442.

Ursing, B.: Clinical and immuno-electrophoretic studies on cerebrospinal fluid in virus meningoencephalitis and bacterial meningitis. Acta Med. Scand. (Supply.) 429:1–99, 1965.

Utz, J. P.: Current and future chemotherapy of central nervous system fungal infections. Adv. Neurol. 6:127–132, 1974.

Vandam, L. D. and Dripps, R. D.: Longterm follow up of patients who received 10,098 spinal anesthetics. Syndrome of decreased intracranial pressure (headaches and ocular and auditory difficulties). J.A.M.A. 161:586–591, 1956.

Vander Ark, G. D., Kempe, L. G. and Smith, D. R.: Pseudotumor cerebri treated with lumbar-peritoneal shunt. J.A.M.A. 217:1832–1834, 1971.

Van Der Meulen, J. P.: Cerebrospinal fluid xanthochromia: An objective index. Neurology 16:170–178, 1966.

Van Deurs, B.: Vesicular transport of horseradish peroxidase from brain to blood in segments of the cerebral microvasculature in adult mice. Brain Res. 124:1–8, 1977.

Van Deurs, B.: Microperoxidase uptake into the rat choroid plexus epithelium. J. Ultrastruct. Res. 62 (2):168–180, 1978.

Vandvik, B.: Oligoclonal IgG and free light chains in the cerebrospinal fluid of patients with multiple sclerosis and infectious diseases of the central nervous system. Scand. J. Immunol. 6:913–921, 1977.

Vandvik, B. and Degré, M.: Measles virus antibodies in serum and cerebrospinal fluid in patients with multiple sclerosis and other neurological disorders, with special reference to measles antibody synthesis within the central nervous system. J. Neurol. Sci. 24:201–219, 1975.

Vandvik, B., Norrby, E., Nordal, H. J. et al.: Oligoclonal measles virus-specific IgG antibodies isolated from cerebrospinal fluids, brain extracts, and sera from patients with subacute sclerosing panencephalitis and multiple sclerosis. Scand. J. Immunol. 5:979–992, 1976.

Vandvik, B. and Skrede, S.: Electrophoretic examination of cerebrospinal fluid protein in multiple sclerosis and other neurological diseases. Eur. Neurol. 9:224–241, 1973.

Van Harreveld, A.: Brain Tissue Electrolytes. Washington, Butterworth, 1966.

Van Harreveld, A.: The extracellular space in the vertebrate central nervous system. In Bourne, G. H. (ed.): The Structure and Function of Nervous Tissue. Vol. 4. New York, Academic Press, 1972, pp. 447–511.

van Rymenant, M., Robert, J. and Otten, J: Isocitric dehydrogenase in cerebrospinal fluid: clinical usefulness of its determination. Neurology 16:351–354, 1966.

van Sande, M., Mardens, Y., Adriaenssens, K. et al.: The free amino acids in human cerebrospinal fluid. J. Neurochem. 17:125–135, 1970.

Vates, T. S., Jr., Bonting, S. L. and Oppelt, W. W.: Na-K activated adenosine triphosphatase formation of cerebrospinal fluid in the cat. Am. J. Physiol. 206:1165–1172, 1964.

Vaughn, G. M., McDonald, S. D., Jordon, R. M. et al.: Melatonin concentration in human blood and cerebrospinal fluid: relationship to stress. J. Clin. Endocrinol. Metab. 47:220–223, 1978.

Veall, N. and Mallett, B. L.: Regional cerebral blood flow determinates by ^{133}Xe inhalation and external recordings: The effect of arterial recirculation. Clin. Sci. 30:359–369, 1966.

Vela, A. R., Carey, B. E. and Thompson, B. M.: Further data on the acute effect of intravenous steroids on canine CSF secretion and absorption. J. Neurosurg. 50:477–482, 1979.

Venes, J. L., Shaywitz, B. A. and Spencer, D. D.: Management of encephalopathy of Reye-Johnson syndrome. J. Neurosurg. 48:903–915, 1978.

Vergara, F., Plum, F., and Duffy, T. E.: Alpha-Ketoglutaramate: increased concentration in the cerebrospinal fluid of patients in hepatic coma. Science 183:81–83, 1974.

Verhas, M., Schontens, A., Demol, D. et al.: Study in cerebrovascular disease: brain scanning with technetium-99m pertechnetate; Clinical correlations. Neurology 25:553–558, 1975.

Verheecke, P.: On the tau-protein in cerebrospinal fluid. J. Neurol. Sci. 26:277–281, 1975.

Vestergaard, P., Sorensen, T., Hoppe, E. et al.: Biogenic amine metabolites in cerebrospinal fluid of patients with affective disorders. Acta Psychiatr. Scand. 58:88–96, 1978.

Victor, M.: The effects of nutritional deficiency on the nervous system. A comparison with the effects of carcinoma. In Brain, W. R. and Norris, F., Jr. (eds.): The Remote Effects of Cancer on the Nervous System. New York, Grune and Stratton, 1965.

Viets, H. R.: Domenico Cotugno: His description of the cerebrospinal fluid with a translation of part of his "De isclude nervosa commentarius" (1764) and a bibliography of his important works. Bull. Hist. Med. 3:701–738, 1935.

Vietze, G.: Malaria and other protozoal diseases. In Vinken, P. J. and Bruyn, G. W. (eds.): Handbook of Clinical Neurology. Vol. 35. Amsterdam, North Holland, 1978, pp. 143–160.

Vincent, F. M.: Granulomatous angiitis. N. Engl. J. Med. 296:452, 1977.

Virmani, V., Rangan, G. and Shriniwas, G.: A study of the cerebrospinal fluid in atypical presentations of tuberculous meningitis. J. Neurol. Sci. 16:587–592, 1975.

Voetmann, E.: On the structure and surface area of the human choroid plexuses: A quantitative anatomical study. Acta Anat. 8 (Suppl.) 10:1–116, 1949.

Vulpe, M., Hawkins, A. and Rozdilsky, B.: Permeability of cerebral blood vessels in experimental allergic encephalomyelitis studied by radioactive bovine albumin. Neurology 10:171–177, 1960.

Walker, A. E. and Adamkiewicz, J. J.: Pseudotumor cerebri associated with prolonged corticosteroid therapy. J.A.M.A. 188:779–784, 1964.

Wallace, G. B. and Brodie, B. B.: On the source of the cerebrospinal fluid. The distribution of bromide and iodide throughout the central nervous system. J. Pharmacol. Exper. Therap. 70:418–427, 1940.

Walsh, F. B.: Papilledema associated with increased intracranial pressure in Addison's disease. Arch. Ophthalmol. 47:86, 1952.

Walshe, J. H.: Observations on the symptomatology and pathogenesis of hepatic coma. Q. J. Med. 20:421–438, 1951.

Walton, J. N.: Subarachnoid Haemorrhage. Edinburgh, Livingstone, 1956.

Waltz, A. G.: Effect of blood pressure on blood flow in ischemic and in non-ischemic cortex: The phenomena of autoregulation and luxury perfusion. Neurology 18:613–621, 1968.

Ward, A.: Atropine in the treatment of closed head injury. J. Neurosurg. 7:398–402, 1950.

Ware, A. J., D'Agostino, A. and Combes, B.: Cerebral edema: A major complication of massive hepatic necrosis. Gastroenterology 61:877–884, 1971.

Watchhorn, E. and McCance, R. E.: Subacute magnesium deficiency in rats. Biochem. J. 31:1379–1390, 1937.

Waterhouse, J. M. and Coxon, R. V.: The entry of glycerol into brain tissue. J. Neurol. Sci. 10:305–311, 1970.

Watson, P.: A slide centrifuge: An apparatus for concentrating cells in suspension onto a microscopic slide. J. Lab. Clin. Med. 68:491–501, 1966.

Wealthall, S. R. and Smallwood, R.: Methods of measuring intracranial pressures via the fontanelle without puncture. J. Neurol. Neurosurg. Psychiatry 37:88–96, 1974.

Weed, L. H.: Studies on cerebro-spinal fluid. III. The pathways of escape from the subarachnoid spaces with particular reference to the arachnoid villi. IV. The dual source of cerebrospinal fluid. J. M. Res. 31:51–117, 1914.

Weed, L. H.: The absorption of cerebrospinal fluid into the venous system. Am. J. Anat. 31:191–221, 1923.

Weed, L. H.: Certain anatomical and physiological aspects of the meninges and cerebrospinal fluid. Brain 58:383–397, 1935.

Weed, L. H.: Meninges and the cerebrospinal fluid. J. Anat. 72:181–215, 1938.

Weed, L. H. and Flexner, L. B.: Cerebrospinal elasticity in the cat and macaque. Am. J. Physiol. 101:668–677, 1932.

Weed, L. H. and Flexner, L. B.: The relations of the intracranial pressures. Am. J. Physiol. 105:266–272, 1933.

Weed, L. H. and McKibben, P. S.: Pressure changes in the cerebrospinal fluid following intravenous injection of solutions of various concentrations. Am. J. Physiol. 48:512–530, 1919.

Weenink, H. R. and Bruyn, G. W.: Cryptococcosis of the nervous system. In Vinken, P. J. and Bruyn, G. W. (eds.): Handbook of Clinical Neurology. Vol. 35. Amsterdam, North Holland, 1978, pp. 459–502.

Weindl, A. and Joynt, R. J.: Ultrastructure of the ventricular walls. Three dimensional study of regional specialization. Arch. Neurol. 26:420–427, 1972.

Weinstein, R. A., Bauer, F. W., Hoffman, R. D. et al.: Factitious meningitis. Diagnostic error due to non-viable bacteria in commercial lumbar puncture trays. J.A.M.A. 233:879, 1975.

Weinstein, M. A., Lederman, R. J., Rothner, A. et al.: Interval computed tomography in multiple sclerosis. Radiology 129:689–694, 1978.

Weintraub, B. M. and McHenry, L. H.: Cardiac abnormalities in subarachnoid hemorrhage: A resume. Stroke 5:384–392, 1974.

Weisberg, L. A.: Benign intracranial hypertension. Medicine 54:197–207, 1975.

Weisberg, L. A.: The syndrome of increased intracranial pressure without localizing signs: A reappraisal. Neurology 25:85–88, 1975.

Weisberg, L. A. and Nice, C. N.: Computed tomographic elevation of increased intracranial pressure without localizing signs. Radiology 122:133–136, 1977.

Weisner, B. and Bernhardt, W.: Protein fractions of lumbar, cisternal and ventricular cerebrospinal fluid. J. Neurol. Sci. 37:205–214, 1978.

Weiss, J. F., Ransohoff, J. and Kayden, H. J.: Cerebrospinal fluid sterols in patients undergoing treatment for gliomas. Neurology 22:187–193, 1972.

Weiss, M. H. and Nulsen, F. F.: The effects of glucocorticoid on CSF flow in dogs. J. Neurosurg. 32:452–458, 1970.

Weiss, W., Figueroa, W., Shapiro, W. H. et al.: Prognostic factors in pneumococcal meningitis. Arch. Intern. Med. 120:517–524, 1967.

Weitzman, S., Palmer, L. B. and Berger, S. A.: Decreased cerebrospinal fluid cyclic adenosine 3', 5'-monophosphate in bacterial meningitis. J. Clin. Microbiol. 9:351–357, 1979.

Welch, K.: The principles of physiology of the cerebrospinal fluid in relation to hydrocephalus including normal pressure hydrocephalus. In Friedlander, W. J. (ed.): Advances in Neurology. Current Reviews. New York, Raven Press, 1975, pp. 345–375.

Welch, K.: Selected topics related to hydrocephalus. In Bito, L. Z., Davson, H. and Fenstermacher, J. D. (eds.): The Ocular and Cerebrospinal Fluid. New York, Academic Press, 1977, pp. 345–375.

Welch, K. and Friedman, V.: The cerebrospinal fluid valves. Brain 83:454–469, 1960.

Welch, K. and Pollay, M.: Perfusion of particles through arachnoid villi of the monkey. Am. J. Physiol. 201:651–654, 1961.

Welch, K. and Pollay, M.: The spinal arachnoid villi of the monkeys Cercopithecus aethiops sabaeus and Macaca irus, Anat. Rec. 145:43–48, 1963.

Welch, K., Sadler, K. and Gold, G.: Volume flow across choroidal ependyma of the rabbit. Am. J. Physiol. 210:232–236, 1966.

Welch, K. M. A., Chabi, E., Bartosh, K. et al.: Cerebrospinal fluid γ-aminobutyric acid levels in migraine. Br. Med. J. 217:516–517, 1975.

Welch, K. M. A., Chabi, E., Nell, J. et al.: Biochemical comparison of migraine and stroke. Headache 16:160–167, 1976.

Welch, K. M. A., Nell, J. Chabi, E. et al.: Cyclic nucleotide studies in migraine. Neurology 26:380–381, 1976.

Weller, R. O. and Wisniewski, H.: Historical and ultrastructural changes with experimental hydrocephalus in adult rabbits. Brain 92:819–828, 1969.

Werner, M. A.: A combined procedure for protein estimation and electrophoresis of cerebrospinal fluid. J. Lab. Clin. Med. 74:166–173, 1969.

Westergaard, E. and Brightman, M. S.: Transport of proteins across normal cerebral arteries. J. Comp. Neurol. 152:17–44, 1973.

Westergaard, E., Go, G., Klatzo, I. and Spatz, M.: Increased permeability of cerebral vessels to horseradish peroxidase induced by ischemia in Mongolian gerbils. Acta Neuropathol. 35:307–325, 1976.

Westergaard, E., Hertz, M. M. and Bolwig, T. G.: Increased permeability to horseradish peroxidase across the cerebral vessels, evoked by electrically induced seizures in the rat. Acta Neuropathol. 41:73–80, 1978.

Westergaard, E., van Deurs, B. and Brondsted, H. E.: Increased vesicular transfer of horseradish peroxidase across cerebral endothelium, evoked by acute hypertension. Acta Neuropathol. 37:141–152, 1977.

Whisler, W. W.: Chronic spinal arachnoiditis. In Vinken, P. J. and Bruyn, G. W. (eds.): Handbook of Clinical Neurology. Vol. 33. Amsterdam, North Holland, 1978, pp. 263–274.

Whitaker, J. N.: Myelin encephalitogenic protein fragments in cerebrospinal fluid of persons with multiple sclerosis. Neurology 27:911–920, 1977.

Whittle, H. C., Greenwood, B. M., Davidson, N. et al.: Meningococcal antigen in diagnosis and treatment of group A meningococcal infections. Am. J. Med. 58:823–828, 1975.

Whitty, C. W. M.: Familial hemiplegic migraine. J. Neurol. Neurosurg. Psychiatry 16:172–177, 1953.

Widal, Sicard, and Ravant: Cytologie due liquide cephalo-rachidien au cours de quelque processes méningés chroniques (paralysie générale et tabes). Bull. Soc. Méd. Hôp. Paris 18:31–32, 1901.

Widell, S.: On the cerebrospinal fluid in normal children and in patients with acute abacterial meningoencephalitis. Acta Paediatr. 47(Suppl. 115), 102 pages, 1958.

Wiederholt, W. C., Mulder, D. W. and Lambert, E. H.: The Landry-Guillain-Barré-Strohl syndrome or polyradiculoneuropathy: Historical review, report on 97 patients and present concepts. Mayo Clin. Proc. 39:427–451, 1964.

Wilfert, C. M.: Mumps meningoencephalitis with low cerebrospinal fluid glucose, prolonged pleocytosis and elevation of protein. N. Engl. J. Med. 280:855–859, 1969.

Wilkenson, A. E.: Fluorescent treponemal antibody tests on cerebrospinal fluid. Br. J. Vener. Dis. 49:346–349, 1973.

Wilkins, R. H. and Odom, G. L.: Cytological changes in cerebrospinal fluid associated with resections of intracranial neoplasms. J. Neurosurg. 25:24–34, 1966.

Wilkins, R. H. and Odom, G. L.: Ependymal-choroidal cells in cerebrospinal fluid. Increased incidence in hydrocephalic infants. J. Neurosurg. 41:555–560, 1974.

Williams, A., Houff, S., Lees, A. et al.: Oligoclonal banding in the cerebrospinal fluid of patients with postencephalitic Parkinsonism. J. Neurol. Neurosurg. Psychiatry 42:790–792, 1979.

Williams, A. C., Mingioli, E. S., McFarland, H. F. et al.: Increased CSF IgM in multiple sclerosis. Neurology 29:996–998, 1978.

Wilson, D. E., Williams, T. W., Jr. and Bennett, J. E.: Further experience with the alcohol test for cryptococcal meningitis. Am. J. Med. Sci. 252:532–537, 1967.

Windisch, R. M. and Bracken, M. M.: Cerebrospinal fluid proteins: Concentration by membrane ultrafiltration and fractionation by electrophoresis on cellulose acetate. Clin. Chem. 16:416–419, 1970.

Wise, B. L.: Effects of infusion of hypertonic mannitol on electrolyte balance and on osmolarity of serum and cerebrospinal fluid. J. Neurosurg. 20:961–966, 1963.

Wise, B. L. and Chater, N.: The value of hypertonic mannitol solution in decreasing brain mass and lowering cerebrospinal fluid pressure. J. Neurosurg. 19:1038–1043, 1962.

Wolf, P., Russell, B. and Jacobs, P.: Immunofluorescence as a diagnostic aid in cryptococcal meningitis. Hum. Pathol. 5:758–760, 1974.

Wolf, S. M.: Decreased cerebrospinal fluid glucose in herpes zoster meningitis. Arch. Neurol. 30:109, 1974.

Wolfe, L. S.: Possible roles of prostaglandins in the nervous system. In Agranoff, B. W. and Aprison, M. H. (eds.): Advances in Neurochemistry. Vol. I. New York, Plenum Press, 1975, pp. 1–50.

Wolfe, L. S. and Mamer, O.: Measurement of prostaglandin F_2 levels in human cerebrospinal fluid in normal and pathological conditions. Prostaglandins 9:183–192, 1975.

Wolff, H. G.: Headache and Other Head Pain. Revised by D'Alessio, D. J. 3rd Ed. New York, Oxford, 1972.

Wolff, H. G. and Forbes, H. S.: The cerebral circulation. V. Observation of the pial circulation during changes in intracranial pressure. Arch. Neurol. Psychiatr. 20:1035–1047, 1928.

Wolfson, W. Q., Levin, R. and Tinsley, M.: The transport and excretion of uric acid in man: I. True uric acid in normal cerebrospinal fluid, in plasma and in ultrafiltrates of plasma. J. Clin. Invest. 26:991–994, 1947.

Wolinsky, J. S.: Progressive rubella panencephalitis. In Vinken, P. J. and Bruyn, G. W. (eds.): Handbook of Clinical Neurology. Vol. 34. Amsterdam, North Holland, 1978, pp. 331–341.

Wolinsky, J. S., Barnes, B. D. and Margolis, M. T.: Diagnostic tests in normal pressure hydrocephalus. Neurology 23:706–713, 1973.

Wolinsky, J. S., Berg, B. O. and Maitland, C. J.: Progressive rubella panencephalitis. Arch. Neurol. 33:722–723, 1976.

Wood, J. H., Glaeser, B. S., Enna, S. J. et al.: Verification and quantification of GABA in human cerebrospinal fluid. J. Neurochem. 30:291–293, 1978.

Woodbury, J., Lyons, K., Carretta, R. et al.: Cerebrospinal fluid and serum levels of magnesium, zinc, and calcium in man. Neurology 18:700–705, 1968.

Woodruff, K. H.: Cerebrospinal fluid cytomorphology using cytocentrifugation. Am. J. Clin. Pathol. 60:621–627, 1973.

Woodward, D. L., Reed, D. J. and Woodbury, D. M.: Extracellular space of rat cerebral cortex. Am. J. Physiol. 212:367–370, 1967.

Woollam, D. H. M.: The historical significance of the cerebrospinal fluid. Med. Hist. 1:91–113, 1957.

Wray, H. L. and Winegrad, A. I.: Free fructose in human cerebrospinal fluid. Diabetologia 2:82–85, 1966.

Wright, E. M.: Mechanism of ion transport across the choroid plexus. J. Physiol. (Lond.) 226:545–571, 1972.

Wright, E. M.: Anion transport by choroid plexus epithelium. In Hoffman, J. F. (ed.): Membrane Transport Processes. Vol. 1. New York, Raven Press, 1978, pp. 293–307.

Wright, E. M.: Transport processes in the formation of the cerebrospinal fluid. Rev. Physiol. Biochem. Pharmacol. 83:1–34, 1978.

Wright, E. M., Wiedner, G. and Rumrick, G.: Fluid secretion by the frog choroid plexus. In Bito, L. Z., Davson, H. and Fenstermacher, J. D. (eds.): The Ocular and Cerebrospinal Fluids. New York, Academic Press, 1977, pp. 149–155.

Wynter, W.: Four cases of tubercular meningitis in which paracentesis of the theca vertebralis was performed for the relief of fluid pressure. Lancet 1:981–982, 1891.

Wyper, D. J., Pickard, J. D. and Matheson, M.: Accuracy of ventricular volume estimation. J. Neurol. Neurosurg. Psychiatry. 42:345–350, 1979.

Yahr, M. D., Goldensohn, S. S. and Kabat, E. A.: Further studies on the gamma globulin content of cerebrospinal fluid in multiple sclerosis and other neurological diseases. Ann. N.Y. Acad. Sci. 58:613–624, 1954.

Yasargil, M. G., Yonekawa, Y., Zumstein, B. et al.: Hydrocephalus following spontaneous subarachnoid hemorrhage. J. Neurosurg. 39:474–479, 1973.

Yen, J. K., Bourke, R. S., Popp, A. J. et al.: Use of ethacrynic acid in the treatment of serious head injury. In Popp, A. J. et al. (eds.): Neural Trauma. New York, Raven Press, 1979, pp. 329–337.

Yen, J., Reiss, F. L., Kimelberg, H. K. and Bourke, R. G.: Direct administration of methotrexate in the central nervous system of primates. Distribution after intracisternal lumbar injection. J. Neurosurg. 48:895–902, 1978.

Young, D. A. and Burney, R. E.: Complication of myelography transection and withdrawal of a nerve filament by the needle. N. Engl. J. Med. 285:156–157, 1971.

Zellweger, H.: Pertussis encephalopathy. Arch. Pedaitr. 76:381–386, 1959.

Zeman, W.: Subacute sclerosing panencephalitis and paramyxovirus infections. In Vinken, P. J. and Bruyn, G. W. (eds): Handbook of Clinical Neurology. Vol. 34. Amsterdam, North Holland, 1978, pp. 343–368.

Ziegler, M. G., Lake, C. R., Foppen, F. H. et al.: Norepinephrine in cerebrospinal fluid. Brain Res. 108:436–440, 1976.

Zilkha, K. J. and McArdle, B.: The phospholipid combination of cerebrospinal fluid in diseases associated with demyelination. Q. J. Med. 32:79–97, 1963.

Ziment, I.: Nervous system complication in bacterial endocarditis. Review. Am. J. Med. 47:593–607, 1969.

Zivin, J. A.: Lateral cervical puncture: an alternative to lumbar puncture. Neurology 28:616–618, 1978.

Zulch, K. J., Mennel, H. D. and Zimmerman, V.: Intracranial hypertension: In Vinken, P. J. and Bruyn, G. W. (eds.): Handbook of Clinical Neurology. Vol. 16. New York, American Elsevier, 1974.

Zupping, R.: Cerebral acid-base and gas metabolism in brain injury. J. Neurosurg. 33:498–505, 1970.

Zupping, R., Kaasick, A. E. and Ravdam, E.: Cerebrospinal fluid metabolic acidosis and brain oxygen supply. Studies in patients with brain infarction. Arch. Neurol. 23:33–38, 1971.

Zwetnow, N. N.: CSF autoregulation to blood pressure and intracranial pressure variations. Scand. J. Clin. Lab. Invest. 22:(Suppl. 102):V:A, 1968.

Zwetnow, N. N.: Effects of intracranial hypertension: Acid-base changes and lactate changes in CSF and brain tissue. Scand. J. Clin. Lab. Invest. 22:Suppl. 103 3:D, 1968.

Zwetnow, N. N.: Effects of increased cerebro-spinal fluid pressure on the blood flow and on the energy metabolism of the brain: An experimental study. Acta Physiol. Scand. Suppl. 339:5–31, 1970.

Zwibel, E. L. and Schwartzman, R. J.: Evaluation of the nitroblue tetrazolium test as applied to polymorphonuclear leukocytes in the cerebrospinal fluid. Neurology 24: 995–998, 1974.

INDEX

Page numbers followed by t indicate tables. Page numbers in *italics* indicate illustrations.

375